EMERGENT
FIELD MEDICINE

EMERGENT FIELD MEDICINE

Michael J. VanRooyen, MD, MPH

Director
Center for International Emergency, Disaster and Refugee Studies
The Johns Hopkins Department of Emergency Medicine
The John Hopkins Medical Institutions
Baltimore, MD

Thomas D. Kirsch, MD, MPH

Vice President and Medical Director
Doctors Community Healthcare Corporation
Attending Physician
Maricopa Medical Center
Phoenix, AZ

Kathleen Clem, MD

Associate Professor
Chief, Division of Emergency Medicine
Department of Surgery
Duke University Medical Center
Durham, NC

C. James Holliman, MD

Professor of Emergency Medicine
Pennsylvania State University
M. S. Hershey Medical Center
Hershey, PA

McGRAW-HILL
Medical Publishing Division

*New York   Chicago   San Francisco   Lisbon   London   Madrid   Mexico City
Milan   New Delhi   San Juan   Seoul   Singapore   Sydney   Toronto*

McGraw-Hill

A Division of The **McGraw·Hill** *Companies*

EMERGENT FIELD MEDICINE

1234567890 DOC DOC 0987654321

ISBN 0-07-135142-6

This book was set in Minion by V&M Graphics.
The editors were Andrea Seils, Kathleen McCullough, and Regina Y. Brown.
The production supervisor was Catherine H. Saggese.
The cover designer was Aimee Nordin.
The illustrations were created by Network Graphics.
The illustration manager was Charissa Baker.
The index was prepared by Kathy Unger.
RR Donnelley & Sons was the printer and binder.

Library of Congress Cataloging-in-Publication Data.

Emergent field medicine / edited by Michael VanRooyen . . . [et al.].
    p. ; cm.
  Includes bibliographical references and index.
    1. Missions, Medical. 2. Emergency medicine. 3. Community health services. I.
VanRooyen, Michael. II. American College of Emergency Physicians.
    [DNLM: 1. Community Medicine. 2. Emergency Medicine. 3. International
Cooperation. 4. Medical Missions, Official. 5. Public Health. 6. World Health. WB 105
E5593 2002]
RA393 .E445 2002
362.1—dc21
                                                                            2001044817

Table of Contents

Contributors

Kathleen Clem, MD
Associate Professor
Chief, Division of Emergency Medicine
Department of Surgery
Duke University Medical Center
Durham, NC

Lynda Daniel-Underwood, MD
Assistant Professor
Department of Emergency Medicine
Loma Linda University Medical Center
Loma Linda, CA

Chayan C. Dey, MD, MPH
Assistant Professor and Fellowship Director
Center for International Emergency, Disaster and
    Refugee Studies
Johns Hopkins Department of Emergency Medicine
Baltimore, MD

M. James Eliades, MD, MPH
Center for International Emergency, Disaster and
    Refugee Studies
Johns Hopkins Department of Emergency Medicine
Baltimore, MD

Timothy B. Erickson, MD
Residency Director
Toxicology Fellowship Director
Associate Professor
University of Illinois Department of Emergency
    Medicine
Chicago, IL

Karen Frush, MD
Assistant Clinical Professor of Pediatrics and Surgery
Duke University Medical Center
Durham, NC

Steven M. Green, MD
Professor of Emergency Medicine & Pediatrics
Director, Emergency Medicine Residency Program
Loma Linda University School of Medicine
Loma Linda, CA

Jeff Hardesty, MD
Associate Professor
Department of Obstetrics and Gynecology
Loma Linda University Medical Center
Loma Linda, CA

Jon Mark Hirshon, MD, MPH
Department of Emergency Medicine
University of Maryland School of Medicine
Baltimore, MD

Richard J. Hoffner, MD
Assistant Clinical Professor of Emergency
    Medicine
Los Angeles County/University of Southern
    California Medical Center
Los Angeles, CA

Teresita Hogan, MD
Director, Emergency Medicine Residency
Resurrection Medical Center
Associate Professor of Emergency Medicine
University of Illinois
Chicago, IL

C. James Holliman, M.D.
Professor of Emergency Medicine
Pennsylvania State University
M. S. Hershey Medical Center
Hershey, PA

Edbert B. Hsu, MD
Center for International Emergency,
    Disaster and Refugee Studies
Johns Hopkins Department of Emergency
    Medicine
Baltimore, MD

Thomas D. Kirsch, MD, MPH
Vice President and Medical Director
Doctors Community Healthcare Corporation
Attending Physician
Maricopa Medical Center
Phoenix, AZ

James Li, MD
Instructor, Division of Emergency Medicine
Harvard Medical School
Mount Auburn Hospital
Cambridge, MA

Mony Mehrotra, MD
University of North Carolina Hospitals
Department of Emergency Medicine
Chapel Hill, NC

Heather Papowitz, MD, MPH
Johns Hopkins Center for International
    Emergency, Disaster and Refugee Studies
Johns Hopkins Department of Emergency
    Medicine
Baltimore, MD

Daniel J. Ross, MD, DDS
Resurrection Medical Center
Emergency Medicine Residency
Chicago, IL

Tamara L. Thomas, MD
Associate Professor
Loma Linda University Medical Center
Department of Emergency Medicine
Loma Linda, CA

John M. Toso, MD
Director
Emergency Services & Travel Medicine Clinic
Austin Medical Center–Mayo Health Systems
Austin, MN

Michael J. VanRooyen, MD, MPH
Director
Center for International Emergency,
    Disaster and Refugee Studies
The Johns Hopkins Department of
    Emergency Medicine
The John Hopkins Medical Institutions
Baltimore, MD

Preface

The International Health Worker: Most doctors, nurses and health personnel who practice abroad begin their work with certain areas of clinical expertise. Soon after their arrival in the field, they find that, regardless of their specialty, they must become the pediatrician, internist, tropical medicine expert, obstetrician and surgeon. Because of limited personnel and resources, they are required to perform a wide variety of tasks, from minor surgery to administrating a clinic; from evaluating an epidemic and conducting immunization programs to training health workers. They are forced to practice outside of their normal scope, and must look at the broad range of health needs around them.

While working in the field, many health workers have discovered the need of a portable, practical textbook to assist them in managing a variety of medical issues and problems. Such a text is not easily found. The practice of medicine varies greatly from region to region. Varied cultural issues, differing disease distribution and limited access to medical supplies create challenges for health workers. Those working in developing systems are forced to rely less on tests and consultants and more on their clinical ability and ingenuity. This book was created to assist all levels of health workers in the day to day practice of medicine in areas with great need and limited resources.

Written from the field: "Emergent Field Medicine" was developed and written by health workers who, while working abroad, found themselves in unfamiliar medical territory. They are among a growing number of doctors, nurses and medical personnel who view the world community as their practice, and seek to provide care to those most in need. The text was designed to be a practical guide for all types of health workers; nurses, doctors, medical assistants and anyone who finds themselves in the position to ease the suffering of people by providing health care.

Attitude of service and contribution to community: The most useful tools in the field are not found in a medical kit, or even a medical text, but in a health worker's motivation to learn and the willingness to listen to the needs of people. This willingness comes from a desire to face head-on the challenges of providing care in remote and sometimes difficult surroundings. Experience in the field tells us that the level of education does not necessarily denote the most able health provider. The most appropriate health care is delivered by compassionate health workers who seek to continually learn to use available resources to best treat their patients.

"Emergent Field Medicine" is intended to be a practical and accessible field guide for health personnel working in remote settings. We have attempted to create a complete resource for basic medical management of injuries and illnesses, as well as information about health systems, community health, hygiene and health education. The authors hope that the book will be as valuable to those working in rural Tanzania as it will be to those working in urban Bangkok.

Low-tech Medicine: One important observation for foreign health workers to make is that timely and appropriate health services can be provided in the field without high tech supplies and expensive tests. With the exception of complex surgical and medical emergencies, most health care can be provided by experienced mid-level health workers with access to modest supplies and medications. The most common missing ingredients are an organized approach to health services and education of health providers.

Simplified methods of diagnosis and treatment of common diseases: "Emergent Field Medicine" is organized by illness types and organ systems, with numerous cross references and tables for differential diagnosis and treatment. The book specifically addresses illnesses which can be confused with others or those prone to misdiagnosis. The diagnosis and treatment protocols are simplified for the purpose of clarity and simplicity. This book is a compilation of many resources, and draws from practical experience as well as a wide variety of books and journals. We have incorporated clinical suggestions from several field manuals, WHO documents, public health/community health resources and recommendations from field health personnel, missionaries, non-government organizations (NGOs), community health providers and indigenous health workers.

Importance of teaching and learning: Throughout the book, references are made to teaching and helping local health workers and community health personnel learn. This is one of the most important and long lasting contributions a health worker can make. If you are a medical practitioner working abroad, you should make every possible effort to involve local health personnel in all aspects of your work. You have much to learn from local health care providers, and much to contribute. Working with indigenous health workers will allow you to make more informed treatment decisions, provide culturally appropriate care, and build important relationships within the community. By teaching local health personnel, your efforts will be multiplied many times in their communities.

We dedicate this book to all health workers in the field, many of whom work in uncomfortable and sometimes unsafe conditions. Your humility, flexibility, sense of service and even sense of humor are the best tools you can bring to the field. We hope this field guide will assist you in exploring ways to provide and teach a balanced, appropriate and effective approach to health care for the families, communities and countries you serve.

MVR

CHAPTER 1

Public and Community Health

Heather Papowitz and Michael J. VanRooyen

EVALUATING COMMUNITY HEALTH NEEDS

Public health is a discipline of health care concentrating on the health status of populations. As opposed to curative care that focuses on the diagnosis and treatment of a single individual, public health is concerned with the diagnosis and prevention of disease within a community. Because curative care solves an immediate problem but doesn't prevent its recurrence, curative care must be coupled with appropriate public health measures to maintain health among communities. Preventive measures can reduce the demand on curative services, impact a large number of people, and provide sustainable improvements to the health of a community.

> **KEY POINT:**
>
> Curative care must be linked with public health services to improve the health of communities.

As a health worker in the field setting, it is essential that you not only treat a patient's illness, but also address the root cause of that illness. This means treating not only the diarrhea, but fixing the contaminated water supply. It is therefore important to understand the interaction between health and the social, cultural, and economic aspects of a community. A poor economy, political instability, cultural and social constraints, and lack of education are factors that can influence community health. A healthy community begins with the awareness and participation of the people brought about by health education. Health education and community participation are neces-

1

sary for programs in water and sanitation, nutrition, maternal and child heath, immunizations, and injury prevention.

COMMUNITY-BASED HEALTH CARE

As a health-care provider, it is extremely important to recognize the importance of community-based health programs and preventive health services. Curative health services from a clinic, dispensary, or hospital without attention to preventive health services will not produce significant improvements in the health of a community. A coordinated, cooperative effort between health workers and the people they serve is essential for improving health for the community.

APPROACH TO COMMUNITY HEALTH DEVELOPMENT

To understand the health needs of a community, you must get to know the people with whom you will be working. If you are an indigenous health provider, you have the greatest resource available: knowledge of the people in your community. If you are an outsider, it is essential to work closely with the community leaders, village health providers, and families in the communities to best understand their unique health needs.

> **KEY POINT:**
>
> Get to know the people in your community—they are your greatest resource.

INVOLVING LOCAL HEALTH PROVIDERS

When you develop a plan for community health and curative care, you need to involve all levels of local health providers from the earliest stages of planning through every subsequent phase. It is not uncommon for foreign health workers to perform assessments and develop plans without consultation with the constituents. Developing solid working relationships (and trust) with your local counterparts is an essential first step (Table 1-1).

THE HEALTH SYSTEM STRUCTURE

Ideally, health systems contain components of preventive health and curative health care. The following elements are the components of such a system (Fig. 1-1):

TABLE 1-1 TYPES OF LOCAL HEALTH PERSONNEL

Community health workers or primary health workers
Maternal and child health worker
Traditional birth attendant
Nurse midwife
Medical assistants
Nurses and nurse assistants
Technical staff (laboratory, radiology, etc.)
Physicians

■ Community health programs are administrated by community health workers, primary health workers, and other local health workers, such as traditional birth attendants. Community health programs serve as the foundation for community health education, sanitation education, immunization programs, and preventive care.

■ Dispensaries are small outpatient treatment facilities where medications are dispensed and where clinicians may perform simple diagnostic procedures, such as microscopy. Dispensaries may serve as community health centers and may be a common site for immunizations and prenatal care.

■ Primary health centers serve as the main outpatient resource for a local region, and may have limited inpatient capability. Primary health centers are typically managed by medical assistants, community health workers, or nurses. The larger ones may have a physician. They refer sicker patients in more advanced services to the district hospital.

■ District hospitals typically have inpatient facilities and some degree of surgical capability, depending on the region and the health-care system in the country. District hospitals serve as the regional catchments for most inpatients.

■ Referral hospitals (regional or national health facilities) take patients with severe injuries, serious health problems, or chronic illnesses. Referral hospitals serve as the accepting center for major medical and surgical emergencies in the region.

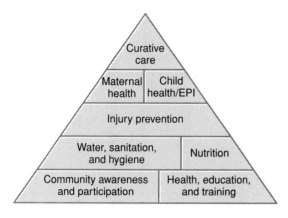

FIGURE 1-1 The healthy community pyramid.

BALANCING CURATIVE CARE WITH PUBLIC HEALTH

Although there are many ways to address the health needs of the community, it is important to first treat the immediate problems of the people. It is impossible for a mother to understand the need for immunizations when her child has meningitis. We must provide prompt and compassionate care to sick and injured patients, but in the long run it is the preventive care that saves the most lives. This means that a balance between preventive and curative care is needed. Physicians and nurses sometimes fail to see the importance of preventive health measures, and place too great a priority on curative care. Conversely, public health workers and community health personnel sometimes criticize the use of resources for curative care.

KEY POINT:

As a health-care provider, it is not only important to treat an illness, but also to learn how to prevent it.

Providing immediate medical care can build relationships and credibility within the community, and can allow the health worker much more influence to improve overall health care. Every time you treat a patient's acute needs, you have the opportunity to address the greater health threats that face them. Always provide care with an eye on working with the community to prevent such suffering in the future through prevention and education (Table 1-2).

TABLE 1-2 INTEGRATING CURATIVE CARE WITH EDUCATION AND PREVENTION: CASE EXAMPLE

You are a village health worker in a rural region of Kenya. Shortly after you arrive, you notice the large number of children who have suffered burns after falling into the family cooking fire at home. Your approach to this issue should take place on several levels:

Curative care: Examples of this are treatment of burns by supportive care, rehydration, debridement, wound care, and prevention of infection. Ensure mechanisms for evacuation of severely burned children to a comprehensive facility. Teach local health providers how to best care for burns and burned patients.

Preventive care: Visit families of burn victims and others in the village. With the input of local community leaders, develop a plan to build a barrier around the fire out of stones and locally made bricks. Teach families to build structures around fires to prevent injuries.

Education: Train community health workers to incorporate prevention of cooking-fire accidents into their community health programs. Recruit local personnel to make house calls on families with small children to assist them in making their cooking fires safe. Arrange for announcements to be made at community gatherings, church services, and markets.

WORKING WITH LIMITED RESOURCES

All countries have some limitations in their capacity to manage the health needs of their population. The limitations in several less industrialized countries are more severe, and there is simply not enough funding for health workers, medications, or supplies. As a health provider, you must always be aware of the limitations and capabilities where you are working and adjust your practice to use resources effectively.

SUSTAINABILITY

One of the primary goals when starting a health program in a developing setting is to make sure that it is sustainable. Complicated or expensive programs can overextend resources and cannot be maintained in the long run without great cost to other aspects of the health delivery system. High-tech, high-cost interventions are tempting, but should be studied carefully.

TIPS AND TRICKS:

If you are thinking of starting a new intervention, you may consider asking yourself, or your team, the following questions:

■ Does it address a real need?
■ Is it sustainable (maintainable) within the community?
■ Are there identified individuals who can manage the program?
■ Will it require long-term funding? If so, who will provide funding?

USE OF APPROPRIATE TECHNOLOGY

Deciding on the level of technology to use is an important part of building a sustainable health program. *Appropriate technology* means using testing and treatment methods within the financial and logistic constraints of the area where you are working. Using equipment or techniques that a community has no hope of sustaining simply creates false expectations. High-tech resources are often expensive and draw financial support away from essential services such as immunizations and maternal child health care. The world is littered with broken ambulances, and nonfunctioning laboratory equipment that helps no one.

STEPS IN ASSESSING OVERALL HEALTH NEEDS

Any health worker who is new to the region needs to understand the health problems of the community. This can be as simple as discussing problems with local health providers and reviewing local and national records. But for new programs, refugee situations, and disasters, it is often necessary to conduct a much more detailed evaluation. The following steps can be used for any assessment process.

STEP 1: GO TO THE COMMUNITY

The first step is to approach the community and find out about their perceived health needs. Learning about health needs from statistics or government officials may be helpful, but nothing replaces the information gathered by walking around a community and hearing first-hand information about the health problems people experience and the way they live. Some of your best information can be obtained from community health workers. Talk to the medical assistant who staffs the dispensary, the community health workers, and traditional birth attendants. Talk to people in the hospital and families in their own homes. The more exposure to the people you aim to serve, the better idea you will get of their health needs.

STEP 2: GATHER DATA

Gathering data does not have to be a confusing or complicated endeavor. Much of the basic health and demographic data may be available for government statistics or in the records of the local health center. A simple regional health survey, like the one in Table 1-3, can provide important information about the community. Some of the information you should obtain is as follows:

- *Size and distribution of the community:* It is important to know the layout of the community. How many people in certain age ranges (<5, <15, >60 years)? Where do people gather? Where do they obtain water and food? What is the main industry and the general economic level of the region? It is possible to make estimates of the proportion of different population groups by using the formula in Table 1-4.
- *Most common illnesses and specific endemic illnesses:* Information such as the number of cases of measles or malaria, or infants with neonatal tetanus, can often be obtained from dispensary notes and records.
- *Preventable causes of death and disability:* The measure of certain sentinel diseases can give an indication of the general health of the population. Obtain information about measles, neonatal tetanus, meningitis, diarrheal illnesses, and certain other illnesses.
- *Current public health efforts and community health initiatives:* Get an idea of the current community-based health efforts and what kind of community resources are available. This includes noting the last immunization campaigns and public health initiatives.
- *Where people seek primary health care:* Look at primary health centers, and evaluate the resources they have and the personnel working there. Talk to individuals who are addressing the day-to-day outpatient needs and find out their level of training and commitment to the community.
- *Availability of medical services options for referral:* Find out where you can transfer critically ill patients, or those requiring surgery or services outside of your capability. It may be that the health center where you work is the end of the line.
- *Health education practices:* Find out about how health practitioners are trained, and if continuing education is integrated into the existing health practice.

TABLE 1-3 COMMUNITY HEALTH ASSESSMENT WORKSHEET

Population, society, and economics
  What is the population of the community?
  How many are under 5 years old?
  What is the level of schooling?
  What is the main source of employment?
  How many babies were born in the community in the last year?
  How many died?
  How many adults died in the last year?
  What caused the deaths?
  Could they have been prevented?
  What kind of illnesses has the family suffered in the last year?
  What kind of injuries?
  What kind of long-term illnesses exist in the community?
  How many children does each family have?

Housing
  In what type of house do people live?
  Do they live with extended family in the house?
  Does the home have adequate ventilation?

Water, sanitation, and hygiene
  Ready access to clean water?
  How many miles to clean water?
  Do families boil water?
  Are there problems with vermin or insects?
  What is being done to prevent them?
  How many latrines or toilets per person in the community?

Nutrition
  What is the main diet?
  Are foods locally grown?
  What percentage of children are malnourished? (perceived by the
    community and measured by arm circumference; see Chapter 5)
  Do mothers breast-feed their babies? If not, why?

Health practices, health care, and health resources
  Do people in the community smoke or use alcohol or drugs?
  How does this affect their health?
  Are there community health personnel to counsel mothers on nutrition?
  Are there traditional birth attendants?
  How many dispensaries, primary health centers, and district hospitals
    are in the region?
  Where do very sick people go for emergency care or surgery?
  How many children have been vaccinated?
  Who gives the vaccinations?
  How much do medications and medical care cost?
  Are health providers accessible to the community?
  Are traditional healing methods used?

TABLE 1-4 TYPICAL POPULATION PROPORTIONS

Population under 5 years	= 1/5 of total
Population under 1 year	= 1/25 of total
Women of fertile age	= 1/5 of total
Women currently pregnant	= 1/25 of total

HIGH-PRIORITY DISEASES Many regions worldwide have high-priority diseases that affect a large percentage of the population and are major causes of death and disability. Examples include malaria in many sub-Saharan African populations, or respiratory and diarrheal diseases in many impoverished or displaced populations, or violence and accidents in much of the Western world. High-priority diseases may require special attention by the health workers, and high-risk groups should be targeted.

STEP 3: DEVELOPING A PLAN

After obtaining information from surveys, you can work with the local health providers and make a health plan based on the needs and capabilities in the community. In evaluating the steps you need to take first, reflect on the most important health priorities and make decisions about where to begin. This will most likely lead you to a combination approach of preventive health care, educational initiatives, and curative health care. Keep in mind the need to address short-term, high-acuity needs.

CRITICAL ACTIONS:

Assigning a priority score to certain identified interventions helps to formulate a plan:

Priority 1. Emergent needs: water supply, cholera epidemic, measles vaccination, traumatic injuries, severe medical conditions
Priority 2. Short-term needs: for example, medical clinic services, maternal and child health services feeding programs
Priority 3. Long-term needs: Expanded Programs on Immunization (EPI) immunizations, tuberculosis (TB) treatment, community health education

---

See Table 1-5 for the components of a community health plan.

TABLE 1-5 COMPONENTS OF
COMMUNITY HEALTH PLAN

Community participation
Education
    Health worker education
    Community education
Prevention initiatives
    Immunizations
    Vector control
    Water and sanitation
Curative care
    Organization
    Level of service
    Referral pattern
        Acute patients
        Chronically ill patients
Health center management
    Staffing
    Supplies and medication
    Maintenance
Interagency cooperation
Health information
    Record keeping
    Surveillance and management of epidemics

STEP 4: IMPLEMENTING THE PLAN

Now that you have worked closely with the community, developed relationships with health providers, and cooperatively developed a plan, it is then time to put the plan into action. The team approach is useful and provides an identified group that can promote the program and evaluate its progress. As implementation of a particular program begins (e.g., a community health education program), a few general considerations should be addressed to make the program successful:

■ Identify a specific group or team to be responsible for a program.
■ Set measurable goals.
■ Make a clear, stepwise plan for implementation.
■ Make sure everyone understands the program.
■ Make sure that everyone involved approves of the plan.
■ Conduct regular coordination meetings of participants.
■ Incorporate training and educational programs into every aspect of the program.
■ Encourage communication between individuals and groups.

STEP 5: MONITOR AND EVALUATE

The evaluation and monitoring of outcomes is an important part of any program to determine the effectiveness of an intervention. Document key indicators of program progress to track effectiveness.

CHILDHOOD HEALTH

Children under 5 years of age are the most vulnerable in the community and are at high risk for disease and malnutrition. Child survival can by enhanced through providing comprehensive primary health-care programs, including the Integrated Management of Childhood Illnesses (IMCI), EPI, treatment and prevention of malnutrition and growth monitoring, and the use of oral rehydration therapy. The discussion of nutrition and growth monitoring in children is discussed in later chapters.

INTEGRATED MANAGEMENT OF CHILDHOOD ILLNESSES

The World Health Organization and UNICEF initiative known as IMCI stresses that a small number of childhood diseases are common in populations and account for a majority of the illness and death among children. The aim of IMCI is to reduce childhood morbidity and mortality and promote childhood growth and development. This is achieved through the integration of curative care with education and prevention in the primary care setting. The majority of this care occurs within a community through the dispensary or health center. Training of primary care providers in IMCI is critical to ensure implementation of quality case management and preventive care.

The Integrated Management of Childhood Illnesses focuses on a few key childhood illnesses: acute respiratory tract infections, diarrhea, measles, malaria, and malnutrition. The program uses algorithms to manage these diseases along with meningitis, anemia, and ear infections. Following training in IMCI, the health worker will be able evaluate child care in the following ways:

- Assess child
  - Recognition of danger signs
  - Review the four major symptoms of cough and difficulty breathing, diarrhea, fever, and ear problems for all children
  - Further evaluate the child if one of the four major symptoms is present
  - Inquire about nutrition and immunization status of all children
- Classify illness
  - Urgent for immediate referral
  - Medical treatment and advice
  - Advice and home management
- Specific treatment
  - Essential treatment before urgent referral

- ■ Treatment plan recommended
- ■ Treatment instructions
  - ■ Instruct mother on administration of medication and rehydration for diarrhea
  - ■ Educate mother to the signs of illness requiring medical treatment
  - ■ Schedule routine follow-up care
- ■ Feeding
  - ■ Assess current feeding methods
  - ■ Counsel mothers on feeding problems
- ■ Follow-up
  - ■ Instructions for various conditions given at point of return to clinic
- ■ Prevention
  - ■ Immunization status updated
  - ■ Nutrition counseling
  - ■ Breast-feeding support

IMMUNIZATIONS AND THE EXPANDED PROGRAMS ON IMMUNIZATION

One of the greatest successes in the history of health care was the eradication of smallpox from the earth in 1979. WHO's EPI developed from that effort and now leads the fight against vaccine-preventable diseases. With the assistance of UNICEF and national governments, approximately 80% of the world's children are now immunized against TB; poliomyelitis; diphtheria, tetanus, and pertussis (DTP); and measles. This translates to a saving of at least 2.7 million lives from measles, neonatal tetanus, and pertussis, and the prevention of 200,000 cases of paralytic polio. Unfortunately, the coverage is not 100%, and vaccine-preventable diseases continue to kill millions of children, accounting for 20% to 35% of all deaths in children under 5 years of age.

DID YOU KNOW?

Vaccine-preventable diseases still account for 20% to 35% of all deaths in children under 5 years of age, and measles alone still kills 1.5 million children annually.

It is important that all health workers promote childhood immunizations and become familiar with the recommendations and delivery of EPI vaccines (Table 1-6). It is likewise important to use routine patient encounters to screen for compliance with routine immunizations. Immunization schedules vary considerably between countries, so individual schedules must be reviewed. Some regions and countries use additional vaccines depending on their local disease epidemiology. These include hepatitis A and B, Japanese B encephalitis, yellow fever, group A meningococcus, mumps, and rubella. Prior to embarking on any international work, health-care workers should familiarize themselves with local immunization schedules (Table 1-7).

TABLE 1-6 WHO'S RECOMMENDED EPI SCHEDULE

DISEASE (VACCINE)	DOSE	AGE
Tuberculosis (BCG)	0.5 mL <1 yr old 0.1 mL >1 yr old	Birth or any time after
Polio (oral or injected)	Two drops	Birth and 6, 10, and 14 weeks (minimum of 4 weeks apart)
Diphtheria, tetanus, pertussis (DTP)	0.5 mL	At 6, 10, and 14 weeks (minimum of 4 weeks apart)
Measles	0.5 mL	At 9 months or soon after
Hepatitis B	0.5 mL	At 6, 10, and 14 weeks
Neonatal tetanus (TT)	0.5 mL	All women of child-bearing age and with each pregnancy (give 1 month prior to delivery)

WHO, World Health Organization; EPI, Expanded Programs on Immunization; BCG, bacille Calmette-Guérin; TT, tetanus toxoid.

KEY POINTS:

- Immunize all children even if they are sick or malnourished.
- All children over 9 months of age must be immunized against measles.
- If the child has been diagnosed with AIDS, do not give BCG (bacille Calmette-Guérin) vaccine. The other vaccines must be given.
- Do not give next dose of DTP vaccine if the child has a severe reaction, such as convulsions or shock. Minor reactions such as fevers, vomiting, or poor feeding should not stop the series.
- For the BCG vaccine to be effective, there must be a swelling, ulcer, or scar at the child's next visit.
- If the polio vaccine was not administered at birth, then start the first dose at 6 weeks.
- Add vitamin A to the immunization schedule to assure coverage.
- Tetanus toxoid (TT) boosters should be administered every 5 years throughout adulthood.

SETTING UP AN IMMUNIZATION PROGRAM

COMMUNITY ACCEPTANCE A successful immunization program requires community acceptance. Communication with the community leaders is critical to gain acceptance and trust from the community as a whole. Outreach and education programs promote awareness of the benefits of an immunization program to the health of the children and the health of their community. There may be cultural beliefs that view injections as dangerous or taboo, but active community education can demonstrate that the benefits outweigh the perceived risks.

TABLE 1-7 CHILDHOOD VACCINES

Polio vaccine
   There are two types of polio vaccines: oral polio vaccine (OPV) and injected polio vaccine (IPV). OPV is the primary recommended vaccine for areas with endemic polio.

   OPV
      Vaccine: live attenuated virus (live organisms that have been made weak); clear pink or orange liquid
      Requires freezing and a strict cold chain
      Dose: Two drops orally

   IPV
      Vaccine: killed virus vaccine that is more heat tolerant than OPV; CDC recommends IPV at 2 and 4 months, then OPV at 12 months and 4 years.

Measles vaccine (see Fig. 2-12)
   Vaccine: Live attenuated virus freeze-dried in a bottle that must be reconstituted with water
   Dose: 0.5 mL subcutaneously
   Site: deltoid muscle of upper arm

BCG vaccine (bacille Calmette-Guérin): protects against tuberculosis
   Vaccine: live bacterial vaccine that comes freeze-dried in dark glass vial to protect it from sunlight; reconstitute in water.
   Dose: 0.05 mL intradermally if <1 yr or 0.1 mL intradermally if >1 yr old
   Site: upper and outer left forearm

DTP vaccine: active against diphtheria, tetanus, and pertussis; comes as a liquid
   Dose: 0.5 mL intramuscularly
   Site: upper outer right thigh
   D = diphtheria vaccine: inactivated toxin or toxoid
   P = pertussis (whooping cough) vaccine: killed bacteria
   T = tetanus vaccine: inactivated tetanus toxin or toxoid

HB vaccine: active against hepatitis B
   Vaccine: comes as a liquid
   Dose: 0.5 mL intramuscularly
   Site: upper outer left thigh

TT vaccine: for use in pregnant women to prevent neonatal tetanus
   Vaccine: tetanus toxoid is an inactivated tetanus toxin that comes as a liquid.
   Dose: 0.5 mL intramuscularly
   Site: deltoid muscle of upper arm

CDC, Centers for Disease Control and Prevention.

ACCESSIBILITY TO THE IMMUNIZATION CENTER Immunizations must be given in an easily accessible area for the whole community. This may require the use of out-reach centers to reach individuals who may not have the means to reach the immunization center.

VACCINATION PROGRAMS

The EPI has been in existence for more than 20 years and has developed a detailed management structure from Geneva, down to individual health centers. At the community level, the EPI must be integrated into the primary health-care system to enable the administration of missed vaccinations and the monitoring of a child's vaccination schedule. A strategy for vaccinating the maximum number of children in the shortest possible time is outlined as follows:

- Start with a rapid mass campaign (if resources and staff allow).
- Provide routine immunization in fixed facilities.
- Use outreach teams to reach dispersed sites.
- Use mobile teams from house to house in a refugee camp or community.
- Immunize refugees upon their arrival at a camp.

> **KEY POINT:**
>
> Use every contact with the health-care system to immunize eligible children. Mild illnesses and fevers are not a contraindication.

MANAGEMENT OF VACCINES

Vaccines are fragile and generally require continuous cooling. Below are some important points to note when handling vaccines:

- Opened vials of oral polio, DTP, TT, and hepatitis B vaccines can be used over if not expired and the cold chain has been maintained; otherwise, discard them.
- Opened vials of measles and BCG vaccines must be discarded after use.
- Discard vaccines if sterile procedures have not been used or if there is evidence of contamination.
- DTP and TT are damaged with freezing. Shake the bottle and let it settle; if thick sediment is seen at the bottom, then the vaccine has been damaged. Throw it away.
- Vaccines are very heat sensitive, so care must be taken to follow the cold chain strictly.

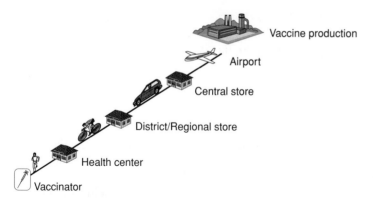

FIGURE 1-2 The cold chain.

THE COLD CHAIN

In order to maintain adequate potency of the vaccine, a cold chain system must be instituted (Fig. 1-2). The vaccines must be kept at their proper temperature from the moment that they are manufactured until they are delivered to the patient. This means that the vaccines must remain in the appropriate temperature range for every step of the journey. The cold chain involves all of the equipment and the people that are involved in this transfer. See Table 1-8 for the recommended temperatures.

> **KEY POINT:**
>
> Most vaccines lose potency when they are exposed to heat. DTP and TT are ruined if frozen.

TABLE 1-8 RECOMMENDED TEMPERATURES AND STORAGE TIME

VACCINE MAXIMUM STORAGE TIME	CENTRAL STORE (UP TO 8 MO)	REGIONAL (UP TO 3 MO)	HEALTH CENTER (UP TO 1 MO)	TRANSPORT (UP TO 1 WK)
Measles BCG OPV	$-15°$ to $25°C$	$-15°$ to $25°C$	$-15°$ to $25°C$	$-15°$ to $25°C$
DTP TT HB	$0°$ to $+8°C$	$0°$ to $+8°C$	$0°$ to $+8°C$	$0°$ to $+8°C$

BCG, bacille Calmette-Guérin; OPV, oral polio vaccine; DTP, diphtheria, tetanus, pertussis; TT, tetanus toxoid; HB, hepatitis B.

REFRIGERATORS Once the vaccines have safely arrived in the health center, they must be appropriately stored for use in vaccination sessions. The vaccines remain in good condition and usable for at least 1 month after arrival, assuming that the refrigerator is functioning and the temperatures are monitored. The following points should be observed regarding refrigeration of vaccines:

- Store vaccines on the top and middle shelves only, not in the door shelves (it is not cold enough here).
- Do not put food or drinks in the refrigerator.
- Throw away expired or contaminated vials.
- Keep the door closed.
- Check the temperature twice daily—the desired temperature is between 0 and +8°C.
- Defrost the refrigerator regularly.
- Read the instructions on your refrigerator and know how it operates.
- Keep backup icepacks and a cold (insulated) box in case the refrigerator breaks.

MONITORING THE COLD CHAIN The cold chain is a dynamic system. Even though the vaccines are safely in the refrigerator, they still need to be monitored at all times.

- Keep a daily or twice-daily record of the temperature in the refrigerator.
- Label the vaccines with the date and make sure that they do not exceed the expiration date and the storage time limit. Some vaccines come with a vaccine vial monitor that is time and temperature sensitive.
- When organizing a mobile immunization clinic, ensure that the vaccines are carried in a cold box or a vaccine carrier to keep them cold during transportation.
- During immunization sessions at the health center, ensure that the vaccines are stored in ice so that they are not exposed to heat for any length of time.

SUPPLIES FOR VACCINATION SESSION

- Syringes: 5 mL, 0.5 mL
- Needles: intramuscular, subcutaneous, and intradermal
- Insulated container of ice to hold vaccines
- If sterilizing needles and syringes, sterilization equipment will be needed.
- National immunization schedule
- Growth charts and immunization cards
- Immunization tally sheet to monitor use

RESOURCES FOR A MASS IMMUNIZATION PROGRAM

For an ongoing immunization program, work with the existing EPI management to order, store, and deliver vaccines. If the community has low immunization rates, a mass immunization can be undertaken to help establish the immunization program and to bring up the immunization rates quickly. Mass immunization of children (9 months to 5 years of age) against measles is also indicated early in crowded refugee situations. If there is a need for a mass campaign during the emergency phase, then the following steps can be taken:

AMOUNT OF VACCINATIONS REQUIRED

- Population size: Estimate the number of people in the community.
  - Example: 100,000 people
- Target group: Calculate the target group for a particular vaccine by multiplying the proportion of the target group in the community by the total population.
  - Example: Target group for polio is all children under 5 years of age, which is 40 per 1,000 population (100,000 × 0.040 = 4,000 children).
- Expected coverage: Assume that the coverage rate will be approximately 80%. Multiply 0.80 by the target group calculation to get the estimate of the expected coverage.
  - Example: 4,000 children × 0.80 immunized children = 3,200 children.

TASKS Before the session:

- Advertise the mass immunization sessions: where, for whom, what days, what times.
- Organize your equipment, human resources, and health center.

At the session:

- Register all children—a community member can do this. Children will receive a growth chart, immunization card, and treatment card if they do not have it already.
- Measuring: Document weight and height. A community volunteer can also do this.
- Screening: A trained health-care provider performs a general physical examination on the child, asks about immunization status, and evaluates the child's nutritional status. The child then either goes right to the immunization station or is treated for possible illnesses.
- Treatment is given if needed by a trained health-care provider.
- Immunizations are given by health workers and recorded on an immunization form. All vaccines used should be tallied.
- Health education and follow-up is recommended.

MONITOR AND EVALUATE Monitor the immunization activities by documenting the number of immunizations given per day, the number of vaccines used, and the temperature charts of the refrigerators.

Monitor the vaccination coverage by calculating the number of children immunized in a target group divided by the number of individuals in that target group multiplied by 100.

Keep in touch with the community and the staff as to how they perceive the program. It is important that the mothers enjoy the visit so they will return and continue to receive vaccinations and preventive child care and education. It is also important that the staff is enjoying the work and they continue to provide a high standard of care to the community.

ORAL REHYDRATION THERAPY

Diarrheal diseases are the leading cause of childhood (<5 years of age) mortality worldwide. Regardless of the cause of the diarrhea, treatment with oral rehydration salts (ORS) is the most successful and cost-effective management (Fig. 1-3). (See also the section on Diarrhea in Chapter 11 for details on the diagnosis and treatment of diarrhea.) Death from diarrhea is directly related to dehydration. Ingredients to formulate the mixture at home are accessible, inexpensive, and available locally. Community health workers should be trained in the use of ORS and provided with tools to educate the community for treatment at home. Once educated, the mother can mix the ORS herself and administer it to her child.

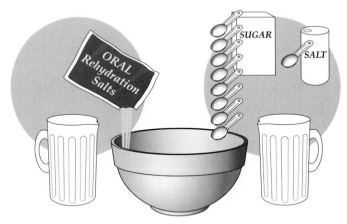

Oral rehydration salt (ORS) solution	Or	Home solution	
3.5 grams sodium chloride		1 level teaspoon	Table salt
20 grams glucose		8 level teaspoons	Sugar
2.9 grams trisodium citrate dihydrate*		Pinch	Baking soda*
1.5 grams potassium chloride		Pinch	Potassium salt*
1 liter of cleanest water		1 liter of cleanest water	
		*if available	

FIGURE 1-3 Oral rehydration therapy.

> **KEY POINT:**
>
> ORS is the most effective treatment for most cases of dehydration from diarrhea.

With the onset of diarrhea, the following protocol is recommended:

- ORS should be given at a dose of half a cup by the teaspoonful every hour or after each loose stool. Rehydration is successful if the child is urinating light-colored urine frequently. Continue to use ORS even if the child is vomiting.
- Increase the amount of breast-feeding, formula feeding, or solid food, depending on prior diet. Reduce the amount of sugar foods such as soda and candy. Reduce the amount of salty foods. Starch, protein, cooked vegetables, and fruits such as bananas are good.
- Seek medical attention if the child has excessively frequent stools or bloody stools, excessive thirst, sunken eyes, severe vomiting, or fever of over 101°F, of if the child is not eating or drinking, or is restless or lethargic.

MATERNAL HEALTH

> **KEY POINT:**
>
> A healthy, educated mother is the best means to ensure a healthy child.

A good public health program should include access to care for all individuals in the community. Women and children often have multiple barriers to accessing care and are therefore more vulnerable to illness. Maternal mortality poses a significant public health problem, with an estimated 500,000 deaths per year worldwide. With the appropriate access to maternal health care, much of this mortality is preventable. A maternal health-care program should include the following:

- Antenatal care
- Delivery care
- Postnatal care
- Family planning, contraception, abortion counseling
- Management and prevention of sexually transmitted diseases (STDs), human immunodeficiency virus (HIV), and acquired immunodeficiency syndrome (AIDS)
- Program for sexual and gender-based violence

ANTENATAL CARE

Prenatal care focuses on education so that each woman can maintain a healthy pregnancy and recognize when complications arise. At least three visits are recommended throughout pregnancy, with the first visit during the first trimester. Below are specific interventions that should be considered when providing prenatal health care at the primary care level.

TETANUS TOXOID IMMUNIZATION Ideally, two doses of TT are given with the first pregnancy. Immunization should be performed at the first visit and at 1 month after, but no later than 1 month before delivery. The woman should receive a booster dose with every subsequent pregnancy (Table 1-9). The administration of tetanus vaccine to the mother is to prevent mortality from neonatal tetanus.

SYPHILIS SCREENING Rapid plasma reagin (RPR) testing of pregnant women is cost-effective and should be routine if the prevalence rate of syphilis is greater than 1% in the community.

MALARIA PROPHYLAXIS Begin at 20 weeks in malaria-endemic regions. The highest risk for low-birth-weight infants is *Plasmodium* infection during the third and fourth trimester. Prophylaxis with chloroquine once a week is recommended. *Plasmodium* resistance for the specific region should be assessed before deciding on antimalarial treatment. See Chapter 9 for details on the diagnosis and treatment of malaria.

NUTRITION

- A balanced diet of 2,300 kcal/day is recommended for women during pregnancy and during lactation.
- Iron supplementation should be given at a dosage of 30 to 60 mg/day if not iron deficient and 120 to 240 mg/day if iron deficient. Check hemoglobin at first visit and at 30 and 36 weeks.
- Folate supplementation of 0.8 mg/day

TABLE 1-9 TETANUS IMMUNIZATION SCHEDULE FOR WOMEN

DOSE	WHEN
TT1	At first contact or as early as possible during pregnancy
TT2	At least 4 wk after TT1
TT3	At least 6 mo after TT2 or with next pregnancy
TT4	At least 1 yr after TT3 or with next pregnancy
TT5	At least 1 yr after TT4 or with next pregnancy

■ Vitamin A may be necessary in areas of vitamin A deficiency. Give 10,000 IU/day or 200,000 IU at time of delivery. Vitamin A–rich local food can also be used, including yellow fruits and vegetables, papaya, carrots, red palm oil, green leafy vegetables, liver, and eggs. Do not treat therapeutically during pregnancy, because excess Vitamin A can be teratogenic. Treat only if the patient is known vitamin A deficient.

■ Vitamin C 500 mg/day should be supplemented with pregnancy and lactation if scurvy is a problem.

COMPLICATIONS Complications of pregnancy should be recognized and managed, including hypertension, anemia, diabetes, malaria, and STDs. Also assess past complications of pregnancy and previous abortions (see Chapter 12).

HEALTH EDUCATION Prenatal visits are a good time to discuss the place to deliver, recognition of major symptoms of complications, who will assist in delivery, and, if the delivery will be at home, the use of clean home delivery techniques. Family planning and STD and HIV/AIDS education also should be addressed.

DELIVERY CARE

Maternal deaths are often caused by complications of childbirth, including hypertensive disease of pregnancy, infection and sepsis, hemorrhage, obstructed labor, and poorly performed abortions. Rapid recognition of these complications, immediate referral, and appropriate treatment will help save lives. Access includes the ability to reach a medical care facility, the availability of trained professionals, appropriate medical supplies, and cultural practices that can delay the woman from seeking care. Prevention is aimed at providing access through the following interventions:

INTEGRATE Through integration of maternal health care into primary care, a system of education and adequate referral methods can be instituted. In this way, a woman can be educated during each of her pregnancies and during her child's well-baby visits.

ACCESS Women must know that maternal health-care facilities exist in order for them to seek medical care. Community outreach and education can encourage early contact with health-care personnel. Culturally sensitive maternal health care can be provided through communication with the community about available resources and how they can be accessed.

Health-care providers must be trained to care for pregnant women. At the level of the primary health center, the providers must be able to recognize complications and stabilize the patient for further care. At the referral hospital, the health-care provider must be trained in how to manage complications and must be proficient in surgical and anesthetic techniques and blood transfusions.

> **KEY POINT:**
>
> Many health-care providers do not know how to manage pregnant patients, and do not know where to refer patients with complicated health problems. Training primary care providers in basic obstetrical care is an important intervention.

Adequate medical supplies must be available at the appropriate level. The health posts must be equipped with clean delivery kits. Health centers should have basic essential obstetric supplies available for the emergency medical treatment of sepsis and eclampsia, labor monitoring, vacuum extraction, removal of retained placenta, and repair of perineal tears. The referral hospital should be equipped with comprehensive essential obstetric supplies, including supplies for surgery, anesthesia, and blood transfusions.

REFERRAL Health centers must be linked directly with nearby referral hospitals for the timely transfer of the patient to the appropriate facilities. Time is often a critical issue in survival, and delay can greatly increase the likelihood of adverse outcomes.

SUSTAINABILITY For programs aimed at reducing maternal mortality from obstetric complications, continuous monitoring and evaluation must be instituted at the start. Accessibility, referral, and appropriate care at the various levels of health-care facilities must be maintained in order to reduce the delay in access to delivery care.

POSTNATAL CARE

Postnatal care is essential to evaluate any postpartum complications, to provide vaccinations and vitamin supplements, and to continue with family planning, education, and breast-feeding. Of importance in the care of the newborn are resuscitative measures, prevention of ocular infections, prevention of cord infection, and documentation of birth weight. Care of the newborn is discussed in further detail in later chapters, along with postpartum complications and family planning.

BREAST-FEEDING Breast-feeding is the best method of providing nutrients to a newborn. Breast-feeding prevents neonatal hypothermia, hypoglycemia, and jaundice. Maternal antibodies in the breast milk protect against infection. Through the use of exclusive breast-feeding, infection also can be avoided through lack of contact with contaminated water and bottles. For the mother, exclusive breast-feeding reduces postpartum hemorrhage, decreases fertility, and allows for child spacing (see Chapter 5 for details).

> **KEY POINT:**
>
> Breast-feeding is the best method of feeding for newborns and infants, and positively impacts the health of both the child and the mother.

WATER AND SANITATION

A well-organized water and sanitation system is crucial for the maintenance of community health. Many of the common diseases in developing countries are transmitted through the fecal-oral route and can be prevented through proper hygiene. Communicable microorganisms follow a simple path to produce disease and epidemics. They are ingested, pass through the gut, exit with the feces, and proceed to spread to others in the community. There are four major environmental interventions:

- Clean water supply
- Management of fecal waste
- Hand washing and personal hygiene
- Vector control

> **KEY POINT:**
>
> The availability of clean water is the single most important measure to ensure the health of a community. Health workers must constantly monitor the availability of adequate supplies of clean water.

WATER

Water is necessary for daily living and personal hygiene. Lack of sufficient water for personal hygiene can aid in disease transmission. The lack of clean water sources spreads vector-borne diseases throughout the community and can result in outbreaks of diarrheal illnesses and significant mortality. Adequate water systems are imperative in the sustainability of a healthy community.

QUANTITY

- Minimum water supply for survival is 3 L/person/day, 6 to 10 L in a hot climate.
- Hygiene (hand washing, bathing, cooking, cleaning) requires another (minimum of) 6 to 10 L/person/day.
- The total minimal amount of water is 20 L/person/day.
- Consider additions for religious and cultural uses of water.

QUALITY *Water quality* refers to the absence of microorganisms and toxins as well as the taste satisfaction of the consumer. Potable water is water that is ready for use for consumption or general hygiene and is relatively safe to use directly from the source. Examples of potable water are ground well water and fresh rainwater. There are three elements of water to consider when evaluating the quality: the presence of microorganisms, chemicals, and the physical attributes.

MICROORGANISMS Significant microorganisms are those that cause disease, including various viruses, *Escherichia coli*, *Vibrio* (cholera), *Shigella*, *Entamoeba*, *Giardia*, and *Schistosoma*. Most of this contamination is from human feces.

How many microorganisms in drinkable water are too many? The amount of human fecal pollution, as measured by fecal coliforms, is the most reliable indication of contamination. Fecal coliforms can be measured with the use of field kits or through the use of local resources. The water should first be filtered through a membrane to retain the bacteria. Incubate the bacteria at 44°C for 14 to 18 hours in a specific culture media. After growth, the colonies can be counted.

CHEMICAL QUALITY Apart from bacterial contamination, there can be an undesirable level of chemical contaminants. Unlike contamination with microorganisms where the water can be treated, the chemical nature of the water is more difficult to resolve, and often a new source of water must be investigated. Chemical contaminants include lead, arsenic, mercury, nitrate, cyanide, chromium, fluoride, and selenium.

DID YOU KNOW?

Salts present in the drinking water can include chloride and sulfates. The salts give the water a bad taste and make it unpalatable and difficult to drink. The chemical quality of water often can be assessed through taste and smell.

PHYSICAL QUALITY The taste, smell, and appearance of water can significantly affect the rate of consumption. Turbid water may be safe to drink, but consumption would be unlikely based on the appearance.

ROUTES FOR WATER-RELATED INFECTION

WATER-BORNE ORGANISMS These are organisms, generally from human feces, that contaminate water. These include organisms that classically cause diarrheal diseases such as cholera, amebic dysentery, shigellosis, giardiasis, salmonellosis, campylobacteriosis, and cryptosporidiosis. Also in this group are other organisms that are transmitted in a similar fecal-oral manner, leading to such diseases as typhoid, hepatitis A, leptospirosis, and poliomyelitis. Prevention is aimed at ensuring adequate quality of water sources.

WATER-BASED ORGANISMS These organisms live part of their life cycle in an intermediate host in a water environment. *Schistosoma* (hosted by a snail) and Guinea worm (hosted by cyclopoids) are common examples. The spread of these organisms can be controlled through improvement of the quality of drinking water and through protection from stepping on schistosomes by wearing shoes.

WATER-WASHED ORGANISMS These organisms are transmitted due to the lack of adequate quantity of water for hygiene. Without sufficient water for hand washing, organisms may be ingested and passed by a fecal-oral route. Diarrheal disease can therefore be transmitted either by a water-borne mechanism or water-washed. Poor personal hygiene from a deficient quantity of water for bathing and washing cloths can leave a community susceptible to infections of the skin and eyes. Most notable are trachoma, which can lead to blindness, skin infections such as scabies and lice, and bacterial and fungal infections. Prevention of water-washed diseases is achieved through supply of adequate water and community education on personal hygiene.

WATER-RELATED INSECT VECTORS Insects that breed in water or bite near water carry diseases that spread through insects. Mosquitoes carry malaria, yellow fever, Japanese encephalitis, and dengue. Flies carry trypanosomiasis and onchocerciasis. Prevention of vector-transmitted disease is achieved through improving surface water management and avoiding the potential for breeding through destruction and maintenance of breeding sites.

WATER SUPPLY The water supply for a community can be obtained from surface water, ground water (springs, bore holes, and wells), and rainwater (Table 1-10). A water source is selected based on required quantity, quality, accessibility, and available technology.

TABLE 1-10 WATER SUPPLY SOURCES

SOURCES	WATER SUPPLY	DISTRIBUTION	SEASONAL FACTORS
Rain water	Simple, off suitable roofs	Individual collection	Seasonal, unlikely to meet total demand
Surface water	Controlled access Organize pumping distant from human activities Treat water	Individual collection or storage tanks Pipe system	Yield may vary seasonally
Ground water Spring water	Simple: controlled access	Individual collection or storage tanks Pipe system	Yield may vary seasonally
Bore-hole	Protect and fix drain-off for surplus water Install electric pump or hand-drawn container	Individual collection or storage tanks Pipe system	Yield may vary seasonally
Well	Protect the well and fix drain-off for surplus water Cover it and install pump	Individual collection or storage tanks Pipe system	Yield may vary seasonally

SURFACE WATER Surface water is accessible in the form of streams, rivers, lakes, ponds, and reservoirs. Surface water, although readily available, is the most contaminated and usually requires complex treatment.

GROUND WATER Ground water is accessible through the use of wells and springs. Ground water from at least 3 meters deep is potable in its pure form. Building a well is the most sustainable form of water supply and the most cost effective.

- The use of a hand pump decreases the potential for contamination.
- A manually operated hand pump should be used in a well that is no more than 7 meters deep.
- If a hand pump is not available, then a rope and bucket can be used. It is essential that there be only one rope and one bucket used. The use of many buckets and ropes from various individuals increases the likelihood of contamination of the water source.
- The well also must be protected from animals and insects.
- To ensure that the drinking water does not come in contact with human waste, the well should be built at a depth of greater than 30 meters and uphill from the latrines if possible.
- If the water source is a spring, the optimal site to obtain the purest water is where the water emerges from the earth.

RAINWATER Rainwater is not a reliable source of water due to its seasonality and unpredictability. It also lacks iodine, so this should not be the only source of water consumed.

TREATMENT All surface water and unprotected ground water must be treated. In areas endemic for Guinea worm, water must be filtered.

STORAGE AND SEDIMENTATION Storage in a covered tank allows time for organic material to fall to the bottom, including helminth eggs and protozoal cysts. In areas endemic for schistosomiasis, water must be stored for 2 days. If the storage container is transparent, then ultraviolet rays can destroy pathogens. Turbid water must be allowed to settle out before treatment with chlorine or filtration.

FILTRATION The use of a slow sand filter is the most convenient and cost-effective water treatment. Local resources can be used, and well maintenance requires little technical expertise. Through the use of a slow sand filter, pathogens can be removed through retention within the layers of sand or at the surface (see Fig. 1-4 for instructions on creating a slow sand filter). The deposit created in the first few layers of the sand is composed of a film of bacteria and plants called the schmutldecke membrane. This membrane forms a very fine filter that collects and destroys microorganisms such as bacteria and viruses as well as eggs and cysts. This layer must never be allowed to dry and should never be exposed to chlorination. The filter must be cleaned every few weeks to a month if the filtration process is too slow. The membrane can be cleaned through removal of approximately 20 mm of sand from the top layer.

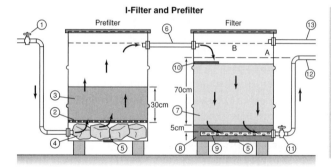

I-Filter and Prefilter

Key

1. Raw water inlet valve
2. Perforated plate (holes about 2mm dia every 5cm)
3. Coarse sand (1-2mm dia)
4. Large stone (e.g. cobbles)
5. Plug holes with plugs
6. Prefilter overflow (towards filter)
7. Fine sand (0.2-0.5mm dia)
8. Gravel
9. Perforated pipe (for collecting filtered water)
10. Flat stone
11. Outlet valve
12. Outlet pipe to distribution
13. Overflow
A. Minimum water level in filter
B. Maximum water level in filter

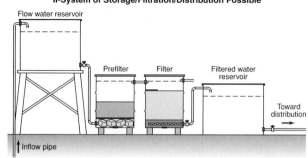

II-System of Storage/Filtration/Distribution Possible

Inputs

– Two 200l drums
– Metal saw, hammer, cold chisel, tape measure
– Drill and bits
– Round and half-round files
– Pipe (PVC or galvanized), 1/2" or 3/4"
– Pipe threader (for galvanized pipe) or solvent and PVC glue
– Teflon tape or mastic and tow (for making joints)
– Elbows and nipples (for fixing pipes)
– Anticorrosion and household paints
– Paintbrush and thinners
– Cobbles (stones)
– Coarse sand (about 1mm dia): about $0.12m^3$
– Fine sand (0.2-0.5mm dia): about $0.3m^3$
– Gravel: about $0.03m^3$

Method

Slow sand filtration allows a highly effective microbiological purification of water in addition to mechanical purification by the sand.
This microbiological treatment is due to the action of a biological layer (called the Schmutzdecke), which develops at the surface of the filter. This layer actively retains and destroys helminth eggs, bacteria, and some viruses.

Construction

1. Paint the insides of two 200l drums. Fix an inlet pipe about 5cm from the bottom of one drum which will be used for the prefilter (as shown in the sketch).
2. Place a layer of large stones on the bottom of this drum (4), making sure there is a plug-hole at the bottom. If there is not, then make one.
3. Place a perforated plate (e.g. the top cut off the drum) on top of the stones (2), to act as a support for a layer of course sand.
4. Place a 30cm layer of coarse washed sand (1-2mm dia) on top of the metal plate.
5. Fix a pipe connecting the two drums near the top, to take water from the prefilter to the filter.
6. Make sure the second drum has a plug-hole in the bottom. Make a hole about 5cm from the bottom and insert a perforated pipe (9). A length of PVC pipe with many slots cut with a saw is suitable.
7. Bury the perforated pipe in a bed of gravel (8), which covers it by at least 5cm.
8. Then add a layer of at least 70cm of washed, sieved, fine sand (7). The ideal diameter is 0.2 to 0.5mm, or in any case, less the 1.5mm. The Schmutzdecke will develop at the surface of this sand.
9. Place a flat stone (10) where the water flows onto the filter so it will not to disturb the Schmutzdecke by its turbulence.
10. Insert and fix the pipework (outlet and overflow). Important: the outlet pipe must rise above the level of the top of the sand, so that the filter surface is always under water, even if the water supply is cut.

Important

– The filter sand should be of uniform size. Sieve it, using mosquito netting for instance.
– Before the first use, fill the prefilter and the filter with a solution of 100mg/l chlorine (10ml of 1% solution per litre); leave it for 12 hours and empty it through the plug-holes. **Never chlorinate after this:** it would destroy the biological layer. Cover the drums to prevent the growth of algae.
– It is vital that the Schmutzdecke at the surface of the sand is always covered with water; again, make sure that the outlet pipe rises above the level of the Schmutzdecke.
– Flow setting: close the outlet valve. Open the inlet valve (not too much, to avoid putting the prefilter sand into suspension); when the filter is full, open the outlet valve so as to have an outflow of about 1l/min.
– The Schmutzdecke is only effective after about 2 weeks, so for the first 2 weeks of service the water is not safe.
– Such a filter can treat 1,000 to 1,400 l/24h. If the needs are greater, several filters may be built in parallel (this also avoids having to cut the supply during maintenance).
– Maintenance: when the yield drops significantly, cut the inflow and undo the plugs of the two drums. Let the water empty completely from the prefilter. Let the water level in the filter fall to 15-20cm below the filter surface; rake the top 1-2cm of sand from the Schmutzdecke. Replace the plugs and put back into service. After this has been done several times, remove about 10cm of sand and put it to one side. Place a layer of clean sand and then replace the 10cm, to bring the total thickness of fine sand back to 70cm.
– If the water is not very turbid (<30 NTU), the prefilter will not be necessary.

FIGURE 1-4 Sand filtration unit.

CHLORINATION Chlorine destroys viruses and bacteria for drinking water. It also can be used as a disinfectant to clean wells, pumps, pipes, and spring boxes. However, it does not destroy protozoal cysts, helminth eggs, or larva. Water must first be filtered to remove these organisms. Chlorine for water treatment comes in a variety of forms, including calcium hypochlorite, chloride of lime, and sodium hypochlorite. For adequate treatment of water there must be a residual of 0.3 to 0.5 mg/L of chlorine in the treated water. The following procedure may be performed to measure the residual:

1. Prepare a 1% solution from the chlorine source available.
2. Fill four nonmetallic containers with water.
3. Add an increasing amount of 1% chlorine solution starting at 1 mL, then increase to 1.5 mL in the second bucket, 2 mL in the third, and 2.5 mL in the fourth.
4. Let the buckets sit for 30 minutes.
5. Measure residual. The appropriate amount of chlorine will be the amount in the bucket with a residual of 0.3 to 0.5 mg/L.
6. The demand dose (or the dose required) is the dose given minus the residual.

WASTE

Fecal contamination is everywhere, particularly in areas with poorly developed waste management. Fecal material on unwashed hands, on animals, or washed into the home by run-off can all be consumed unknowingly. Proper waste disposal is important in order to remove all fecal waste from the vicinity of the home. To prevent this continuum of infection, a strong mechanism of waste management must be established, as described below.

> **KEY POINT:**
>
> Fecal contamination is the most serious threat to a community's water supply. Take every available precaution to ensure the safety of the water supply.

LATRINES Latrines are fecal disposal systems that come in many varieties. The appropriate latrine can be chosen with respect to the resources available, environmental constraints, and the cultural nuances of the community. An effective latrine has the following qualities:

■ Accessibility: If a latrine is not accessible, it will not be used, and disease transmission is inevitable. The latrine must be close to the home but far away enough to ensure that no contamination of the home or drinking water occurs. It must be in a safe place by day or night and easy to reach for children and the elderly. It also must ensure adequate privacy.

■ Respect for local culture: The use of squat versus sit-down versions of latrines should be chosen based on community customs. The structure of the latrine also should be adapted to fit traditional styles.

- Removed from water source: The latrine should be located at least 30 meters from the community water source. The depth of the latrine should be 2 meters above the water table to avoid contamination of ground water.
- Free from insects: Apart from the aesthetic discomfort of insect infestation of latrines, insects can carry disease and aid in communicable disease transmission.
- Maintenance: The latrines must be monitored and maintained. Through community education on the use and maintenance of the latrines, a sustainable waste management program can be implemented.

Types of latrines are as follows:

- The pit latrine is a standard simple latrine structure. It is 3 meters deep and 1 meter wide, and has a platform and a superstructure (see Fig. 1-5 for construction directions).
- The ventilated improved pit latrine uses a ventilation system to avoid infestation by flies and to improve the air quality within the superstructure (see Fig. 1-6 for construction directions).

To estimate the necessary volume for the pit of a new latrine, see Table 1-11.

WASTEWATER Wastewater from washing or cooking should be discarded far from the home and the clean water source. Wastewater can carry disease and can supply a breeding ground for disease-carrying vectors. Wastewater also can pollute the environment and threaten the lives of animals through deposition of chemicals such as detergents.

- Wastewater should be allowed to pass through soil to be naturally filtered.
- The water should be at least 2 meters away from a clean water source and the water table.
- If possible, pass detergent-laden water through grease traps to clarify it.

DISPOSAL OF REFUSE Garbage that is not discarded properly can supply a desirable habitat for insect vectors to breed and rodents to survive. It is important that solid waste be contained and discarded regularly. Neglect of solid waste management can lead to spread of epidemics through infestation of vectors.

- Storage: Store solid waste in refuse containers that are covered and inaccessible to rodents and insects. Metal tins are standard if available, with a small hole in the bottom for drainage of decomposing organic matter. Place these containers near the home and within easy reach for collection.
- Collection: A system of collection should be instituted that is convenient and easy to maintain.
- Disposal: Waste disposal can be in the form of burial (avoid water level and clean water supplies), incineration, composting, reuse, and recycling.
- Education: The community must be educated to the importance for refuse disposal and collection procedure. The whole community must be active in maintenance of the system in order to avoid potential disease epidemics.

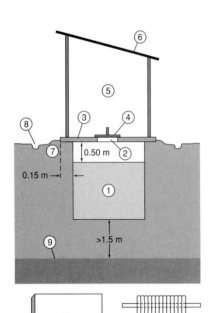

Key

1. Effective volume of pit
2. Defecation hole
3. Slab
4. Cover
5. Superstructure
6. Roof
7. Slab seating
8. Drainage channel
9. Water table
10. Example of concrete slab (see brief)
11. Possible alternative: slab of logs (covered with soil to make maintenance easier: quality of wood is important: aging + termites = danger

Inputs

- Shovel, pick, miner's bar
- Slab (see technical brief)
- Cover (wood, metal or concrete)
- Material for superstructure and door

Method

The simple pit latrine is one of the simplest and cheapest means of disposing of human wastes.
If well designed and built, correctly sited and well maintained, it contributes significantly to the prevention of fecal-orally transmitted diseases.

Construction

1. Choose a site downhill from groundwater abstraction points and at least 30m away; the latrine (or group of latrines) should be not less than 5m and not more than 50m from the dwellings
2. Dig a pit, assuming that the solids accumulation rate will be about 0.4m³ per person per year. Thus, for a group of 25 people (the maximum number per latrine recommended by WHO), it needs a pit of at least 0.04 × 25 = 1m³ per year of use.
3. If a cement slab is to be used, it should extend at least 15cm beyond each side of the pit to ensure a secure seating.
4. Make a slab (see technical brief *Latrine slab*), and place it over the pit. If the soil is unstable it may be necessary to build a foundation to strengthen the pit walls before placing the slab.
5. Construct the superstructure. It may be built with bricks, earth, wood, plastic sheeting, etc., but preferably local materials. The superstructure should have a door if local habits dictate. Otherwise a spiral form may be used.
6. Fix a roof with the slope towards the back if the structure.
7. Dig a drainage channel around the latrine to prevent run-off entering and to protect the walls of the pit.

Important

- Try to ensure that the cover is always replaced to avoid breeding of flies and bad smells around and inside the latrine.
- The slab and surroundings should be cleaned every day.
- If possible, provide lighting for use at night.
- Never put disinfectants (chlorine products, Lysol, etc.) in the pit: this only serves to inhibit the natural decomposition of fecal material. The only situation in which it is recommended to pour disinfectants into a latrine pit is during a cholera epidemic.
- On the other hand it is recommended that fire ashes are put into the pit after each use. This gives a perceptible reduction of odors and accelerates decomposition.
- When the pit is nearly full (50cm from the surface), demolish it, or move the superstructure and slab to a neighboring place and fill the pit with soil. Do not dig this place again for at least 2 years.
- Important; allow for the spare 50cm of depth in the calculation of pit size. It is not part of the effective pit volume.
- Alternative method: if the subsoil is very rocky or the water table is very high and it is not possible to leave 1.5m between the bottom of the pit and the groundwater level, the pit may be partially dug in a very well compacted earth mound. In this case the above-ground part should be lined with bricks or stones.
- Improvements: ventilated improved pit (VIP) latrine, twin pit latrine (see corresponding technical briefs),

FIGURE 1-5 Pit latrines.

MEDICAL WASTE All medical waste should first be incinerated and then deposited in an on-site pit. Anatomic waste should be buried far from homes and water sources or deposited in a pit on-site.

PERSONAL HYGIENE

Personal hygiene is an important point at which disease transmission can be controlled. Through proper hand washing with soap and water, regular bathing, and cleanliness of clothing and bed sheets, transmission of organisms can be minimalized. Education on

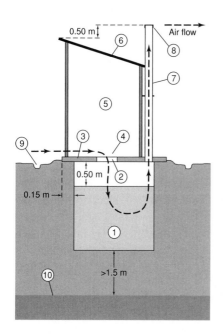

Key
1. Effective pit volume
2. Defecation or squatting hole.
3. Slab
4. Absence of cover
5. Superstructure
6. Roof
7. Ventilation pipe (internal diameter: 150mm)
8. Mosquito netting
9. Drainage channel
10. Water table

Inputs
– Shovel, pick, miner's bar
– Special VIP slab
– Mosquito netting (preferably nylon)
– Pipe of PVC or building material
– Material for superstructure and door

Method
The VIP uses the movement of air across the top of a ventilation pipe to draw odors up the pipe and out of the latrine.
Flies entering the pit are attracted to the light at the top of the pipe and die trying to escape through the mosquito netting.

Construction
1. Choose a site downhill and at least 30m distant from groundwater points; the latrine (or group of latrines) should be not less than 5m and not more than 50m from the dwellings.
2. Dig a pit, assuming that the solids accumulation rate will be about 0.4m³ per person per year. Thus, for a group of 25 people (maximum number per latrine recommended by WHO), it needs a pit of at least 0.04 × 25 = 1m³ per year of use. If possible make the pit big enough to last 5 years.
3. If it is planned to use a concrete slab, it may be necessary to build a foundation on the upper right part of the pit to support it.
4. Cast a slab and place it over the pit. The slab should have a second hole behind the defecation hole with a diameter of about 150mm to fix the ventilation pipe.
5. Construct a superstructure of brick, stone, wood, plastic sheeting, etc., but preferably using local materials. A spiral form maybe suitable, if it is acceptable to the population; this saves having to fit a door. The superstructure should provide a minimum of darkness so that when flies leave the pit they are attracted to the light coming from the ventilation pipe and not coming from inside the superstructure.
6. Fix the ventilation pipe at the back of the latrine. It may be round or square, made of PVC, metal, bricks, reeds with earth plaster, etc. It should be vertical, with an internal diameter of about 150mm. A screen of mosquito netting is fixed to the top of the pipe to prevent the entry and exit of flies. Fit a roof to the superstructure with a slope carrying rainwater towards the back. Important: the ventilation pipe should extend 50 cm above the highest part of the roof.
7. Dig a drainage channel around the latrine to prevent erosion of the pit walls.

Important
– The slab and surroundings should be cleaned every day.
– If possible, provide lighting for night use.
– Never put disinfectants (chlorine products, Lysol, etc.) in the pit: this only serves to inhibit the natural decomposition of fecal material. The only situation in which it is recommended to pour disinfectants in a latrine pit is during a cholera epidemic.
– On the other hand it is recommended that fire ashes are put into the pit after each use. This gives a perceptible reduction of odors and accelerates decomposition.
– When the pit is nearly full (50cm from the top), demolish it, or move the superstructure and the slab to a neighboring place and fill the pit with soil. Do not dig this place again for at least 2 years.
– Alternative method: if the subsoil is very rocky or the water table is very high and it is not possible to leave 1.5m between the bottom of the pit and the groundwater level, it is possible to dig the pit partially in a very well compacted earth mound. In this case the above-ground part should be lined with bricks or stones.
– Do not use a cover on the defecation hole: this prevents the circulation of air.
– Do not forget the mosquito netting which traps flies at the top of the pipe where they die. Use a synthetic or painted metal mesh because the gases which escape via the pipe are corrosive to metal.
– The VIP latrine should be built in a clear space, away from trees which impede air movement. Pay attention to the wind direction so as not to cause an odor nuisance.

FIGURE 1-6 Ventilated improved pit latrines.

personal hygiene is imperative and should be established as a priority in the primary health-care setting and as part of community education programs.

CRITICAL ACTION:

Frequent hand washing by health-care workers is the most important way for health-care workers to prevent disease transmission.

TABLE 1-11 ESTIMATING THE SIZE NEEDS OF A PIT LATRINE

$V = N \times S \times Y$
V = Effective volume in cubic meters (m³)
N = Number of users of the latrine
S = Solids accumulation rate of approximately 0.02–0.04 m³/person/year.
Y = Lifetime of latrine in years approximately 5–10 years suggested.

Free space of 0.5 m is added for the extra space at the top.
Add 30–50% more volume if bulk cleansing material is used (such as corn husks).

VECTOR CONTROL

Essential in the prevention of disease in communities is the control of vectors that carry disease. Insects that carry disease include mosquitoes, flies, fleas, lice, and ticks. Vector control also includes reducing the hosts that allow survival of the vectors, such as rats and mice.

Personal protection can be achieved with the used of mosquito netting and the use of protective clothing. If epidemics are of concern, then the implementation of mass insecticide use is warranted. Community involvement and education about vector control is critical for sustainable preventive measures. Community ownership of the program is essential for the control measure to work. Table 1-12 lists common vectors, the diseases they carry, and the methods of control and disease prevention.

INJURY PREVENTION

With the increase in urbanization and introduction of new technology, injury is becoming an increasing cause of concern in developing communities. Injuries have multiple causes, from motor vehicle collisions, to household accidents, to intentional violence. The impact of injuries is felt broadly. An injury to a provider can be devastating to an entire family. Injuries are not "acts of God": they are predictable and preventable. Injuries are either unintentional (unintended) or intentional (including assault, homicide, and suicide).

Injury is a preventable phenomenon. When approached as such, diagnosis, treatment, and prevention strategies can be implemented. Like any other disease, the following path toward disease control can be established:

- Identify the problem: Review local medical records and data to identify which injuries are most prevalent, whom they affect, and where they occur.
- Risk factors: Identify the risk factors and the points of intervention at each stage. The risk factors can involve the host, the vector, the agent, or the environment (Table 1-13). Each of these points or a combination of any can put the individual and the community at risk for injury.

TABLE 1-12 COMMON VECTORS AND THEIR CONTROL

Aedes aegypti: Mosquito
  Disease: dengue and yellow fever
  Site: open containers of water near human habitation
  Control: Cover open containers and continuously empty containers of water at least once a week.

Culex: Mosquito
  Disease: Japanese encephalitis
  Site: stagnant water
  Control: Eliminate stagnant water sources in the community through disposal of waste water and
    refuse.

Anopheles: Mosquito
  Disease: malaria
  Site: stagnant water
  Control: Eliminate stagnant water sources in the community through disposal of waste water and
    refuse.

Flies:
  Diseases: tsetse fly, trypanosomiasis; black fly, oncocerciasis
  Site: households, refuse, animal excreta, spoiled food, waste water, and latrines
  Control: Keep house clean and free of spoiled food and refuse. Cover and dispose of refuse
    properly. Keep animals out of the house and away from the immediate vicinity of the home.
    Implement proper methods of waste water disposal.

Lice:
  Disease: typhus
  Site: human body, clothing, and bedding
  Control: personal hygiene and avoidance of overcrowding. Treat with powdering of body, clothing,
    and bedding if lice detected. The whole household should be treated. Malathion or permethrin
    powder can be used and a shampoo can be made with use of a detergent; 30 g per person is
    indicated.

Fleas:
  Disease: plague and endemic typhus
  Site: rodents, humans, and within homes
  Control: rodent control, insecticide powder (as above) for treatment of infected human, cloths,
    and bedding

Ticks:
  Disease: encephalitides
  Control: rodent control; avoid animals within the home.

Rodents:
  Rodents carry diseases as mentioned above.
  Control: proper packaging and storage of food and disposal of household refuse; block openings
    to home that are >6 mm with cement or metal netting 1 mm wide, discs on cables between
    roofs, bands on walls 1 m from the ground to prevent walking up walls, and fix galvanized sheets
    at the bottom of doors and on skirtings. Poisons are necessary for control at epidemic levels.

TABLE 1-13 INJURY EPIDEMIOLOGY: HOST, AGENT, VECTOR, ENVIRONMENT

Host: Individual risk factors include alcohol and substance abuse as well as age, sexual practices, disabilities. These characteristics can put the individual at risk for certain injuries.

Agent: The agent of injury is the energy that causes the tissue damage. These include mechanical, chemical, thermal, electrical, and radiant energy sources. Tissue damage results from the rapid transfer of energy to the body or the body's inability to cope with this energy transfer.

Vector: The vector is what carries the agent. For example, in the case of malaria the mosquito is the vector that carries the *Plasmodium*. In the case of injury, the vector can be a motor vehicle, a machine, or a falling object.

Environment: The environment is the place and the external mechanisms that facilitate injury. These can include poor road conditions, poor lighting on the roads, and the lack of safety equipment with use of machinery.

- Intervention and prevention: Interventions for the prevention of injury can occur at three different time periods:
  - Preevent: Before the injury occurs, the environment can be modified to prevent an injury event. Examples include improving road conditions to avoid traffic collisions or modifying cookstoves to prevent burns.
  - Event: During the injury event (crash, fire, etc.), the severity of injury to the affected person can be reduced by modifying the vector or environment. Seatbelts and airbags are the best example of this.
  - Postevent: Once the injury has taken place, the only impact on outcome is from the rapidity and quality of the health-care system. In areas with limited resources, the ability to care for severely injured persons is greatly limited.

> **KEY POINT:**
>
> If you are treating a patient after an injury, use this opportunity to reinforce the need for prevention.

The most effective injury prevention interventions occur in the preevent phase and are passive protection. Some examples are improvements in roads, providing walkways adjacent to roads for pedestrians, covering electric fuses, and child-proofing houses to prevent childhood injuries. Active protection is also important in implementing a public health policy. Community education as to the risks of injury, preventive measures, and access to emergency care is a critical part of injury prevention. Behavioral change can be challenging, especially changing risky behavior and substance abuse. Education should be an integral part of every health-care visit as well as part of community outreach programs.

CHAPTER 2
Health Education Techniques

Tamara L. Thomas and Kathleen Clem

INTRODUCTION

Health education is more than conducting seminars and classes when working abroad; it is a philosophy or practice that promotes teaching at all levels and during all activities in the health field. Teaching gives us the opportunity to multiply the effect of our clinical work, and should be incorporated into every aspect of the care we provide. This chapter discusses the approach to health education on a variety of levels.

Key Points
- Learn about and be sensitive to the culture you are working with.
- Respect the expertise of foreign colleagues and keep exchanges two-way. Remember you can learn a lot from local providers.
- Set realistic goals and objectives in advance.
- Address sustainability of your project through these goals.
- Address local needs through a needs assessment. Match topics to your audience.
- Investigate the local "wants" and ask "who cares?" when planning programs.
- Keep it interesting and fun.

COMMUNITY HEALTH EDUCATION IN A CULTURAL CONTEXT

Goals for Teaching in the International Setting
- Remain culturally sensitive.
- Build on local customs, ideas, and methods currently in use.

- Help people stay open to new ideas (including yourself).
- Encourage independence—you as a visiting teacher want to be dispensable.
- Create self-sustaining programs.

CULTURAL ISSUES

Introducing new ideas that challenge current practice can be encouraging but also may be threatening to local health workers. Reinforce pride in local culture and practices by building on current resources. Don't focus on what is wrong with medical care; focus on what local health-care workers are doing right. Help students explore and find their own answers.

Avoid being an "ugly foreigner." Remember there is more than one right way to do things. Implementing change in another culture is challenging as well as controversial. Medical care is multidisciplinary and is affected by education, training, culture, customs, and local beliefs. Forcing change onto a culture without a comprehensive assessment and local involvement is a waste of time and may be detrimental.

"Buy-in" by local medical workers is essential to a program's success. When teaching in the international setting, do not push ideas and changes on local providers. People change when they are convinced there is a need to do so.

LANGUAGE Take special care to ensure that the student understands the lecture or discussion. If the lecture is given in the second language of students, speak slowly to give time for understanding and comprehension. Be respectful of professional colleagues. Use a translator if your language skills are elementary, and allow extra time allowance for translation. Check to make sure your translated medical terms are understandable.

TONE International education courses conducted by "outsiders" have a cultural gap that may or may not be exacerbated by an educational gap. Acknowledge these differences, but in the process validate local expertise. It is very easy to take the wrong approach in another culture unless you ask a lot of questions first about local medical customs and practices. Put yourself in the local providers' shoes by observing how they practice, work, and live. Incorporate your teaching with local instruction.

FOCUS Avoid aligning yourself with one political group. Attempt to be the person without the political agenda. Foreign health-care policy planners often change with the political climate. Focusing on education can help you maintain programs.

Explore your own expectations as an instructor. Identify expectations of other teachers and students. Why are they there? Communicate with local providers in order to estimate local expectations. Your goal is to be dispensable. Long-term goals should be to create self-sustaining programs.

The "teach the teacher" model has been effective historically in this setting. It allows the continuation of the educational program to continue long beyond your presence. Teach a defined curriculum to health workers. Follow this with an instructor course to selected students. A second course can be set up to allow local instructor candidates and original instructors to teach together. Local instructors should be able to continue the course after you have gone home.

Pitfalls to Avoid
- Trying to teach it all
- Failing to assess true needs
- Trying to inject the system you are familiar with into another culture
- Failing to involve local providers
- Failing to establish effective communication methods with the host country

TEACHING TECHNIQUES AND APPROACHES

WHAT DO STUDENTS WANT FROM A TEACHER?

Students want a teacher that is both interested and interesting. Effective teachers are enthusiastic and stimulating; they establish rapport with students and actively involve them. An ideal teacher provides direction, but is always looking for feedback for improvement.

> Steps to effective teaching—incorporate the following:
>
> Organize
> Prepare
> Select a form of instruction
> Establish positive relationships
> Knowledge—know your stuff

ORGANIZATION

Setting practical and realistic goals is the most important preliminary step. Few talented teachers can "ad lib" in the classroom. Effective teachers plan their objectives and organize prior to arriving in the classroom. Planning a course or teaching program in the international setting requires not only organization of the topics but numerous additional items as well. Communication and trip logistics must be planned, because local and traveling instructors as well as students will depend on your organizational skills.

> **A COMMON PITFALL**
>
> Trying to "teach it all" in a short amount of time. This is confusing and overwhelming to the student. Set realistic goals.

PREPARATION

Courses are often planned without local information or input. For a course to be useful, local resources, practices, and customs should first be considered.

NEEDS ASSESSMENT In order to prepare your teaching for a specific area, understand the local health needs. An assessment of the local health resources is mandatory to effectively prepare an education program for a location foreign to you. Investigate how medical education is organized. Is education planned locally or centrally?

WANTS VERSUS NEEDS A useful course achieves a balance between local wants and needs. In addition, it should be both technologically and culturally appropriate. This can be difficult, because the most desired interventions to receive and give are cutting edge technology. However, should intubation skills and equipment be the teaching priority in an area where there are no ventilators?

DILEMMA

You are a first-time visitor to a country where teaching is needed. You feel that they need a course on triage and they wish to have a cardiac care course. What do you do? Remember, you are the visitor. Involve the local health providers in the process. Try to plan education with local needs and wants in mind.

PURPOSE Define the purpose of your course. The purpose may be to transmit information they do not have access to elsewhere. In addition, you may wish to teach students an important concept, a specific skill, or simply to motivate them.

IDENTIFY AUDIENCE Identify early who your audience is going to be. At times you will have the challenge of speaking to an audience with a variety of skill levels. This is difficult, because you want to engage all members of the audience.

LOCAL RESOURCES Investigate the local resources at your disposal. Involve local health-care providers in both planning and teaching the course.

INTEREST—"WHO CARES?" After selecting the topic ask yourself, "Does anyone care about this topic?"

- Is the topic relevant to the students?
- Is the topic interesting to the students?
- Is the topic practical to the students?

There should be buy-in on the selected topic from the local health authorities and from the student.

APPROACHES TO INSTRUCTION

Select a form of instruction. Think about different ways to present your topic.

INSTRUCTION OPTIONS

Explain	Discuss
Demonstrate	Small groups
Case studies	Use teaching aids
Simulations	Stimulate thinking
Role playing	

Simply relating facts is not as valuable as engaging the students in their instruction process. Learning should be both active and experiential.

Your options may be limited if the teacher-to-student ratio is large, but keep things fun and interesting. Involve the students in your discussions. Give examples the students can relate to. Divide into smaller groups when possible.

RELATIONSHIPS

The way you relate to the students you teach is important. Personal characteristics for effective instructors include enthusiasm and showing genuine interest in both your topic and the students. Keep things fun and keep your sense of humor. Long-term sustainability is as much due to positive relationship building as to successful educational components.

Caution—Don't have blinders on. Teachers can focus on their agenda to the exclusion of student considerations.

KNOWLEDGE

DEVELOPING EXPERTISE Content-based learning allows you to get through more material in a shorter amount of time. However, it may be difficult to keep the students' attention and help them retain the information.

The problem-centered plan teaches major concepts and principles rather than transmitting factual information. You may begin with an open statement of the problem or real-life situation and lead students through a variety of possible solutions. This allows effective participation.

CONTINUING MEDICAL EDUCATION IN THE FIELD

SETTING UP AN EDUCATIONAL COURSE

Several basic questions should be answered during general preplanning and again in the actual course planning. Historically, international courses are planned with little local input or considerations of local needs. Often they are planned backward. The place, time, contents, and instructors are decided before students, resources, needs, local strengths, and weaknesses are considered.

The	*What?*		*Who?*
	How?	determines the	*Where?*
	When?		*How long?*
			Why?
	Logistics		Purpose

Therefore, the logistics of the course drive the purpose of the course. General preplanning is outlined in Table 2-1.

WHY?

Why are you teaching a course? Why does the country/city/hospital want the course?

WHO?

Who are you planning to teach? Acquaint yourself with the range of skill levels. Identify groups providing medical care (physicians, nurses, prehospital care providers, health-care workers). Identify members of the existing health-care system and how they work together, including the Ministry of Health, regional medical care, and local health care. Whose needs will the training program be designed to meet? How does your course affect/change the existing health-care system? Identify parties that need to be involved in the planning process. Ensure local health-care provider involvement early. Who needs to be notified of the planning process? Who will/should make the planning decisions?

WHAT?

Identify needs, analyze needs, and then prepare to meet the needs. Communicate with local/regional/government resources. Identify expectations of involved groups. Set your goals and objectives. Does it encourage independence/self-reliance? Is your plan self-sustaining?

TABLE 2-1 HEALTH-CARE TEACHING IN AN INTERNATIONAL SETTING:
                PRECOURSE PLANNING CHECKLIST

Invitation
  Obtain appropriate permission on conduct course
    Investigate level of permission/notification required
    Local hospital, regional medical care, or ministry of health
    Is there "buy-in" of the course with all parties involved?
Precourse communication
  Identify available avenues of communication for precourse planning
  Identify individual in host country that you will communicate with
  Identify communication responsibilities
  Notify hospitals and physicians to be invited to the course
  Notify course faculty
General background information
  Identify target group members and size
    Identify health-care system and general medical practice as well as local practices
    Classify wants and needs of target group through a basic needs assessment
    Identify short- and long-term goals and objectives
Course Details
  Evaluate potential topics through the local health leaderships', students', and your
    point of view
  Choose an appropriate teaching style—lectures, small groups, skill stations
  Choose a topic that fits both wants/needs
  Select faculty/instructors
    How many instructors are needed for the number of students?
    Are local instructors available?
    How many visiting instructors are needed?
    Select Medical Director and local counterpart
    Select a course coordinator and local counterpart
    Equipment
    Teaching materials, audiovisual, skill station materials needed
Logistics
  Scheduling (bilateral agreement)
    Ask the local counterparts to list several options for dates
    Set dates well in advance and reconfirm to avoid misunderstandings
    Develop a time-line for course planning that includes several time spots for
      reconfirming course plans
  Select a set for the course
    Identify facility necessities
      Lecture room (adequate seating, microphone, and audiovisual capabilities)
      Space for small groups if needed
      Security for equipment
  Develop a tentative budget

Investigate local medical problems. Identify the most common local illnesses as well as public health and social issues. Classify health-care levels of training. Acquaint yourself with previous educational programs.

Identify local resources available for health-care education. In addition, research potential outside resources available. Contact individuals with an interest in the area, particularly if they have planned previous trips to the site. Ask about the "perils and pitfalls" of previous expeditions.

Research potential economic resources. Are there special interest groups or individuals interested in the area you will be visiting? What types of course or educational intervention are you planning based on both existing resources and local needs? Set the general goals and objectives for your program.

WHERE?

Where are the ideal locations for local medical workers to meet? Are there "neutral" areas to meet for multiple groups? Are the areas accessible to outside instructors?

WHEN?

What are tentative times convenient for the local providers? Are there conflicts with other programs in the area? Are both visiting and local instructors available?

Prioritize and fine-tune goals and objectives. Make sure your target group is identified. List and prioritize needs, then match needs to available resources. List program possibilities and get input from local medical workers. Do these program options coordinate with your planned objectives? Be specific in precourse planning.

WHO?

Students: Whose needs is the training program designed to meet? Ascertain the number of students and backgrounds/education levels.

Instructors: Who will be teaching?

Select a medical director and a course coordinator. Planning an educational course at home is time consuming; planning one abroad is doubly so. Dividing the planning between two people facilitates planning. A course coordinator may help with the logistics of the course such as coordinating reservations, making travel arrangements, and helping with troubleshooting.

A medical director should understand local needs and resources. It is essential to identify a local counterpart who is invaluable for planning. He or she can guide you through local politics, assist with local promotion of the course, and help you to focus education efforts. Confirm your dates with your local contacts early.

WHAT?

Timing: What time of year is best? Will the course be continuous or divided into short blocks of time?

Funding: What are potential funding sources? What should be the balance between local and outside sources? What are advantages and disadvantages of the local community sharing the cost? Sources of funding may affect where control of the course is.

Budget potential costs: How can costs be contained? Meet with local counterparts and clearly identify what financial responsibilities will go to each group (local and outside).

Course specifics/topics: Create a list of topics that meet the needs, goals, and objectives and receive local input. Define an appropriate time frame to adequately cover selected topics. Select a balance between classroom and practical instruction.

WHERE?

Where will the course take place?

Does lodging need to be arranged for instructors and students?

Is a preliminary site visit necessary for preplanning?

WHEN?

Identify time needed for preparation, travel, and teaching.

Prepare a course time-line to include preplanning items as well as a timetable for the course (Table 2-2).

Set course dates and confirm with local providers.

Define length of course.

Plan for the local cultural definition of time to avoid frustration and misunderstandings.

> **DID YOU KNOW?** Many Latin American countries do not start education courses at the "break of day"? Therefore, do not tightly schedule lectures starting at 7:00 A.M.
>
> Many tropical countries have a longer mid-day break during the warm season.

POTENTIAL OBSTACLES

Look at the history of previous projects and problems that occurred. Define language issues for lectures and teaching materials. Precourse communication between you and local providers is essential. Many obstacles may be avoided with effective communication. Work out a plan for effective communication. E-mail is invaluable if it is available. Fax machines seem to be available in many remote areas. Identifying how communication is going to take place is essential to the success of the course. Communication "etiquette" varies in different parts of the world, and it is helpful to acquaint yourself with ways to effectively communicate. Mail service in some countries is unreliable, and you may need to fax all letters.

TABLE 2-2 PREPARATION TIME-LINE

This time-line is somewhat arbitrary. Precourse planning helps to systematically identify your planning needs. Certain locations will require 6 to 12 months to adequately prepare and effectively put on a course, whereas in other areas a course could easily take place with 3 months' preparation. However, a preparation time-line process is valuable.

4–6 mo prior to course

Select target group of students
Select site and date
Contact faculty
Develop a tentative budget
Inventory equipment
Visit sites and confirm dates
Course outline finalized

3 mo prior

Reserve faculty/staff accommodations
Educational materials/equipment
  Topics—lectures, small groups, skill stations
  Are copying facilities available?
  Skill station supplies
  Teaching tools
    Are LCD, slide, or overhead projectors available?
    Do you have a backup system if a problem occurs?
  Precourse student materials
  Testing/certificate for those completing the course
  Faculty acknowledgment with course dates/reply cards
    for confirmation
  Set clear expectations for reimbursement
  Reconfirm site and dates with local planners

2 mo prior

Prepare faculty roster/assignments
Contact faculty: acknowledgment
Lecture/slides if preassigned
Course schedule
Faculty assignments/lecture, skill station, patient assessment
  station
Precourse student packet
  Student study packet
  Map
Equipment transport issues

2 wk prior

Final candidate roster
Confirm
  Final schedule
  Equipment
  Facility
Final agenda
Photocopy skill stations

1 wk prior

Receive all lectures on disc (or electronically)
  so you have a backup if lecturers have travel
  conflicts. Bring extra overhead transparencies to
  print out lectures.

1 day prior

Take equipment to facility, label, secure
Set up and check audiovisual equipment
Backup 35-mm projectors, extra carousels
Extension cord (correct voltage)
Meet with faculty for
  Final assignments
  Schedule
  Skill station/equipment

Postcourse

Thank faculty/support people
Check receipts/reimbursements
Evaluate form from participants and instructors
Debriefing session with course planners and
    instructors at the end of the course
  Discuss ways to improve things that did and
    didn't work, and express appreciation to all
    those who helped
Future plans

COURSE PLANNING

Prioritize areas needs and involved parties' wants and try to achieve a balance.
What can you achieve in the time frame allotted?
Organize subject material
Choose general topic with specific areas of emphasis. Do topics match up with needs? Prioritize items that are wanted/needed.
Is the time appropriate for topic? Do not overextend yourself by trying to teach it all.

Select appropriate teaching methods for selected topics and audience. Strive for a balance between classroom and practical applications.

- Classroom—lecture, small groups, video
- Practical applications—case scenarios, actual patients, patient simulations, skill stations
- Tests/examinations
- Number of students per instructor
  - Lectures
  - Small groups
  - Skill stations
- Schedule—detailed planning of classes and activities
- Supplies

PREPARING FOR THE FUTURE

The primary evaluation of training should focus on how easily people can put the training into sustained practice. Choose a form of evaluation (formal/informal) prior to the course. Review your goals and what you want to accomplish. Identify accomplishments and address problems, difficulties, and ways to improve. Provide feedback to instructors and students. Schedule a debriefing session for all course planners and instructors before everyone goes home to gather feedback helpful for the future.

TEACHING METHODS: CLINICAL ROUNDS

Unique aspects of clinical teaching include the mixture of work and education and the immediate practical application of the knowledge. You are able to demonstrate your teaching points on the spot, and teach problem solving, not just facts. Bedside teaching motivates students and stimulates interest and curiosity.

Tips for Effective Clinical Teaching
- Limit amount of information given (develop "take-home" items).
- Give the most important information first and tell why it is important.

- Confirm that information is understood.
- Use repetition for emphasis.
- Use all visual examples possible.
- Verbally work through clinical problems.

METHODS

Goals for clinical teaching are critical thinking and problem solving. It is helpful for students to learn these in a "safe" environment. Examples are role playing and patient simulation.

ROLE PLAYING

Have student #1 act out an angry parent while student #2 is an ill, misbehaving child. Student #3 is the physician who deals with both.

This scenario helps all students:

Explore control issues.
Identify different manners in which fear is expressed.
Learn to be nonjudgmental.
Realize that when you are treating sick children you have more than one patient.

SIMULATION

Have an unhappy (simulated) patient telephone the classroom; put the patient's call on speakerphone. A student can then attempt to resolve the conflict. Give several students an opportunity to resolve the conflict in different ways. Afterward, have the entire class discuss the advantages and disadvantages of the varying solutions.

Procedures also can be simulated. Many models for clinical procedures have been developed. These simulated situations allow the student to experience problems in both "real-time" and a safe environment for learning.

BEDSIDE TEACHING

Base teaching on information about the patient with a consideration for his or her dignity. Actively demonstrate ways to discover physical findings and establish a comfortable rapport with students to encourage participation. Continuously provide them with feedback.

SKILLS TEACHING

A common traditional approach is to "see one, do one, teach one." This does not always focus on successful learning. Seeing a procedure does not give the student the skills to successfully complete the task. This leads to another variation: "see one, screw one, do one" (see Konner). This approach focuses on "how" to do, not "why." Also, it may be difficult for a teacher to teach a skill that is too familiar. The instructor may not be conscious of the step-by-step process necessary for successful procedure completion.

Steps in Skills Teaching (see Wainscott)
    Assess learner (define needs and a starting point)
    Develop learning plan
    Identify resources (patients, mannequins, video, written materials)
    Demonstrate skill
    Provide a way to practice
    Observe learner
    Provide feedback

IDENTIFY EVALUATION TOOLS

Provide nonjudgmental, constructive feedback that seeks to correct without belittling. Give meaningful positive as well as negative feedback, and put feedback in positive language. Give feedback in real time as much as possible.

    Keep yourself open to new ideas; remember that every question does not have only one correct answer. Try to break up skill into separate components. It is difficult for an instructor to break up a complex skill (which is unconscious to them) into simpler components.

TEACHING METHODS: CLASSROOM AND SMALL GROUP

Small groups may be very useful if a clear focus and defined purpose is identified. Discourage getting off the point and keep the group on track. Advantages of small groups are that they allow students to listen, speak, and debate, and they give them the opportunity to analyze, criticize, problem solve, and make decisions.

    The size of the group should be such that everyone can participate. Five to eight people is an ideal size for an effective working group, although a group of this size may not be practical. Use your creativity for "small groups" of larger sizes. Dividing into separate "discussion groups" may break the monotony as well as add interest. For larger groups you may want to assign tasks to subgroups.

TEACHING METHODS: DEMONSTRATIONS AND TECHNIQUES FOR LARGE GROUPS

Lectures are the most common form of teaching to large groups, partially due to tradition. In addition, lectures are the most practical method for one teacher in the international setting to teach a large group of students.

BENEFITS OF LECTURES

Lectures can synthesize information from multiple sources. The learners may not have the time, resources, or skills to do this.

TABLE 2-3 THE WAYS LECTURES WAVER (KROENKE)

- Don't be complete.
  You can't say it all, give key pearls to work from. Process information (get rid of chaff).

- Don't mention anything once.
  Tell them what you're going to say, say it, and tell them you said it.

- Don't restate. Create.
  The audience should be both educated and entertained.

- Don't be democratic, be a leader.
  Have a definite agenda.

- Don't apologize.
  "Sorry, I'm going past the hour" or "Forgive this busy slide."
  Delete busy slides, don't go overtime.

- Don't talk about molehills to mountaineers, match topic to audience.
  Don't talk specifics to generalists and vice versa.

- Don't extemporize. Organize.
  Don't waste your audience's time with ad libbing. Facts are only one element of a good lecture. Remember repetition, selectivity, creativity, leadership, and proper topic requires careful preparation.

- Don't confess. Profess.
  Have lecture complement the literature. (Use personal experience, expert opinion, and anecdotes.)

- Don't dwell, don't defer.
  The speaker should feel a need to keep moving. Deferring a message leads attention astray from the present subject.

- Start and finish.
  Don't try too hard.

DRAWBACKS OF LECTURES

Lectures are a form of passive learning. Students may not assimilate facts or be able to apply them to the practical things that they do. Here are some ways to maximize lecture-based learning (see also Table 2.3):

Grab attention by presenting an anecdote, dilemma, or question.
Be organized.
Define lecture plan to the audience and stick to it.
Respect your audience's time. Choose the amount of material students can learn in amount of time provided.
Leave time for questions.

QUALITIES OF A GOOD LECTURER

Is organized
Stimulates thinking
Explains clearly
Uses eye contact and body language
Knows and is enthusiastic about subject

SUMMARY

Providing health care in any setting should always be blended with teaching efforts, whether it is nurse to patient, doctor to medical assistant, or in classroom or clinical setting. Actively look for ways to teach and instruct in the classroom, clinic, or hospital.

SUGGESTED READINGS

Irby DM, Rakestraw P. Evaluating clinical teaching in medicine. *J Med Educ* 1981;56:181–186.
Konner M. *Becoming a Doctor.* New York: Penguin Books, 1987.
Kroenke K. The lecture: where it wavers. *Am J Med* 1984;77:393–396.
McLeisch J. The lecture method. In: Gage NL, ed. *The Psychology of Teaching Methods.* Chicago: University of Chicago Press, 1976.
Schwenk TL, Whitman N. *The Physician as Teacher.* Baltimore: Williams & Wilkins, 1987.
Whitman N. *Creative Clinical Teaching.* Salt Lake City: University of Utah School of Medicine, 1990.

CHAPTER 3
Refugee Health Needs

Chayan C. Dey

INTRODUCTION

In the past decade, public health emergencies involving displaced populations have occurred with greater frequency. Since 1984, the number of refugees dependent for their survival on international assistance has more than doubled to a current estimate of approximately 20 million persons. Most of these refugee displacements involve developing countries, where the local infrastructure may be ill equipped to handle the influx.

When a population is forced to migrate, they usually end up in camps or urban slums characterized by overcrowding, poor sanitation, substandard shelter, and limited access to health services. Refugees are exposed to many factors that increase the risks of disease. It is important to minimize the effects of these hazards, and deliver an appropriate level of health care to reduce morbidity and mortality.

Refugee health care must include both preventive and curative measures. Diagnostic techniques and treatment of the major diseases should be simplified, standardized, and appropriate. Most health problems should be managed at the community level by local health-care workers, preferably from the refugee population. The more complicated cases should be referred to local health centers. Health workers also must spend time among the community to identify individuals most in need of medical attention. Special attention should be given to vulnerable populations, such as pregnant women and young children.

Refugee health care is divided into three phases: emergency, post-emergency, and repatriation. The needs and services change according to the different phases. Death rates are highest in the emergency phase (>1/10,000/day) and require emergent intervention. This chapter focuses primarily on the emergency phase.

CRITICAL ACTIONS

Médicins Sans Frontières recommends the top ten priorities in refugee health care:

1. Initial assessment
2. Measles immunization
3. Water and sanitation
4. Food and nutrition
5. Shelter and site planning
6. Health care in the emergency phase
7. Control of communicable diseases
8. Public health surveillance
9. Human resources and training
10. Coordination

ASSESSMENT OF REFUGEE HEALTH NEEDS

Rapid health assessment of an acute population displacement is conducted to

1. Assess the magnitude of the displacement
2. Decide whether or not to intervene
3. Determine the major health and nutrition needs of the displaced population
4. Implement program priorities
5. Initiate a health and nutrition surveillance system
6. Assess the local response capacity and immediate needs

The purpose of an assessment is to gather information in order to make timely decisions. An initial assessment of the situation and needs must be carried out on the spot as soon as it is clear that a refugee emergency may exist. The assessment helps identify the most vulnerable groups, the most urgent food and medical needs, and the capabilities of the local community, and helps establish the foundation for further monitoring. The assessment should seek the advice from qualified personnel such as epidemiologists and health-care workers, as well as local health personnel.

TABLE 3-1 REFUGEE SITUATION ASSESSMENT

The displaced population
The geopolitical context, the background to displacement
The environment in which the refugees have settled
The major health problems
The security situation
The human and material resources requirements
The involved operating partners

TABLE 3-2 REFUGEE NEEDS ASSESSMENT

Information on refugees
   Number of refugees
   Location of refugees
   How many more may be coming
   How are they arriving
   Proportion each gender and age group
   Sanitation and shelter customs
   Ethnicity
Health status
   Number and type of injuries
   Malnutrition
   Mortality and morbidity rates
   Current health situation
   Condition prior to refugee status
Material status
   Sufficient clothing and blankets
   Food
   Shelter material
   Funds
Location characteristic
   Security
   Accessibility
   Water
   Soil topography
   Soil drainage
   Vegetation
Current assistance
   Logistic needs
   Local infrastructure to help
   Local health-care status
   Current assistance provided

The initial assessment is composed of the situation assessment and needs assessment. The situation assessment gathers information on the magnitude of the refugee displacement and impact on the local community (Table 3-1). The needs assessment identifies resources and services for immediate emergency measures to help the affected population (Table 3-2).

These common problems can be measured using some of the analytical tools listed in Table 3-3. This is described in further detail in later sections and requires familiarization with some basic epidemiologic techniques.

Refugee situations have multiple problems that cannot all be addressed immediately. It is essential to establish a priority list of the problems to be addressed. Key factors in establishing priorities are the extent of the problem and their urgency. However, a problem should not become a priority unless an intervention is possible.

The priority list must take into account the feasibility of the solution and possible barriers to its implementation. Examples of these barriers include political, logistical,

TABLE 3-3 MEASUREMENT TOOLS

Standard survey techniques
Direct interview
Aerial assessments
Questionnaires
Checklists

and financial constraints, such as lack of security, storage and communication problems, and high cost of delivering the product. Establishing priorities is dependent on a combination of identifying the extent of the problem and urgency, evaluating the technical feasibility, and being able to work through possible barriers to implementation.

Health sector issues to be addressed are the immediate health care needs and capabilities of local authorities to handle the situation. If the initial assessment indicates specific problems, measures must be taken to organize specific data collection. A sample checklist for rapid health assessment and sample assessment form are provided in Tables 3-4 and 3-5.

TABLE 3-4 CHECKLIST FOR RAPID HEALTH ASSESSMENT

CATEGORY	INFORMATION NEEDED	POSSIBLE SOURCE
Preparation	Obtain refugee information	Host countries' ministries, other organizations
	Obtain available maps	Local ministries or aerial photographs
	Obtain demographic and health data	International organizations, local government
Field assessment	Determine total displaced population	A. Mostly through field assessments
	Determine age and sex breakdown of population	B. Sometimes international organizations might have data
	Identify groups at increased risk	C. Rarely, the local government will have data
	Determine average household	
Health information	Identify primary health-care problems in country of origin	Local data bank or international organizations
	Identify previous sources of health care	
	Ascertain important health beliefs and traditions	Local data bank or interviews with refugees
	Determine existing social structure	Local data bank or international organizations
	Determine the strength of public health programs in country of origin	

TABLE 3-4 CHECKLIST FOR RAPID HEALTH ASSESSMENT *(continued)*

CATEGORY	INFORMATION NEEDED	POSSIBLE SOURCE
Nutritional status	Determine prevalence of malnutrition in under 5 population	See malnutrition section
	Determine prevalence of micronutrient deficiencies in under-5 population	
	Ascertain prior nutritional status	Local health data or international organizations

Mortality rates	Calculate
	   Crude rate
	   Age-specific rate
	   Sex-specific rate
	   Cause-specific rate
		See Epidemiology section

Morbidity rates	Determine	See Epidemiology section
	Age- and sex-specific incidence rates of disease that have public health importance	
Environmental conditions	Determine climatic conditions	A. Information from local sources and interviews B. Ministry of Health C. Ministry of Commerce or Finance
	Identify geographic features	
	Identify water resources breakdown of population	
	Ascertain local disease epidemiology	
	Assess availability of local materials for shelter and fuel	
	Assess existing shelters and sanitation arrangements	
Resources available	Assess food supplies and distribution systems	Local information from direct observation and interviews
	Identify and assess local, regional, and national food sources	
	Assess logistics of food transport and source	
	Assess feeding programs	
	Identify and assess feeding programs	
	Assess camp health services	

TABLE 3-5 SAMPLE INITIAL ASSESSMENT FORM

Location:
Disaster type:
Date:
Method (survey, mapping, interviews):

Summary of event:	(Summarize the findings of disaster)
Disaster current response:	
Determine area affected:	(Portion of city, villages, or large part of country

Population profile

Number of displaced population:	
How many are arriving per week:	
How are they arriving:	
Number of men:	
Number of women:	
Number of children:	
Number of children under 5:	
How many deaths/10,000 persons/day in past week:	
How many under 5 children deaths/10,000/day in past week:	
Main cause of death:	
Most common diseases in adults and children:	
Percentage of children vaccinated:	
Incidence of diarrhea in adults and children:	
Number and types of blanket needed:	
Food type and consumption pattern:	

Shelter, water, and sanitation issues

Determine amount of liters of water per person per day:	
Source and quality of the water:	
Determine availability of additional sources of safe water if required:	
Determine the number and placement of latrines:	
Determine number requiring shelter and whether it is temporary or for an indeterminate time:	
Determine average household:	
Determine existing structures that could be used:	
Number of health-care workers and type	

EPIDEMIOLOGY AND SURVEILLANCE IN A REFUGEE SETTING

Epidemiology is the study of health problems in populations. In the refugee population, epidemiologic studies help determine the incidence of health problems, the population they affect, and the severity of these problems. Epidemiologic studies also allow us to determine the capabilities of the local community to handle the current health problems.

An epidemiologic study can yield a long list of information, and it would be unwise to try to collect all the data possible in an emergency situation. It is better to focus on a few key indicators that are more relevant and will help with monitoring of the progression of the refugee situation. These key indicators can be broken down into the following components:

HEALTH STATUS INDICATORS

Mortality (Table 3-6)
- Most specific indicator for measuring the health status of the population and monitoring any intervention
- Estimated retrospectively from community-based surveys, hospital records, or burial records; prospectively from 24-hour burial site surveillance

TABLE 3-6 COMMON INDICATORS FOR DESCRIBING MORTALITY

HEALTH INDICATOR	NUMERATOR	DENOMINATOR	EXPRESSED PER NUMBER AT RISK
Crude mortality rate (CMR)	Total number of deaths reported over a given period of time	Estimated mid-period population	1,000 or 10,000
Under 5 specific mortality rate	Number of under-5 deaths reported over a period of time	Estimated mid-period under-5 population	1,000 or 10,000
Case fatality rate	Number of individuals dying during a specified period of time after disease onset or diagnosis	Number of individuals with the specified disease	Out of 100%
Cause-specific mortality rate	Number of death attributed to a specific cause over a period of time	Estimated mid-period population	1,000 or 10,000

- Rates are often underestimated due to inaccurate denominators, lack of standard reporting procedures, population size exaggeration, and underreported death counts
- Mortality rates should not exceed 1.5 times those of the host population
- Initial high mortality rates should fall to or below 1 per 10,000 per day within 6 weeks of beginning a basic support program
- Mortality rates above 2 per 10,000 per day indicate a serious situation, and immediate action should be taken

Morbidity (Table 3-7)

- Information should be attained from health facilities and feeding centers
- Each disease reported should have a case definition
- Morbidity data allow for the efficient planning of interventions and the effective use of resources by identifying the major causes of illness and the groups in the affected population that are at greatest risk

Nutritional Status

- The prevalence of acute malnutrition acts as an indicator of the adequacy of the relief ration
- Allows evaluation of the general health of the population and the impact of any intervention
- A high prevalence of malnutrition in the setting of adequate average daily ration may indicate problems in food distribution, micronutrient deficiencies, or high rates of communicable diseases.
- Weight is more sensitive to nutrition changes than height; thus, weight for height is the assessment tool that should be used to measure acute malnutrition

TABLE 3-7 COMMON INDICATORS FOR DESCRIBING MORBIDITY

HEALTH INDICATOR	NUMERATOR	DENOMINATOR	EXPRESSED PER NUMBER AT RISK
Incidence rate	Number of new cases of a specified disease reported over a given period of time	Number of persons at risk of developing the disease during that period of time	1,000, 10,000, or 100,000
Prevalence rate	Number of cases, new and old, of a specified disease at a given point of time	Number of persons in in the population at that specified time	1,000, 10,000, or 100,000
Attack rate	Number of new cases of a specified disease reported over the duration of the epidemic	Total population at risk over the same period	1,000, 10,000, or 100,000

■ The best way to measure the nutritional status of the population is to measure the subgroup most acutely affected by undernutrition—children under 5 years of age
■ An alternative measurement, the mid-upper arm circumference (MUAC), also may be used for rapid nutritional screening

OTHER INDICATORS

Physical Environment
■ Water and sanitation status
■ Information on housing capabilities, local infrastructure, and climate

Health-Care Services
■ Number of personnel and services are available
■ Number of patients hospital can handle
■ Quality of care available

Socioeconomic Situation
■ Local food storage and delivery capabilities
■ Local customs and the political environment

The key to an effective assessment and surveillance program is good information. The information required to formulate these indicators can be obtained from several sources, including the refugee population, local community health services, humanitarian organizations, and national government.

Information can be collected by observation or from health workers. Sample surveys reveal symptoms and disease patterns and indicate distribution in the community. If possible, mass screening on arrival is the most effective method and can sometimes be conducted at a camp during the registration process. It is important to realize which groups would be most helpful in providing the correct information for the indicator chosen. Sometimes a combination of methods must be used (Table 3-8).

EARLY INTRODUCTION OF A SURVEILLANCE SYSTEM

A surveillance system helps monitor health and nutritional status. Continued monitoring allows the health service resources to be allocated properly. The form of surveillance should be simple but effective in emergencies. Overly detailed and complex reporting is ineffective. The system should be centrally coordinated. (A sample surveillance form is provided in Table 3-20.)

Information that is not immediately useful should not be collected during the emergency phase of a refugee relief operation. The most valuable data are generally simple to collect and analyze. The data collected will fall into one of the key health status indicators as listed above.

TABLE 3-8 DATA COLLECTION METHODS

METHOD	OBJECTIVE	EXAMPLE
Visual inspection and direct interviews	Achieve rapid appraisal of area damage	1. Flying over the area 2. Direct observation
Automatic initial assessment	Achieve appraisal from key elements in the system	1. Preplanned damage report from civil authorities 2. Military unit reports
Simple random sampling	Sample specific characteristic of affected population	Every member of target population is equally likely to be chosen
Systematic random sampling	Sample specific characteristic of affected population	Choosing every 5th, 10th, or nth member on a numbered list
Stratified random sampling	Sample specific characteristic of affected population	Divide the population in categories and then use the simple or systemic method
Cluster sampling	Sample specific characteristic of affected population	1. Restricts sample to limited number of geographic areas 2. In each area, select a sample by simple or random sampling 3. Combine these samples to get an overall sample
"Sentinel" surveillance	Detects early signs of particular problems at specific site	Reporting system
Detailed critical sector assessments by specialist	Technical inspections and assessments by experts	Usually required in sectors such as health and nutrition food, water supply, and other infrastructure systems
Regular "polling" visits	Continuing surveillance	Direct interviews
Routine reporting	Continuing surveillance	Reporting by the population of events
Interviews with key informants	Continuing surveillance	1. Government interviews 2. NGO interviews 3. Local community leader interviews

The basic steps in forming a simple surveillance system are as follows:

1. Use the initial assessment data base
2. Central coordination—one person in charge of information collection, analysis, and feedback
3. Decision on information collection and action; develop test forms and definitions
4. Establish case definitions for common diseases—diarrhea, dysentery, cholera, malaria, acute respiratory infection (ARI), measles, etc.
5. Select data sources—hospitals, clinics, community, etc.
6. Design quality checks for information
7. Program objectives—coverage and access to services
8. Train personnel to collect and analyze
9. Establish data analysis process
10. Feedback process—informal, meetings, or frequency during epidemics
11. Data dissemination
12. Implementation of community education and prevention programs
13. Review of surveillance system based on continuing needs

SPECIFIC EMERGENCY HEALTH NEEDS OF REFUGEES

Refugees must have easy access to treatment. Often the local health system becomes overburdened with common illnesses. It is important to establish a community-based health service that both identifies those in need of health care and provides appropriate care. The health system should be developed so that most patients can be taken care of locally, with complicated cases referred to a district hospital.

SPHERE PROJECT

The SPHERE project (Steering Committee for Humanitarian Response) provides a set of universal standards in core areas of humanitarian response. When developing interventions for refugee health, it is useful to consider SPHERE guidelines in the planning and delivery of services. Several of the SPHERE standards are described below.

INITIAL HEALTH-CARE PRIORITIES

FOOD   For the population totally dependent on food aid, a general ration of at least 1,900 kcal/person/day is required (Table 3-9).

Each of the rations should provide at least minimum quantities of energy, protein, and fat. The calculation of rations should be increased accordingly 1% per degree of temperature below 20°C. The calculation of rations should be adjusted for the underlying health status of the population and the relative activity levels of the community.

TABLE 3-9 CHARACTERISTICS OF A GENERAL RATION

FOOD	NO. OF KCAL	COMMENT
Cereal, grains (rice, corn, oats, etc.)	350	Main source of both energy and protein in most diets
Legumes and oilseeds (beans, peas, soya, etc.)	350–750	Useful when eaten with cereals as the protein complements each other
Whole tubers and roots (yams, cassava potato, etc.)	75–110	Bulk and low protein content makes them unsuitable as staple foods in emergencies
Milk, meat, eggs, and dairy products	150–550	Usually consumed in small quantities in normal times
Fats and oils	900	Useful way to increase energy without increasing bulk of diet

However, absolute priority must be given to the delivery of the staple food. The assured delivery of a few items is better than a complex ration.

The first level should be the community health worker, preferably a refugee, working among the population. The main function of this worker is to identify and treat common diseases, recommend preventive measures, and provide public health education. If this is not possible, he/she should refer the more difficult cases to the clinic for evaluation. The clinic, based as 1 per 5,000, should have facilities for consultation, clinical procedures, and a small pharmacy. In support of the clinics, there should be a health center for each refugee settlement.

The food should be distributed in a community setting on a regular basis. This should solve the problem of food distribution to a dispersed population, where the local population may be intermingled with displaced populations. Distributed food should be culturally acceptable and should complement, not replace, any food the refugees are able to provide for themselves. Adequate fuel and utensils should be provided if the rations need to be cooked. If fresh fruits and vegetables are not available, fortified blended foods should be provided. Lactating women should be provided with extra sources of calories and protein. Breast-feeding should be encouraged, and bottle-feeding should be discouraged.

Dry ration has major advantages over cooked food distribution. Dry ration distribution allows families to prepare their own food as they wish and is generally more culturally and socially acceptable. The dry rations are usually distributed in 7- to 14-day intervals.

The wet ration method requires centralized kitchens, fuel, and trained personnel. At least two meals must be provided per day. Although this may be necessary during the initial stages of a population displacement, this method requires more organization and may be difficult in large refugee settings.

WATER   Water needs demand immediate attention from the start of a displaced emergency. The goal is to assure availability of enough fresh water to allow unrestricted distribution and safe drinking. Special arrangements might have to be made for extraction, storage, and distribution. Additional measures, such as treatment, might be required to protect the water from contamination. The eventual goal is to provide safe water for consumption in the home.

An on-the-spot assessment of water sources by local authorities and experts is important. This involves identifying sources of water, appropriate supply/distribution methods, and seasonal factors that effect the water supply (Table 3-10). Water sources must be protected from contamination. If the local available water supply is insufficient, water must be bought in by truck. Meanwhile, other sources of water such as surface water, ground water, and rainwater should be sought. To properly meet emergency needs, a long-term water supply system needs to be established.

Although the quantity of water may meet minimum needs, the quality of the drinking water is even more important. Water must be safe to drink. The most serious threat

TABLE 3-10 WATER SUPPLY METHODS IN REFUGEE SETTLEMENTS

SOURCE	WATER SUPPLY	DISTRIBUTION	SEASONAL FACTORS
Rain water	Simple; off suitable roofs	Individual collection	Seasonal, unlikely to meet total demand
Surface water	1. Controlled access 2. Organize pumping from human activities 3. Treat water	1. Individual collection or storage tanks 2. Pipe system	Yield often varies seasonally
Spring water	Simple: controlled access	1. Individual collection or storage tanks 2. Pipe system	Yield may vary seasonally
Bore-hole	1. Protect and fix drain-off for surplus water 2. Install electic pump or hand-drawn container	1. Individual collection or storage tanks 2. Pipe system	Yield may vary seasonally
Well	1. Protect the well and fix drain-off for surplus water 2. Cover it and install pump	1. Individual collection or storage tanks 2. Pipe system	Yield may vary seasonally

to the safety of a water supply is contamination by feces. Once contaminated, it is hard to purify water quickly in emergency conditions. Thus, the quantity of fecal coliforms in the water is one of two important water quality indicators, the other being amount of free chlorine.

SHELTER The overall goal is to provide protection from the elements, space to live, and privacy. This is one of the most important determinants of general living conditions, and the lack of shelter can have a major adverse affect on health. This is especially true in cold climates, where additional provisions such as blankets, clothes, or heaters will have to be offered. Although the basic need for shelter is similar in most emergencies, multiple factors such as type of housing, materials, and length of time needed will be different.

Shelter is a high priority and must be available before other services can be developed properly. Although the ideal solution would be to build housing at a known location, forming a displaced camp is often unavoidable. A temporary camp often becomes permanent. Therefore, it is important to take into account the social and cultural background of the displaced prior to camp selection.

The single most important site selection criterion is the availability of an adequate supply of water throughout the year. Do not assume that water can be acquired by drilling or hauling for long periods of time. When that site is chosen, its relationship to the water table is important.

The entire camp should be placed at least 3 meters above the water table to ensure adequate drainage. Flat sites and marshes should be avoided because they may become problematic during the rainy season. Other considerations to take into account are listed in Table 3-11.

The best way to meet emergency shelter needs is to provide materials or shelter similar to those used by the displaced or the local population. Whenever possible, emergency shelter should be reusable for construction of improved housing. The key to providing adequate shelter is the provision of a roof. Tents can provide temporary shelter, but they are difficult to live in and provide little protection from temperature changes. This should be the choice of last resort.

TABLE 3-11 WORLD HEALTH ORGANIZATION RECOMMENDATIONS FOR SHELTER

WHO MINIMUM CRITERIA	HEALTH PROBLEMS	OTHER CONSIDERATIONS
1. 30 square meters per person per person 2. 3.5 square meters of floor space per person	1. Overcrowding has negative health implications 2. Communicable diseases increases in communal shelters	1. Road access 2. Environmental hazards 3. Climate conditions 4. Soil for water absorption

Whenever possible, the displaced population should have significant input into building the shelter. This ensures that the shelter will meet their particular needs and reduce their sense of dependence.

SANITATION Indiscriminate disposal of human and other waste poses serious threats to the health of the refugees. In a displaced population, latrines are often unavailable and people may contaminate the water supply. It is important to establish an effective waste disposal system. After establishment, a publicity campaign will be required to encourage the population to use specified areas and not defecate near dwellings or the water supply.

Advice from local experts is needed to develop the most appropriate waste disposal system. The most common cause of complete failure of a sanitation system is the establishment of the wrong system. Good sanitation depends primarily on the attitudes of the community and the people who manage the system.

In an emergency situation, time is critical. The pollution of the environment by human excreta cannot be stopped without immediate sanitation measures. Thus, the initial choice is limited and usually dictates the use of trench latrines. These can be dug quickly and are very effective for short-term use.

Once a temporary system has been established, more time should be used to establish the most appropriate waste disposal system. The two main factors to consider are traditional sanitation practices of the displaced people and the physical characteristics of the settled area (Table 3-12). Failure to take proper account of either factor can cause the system to become a health hazard. However, the cleanliness of latrines and their ease of access will determine whether or not they are used.

Expert advice should be elicited prior to establishing a long-term waste disposal system. To determine the most appropriate latrine style, consideration must be given to the factors listed in Table 3-13.

IMMEDIATE MEDICAL PRIORITIES

The most common medical diseases among refugees are the same as those normally expected in any community in a developing country. However, the conditions likely to be encountered, such as overcrowding, malnutrition, and poor personal hygiene, lead

TABLE 3-12 FACTORS TO CONSIDER FOR WASTE DISPOSAL

TRADITONAL PRACTICE ISSUES	PHYSICAL CHARACTERISTICS OF AREA
Method of anal cleaning	Geology
Preferred position	Availablility of water
Previous sanitation system	Rainfall
Previous sanitation practice	Drainage of water

TABLE 3-13 THINGS TO CONSIDER FOR BUILDING A LATRINE

Number and siting of latrines
   One latrine should be provided for every 20 people
   Latrines should be located at least 6 meters from dwellings, 10 meters from
      health centers, and at least 15 meters from water source
   Latrines should not be located more than 50 meters from users
Population density—camp layout should be determined by the needs of the
      most suitable sanitation system; avoid overcrowding
Soil type variation
   Rocky soil may prevent pit digging
   Sandy soil will require special measures to guard against collapse
Seasonal water table differences
   High water table may cause seasonal contamination from seepage
Available water
   Will determine if disposal system requiring water is a possibility
   Where appropriate, water should be available for anal cleaning
Drainage—consider surface run-off, cut-off ditches, and flooding
Construction materials
   For walls and roofs
   Squatting or sitting slabs for wet system
   Cover slab

to a higher-than-normal incidence of communicable disease. Those at highest risk are the poor, elderly, women, and young children. In addition, the interaction between malnutrition and infection in these populations leads to the high rates of morbidity and mortality from communicable disease, which account for 60% to 95% of all deaths.

The goal is to prevent, detect, and treat diseases. Diarrhea, in particular, poses a major threat to a refugee's health during the first weeks of a settlement's life. This is usually a consequence of new surroundings, poor environmental services, and deterioration of communal services, such as contamination of the water supply. The greatest impact on prevention is improving the environmental conditions.

Despite the best preventive measures, an outbreak of a disease may begin in the population. It is important to identify the source in order to limit its effect on the refugee population. The quickest way to accomplish this is by doing a rapid assessment during the disease outbreak (Table 3-14).

IMMUNIZATION The only immunization indication in the early weeks of an emergency is of young children against measles. Even though there is considerable pressure for immediate mass immunization, there are medical and practical reasons for this to be avoided. Most illness are due to infectious diseases and malnutrition, which cannot be prevented by immunization. Also, mass immunizations require tremendous staff and resources that are often unavailable.

After the acute phase, children should be immunized within the framework of the national immunization program.

TABLE 3-14 ASSESSMENT OF AN EPIDEMIC

Epidemic: the occurrence in a community of an illness, clearly in excess of normal expectancy, and derived from a common or propagated source

1.	Confirm the existence of an epidemic Compare for week or month to month variability
2.	Confirm the diagnosis: identify the agent Clinical basis (measles) or laboratory studies (serum, feces, etc.)
3.	Determine the number of cases and case definition Separate between suspected, probable, and confirmed
4.	Establish time, place, and person Epidemic curve, map, and chart of age and sex
5.	Determine who is at risk Age: young vs. old Sex: male vs. female
6.	Evaluate transmission/risk factors (resistance, serotype, mode of transmission, etc.). Might need to do Case control studies Retrospective epidemiologic surveys Environmental assessments
7.	Document findings
8.	Establish priorities and select alternatives

Reduce source of infection	Protect susceptible groups	Interrupt transmission
Treatment of cases	Immunization, chemoprophylaxis	Vector control and disinfection

9.	Establish treatment program
10.	Information source and public education

IDENTIFYING THE LEADING CAUSES OF ILLNESS AND DEATH Table 3-15 provides information on diseases common to refugee situations. It includes information on the symptoms, transmission, and possible measures that can be introduced for these diseases.

In refugee health, it is advisable to identify case definitions for the most common illnesses in order to identify them properly (Table 3-16).

CHILDREN

MALNUTRITION Malnutrition can be recognized by certain clinical signs and body measurements. The clinical signs include marasmus, kwashiorkor, and marasmic kwashiorkor, which is a combination of the two former conditions and is often seen in refugee settings.

TABLE 3-15 DISEASES COMMON TO REFUGEE SITUATIONS

DISEASE	TRANSMISSION	SYMPTOMS	MAJOR CONTRIBUTING FACTORS	PREVENTION	TREATMENT
Diarrhea	Contaminated water and food	1. 3 or more loose bowel movements a day 2. If watery stool, suspect cholera 3. If bloody stool, suspect invasive diarrhea	1. Overcrowding 2. Malnutrition 3. Change in living environment	1. Adequate living space 2. Good personal hygiene 3. Safe water—purify water and check for fecal contamination 4. Safe sanitation	1. Usually self-limited 2. ORS is important 3. IV fluids for severe cases 4. Antibiotics for bloody diarrhea
Acute respiratory infection	Aerosol and coughing	1. Fever 2. Cough 3. Shortness of breath	1. Poor housing 2. Lack of clothing and blankets 3. Malnutrition 4. Poor crowding and ventilation	1. Shelter 2. Clothing 3. Blankets 4. Minimum living space standards 5. Child immunization	1. Antibiotics for severe cases
Malaria	Infected mosquitoes	Early stage: 1. Fever 2. Chills and sweats 3. Headaches Late stage: 1. Liver and kidney failure 2. Shock 3. Coma	1. Nonimmune strains in new environment 2. Stagnant water 3. Breeding sites	1. Destroy breeding sites 2. Spraying 3. Nets 4. Vector control	Drug prophylaxis
Neonatal tetanus	Spores through open wounds	1. Muscular contractions (jaw and neck muscles) 2. Respiratory depression (late stage)	Poor obstetrical care: 1. Unsterile cord cutting 2. Unsterile covering of cord stump	1. Immunization of pregnant woman 2. Training of midwives 3. Clean equipment 4. Sterile practice	Supportive care
Measles	Highly contagious by airborne particles or direct contact	1. Fever, cough, red eyes, and runny nose 2. Followed in 3–7 days by blotchy red rash that starts in face and then over to rest of body	Overcrowding	1. Immunization of children 9 months to 5 yrs 2. If vaccine limited, priority to malnourished and hospitalized children	Self limited
Tuberculosis	Airbone particles	Fever and cough that persists for at least 3 weeks	Overcrowding	1. Minimum living standards 2. Endemic areas will continue to have problems	1. 6 months of treatment with antituberculosis medication 2. BCG vaccination in children under 1 yr

TABLE 3-16 CLINICAL CASE DEFINITIONS FOR COMMON ILLNESSES

ILLNESSES	DEFINITION
Common diarrhea	3 or more liquid watery stools per day
Dysentery	3 or more liquid stools per day and presence of visible blood in stools
Acute respiratory infection	Fever, cough, and rapid breathing (>50/min)
Malaria	Temperature >38.5°C and absence of other infection
Malnutrition	Weight for height index −2 Z-scores or kwashiorkor
Measles	Generalized rash lasting >3 days and temperature >38°C and one of the following: cough, runny nose, red eyes
Neonatal tetanus	1. Normal suck and cry for the first 2 days of life 2. Onset of illness between 3 and 28 days of life 3. Inability to suck, followed by stiffness and/or convulsions
Meningitis	Sudden onset of fever >38.9°C and stiff neck or purpura
Tuberculosis	Fever and cough that persists >3 weeks

The two most common body measurements that can be used for the objective assessment of nutritional status are weight for height (WFH) and the MUAC (Table 3-17).

If severe malnutrition exists, therapeutic feeding programs will need to be initiated. This is the main method of saving the lives of infants and children with severe malnutrition. However, it is important to remember that there should always be some sort of supplementary feeding program in place prior to establishing the therapeutic program. Otherwise, less malnourished children will deteriorate until they need stronger intervention (Table 3-18).

DIARRHEAL DISEASE This is the most common fatal childhood disease worldwide. This is also a major cause of morbidity and mortality among refugee populations because of the inadequacy of the water supply and inefficiently maintained sanitation facilities. Although the etiology of diarrheal disease during refugee emergencies has not been well documented, the responsible pathogens are most likely to be the same agents that cause diarrhea in the normal populations in developing countries. Malnourished individuals are particularly prone to diarrhea, and the complications can result in dehydration and shock.

ACUTE RESPIRATORY INFECTION Acute respiratory infection is among the leading causes of death among refugee populations. ARIs are caused by a variety of viruses and bacteria. Signs and symptoms may be mild initially but may progress rapidly to death.

TABLE 3-17

WEIGHT FOR HEIGHT (WFH)	MID-UPPER ARM CIRCUMFERENCE (MUAC)
Preferred method	Less sensitive
Best indicator of acute malnutrition	Quicker than WFH
Can be monitored to assess individual progress	Measures area that does not change with age but wastes rapidly in malnutrition
	Cannot be monitored to assess individual progress
Two methods	
% scale method	MUAC method
Weight as % of a international reference medium for height:	Children between ages 1 and 5 by random or cluster sample
<80% = malnourished	If age uncertain, check for more than six teeth but stand less than 115 cm in height
<70% = severely malnourished	Eliminate from study any child with edema but report in final results
Z-score method	
Z is the median score for the children	Kwashiorkor
Z-score is number of standard deviation above/below the median	MUAC <13.5 cm = mild malnutrition
Z-score < −3 = severely malnourished	MUAC <12.5 cm = severe malnutrition
	Calculate amount and degree of malnutrition as % of sample

MALARIA This is a major health problem in many areas that host large refugee populations. Malnutrition may be directly related to recurrent or persistent malaria infection, and may compound the effects of malaria and lead to high mortality. The transmission of malaria is more likely to occur when the displaced population travels through or into an area of higher endemicity than its region of origin. In some camps, malaria outbreaks have been caused by the emergence of chloroquine-resistant organisms.

In an area known to have falciparum malaria, any signs such as fever, delirium, disorientation, or coma should be assumed to be malaria and treated promptly. In other scenarios, if malaria is suspected, the following measures should be taken:

1. Attempt to confirm the diagnosis via blood smears or symptom analysis
2. Assess the risk of disease
   A. Find out about the prevalence of malaria in refugees' homeland
   B. Find out if they traveled through any malaria-infected area
   C. Obtain information regarding malaria in the camp area
3. Assess prevalence and severity
   A. Use case definition to test for malaria in patients by doing blood smears
   B. Determine the number of smears done and the number positive, and the identification of the organism
   C. Check morbidity and mortality records to assess the prevalence of the disease in the camp

TABLE 3-18 ESTABLISHING A FEEDING PROGRAM

Goals:
To provide extra high energy, high protein, and low bulk extra meals 1–2/day to those who need it

Target groups		
Acutely malnourished children <5 yr	*Pregnant or lactating women*	*Elderly*

Program is needed when:

General ration <1,500 kcal/person
>20% acute malnutrition
High incidence of measles or diarrheal disease

Supplementary Program	Therapeutic Program
On-site feeding is preferred (can be observed and supervised)	Inpatient basis always at least 150 kcal diet with 3–4 g of protein/kg/day
Provide at least 500 kcal and 15 g protein/day in 1–2 feedings in addition to regular rations	Given during 5–7 meals at 3-hour interval/24 hour
	Admission criteria
	Severe edema or marasmus
Food should be easily digestible (soup or porridge); can be eaten by all ages	WFH <70% or Z-score <−3
	Should be discharged to supplementary program after >80% WFH or without
Children to be discharged only after >85% WFH for at least 1 month as % of sample	edema

WFH, weight for height.

4. Decide whom to treat. The three main options are
   A. Treat all fever cases
   B. Treat all clinical cases according to clinical case definition
   C. Treat only cases confirmed by blood smears
5. Institute control measures
   A. Malaria outbreak will be a problem if refugees are in a highly endemic area and come from a less endemic region.
   B. In an outbreak of fever-producing illness, blood smears will confirm or exclude malaria epidemics
   C. If outbreak is suspected:
      i. Health services providing prompt diagnosis and treatment of cases should be reinforced
      ii. Treatment is given to all patients with fever
      iii. Active case finding and prompt referral should be initiated by community health workers

    iv. Control measures, like spraying or vector control, should be initiated, and monitoring of malaria should be instituted

    D. If malaria is already a problem, the situation is more urgent

Prophylaxis with antimalarial drugs for the entire population should be considered until mosquito abatement programs can be instituted.

NEONATAL TETANUS Neonatal tetanus is usually caused by unclean delivery techniques during birth or lack of immunization in women of childbearing age. In the emergency phase, the focus is toward providing traditional birth attendants with basic training in clean delivery techniques.

All women between the ages of 15 and 44 should receive a full schedule of tetanus toxoid vaccination. This should be part of standard antenatal care. Female health workers should be employed to educate women about the need for the tetanus toxoid vaccination and to refer pregnant women to the antenatal care clinic.

WOUND-RELATED TETANUS Wound-related tetanus infection can be prevented by early and adequate excision of dead tissue, administration of penicillin as soon as possible, and administration of antitetanus serum and tetanus toxoid simultaneously.

MEASLES Measles represents one of the leading causes of death among children in refugee camps. This is due to the coexistence of low levels of immunization coverage and high rates of undernutrition. Such outbreaks have played a critical role in the spread of measles and the mortality within some refugee camps. In addition, measles has contributed to high mortality rates among those who have survived the initial illness, because of susceptibility to other illnesses. Mass immunization campaigns have been shown to be effective in reducing the morbidity and mortality associated with measles, especially in areas where previous immunization coverage is low (Table 3-19).

TUBERCULOSIS Tuberculosis is a well recognized health problem among refugee populations. This is due to the crowded living conditions and underlying poor nutri-

TABLE 3-19 STEPS IN CONDUCTING A MEASLES IMMUNIZATION PROGRAM

1. Estimate the size of target population (initial assessment data)

2. Obtain map of the site

3. Strategy: vaccinating the maximum number of children in shortest possible time
   A. First and rapid mass campaign
   B. Followed by routine immunization in fixed facilities

Mass immunization by outreach teams at dispersed sites	Immunization at refugee arrival	Mobile teams from house to house

Once target population is reached, a system of maintaining immunizaton should be established.

tional status of refugees. Although not a major cause of mortality during the acute emergency phase, tuberculosis often becomes a critical problem once measles and diarrheal disease have been adequately controlled.

In very young children, tuberculosis can be a rapidly fatal disease in the form of disseminated tuberculosis or tubercular meningitis. Treatment is complicated in refugee situations because regimens usually cannot be completed due to uncertain duration of stay, frequent changes in camp locations, poor camp organization, and lack of personnel to supervise treatment.

If tuberculosis is suspected, the following measures should be taken:

1. Confirm the diagnosis
   A. Sputum smears
   B. Patient history of fever and cough for at least 3 weeks (when laboratory analysis is not available)
2. Determine the magnitude of the disease
   A. Determine the percentage of smears positive for tuberculosis
   B. Confirm morbidity and mortality data to assess number of deaths due to tuberculosis
   C. Check the number of patients reporting to health services with fever and cough
3. Establish control programs if sputum tests are positive or if symptoms are consistent with tuberculosis
   A. Prior to starting any program, make sure that basic health priorities have been addressed and the population is expected to remain stable so patient can finish treatment
   B. Then define clear protocols with
      i. Case definition
      ii. Treatment regimens including specific cases
      iii. Data collection
      iv. Evaluation
   C. Monitoring and evaluation organized from the beginning
   D. Proper laboratory and sufficient supply of drugs
   E. Direct observed treatment plan (DOTS) (patient takes medication in front of health-care worker)
   F. Should be in coordination with national authorities
4. Bacillus Calmette-Guérin (BCG) vaccination program in children less than 1 year old should be considered because it provides a high degree of protection against serious forms of disease in children. It is recommended for all children at birth or soon after, unless they have signs of immunodeficiency (e.g., clinical AIDS)

OTHER ACUTE INFECTIONS Other acute infections, such as meningitis, skin infections, HIV, and other sexually transmitted diseases, may be observed. Meningococcal outbreaks in refugee populations have been due to overcrowding and limited access to medical care. The disease tends to affect all age groups, although children under age 5 are at greatest risk for meningitis.

TABLE 3-20 EXAMPLE OF SURVEILLANCE FORM

Location:
Start Date:
End Date:
Source:
Summary:

Population	End of last week (A)	New arrivals	Departures	End of this week (B)	Population average (A + B)/2
Under 5					
All age					

Causes of Mortality

Diseases	<5 years			>=5 years			Total			%
	M	F	T	M	F	T	M	F	T	
Bloody diarrhea										
Nonbloody diarrhea										
Fever										
Suspected malaria										
Measles										
Malnutrition										
Others										
Total										

Mortality Summary

	Total Deaths			Rate/10,000/Day		
	Male	Female	Total	Male	Female	Total
<5 years old						
All age						

Morbidity Summary

Disease	<5 years	>=5 years	Total	Incidence
Bloody diarrhea				
Nonbloody diarrhea				
Fever				
Suspected malaria				
Measles				
Malnutrition				
Others				

Skin infections, such as scabies and impetigo, are also of concern but are of lower priority in emergency situations. Scabies, caused by a mite, and impetigo, caused by a streptococcal infection of the skin, are common for individuals living in crowded conditions with inadequate water supply for washing. If skin infections are a problem, the following measures should be taken:

1. Check that there is enough soap and water for washing
2. Specific treatment for both can be given
3. Clothes worn prior to infection must be washed thoroughly

There has been no evidence that the incidence of sexually transmitted diseases or HIV in camps is any higher or lower than in nonrefugee populations. Table 3-20 provides a sample surveillance form for recording health problems in a refugee setting.

VIOLENCE The violence associated with forced migrations contributes to the health problems experienced by displaced persons. It is important that an adequate security force be in place in order to reduce violence within the refugee population. The security force also plays a critical role in protecting the refugees from outsiders that might try to benefit from the situation. They provide a safe atmosphere where people can live with relative peace of mind.

CHAPTER 4
Culture and Health

Tamara L. Thomas

INTRODUCTION

Culture has no single definition but is a complex whole of beliefs, practices, likes, dislikes, rituals, and habits. Culture is a set of rules we use for living where we do in the world. The rules change with each location. The local culture affects how we, as local health-care workers, communicate and practice. It also influences the patient's interpretation of what we do and say. In order to effectively care for the whole patient we must be aware of the culture in which we are working.

ABCs OF CULTURAL AWARENESS

A—Ask
- If you are uncertain where to proceed, communicate this.
- Discreetly asking a contact person can save you more trouble than allowing your ego to take over.

B—Balance Your Views With Local Views
- See issues from the other person's viewpoint and cultural background.
- Remember that you are the visitor and your way may not work here.

C—Courtesy
- Many cultural faux pas can easily be smoothed over by simply remembering common courtesy.
- Treat colleagues as you would wish to be treated.

COMMUNICATE RESPECT

The opportunity to work with a variety of cultures is a unique privilege, and communication is imperative to performing effective health care. Start by showing the patients that you respect their views. Health workers in other countries and cultures take pride in the work they are doing, despite limitations in supplies and technology, and may feel embarrassed at the resources they have available. When working with your foreign colleagues, it is important to be as complimentary as you can, and wait until you have established a relationship before offering suggestions for improvement.

AVOID PATERNALISM

A pitfall to avoid when working transculturally is to assume "I know what you need." Be open minded and remind yourself that you are in a different country and culture. Many medical personnel have alienated themselves by being paternalistic and giving the appearance of superiority. Although you have different ideas, opinions, and ways of living, strive to be open minded and respectful.

KEY POINTS:

- Remember that you are the visitor.
- Establish a positive relationship before making suggestions for improvement.
- Allow your views of the way things should be done to be flexible.
- Avoid judgmental statements.
- Be patient and tolerant of cultural barriers imposed by verbal and nonverbal communication.
- There are many ways to complete a task. Doing something different does not translate to it being wrong.

PREPARATION FOR INTERNATIONAL WORK

IDENTIFY YOUR PRECONCEIVED PERCEPTIONS

It is important to recognize how your personal background and culture affect your views of others. As a health-care provider you have a culture of medicine with its own set of beliefs, practices, likes, dislikes, norms, and language. Remember that your "medicine culture" affects the way you practice. Workers from countries with more developed health-care systems rely on abundant technology and resources in daily practice, whereas people with fewer resources rely on their examination skills and experience.

Suppose a mildly dehydrated child with diarrhea is brought into a medical clinic for care:

- A local health worker in a developing country would safely and effectively treat with oral rehydration solution and give instructions to the parent.
- A hospital-based health-care worker from a more developed country may have electrolytes drawn and an intravenous line placed. This wastes the time of the health worker, patient, and family, and unnecessarily uses scarce supplies and resources. In addition, this overly invasive approach may create an unnecessary dependence by local populations on health resources.

IDENTIFY THE LOCAL STANDARD OF CARE

Investigate what is currently working well in local health care and build upon this. Identifying and understanding the local medical practices will help to avoid raising expectations and providing inappropriate levels of technology. Define local capabilities and do not overextend these resources. A common pitfall is trying to do it all and creating dependency.

KNOW YOUR HISTORY

Find out as much as you can about the recent and distant history of the country in which you are about to work. Research into the social customs and behaviors of people can give you important information about

Ethnic groups and potential conflicts
Authority structure
Geographical distribution and resultant access to health care
Religious groups and controversies over religion
Political tensions

UNDERSTAND HOW THE PATIENT AND HIS FAMILY VIEW YOU

It is useful to explore what local health workers and the patients expect of you. Remember that expectations come from the patient, his family, the local community, health workers, and you. A patient's treatment success is dependent on both his faith in the practitioner and faith in his treatment.

BELIEF HAS A STRONG HEALING POWER

The placebo effect has demonstrated that if patients believe in their treatment, they often will get better because of this belief. Remember that you are there to provide health care to the patient. You may need to adjust your approach to coincide with the patient's beliefs, whether he or she is knowledgeable about the cause of disease, how it should be treated, what behavior is appropriate, and how the body is viewed. Working in cooperation with traditional healers when possible will help the patients have confidence in their treatments.

DID YOU KNOW? . . . that just as a patient's belief can make him well, a patient's belief can also make him sick? For example, the evil eye is a spell cast upon another by a powerful individual within the culture. It can affect how a patient or his family member views illness and treatment. Belief in the evil eye is a superstition that is widespread in parts of North Africa, Southern Europe, and the Middle East. A reported 36% of the world's population believes in the evil eye. The nature of the evil eye differs in how it is given, who can give or receive it, and the degree of power it has.

SOCIAL AND CULTURAL CONSIDERATIONS IN HEALTH CARE

Social and cultural issues influence everything we do. Our health practices, diet, and methods of seeking health care are all dependent on cultural morays. Certain cultural phenomena affect health:

- Environmental: Local culture can control environmental health factors. Developing rickets can be affected by environmental factors of both diet and exposure to sunlight.
- Biologic: People from one cultural group may differ biologically from members of other groups. There may be physical differences in body type and skin color. Genetic differences occur in susceptibility to disease and enzyme abnormalities.
- Social organization: Social groups and organizations, particularly religious and ethnic groups as well as family units, affect how health is perceived.
- Communication: The language a person speaks obviously affects health and a patient's ability to access the health-care system. In addition to verbal behavior, culturally specific nonverbal gestures also can be misunderstood.
- Space: Personal space is influenced by culture. There is a personal distance, a social distance, and a public distance, all of which vary between cultures.
- Time: Individual perception and management of time differs between cultural groups. Present, past, and future time may be viewed differently. Planning education/training courses can be chaotic and frustrating when people perceive time differently.

KEY POINTS:

Consider the following attributes to see if there are barriers to effective communication:

Greeting: How do you say hello?
Respect: Who should be shown deference and respect?
Physical contact: What is expected when you greet someone?
Gender: What are opinions and social norms toward the opposite sex?
Attitude about drugs and alcohol
Attitude about work
Time: Are people punctual or routinely late?
Attitude about religion and spirituality
Social hierarchy: Who makes decisions?
Roles of males and females in the culture

CULTURAL BARRIERS TO CARE

Communication is one of the most obvious and important issues in transcultural medicine. We communicate through words, gestures, music, art, work habits, or whatever culture creates as a way of communicating ideas between people. Difficulties in communicating cross-culturally can occur for a variety of reasons (Table 4-1).

TABLE 4-1 PROBLEMS IN CROSS-CULTURAL COMMUNICATION OCCUR BECAUSE

People stand
  Too close
  Too far away
People show up
  Too early
  Too late
  Without appointment
People talk
  Too much
  Too little
  Too fast
  Too slow
  Too loud
  Too soft
People show
  Too much emotion
  Too little emotion

Learn native languages whenever possible. If you are not fluent in the native language, remember to use interpreters as much as possible to avoid misunderstandings. When you are teaching a group of native health-care professionals, don't overestimate your language skills. Would you like to have a lecture given to you in first-grade language?

Nonverbal communication can have a profound impact on others. Gestures and body language are powerful communicators. Cultures have more unique gestures and nonverbal cues than they do verbal expressions. To add to the confusion, some simple gestures have completely different meanings in different cultures, even a simple greeting.

DID YOU KNOW? . . . that the thumbs-up sign has different meanings for different cultures? North Americans flash this sign when they want to communicate "good job" or "okay." However, it may be considered a rude gesture in many parts of the world. It may signify counting in Japan or Germany, and may be saying "up yours" in several African countries.

Direct eye contact can be interpreted as confident and positive in some areas or arrogant and rude in others. In the Native American population, direct eye contact and a firm handshake is seen as aggressive, and may cause the recipient to become withdrawn (Table 4-2).

Personal space varies depending on where in the world you are. Standing "toe to toe" may be comfortable for a Latin American, slightly uncomfortable for a North American, and very uncomfortable for Japanese. However, in crowded U. S. elevators or Japanese subways, it is acceptable to stand shoulder to shoulder. This public closeness is handled by looking straight ahead, avoiding eye contact, and drawing into oneself (Table 4-3).

Gestures are shortcuts in communication. Make sure your gestures are understood. Don't interrupt others' gestures when you are in the international setting (Table 4-4). Getting someone's attention can be done in many different ways. However, gestures to beckon someone may be misinterpreted.

TABLE 4-2 EYE CONTACT

CATEGORY	PRESENT	ABSENT
North America	Positive: Direct eye contact shows strength	Negative: Sign of shyness, lack of warmth, weakness
Japan and Korea	Negative: Intimidating, may indicate sexual overtones	Positive: Lack of eye contact shows respect

TABLE 4-3 PERSONAL "BUBBLE" OR SPACE

AREA OF THE WORLD	PERSONAL SPACE
Latinos Middle East	Toe to toe
United States	Arms length
Japan	Longer than the arm

TABLE 4-4 GESTURES

GESTURE	COUNTRY	MEANING
Thumb forming a circle with first finger and other fingers extended	United States France Brazil	Okay Zero, worthless Rude, female genitalia
Wave	United States Europe	Goodbye, get attention May mean "no"
Pointing	United States Japan Germany	Identifying an object or making a point Impolite May mean "2"; thumb is used in counting
Motioning with crooked index finger with palm up	United States Malaysia/Yugoslavia Indonesia, Australia	"Come here" Used to "call" animals Summon a prostitute
Moving hand from side to side with palm down	Europe, Latin America, Greece United States Certain parts of Europe	"Come here" So so, maybe May be confused with waving goodbye
Hand clapping	Worldwide	May be taken for applause or to get someone's attention
Showing sole of foot	Middle and Far East	Rude
Eye contact and nod	Europe, United States	Greeting, acknowledgment, intention to say something
Kissing sounds	United States, parts of Mexico	Taunting or sexual advances

SOCIAL DIFFERENCES IN THE APPROACH TO HEALTH CARE

Health is multidimensional. It includes physical, psychological, social, and religious factors. It is helpful to realize the difference between disease and illness. Disease is the causative agent, and illness is represented by the effects of the agent on a person's health. Health workers often refer to a disease state or "what's wrong" with the patient. Illness is how a person experiences a disease state, and is mingled with cultural overtones and social norms. The majority of people's perceptions of health and illness are influenced primarily by local (indigenous) factors, yet health-care workers have little understanding or training in these concepts.

MENTAL ILLNESS

In no other disease state is there such broad variation in cultural interpretation than in mental illness. The key to diagnosing mental illness depends on what is considered normal, culturally appropriate behavior. Psychiatric conditions may not be recognized in certain cultures or may be attributed to other causes.

Mental illness is highly stigmatized in many cultures. Certain Japanese psychiatrists may have difficulty disclosing a schizophrenic diagnosis to a patient due to the stigma attached. In parts of Asia, psychotherapy is reserved for severe mental disabilities. Psychiatric interventions for milder disorders can be difficult to arrange because patients may feel that they will bring shame to their family. They may not seek necessary treatment because they do not feel they can discuss "private" matters with strangers and feel that problems should handled within the family.

Mental illness definitions vary between different cultural groups. For instance, a Mexican boy hearing voices felt that he was destined to be a *curandero* (a traditional healer), whereas health-care workers diagnosed him as psychotic. His family felt these voices were a sign of something great for their son.

AGE AND GENDER

Age signifies authority in many cultural groups, particularly in Asian cultures. Elder family members may expect medical information to be addressed to them primarily, before addressing the younger patient. Gender also plays a strong role in the exchange of medically pertinent information. Many countries have a largely male-dominated culture, and female patients belonging to certain Middle Eastern, Asian, Hispanic, or gypsy groups may defer all health-care decisions to a husband or father. This may also take the form of preferentially seeking medical care for male children and considering female children subordinate.

Many of these well-established traditions of male authority may raise cross-cultural conflicts between male physicians and female patients. Conflicts also occur for female physicians when a patient's family feels that male doctors whom they trust should manage important decisions. In contrast, Navajo Indians are a matriarchal society with authority lying with the most elderly females.

PURITY AND SEXUALITY

Middle Eastern and Muslim countries value female purity. Men may not allow their veiled wives to undress in front of a male physician. Same-sex caregivers are most effective. Casual touch of the opposite sex can offend and cause misunderstandings. Traditional Chinese men are not allowed to touch females who are not family members. Medical diagnosis can be made by indirectly "examining" a patient by attaching a ribbon to the female patient's wrist. An alabaster figurine may be provided for the patient to point to affected body complaint areas.

In many parts of the world, female circumcision is performed as a rite of passage into female adulthood, and may be intended to help females control strong sexual urges and maintain family honor. Female circumcision, in distinction to male circumcision, is a debilitating procedure that leads to many severe health complications. Although practices of female circumcision, also known as female genital mutilation, have been outlawed in many countries, the practice still occurs throughout Northern Africa and parts of the Middle East (see Table 4-5).

CHILDBIRTH

Customs vary greatly for the attendance of women in labor. Traditional birth attendants exist in almost every culture. The role of men in assisting in the labor process is limited in many cultures. For example, in Mexico it is inappropriate for a husband to attend a wife at birth. The patient's mother is a more appropriate choice.

TABLE 4-5 FEMALE CIRCUMCISION: TRADITION OR TORTURE?

What does it claim to do?
Keep women "pure."
Does the practice of female circumcision cause direct harm?
Yes, it distorts anatomy, causes pain, loss of normal function, and may create disfigurement and genitourinary dysfunction.
Does this serve a function in the community?
Yes, it serves a social function in some societies that signifies entering womanhood as well as preparation for marriage. There may be consequences for women not undergoing the ritual—both social and economic (dowry).
Does it affect how individuals see themselves?
Yes, this affects the way women see themselves as individuals and as part of the group.
Does it have a spiritual connotation?
The spiritual connotation of female purity is a consideration in some cultures.

DID YOU KNOW? . . . the healthy Chinese person needs a balance between yin (cool) and yang (heat). After childbirth, a sudden loss of yang that must be restored, women must remain at bedrest for 7 to 10 days, and they must not bathe, eat, or open windows for circulation.

DEATH AND DYING

Today many people die in hospitals, whereas in previous times most died at home, cared for by their family. There are many cross-cultural differences in dealing with death and the issues surrounding it. These issues include how people grieve, how health-care workers inform patients and family of a terminal illness, last rites rituals, and views on life support.

KEY POINT:

It is not uncommon for the family to insist that a terminal diagnosis be withheld from the patient. This raises conflicts when weighing a patient's "right to know" versus a cultural tradition of protecting patients from the stress of their illness that may hasten their death as is felt in areas of Mexico.

Expressions of grief may vary. Some cultures value emotional restraint, whereas others feel that loud expressions of emotion appropriately illustrate a family's grief and help the deceased into the afterlife. Wailing is an important cultural ritual in certain Middle Eastern cultures. In Native American culture it is important to allow "the spirit to leave" after death by opening windows in the room. The Chinese have a deep respect for their bodies and may wish to die with their body intact. This may lead them to refuse to give consent for surgery and accept a terminal prognosis.

DID YOU KNOW? . . . the number 4 is unlucky in some Asian cultures and may be associated with death. Dates, room numbers, and other items associated with the number 4 may want to be avoided.

PAIN PERCEPTION

Some cultures value emotional expressiveness, whereas others value stoicism. This may cause one patient to ask for pain medication frequently, but another to suffer and wait to be offered medication. It is helpful to understand the amount of outward expression that a particular culture values. Do not overgeneralize or stereotype patient responses because of culture.

HOME REMEDIES AND ALTERNATIVE HEALING

Home remedies have both tradition and value. Learn to respect these traditions. Many home and traditional therapies are inexpensive and effective. Encourage healthy practice of home remedies, and avoid instructing patients to seek medical care for all complaints. Build on these cultural practices, reinforcing those that are positive and promoting change only if they are harmful (Table 4-6).

TABLE 4-6 TRADITIONAL HOME REMEDIES

Colds	Garlic
	Thyme
	Rosemary
	Honey and milk
	Witch hazel
	Sweetflag
	Plasters—onion, mustard
	Goose fat rubbed onto chest
	Cod liver oil
Cough	Hot lemonade with whiskey
	Few drops of turpentine and sugar
	Onion poultice
Sore throat	Eucalyptus
	Bayberry gargle
	Goldenrod leaves
	Comfrey
	Salt water gargle
	Chicken soup
	Onion
Fever	Chamomile
	Chestnut bark
	Blessed thistle
	Cool compresses
	Cool patient
	Cooling blanket
	Cold drinks
	Ice
	Warm patient
	"Sweat it out"
	Blankets
	Hot drinks
Wound care	Abscess
	Ivy leaf poultice
	Boils
	Sulfur water
	Sand sagebrush
	Wounds
	Turpentine
	Globe mellow

EVALUATING FOLK REMEDIES

When evaluating the value and consequences of traditional healing and folk remedies, the most important consideration is the potential for causing harm. Most cultural practices are not dangerous, and many are helpful. Some, however, cause injury or disability, or may lead to health complications. Other practices may not be inherently harmful, but may cause a delay in seeking medical attention for serious health problems. For example, serious infections are more effectively treated with modern antibiotics, and time can be wasted in treating first with home remedies and delaying care of a treatable illness. If a medical condition is not serious and the remedy is harmless, you may encourage traditional remedies.

When evaluating traditional health practices, consider asking these questions:

- What does it claim to do?
- Does the practice or remedy cause direct harm or health risk?
- Does it have a function and value within the community?
- Does it affect how individuals see themselves?
- Does it have a spiritual connotation?

SOME EXAMPLES OF TRADITIONAL REMEDIES

- A villager places animal feces on a baby's skin rash or newborn's umbilical cord.
  - Is this harmful?
    Yes, this treatment can cause tetanus and you must discourage the practice.
- A patient with a viral cough is given herbal tea.
  - Is this harmful?
    No, you do not need to discourage this practice.
- A patient with a minor skin burn is treated topically with the nectar from an aloe vera plant.
  - Is this harmful?
    No, you do not need to discourage this practice.

WORKING WITH TRADITIONAL HEALERS

LOCAL RESOURCES

Indigenous medical workers include a wide variety of individuals performing a broad array of functions that may vary greatly between cultures. Many traditional health workers have unique roles, responsibilities, and positions in their communities. China and India have strong indigenous health systems that are popular and legitimate, and many people simultaneously seek both conventional medical care and traditional medicine.

Traditional healers may serve a variety of functions as herbalists, traditional birth attendants, witch doctors, shamans, or *curanderos*. Most folk healers share the cultural values and worldview of the community where they live, as well as a similar belief of the origin and treatment of illness. There are several advantages and disadvantages to working with traditional healers.

Advantages of Traditional Healers
- Shares the patient's community and views of the world
- Frequently involves the family in diagnosis and treatment
- Treatments may be effective, practical, and inexpensive
- Greater understanding of a person's fears and perceptions
- Holistic: they treat the whole person—body, mind, and spirit

Disadvantages of Traditional Healers
- Some practices may be harmful, such as painful scarification, incision, and mutilation
- Spreading infections and blood letting
- They are often panaceas and may delay treatment

DID YOU KNOW? . . . that certain East African mothers believe that "plastic teeth" cause chronic intermittent diarrhea in their babies. These "teeth" are believed to show up prior to "milk teeth" and are treated by

- Rubbing gums with plant leaves
- Vigorous rubbing with a millipede wrapped in a leaf
- Extracting plastic teeth from gums with sharp objects like a homemade knife that can lead to infection, discomfort, and poor feeding by the child
- Mothers rarely bring their infants to medical workers for this problem because they know that "plastic teeth" are not recognized by anyone other than indigenous workers

---

UNDERSTANDING THE ROLE OF HEALERS IN SOCIETY

One of the first steps in working with traditional health practitioners is to identify the role they play in the community. By understanding their practice, you can learn how to recognize the benefits of traditional methods and develop creative solutions for patient care.

WORKING TOGETHER A *curandero* is a traditional holistic healer in many Latin American countries. In addition to treating with herbs, the *curandero*'s treatment often has a religious component. A Mexican boy experiencing hallucinations was felt by health-care personnel to need antipsychotic medications. Both the boy and his parents were reluctant to start medication. Hospital personnel brought in a *curandero* who initiated traditional treatment. The boy and his parents were comfortable and started medication in addition to traditional therapy. Cooperation between the traditional and curative therapies gave the patient the best care.

TRADITIONAL MEDICINE TECHNIQUES AND COMPLICATIONS

Many traditional practices have gained scientific acceptance. Traditional herb and plant therapy is becoming increasingly recognized in more industrialized countries. Here are a few examples of traditional treatments you may encounter:

Herbalists: Herbal therapy is well established in Native American, Chinese, and Bedouin cultures. Many medications are based on traditional herbal remedies.

Coining: Coining is a traditional Asian form of healing described as rubbing a coin firmly on the skin, eliciting red welts to draw illness out of the body. The red welts show only on ill people. Health workers unfamiliar with this practice may misdiagnose these welts as child abuse.

Cupping: Another remedy resulting in red marks on the body occurs from heating glass cups and placing them on the body, creating suction. This therapy is thought to be particularly successful for treating muscle pain.

Acupuncture: Traditional Chinese therapy uses fine needles that are inserted into areas known as meridians. The goal is to restore the balance between yin and yang. This is accepted as a legitimate method of healing in both the Eastern and Western world.

Moxibustion: This Chinese treatment is based on the therapeutic value of heat and is used for disease with an excess of yin. Heated, pulverized wormwood is applied to the skin in a specific meridian.

Fire Doctor: Traditional Bedouin healers in the Middle East use fire as a form of therapy. Fire is used at certain skin points, followed by application of a medicine at these points.

Bush thoracotomies: In Papua New Guinea, patients may be told by their bush doctor that their disease is caused by evil. Treatment includes piercing the chest wall with a sharp pandana leaf and packing the chest cavity with leaves. They are told that the evil will drain from them in several days. Serious empyema results from this treatment.

SUMMARY

Working with people from different cultures is one of the most interesting aspects of working internationally. Local customs may vary greatly from your own. It is important to treat all individuals and traditions with respect and a spirit of helpfulness. Recognizing the importance of cultural issues can be the key to successful and productive health work abroad.

CHAPTER 5

Field Assessment of General Health and Nutrition

Kathleen Clem and John M. Toso

EVALUATION OF NUTRITIONAL STATUS

A good nutritional state is one of the backbones of good health in all cultures. For any health worker, it is important to assess the general nutritional status in each patient you see. Poor nutrition can lead to various forms of malnutrition, and can cause or contribute to many illnesses. A poor nutritional state can cause a child or an adult to be more susceptible to infections, such as tuberculosis or pneumonia. Malnourished children are far more prone to die from diarrhea and respiratory infection.

People at high risk for developing health problems related to malnutrition include

Young children
Pregnant or breast-feeding women
Elderly patients
Children or adults with preexisting illness
Refugees and displaced people
People with chronic underlying medical conditions

Before examining a patient, ask him questions about the food he eats. It is particularly important to ask nursing mothers and mothers caring for young children about the types of food they are eating, and the need for a balanced diet with enough protein, fat, and carbohydrates. Also ask about the following:

Loss of energy
Failure of a child to grow

Frequent diarrhea or respiratory illnesses
Hair loss or thinning
Failure of sores to heal properly
Rashes or dry, cracked skin

All levels of health-care workers should be familiar with signs and symptoms of malnutrition. As a routine part of any physical examination, be sure to examine your patient for signs and symptoms of nutritional deficiency.

HOW TO PERFORM A RAPID NUTRITIONAL STATUS EXAMINATION

- Expose: Remove enough clothing to examine the patient well
- Touch: Skin turgor, warmth, texture, and moisture
- Look: Color, rashes, and overall condition
- Listen: Respiratory, circulatory, and gastrointestinal system
- Test/measure: Physical measurements such as middle upper arm circumference and weight for height score

> With practice, health-care workers will be able to recognize poor nutritional states. Most of the assessment can be done quickly at a glance. By starting at the head and working down, important nutritional deficiencies can be identified.

Physical examination: Look for these signs of malnutrition when examining a patient

HEAD AND NECK

Hair: Thinning, straightening, or color changes may signify marasmus or kwashiorkor.
Eyes: Check for corneal edema, Bitot's spots (patches of small gray bubbles on the sclera), complaints of night blindness, and xerophthalmia. This can progress to corneal ulcers/scarring and represents vitamin A deficiency. One cause of cataracts and glossitis is riboflavin deficiency.
Mouth: Tooth loss and dental caries represent a diet too high in sugar or protein-energy malnutrition (PEM). Dermatitis around the eyes and mouth can be caused by pyridoxine deficiency. Pyorrhea and gingivitis signal a diet low in vitamin C.
Nose: Frequent nosebleeds may be caused by a diet low in vitamin C.
Neck: Goiters may represent a diet lacking iodine.

CARDIOVASCULAR Tachycardia and dyspnea may represent anemia. Edema can be caused by low protein intake.

GASTROINTESTINAL Organomegaly may represent kwashiorkor. Abdominal distention can be caused by intestinal parasites and malnutrition.

SKELETAL Rickets in children is caused by lack of vitamin D. Adults get osteomalacia.

SKIN Pellagra is due to malnutrition and can be associated with kwashiorkor. Dry, cracked skin may show vitamin A or B1 deficiency. Peeling skin with light and dark patches (flaking paint rash) indicates kwashiorkor. Open sores that don't heal well can be caused by lack of vitamin C. Vitamin B2 deficiency can cause skin atrophy. Candidiasis is found more frequently in those who are not well nourished (Figs. 5-1 and 5-2).

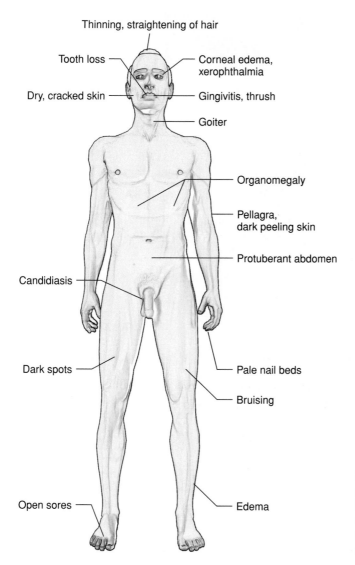

Thinning, straightening of hair

Tooth loss

Corneal edema, xerophthalmia

Dry, cracked skin

Gingivitis, thrush

Goiter

Organomegaly

Pellagra, dark peeling skin

Protuberant abdomen

Candidiasis

Dark spots

Pale nail beds

Bruising

Open sores

Edema

FIGURE 5-1 Quick visual assessment for signs of malnutrition and deficiency syndromes.

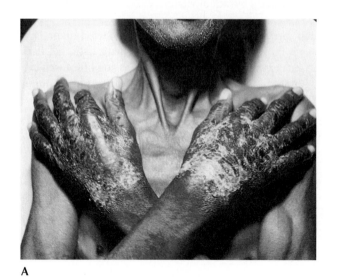

A

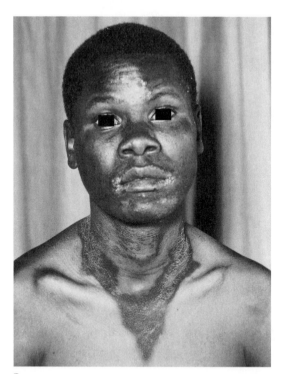

B

FIGURE 5-2 Signs of pellagra. **A**: Glove, or gauntlet, exudation and crusted lesions of the hands. **B**: Casal's necklace on the neck with facial involvement. (Reprinted from Freedberg IM, Eisin AZ, Wolff K, et al., eds. Fitzpatrick's *Dermatology in General Medicine.* Vol 2. New York: McGraw-Hill, 1998.)

IDENTIFICATION OF MALNUTRITION

Many patient complaints and signs or symptoms point to nutritional deficiency or diseases. Specific signs and symptoms determine types of nutritional deficits. For example, people with anemia may appear pale, complain of heart palpitations, and have decreased levels of energy. Low levels of vitamin D and calcium lead to broken bones, bowed legs, and leg cramps. Vitamin A deficiency can cause dry eyes (xerophthalmia), night blindness, and corneal ulcers. Children with low-protein diets have large protuberant abdomens and skinny, small arms (Table 5-1).

Children with nutritional deficiency usually present with multiple symptoms or syndromes. Two common presentations are marasmus and kwashiorkor. These may also present as a mixed picture.

Infants and children with marasmus (starvation) (Fig. 5-3) have the following features:

Normal or thinning hair
Potbelly
No body fat

TABLE 5-1 SOME NUTRITIONAL DISEASES, THEIR SIGNS AND SYMPTOMS, AND COMMON ETIOLOGIES

DISEASE	SIGN OR SYMPTOM	COMMON CAUSES
Anemia	Pale skin Fatigue Pica	Poor iron intake Niacin deficiency Malaria Folic acid deficiency
Beriberi	Neuritis Cardiovascular changes Edema	Alcohol abuse Thiamine deficiency
Hypothyroidism	Goiter, bulging eyeballs Tremor Tachycardia Vomiting/diarrhea	Lack of iodine, goitrogens
Kwashiorkor	Protuberant abdomen Skinny arms Swollen hands, feet, and face Peeling sores, large liver Thin, straight, or light hair	Protein deficiency
Marasmus	Cachexia	Starvation
Pellagra	Adults: Dry, cracked skin Children: Peeling sores and dark marks, swollen ankles and feet Sores in the corners of the mouth Diarrhea	Niacin deficiency

TABLE 5-1 SOME NUTRITIONAL DISEASES, THEIR SIGNS AND SYMPTOMS, AND COMMON ETIOLOGIES *(continued)*

DISEASE	SIGN OR SYMPTOM	COMMON CAUSES
Pernicious anemia	Muscle weakness (neural etiology) Macrocytic red blood cells	Vitamin B_{12} deficiency
Retinal changes	Night blindness Xerophthalmia Corneal ulcers Poor skin turgor	Vitamin A deficiency
Rickets	Long bones curved and prominent at extremities Slight fever at night Hepatosplenomegaly Kyphosis, lordosis, or scoliosis Nodules at sternal end of ribs	Vitamin D deficiency Calcium deficiency
Scurvy (Barlow's disease in infants)	Easy bruising Bleeding gums/gingivitis Abnormal formation of bones and teeth Anemia Loss of energy Brawny induration of muscles	Vitamin C deficiency
	Slow learning, nervousness Loss of muscle control Leg cramps Edema Dermatitis around mouth and eyes Anorexia, nausea/vomiting	Vitamin B_6 (pyridoxine deficiency

Skinny
Wasted
Wrinkled skin
Face of an old man
Grossly underweight
Always hungry
Lethargic
Gross muscle wasting

Infants and children with kwashiorkor (protein deficiency) (Fig. 5-4) may have the following features:

Swollen moon face
Stopped growing
Underweight
Anemic
Thin shoulders and upper arms

Wasted muscles (but may have some fat)
Skin with light and dark patches with cracking, peeling, and sores
Thin pale hair
Abdominal distention
Anorexia

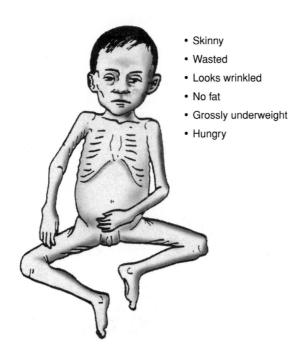

- Skinny
- Wasted
- Looks wrinkled
- No fat
- Grossly underweight
- Hungry

FIGURE 5-3 Signs and symptoms of pellagra.

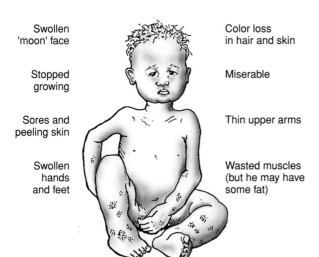

Swollen 'moon' face

Stopped growing

Sores and peeling skin

Swollen hands and feet

Color loss in hair and skin

Miserable

Thin upper arms

Wasted muscles (but he may have some fat)

FIGURE 5-4 Signs and symptoms of kwashiorkor.

ADDITIONAL TESTS TO ASSESS NUTRITIONAL STATE

PHYSICAL EXAMINATION AND LABORATORY TESTS

In assessing the nutritional status of an adult or child, usually a simple examination is enough. You may wish to send a hemoglobin sample for analysis and to perform a few other tests, but the best tests are those you can do yourself and do not require expensive equipment or a lot of time. Use available laboratory tests sparingly. Some tests may require blood to be sent to a laboratory in another part of the country and may be too expensive for the resources available.

Some good measurements and low-cost tests include

- Height
- Weight
- Physical examination (see above)
- Arm circumference
- Hemoglobin/hematocrit (H&H)
- Urine dipstick
- Glucose stick

USING A GROWTH CHART

Recording a child's weight frequently and plotting it out on a growth chart is the best way to make sure the baby is well nourished and growing normally.

> Record the weight of children every month the first year of life, then every 3 months.

The World Health Organization (WHO) and other organizations publish a chart for following the growth of children (Fig. 5-5). All primary health workers should be familiar with this chart, and all children should have this as part of their health record. Plot a child's progress by
1. Doing a careful examination when you see the child for the first time
2. Weighing the child (Fig. 5-6)
3. Plotting the weight on the growth chart
4. Marking any notes or dietary recommendations right on the growth chart
5. Looking for a normal growth trend and watching for declining weight for age

SCREENING FOR MALNUTRITION

There are two common ways to check for malnutrition: taking weight-for-height measurements and measuring the mid-upper arm circumference (MUAC). Height for weight

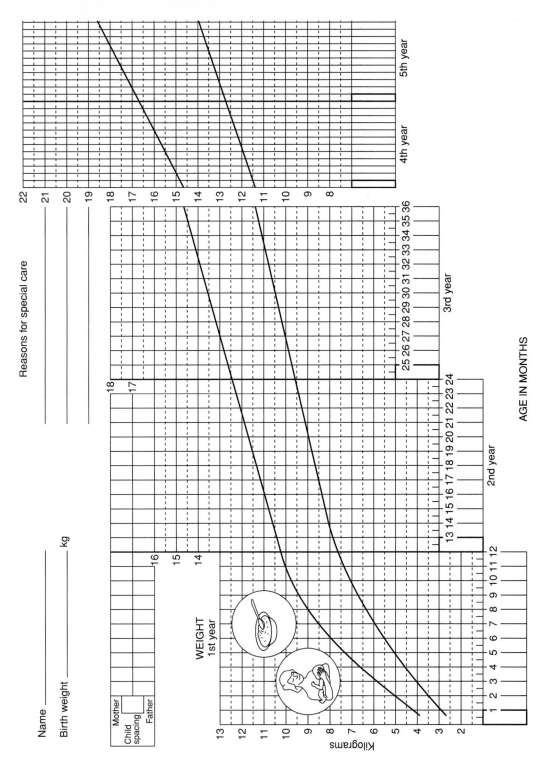

FIGURE 5-5 World Health Organization prototype growth chart.

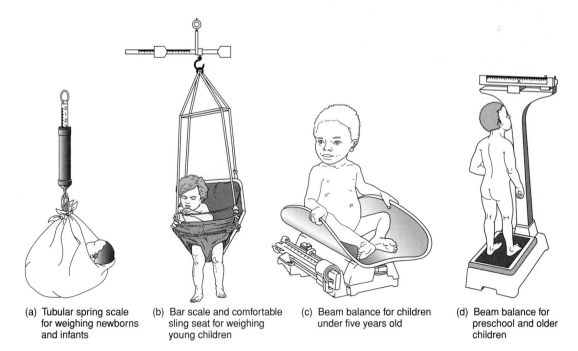

(a) Tubular spring scale
for weighing newborns
and infants

(b) Bar scale and comfortable
sling seat for weighing
young children

(c) Beam balance for children
under five years old

(d) Beam balance for
preschool and older
children

FIGURE 5-6 Types of scales. **A**: Tubular spring scale for weighing newborns and infants. **B**: Bar scale and comfortable sling seat for weighing young children. **C**: Beam balance for children under 5 years of age. **D**: Beam balance for preschool and older children.

can be plotted on the WHO chart (as above). A Z-score can be calculated to determine severity of malnutrition using a scoring table. This is more accurate but also more complicated and beyond the scope of this text.

Measuring MUAC is a useful way to screen for malnutrition, although not as accurate as Z-scores. Another similar method of screening include the Quaker arm circumference stick, but MUAC is still widely used in emergency settings for children 1 to 5 years of age. At 1 year of age a child's upper arm should measure at least 13.5 cm. If it measures less than 12.5 cm, the child is probably severely malnourished, even if the rest of the child appears "fat".

> Rule of thumb: Children's arm circumference should be at least 13.5 cm.

Steps to measure MUAC (Figs. 5-7 and 5-8):
1. Choose the half-way point on the child's arm between the shoulder and the elbow.
2. Let the child's arm hang down with the elbow straight.

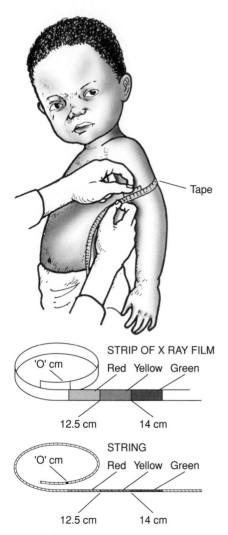

STRIP OF X RAY FILM

'O' cm   Red   Yellow   Green

12.5 cm   14 cm

STRING

'O' cm   Red   Yellow   Green

12.5 cm   14 cm

FIGURE 5-7 How to measure the circumference of a child's arm.

3. Pull the tape firmly but gently around the arm, without creating wrinkles in the skin.
4. Use the tape measure to measure the circumference (in centimeters).
5. If greater than 14 cm, the child is probably well nourished; if between 12.5 and 13.5 cm, the child is moderately malnourished; if less than 12.5 cm, the child is severely malnourished.

Use these parameters to decide on the need for supplemental feeding programs or dietary supplementation. Remember, MUAC is only helpful in children ages 1 and 5.

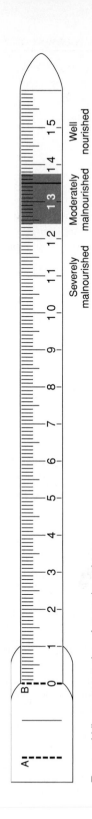

To use middle upper arm circumference (muac) tape:
1. Cut this out of the page
2. Make a cut along perforation A and B
3. Measure muac

FIGURE 5-8 Middle upper arm circumference (MUAC) tape

VITAMIN DEFICIENCY SYNDROMES

See Table 5-2 for a listing of nutrients and common food sources.

ANEMIA

Anemia occurs due to blood loss (wounds, bleeding ulcers, childbirth, dysentery, hookworm in children), red cell destruction (malaria), or inadequate blood production (iron deficiency, blood disorders). Signs and symptoms of anemia include paleness, heart palpitations, and decreased levels of energy. Treatment of mild anemia includes adding meat and fish to the diet. If anemia is moderate or severe, iron supplements may be necessary.

VITAMIN A DEFICIENCY

Vitamin A comes from some animal foods such as liver and foods rich in beta carotene, such as yellow fruits and vegetables. Vitamin A deficiency causes damage to the retina and conjunctiva. Night blindness may occur, and the child may not be able to see well

TABLE 5-2 NUTRIENTS AND COMMON FOODS SOURCES

NUTRIENT	SOURCES
Vitamin A	Animal fats, butter, cheese, cream, egg yolk, whole milk, fish liver oil, liver, green leafy vegetables, carrots, yams
Thiamine (vitamin B_1)	Whole grain cereals, peas, beans, peanuts, oranges, organ meats, fruits nuts, wheat germ
Riboflavin (vitamin B_2)	Eggs, green vegetables, liver, kidney, milk, wheat germ
Niacin	Yeast, lean meat, fish, legumes, whole-grain cereals, peanuts
Viatamin B_{12}	Liver, kidney, dairy products
Vitamin C	Fresh fruits and vegetables, especially citrus fruits, tomato
Vitamin D	Butter, egg yolk, fish liver oils, salmon, tuna, herring, sardines, liver, oysters, sunlight on skin
Vitamin E	Lettuce, green leafy vegetables, wheat germ oil, margarine, rice
Vitamin B_6	Molasses, meat, cereal grains, wheat germ
Folic acid	Glandular meats, yeast, green leafy vegetables
Protein	Legumes, nuts, meat, dairy
Fats	Oils, seeds, nuts, meats, butter, whole milk, lard, coconuts, olives
Iodine	Iodized salt or 1 drop of iodine in glass of water per day
Carbohydrates	Cereals and grains, cassava, potatoes, taro, yams, bananas, plantain, breadfruit, sugar, honey, molasses

in the dark. Xerophthalmia is the drying of conjunctiva, leading to a dull, dry cornea. Bitot's spots are frothy white lesions that can be removed by wiping with a soft cloth. Untreated, this can lead to keratomalacia and destruction of the cornea, ocular scarring, and eventually blindness. Vitamin A deficiency is a nutritional emergency and needs prompt treatment before irreversible damage occurs. Treat with vitamin supplements, one capsule of vitamin A every 6 months (no more), and green leafy vegetables and yellow fruits and vegetables in the diet.

GOITER

Low iodine intake in adults can lead to goiter. Goiter is the abnormal swelling of the thyroid gland, due to inadequate intake of dietary iodine. Cretinism occurs in children born to mothers with iodine deficiency, resulting in mental retardation, jaundice, and deafness. Goiter and cretinism usually occur in regions with low iodine content in the soil. This can easily be remedied by adding iodine to the diet by using iodized salt.

PELLAGRA

Pellagra is caused by a lack of nicotinic acid. This is common in regions where people eat maize and little else. Usually adults or children with pellagra are malnourished. Skin findings include a dark, rough, scaly rash on the forehead, cheeks, and sun-exposed surfaces of the arms and legs. Treatment is vitamin B supplementation and improved diet (higher protein).

RICKETS

Rickets are bony deformities that include bowed legs, curved long bones, and joint swelling, and is caused by vitamin D deficiency. This occurs in children who are malnourished and rarely exposed to sunlight. Vitamin-fortified milk or vitamin supplements may help, but the best cure is daily exposure to sunlight.

MAKING NUTRITIONAL RECOMMENDATIONS

In general, it is best to recommend variety in a diet. This includes a combination of main foods (such as grains and cereals) and helper foods—foods rich in proteins, carbohydrates, and vitamins and minerals (Table 5-3). Certain groups of people are more prone to malnutrition and vitamin deficiencies. As a health worker, your role is to identify those most at risk and give advice about how to treat nutritional problems. This will involve talking to pregnant women, parents of young children, sick and elderly patients—children because their nutritional requirements are higher for growth and

TABLE 5-3 NUTRITIONAL PRINCIPLES FOR EATING FOR GOOD HEALTH

Main foods* (provide most of the body's needs):
  Cereals and grains (wheat, maize, rice, millet, sorghum)
  Starchy roots (cassava, potatoes, taro)
  Starchy fruits (bananas, plaintain, breadfruit)
Helper foods (needed in addition to main foods to keep the body healthy)
  Go foods (energy helpers):
    Fats (vegetable oils, butter, ghee, lard)
    Foods rich in fats (coconut, olives, fatty meats)
    Nuts (cashews, groundnuts, almonds, walnuts)
    Oil seeds (pumpkin, melon, sesame, sunflower)
    Sugars (sugar, honey, molasses, sugarcane, jaggery)
  Grow foods (proteins or body-building foods):
    Legumes (beans, peas, lentils)
    Nuts (cashews, groundnuts, almonds, walnuts)
    Oil seeds (pumpkin, melon, sesame, sunflower)
    Animal products (milk, eggs, cheese, yogurt, fish, chicken, meat, small animals such as mice
    and insects)
  Glow foods (vitamins and minerals or protective helpers):
    Vegetables (dark green leafy plants, tomatoes, carrots, pumpkin, sweet potato, peppers)
    Fruits (all kinds)

Remember: Feeding children enough and feeding often (three to five times a day) is usually more important than the types of food they are fed.
*Main foods are cheap sources of energy. The cereals also provide some protein, iron, and vitamins and at low cost.

development, and elderly because they may lose their taste for food and may not have the dentition necessary to chew well. Pregnant women are also at risk due to their greater nutritional requirements.

Patients who are ill also have greater nutritional requirements. This can be a challenging situation because the patient's appetite is often diminished, and he or she may be unable to obtain food or prepare it.

Recognize the need to treat specific vitamin deficiencies (Table 5-1) and use know food items that are available to help supplement a patient's diet (Tables 5-2 and 5-3).

DEHYDRATION

Children and adults who are malnourished are more prone to severe forms of diarrhea and other infections leading to dehydration. In assessing the nutritional status of a patient, a health worker must recognize and treat dehydration.

Signs of dehydration include

■ Tachycardia
■ Weak pulse

- Hypotension
- Dry mucous membranes
- Sunken eyes
- Poor urine output
- Listlessness
- Poor skin turgor (skin tents when pinched together lightly on the back of the hand)
- Poor capillary refill (greater than 2 seconds)

If you notice children or adults who are dehydrated or at risk for dehydration, you can teach their families to treat them by providing oral rehydration. Recommend to patients to drink as much fluid as possible (at least two big cups six times a day), particularly when they are ill and not taking much food. In general, any fluid is fine, including tea, water, coconut water, sugar water, or oral rehydration solution.

In some countries packets of electrolyte solutions called oral rehydration salts (ORS) are sold to make rehydration drinks. These are inexpensive and can be used when available. Be sure to follow the mixing instructions carefully.

If you need to make your own, one recipe is

- 1 liter of boiled/cooled water
- ½ teaspoon of salt
- 8 teaspoons of sugar (can also use raw sugar or molasses)
- ½ cup of fruit juice, mashed banana, or coconut water

For longer use when added nutrition is needed mix:

- 1 liter water
- ½ teaspoon of salt
- 8 heaping teaspoons of one of the following:
  - Powdered rice cereal
  - Ground maize
  - Wheat flour
  - Cooked and mashed potatoes

Boil together for about 5 minutes, then cool. This mix will spoil in a few hours in hot weather, so only make what you can use promptly.

If the patient is too ill to drink enough, and is showing signs of severe dehydration, start intravenous fluids. One method in adults is to give 2 liters of normal saline wide open, then 1 liter every 2 hours until signs of dehydration have resolved, or the patient is able to take fluids by mouth. If the patient is still not able to drink, begin maintenance fluids (1 liter D5½NS every 6 hours). If you have trained staff and know that intravenous fluid administration will be observed closely, add 20 to 40 mEq of KCl to each liter.

FOOD GUIDELINES FOR ACUTELY ILL PATIENTS

Once the patient is able to eat, feed small frequent meals with a high nutritional content. Patient preferences should be tolerated. It is better that they eat something than push away a nutritionally better choice. Spoon feed the patient if necessary. Nasogastric feeding can be done as a last resort if long-term feeding is necessary. This should only be done by trained health-care workers due to the risk of aspiration.

Pureed food using locally available items can be made and should include the following:

- Staple: rice, sweet potato, taro, yam, or cassava, cooked and mashed
- Vegetables and fruits: cooked and mashed if necessary
- Protein: beans, nuts, fish, meat, or eggs, cooked and mashed
- Fats: cooking oil
- Can also add milk and sugar
- Adequate water for hydration

DIETARY NEEDS OF INFANTS AND CHILDREN

Young children between the ages of 6 months and 3 years are at most risk of undernutrition. Inadequate feeding is one of the immediate causes. To prevent malnutrition

- Teach the family about good dietary habits.
- Encourage breast feeding
- Identify and overcome problems that prevent a child from eating enough.
- Chart the child on a growth chart to check progress and keep checking them.

NUTRITIONAL ASSESSMENT

Young children have small stomachs. To get enough nutrients from the amount they can eat, meals should be rich in energy and nutrients. The amount of food a child needs at each meal depends on the energy and nutrient density of the food, feeding frequency, age, and amount of breast milk taken. Give as much food as the child can eat when actively encouraged, then regularly use a growth chart to show if the child is growing to a healthy weight.

Plot the age and weight to follow the child's progress. If the age of the child is not known, his or her age can be estimated by counting the teeth. If the child has 19 teeth or less, then the approximate age in months equals the number of teeth plus six.

> Approximate age in months = number of teeth + 6.

If the child refuses to eat enough food, is not gaining weight well, or the mother is unable to produce enough breast milk

■ Ensure that the mother is well fed and healthy.
■ Assess the child's general health (don't forget to check for intestinal parasites).
■ Begin supplemental feedings six times a day. These can be commercial formulas or they can be made.

If the child is sick, encourage oral feeding by

■ Making sure the child is clean and comfortable before feeding
■ Giving small meals using foods that are easy to swallow
■ Feeding small, frequent meals
■ Increasing the amount of between-meal fluids
■ Teaching the parent that the child needs extra food during the recovery period to regain lost weight

Help children develop healthy eating habits by

■ Providing positive reinforcement when the child eats well
■ Making mealtimes peaceful and happy
■ Not hurrying the child (he may play between bites)
■ Feeding the child when he is hungry, not tired
■ Giving the child foods he can feed himself
■ Providing a variety of healthy foods and mixing the foods together so it is more difficult to pick out favorites
■ Not force feeding

AMOUNTS TO FEED AND PROGRESSION OF FEEDING

There are no firm rules, but a suggested feeding schedule is

■ Birth to 4 to 6 months
  ■ Breast-feed on demand at least eight times in 24 hours
■ 6 months
  ■ Breast-feed at least eight times in 24 hours
  ■ Start complementary foods once or twice daily after breast-feeding
■ 6 to 12 months
  ■ Breast-feed on demand
  ■ Feed complementary foods three to four times daily (five times a day if weaned)
■ 12 to 23 months
  ■ Breast-feed on demand
  ■ Feed complementary foods four to five times per day
■ Over 2 years
  ■ Feed three meals and two snacks per day

TABLE 5-4 MILK-OIL FORMULA

Milk powder	250 mL
Sugar	150 mL
Cooking oil	50 mL
Cooled boiled water	1,000 mL

Complementary foods are given in addition to breast milk. They can be specially prepared foods or family foods. Start complementary foods when the child seems hungry after breast-feeding, is not gaining weight, or when he or she shows an interest in other foods. If a mother has poor milk production, encourage her to keep trying to breast-feed, eat well, and supplement the infant's diet with boiled milk formula (Table 5-4).

SPECIAL NEEDS OF PREGNANT AND LACTATING WOMEN

The most important factor in promoting the nutritional health of the mother and of her unborn child is to have a well-balanced diet. The mother should be encouraged to eat plenty of fruits, vegetables, grains, and protein foods (Table 5-5).

The importance of a diet high in folate should be stressed even before the woman becomes pregnant. An inadequate supply of folate at the time of neural tube closure (about 28 days after conception) has been shown to increase the risk of neural tube defects. Some developing countries recommend supplemental folic acid to women in the first trimester or who may become pregnant. A suggested dose is 400 μg/day.

Iron deficiency anemia is the most common cause of malnutrition in pregnant and lactating women. Extra iron is needed for the development of the fetus and placenta, and as a reserve for blood loss during delivery. The cause of anemia is usually multifactoral.

> The hemoglobin or hematocrit should be checked when the woman first learns she is pregnant, at 28 to 32 weeks, and again at 36 weeks.

If supplementation is needed, the dose to start is usually ferrous sulfate 400 mg/day. Also, check for intestinal parasites and malaria.

NUTRITIONAL GUIDELINES IN PREGNANCY

- Eat a varied, balanced diet based on healthy eating guidelines (Table 5-5).
- Eat regular meals and drink enough water.
- If the quantity of food consumed is reduced due to illness, ensure that the foods that are eaten are of good nutritional quality.

TABLE 5-5 FOOD GUIDELINES IN PREGNANCY

FOOD GROUP	SERVINGS PER DAY
Bread, cereals, rice, pasta, potatoes	4–6
Fruit and vegetables	5
Milk and daily products	2–3
Meat, fish, eggs	2

- Observe strict food hygiene.
- Avoid alcohol.

In pregnancy there are particular risks from certain food-borne infections, including listeriosis, salmonellosis, and toxoplasmosis. Eating cheeses made from unpasteurized milk or drinking unpasteurized milk can cause listeriosis. Salmonellosis can result from the consumption of raw eggs. Toxoplasmosis can be contracted from contact with cat feces, soil, and raw meat. Preventive measures include cooking food well, washing hands, and practicing good personal hygiene.

CHAPTER 6
Adult Resuscitation

Thomas D. Kirsch

Recognizing life-threatening signs and symptoms in an acutely ill patient and initiating treatment is the first priority for any health worker. It is important to begin resuscitation even before the cause or diagnosis is identified. This chapter reviews the first and most critical steps in the management of acute, life-threatening emergencies. The priorities of airway, breathing, and circulation (ABCs) will be repeatedly stressed.

CRITICAL ACTIONS

1. Assess responsiveness. If unresponsive,
2. Assess and treat the ABCs
3. Begin resuscitation prior to completing diagnostic tests
4. Decide if referral to a more advanced health-care facility is needed

ASSESSMENT OF THE ACUTELY ILL PATIENT: THE ABCs (and D)

A systematic, step-by-step approach helps to ensure the best possible actions in a high-stress situation. The ABCs should be the initial examination for all patients, no matter how stable they initially appear. Assuring the function of the ABCs enables you to proceed with the complete examination.

> **KEY POINT:**
>
> The key to successful ABC management is to correct the problem as soon as it is identified. Treat before making the definitive diagnosis.

Be consistent in following the ABCs. First assess the patient's responsiveness. If unresponsive, the following specific steps should be taken:

- Airway: Open the airway with the head tilt or chin lift, maintain c-spine immobilization
- Breathing: Bag-valve-mask or mouth-to-mouth breathing once every 5 seconds for nonbreathing patients.
- Circulation: Begin chest compressions (100–120/min) if pulseless.
- Disability and Defibrillation: Shock patients with ventricular tachycardia (VT) and ventricular fibrillation (VF) as soon as they are diagnosed (don't wait for drugs).

PRELIMINARY ASSESSMENT

The first look at a patient can give many clues about the stability of their ABCs. Unconscious and unresponsive patients are readily identifiable. The condition of awake patients is more subtle. The position the patient assumes, age, alertness level, respiratory pattern and color, and any sign of trauma are all signs about the severity of the patient's condition and possibly its cause. For example, an anxious child sitting up and leaning forward in respiratory distress may have acute epiglottitis, whereas an elderly man in the same position in respiratory distress may have an exacerbation of congestive heart failure (CHF) or chronic obstructive pulmonary disease (COPD).

A rapid, preliminary assessment of the ABCs can be accomplished in seconds by simply asking the patient a question (e.g., "Can you speak?" or "What is your name?") while simultaneously palpating for a pulse and observing the response. Patients who speak in full clear sentences without difficulty and have a palpable pulse have initially stable ABCs, so a more complete evaluation can proceed (Table 6-1).

UNIVERSAL EMERGENCY ASSESSMENT ALGORITHM

This is a brief outline of the basic assessment steps for all patients who appear unconscious. More details on each of the steps are provided throughout this chapter.

1. Assess the patient's responsiveness to voice and pain.
   - If the patient is unresponsive, call for help and a defibrillator (if available).
   - If the patient is responsive, protect the airway if needed and determine the cause of the mental status changes.

TABLE 6-1 GENERAL GUIDELINES FOR THE RAPID ASSESSMENT OF THE ACUTELY ILL ADULTS USING THE QUESTION, PULSE, AND OBSERVE METHOD

VERBAL RESPONSE	INTERPRETATION	CRITICAL ACTION
Speaks clearly and coherently	Clear airway Good ventilation Adequate cerebral circulation Normal mentation	None
Muffled/garbled voice	Partial airway obstruction	Examine the airway Heimlich maneuver Finger sweep Possibly intubate
Confused speech	Hypercarbia/hypoxia (airway obstruction?) Hypotensive (low cerebral perfusion?) Head trauma	Ventilate (bag) Intubate Fluid resuscitation Assess for trauma Cervical spine stabilization
Unresponsive	Same as above Cardiac arrest Postictal seizure Massive CVA	Same as above

PULSE FINDING	INTERPRETATION	CRITICAL ACTION
Radial pulse strong	SBP >100 mm Hg	Check the patient's BP
Weak radial pulse	SBP 80–90 mm Hg	Check the patient's BP Prepare for an IV
No radial pulse	SBP <80 mm Hg	Check femoral and carotid pulses Start an IV with NS or LR
Femoral pulse palpable	SBP 70–80 mm Hg	Start an IV with NS or LR Look for causes Check the patient's BP
Carotid pulse palpable	SBP 50–70 mm Hg	Start an IV with NS or LR Look for causes Check the patient's BP
No carotid pulse	SBP <50 mm Hg	Start CPR Cardiac monitor ACLS protocol

CVA, cerebrovascular accident; SBP, systolic blood pressure; NS, normal saline; LR, lactated Ringer's solution; CPR, cardiopulmonary resuscitation; ACLS, Advanced Cardiac Life Support.

2. Assess the airway and breathing (open airway, look, listen, feel).
   - ■ If the patient is not breathing, give two slow breaths by bag or mouth, look for an obstruction, and then support breathing.
   - ■ If the patient is breathing, protect the airway and support breathing as needed.

3. Assess circulation.
   - ■ If no pulse, start chest compressions and look for a ventricular dysrhythmia.
   - ■ If there is a pulse, manage airway and breathing. Monitor the rhythm if possible.

4. Is the patient in VF or VT?
   - ■ If yes, defibrillate immediately (or give a chest thump with your fist).
   - ■ If no, continue defibrillating.

5. Intubate or use other airway techniques if indicated.

6. Start an intravenous (IV) line to deliver fluids and drugs.

7. Determine the cardiac rhythm and treat as indicated.

AIRWAY: EVALUATION AND TREATMENT

The airway is always first in resuscitations. Even with no equipment, there are many ways to fix an obstructed airway.

First, look, listen, and feel to identify the problem. Causes of airway obstruction include the following:

- ■ The tongue is the most common cause of obstruction in an unconscious person (especially if the individual is lying on his or her back)
- ■ Foreign bodies such as food, dentures, toys
- ■ Trauma to the neck or face
- ■ Anatomic problems such as pharyngeal infections (epiglottitis) or cancers

FIXING AIRWAY PROBLEMS

Act immediately to provide a patent airway in the unconscious patient. In the unconscious and supine patient this is accomplished via several techniques of head/jaw positioning.

CRITICAL ACTION:

Always reassess after every intervention to see if it was successful. If not, try again, or try a different intervention.

HEAD-TILT/CHIN-LIFT MANEUVER This technique cannot be used on an injured patient because it hyperextends the neck, which can cause paralysis if spine injuries are present. To perform the maneuver (Fig. 6-1)

- Position yourself above the head of a supine patient.
- Assess for any possible injuries to the head or neck.
- Place one hand on the victim's forehead, and apply pressure to tilt the head back.
- With the second hand, lift from behind the patient's neck to further extend the chin.
- Assess to see if the patient begins breathing.

If this is not successful in opening the airway, the following further actions may be taken:

- Grab the patient's lower teeth with the thumb and forefinger of the second hand and lift the jaw forward until the teeth are almost occluded.
- Look or sweep your fingers through the mouth for a foreign body.
- Assess for breathing.

Don't press your fingers into the soft tissues of the chin and occlude the airway when performing this maneuver.

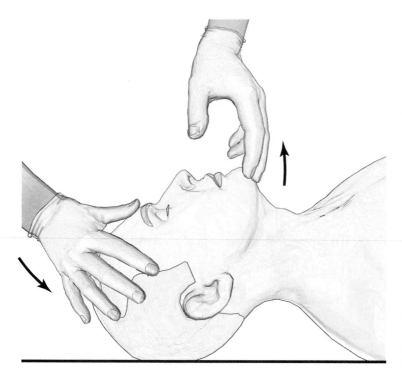

FIGURE 6-1
The Head-tilt/chin-lift maneuver.

JAW-THRUST MANEUVER This method is the safest for a patient with suspected cervical injury, but is more difficult and tiring to perform (Fig. 6-2).

■ Position yourself above the head of a supine patient.
■ Place both hands behind the angles of the patient's mandible.
■ Place elbows on the surface that the patient is on to assist in leverage.
■ Press the mandible forward with the fingertips without moving the head.
■ Assess for breathing.

ARTIFICIAL AIRWAYS For the unconscious but breathing patient, oropharyngeal and nasopharyngeal airways provide longer-term airway support (if the patient will not be intubated). Both airways help ventilation but do not prevent air from entering the stomach, which can lead to gastric distention, vomiting, and possible aspiration. In addition, an oropharyngeal airway itself can cause gagging and vomiting in a partially conscious patient, or one who may become conscious (such as after a seizure).

OROPHARYNGEAL AIRWAY The oropharyngeal airway is a rigid plastic tube that holds the patient's tongue forward (Fig. 6-3A) This airway should be used only in unconscious patients. To insert an oropharyngeal airway, stand at side of supine patient.

■ With one hand, open patient's mouth and look for foreign bodies.
■ Insert the airway with the outside curve (convex side) against the tongue, and the end pointing into the roof of the mouth.
■ Slowly slide the tube into the mouth, making sure not to push the tongue back.
■ At the halfway point, rotate the airway 180 degrees so that the curved section hooks over the tongue and the tip goes behind the tongue.

NASOPHARYNGEAL AIRWAY The nasopharyngeal airway is a soft, flexible tube that is inserted through the patient's nose to the back of the throat (Fig. 6-3B). It can be used in unconscious and conscious patients, but it may be very uncomfortable.

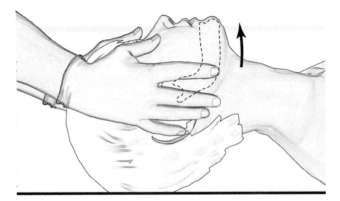

FIGURE 6-2 The jaw thrust maneuver.

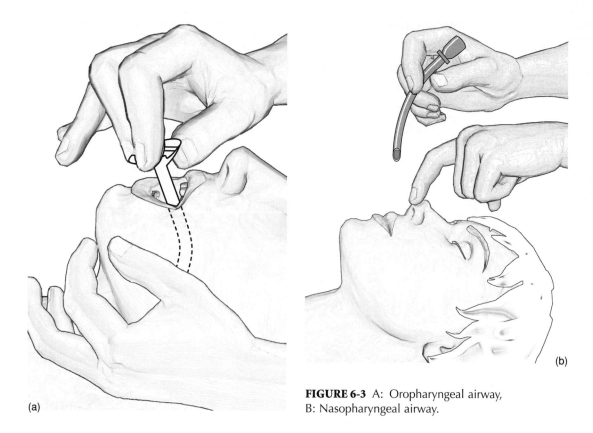

(a)

FIGURE 6-3 A: Oropharyngeal airway,
B: Nasopharyngeal airway.

(b)

Unlike the oropharyngeal airway, it does not prevent the tongue from falling back, so proper head position is still important. It should also not be used following facial trauma.

- Lubricate the tube with surgical jelly or viscous (gel) lidocaine.
- Provide anesthesia to the patient's nasal passages if possible. Squirt liquid or viscous lidocaine or other agent into the nose.
- Hold the lubricated nasopharyngeal airway with the beveled end facing toward the nose. Insert the tube gently into the nose until its end is flush against the skin.
- If the tube does not pass, partially withdraw the tube, reposition it (rotate the tube), and try again.

CHOKING (AIRWAY OBSTRUCTION WITH A FOREIGN BODY)

The most common foreign body obstruction of the airway of an adult is food. For children under 4 years of age, obstruction can be due to any small object. If an individual is found unconscious and you cannot get air into the lungs by mouth-to-mouth or bag-valve-mask (BVM) ventilation, then that person has an airway obstruction.

AIRWAY OBSTRUCTION IN THE UNCONSCIOUS PATIENT: ABDOMINAL THRUSTS
In the unconscious patient, abdominal thrusts (Fig. 6-4) are performed as follows:

■ Lay the patient supine on a hard surface.
■ Look in the mouth for any obvious foreign bodies; remove if present.
■ Straddle the patient, facing the head, with your knees on each side of the patient's abdomen.
■ Place the heel of one hand on the patient's abdomen above the umbilicus but below the xiphoid.
■ Place the second hand atop the first.
■ Give several quick upward thrusts.
■ Use a finger to sweep the mouth. Open the mouth with one hand and use the other index finger to dislodge and remove any objects.
■ Assess to see if the patient starts breathing.

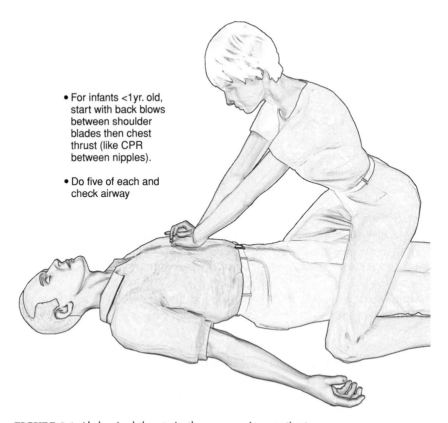

• For infants <1yr. old, start with back blows between shoulder blades then chest thrust (like CPR between nipples).

• Do five of each and check airway

FIGURE 6-4 Abdominal thrusts in the unconscious patient.

If this attempt is unsuccessful, the sequence of abdominal thrust/finger sweep should be repeated in the ratio of six to ten thrusts before each finger sweep. If you have equipment you can

- Use a laryngoscope to look all the way down to the vocal cords for foreign bodies.
- Use any kind of clamp (although a McGill forceps works best in the airway) to grasp and remove the foreign body.
- Attempt an emergency cricothyrotomy or tracheostomy.

CHEST THRUST Use chest thrusts in situations where abdominal thrusts are difficult to perform, such as in patients who are pregnant or markedly obese. The technique is the same as for abdominal thrusts, but the thrusts are delivered to the chest above the xiphoid.

AIRWAY OBSTRUCTION IN THE CONSCIOUS PATIENT Patients who have aspirated an object (usually food) will be in obvious distress. They usually cannot speak and may be clutching at their throat. Audible stridor or muffled sounds may be heard.

The treatment of the conscious patient with an airway obstruction depends on the degree of obstruction. Patients with a partial airway obstruction who can still breathe are best left to allow them to clear the airway themselves. If they cannot cough out the foreign body then attempt the standing abdominal thrust maneuver as patient is exhaling (Fig. 6-5).

- Stand behind the upright patient
- Wrap your arms around the patient's waist with the fist of one hand on the abdomen below the xiphoid and the second hand over the fist.
- Deliver quick upward thrusts by pulling inward and upward against the abdomen. Continue the thrusts until the airway is cleared or the patient becomes unconscious.
- If the patient becomes unconscious, then lay him or her supine and use the methods for the unconscious victim.

Once the airway is open, always assess the patient's breathing by looking for chest rise and listening for breath sounds. If no breathing is noted, begin artificial respiration.

ADVANCED AIRWAY MANAGEMENT: INTUBATION

Endotracheal intubation is an advanced airway and breathing management technique that may not be available to all providers and all patients (Appendix 6.1). When working in a situation with limited resources, there are two important considerations to making the decision to intubate a patient.

First, before a critical situation even arises, you must decide if intubation will even be attempted, and if so, on which patients. This decision must address the scarcity of resources and the proximity of more advanced care. It is both a moral and clinical decision. The resource issue has the greatest effect on this decision. For example, if no mechanical respirator is available, is there a way to ventilate a patient for a

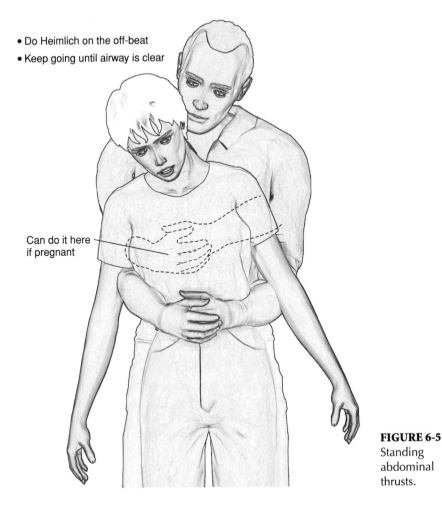

- Do Heimlich on the off-beat
- Keep going until airway is clear

Can do it here if pregnant

FIGURE 6-5
Standing abdominal thrusts.

long period of time? Can advanced life support be provided without monitoring equipment and a limited supply of drugs? Does the staff have the skills and supplies to intubate and provide critical care?

> **KEY POINT:**
>
> The entire health-care team should make decisions about resuscitation before a critical case occurs so that they can be comfortable with the plan and care can be delivered.

The second decision involves deciding when and how to intubate individual patients. In general, if a patient's condition is critical enough that you are considering intubation, and you have the skills and equipment, then the patient probably should be intubated. Delays can lead to more complications. This is especially true for patients who have suffered significant trauma. For example, patients with neck trauma potentially have expanding hematomas that are rapidly occluding the airway. The sooner the airway is secured, the less obstruction will be encountered when inserting the endotracheal tube (ETT).

BREATHING: EVALUATION AND TREATMENT

Once an airway is clear, then resuscitation efforts turn to providing adequate ventilation (breathing). Sometimes just giving oxygen by nasal cannula or facemask is sufficient to correct poor oxygenation. Other artificial respiration methods, in order of increasing complexity of equipment and technique, are mouth-to-mouth breathing, BVM ventilation, and endotracheal intubation.

ASSESSING BREATHING PROBLEMS:
Look, listen, and feel are also used to assess breathing:

- Look at the chest to see it expand (expose the chest first).
- Look and listen at the mouth and nose for signs of breathing.
- Listen with a stethoscope to both sides of the chest. It is best to listen laterally and high in the axilla to lessen the chance of hearing breath sounds transmitted from the other lung.
- Place both hands over the anterior chest to feel the chest expand.

TREATMENT OF BREATHING PROBLEMS

ARTIFICIAL RESPIRATION Artificial respirations can be given by either mouth-to-mouth or BVM if it is available (Fig. 6-6). BVM is preferred because it delivers higher oxygen content and it does not expose the health-care worker to infectious diseases. If mouth-to-mouth or mouth-to-nose is to be attempted, a barrier should be used. With either method, the technique is the same:

- A good seal is essential to get air into the lungs.
- Give two long, deep breaths in a row.
- If the chest does not rise and fall with each breath, then an airway obstruction is present.
- Begin ventilations at 12 to 20 per minute. If the patient is receiving cardiopulmonary resuscitation (CPR), the rate is one breath for every five chest thrusts.

BAG-VALVE-MASK VENTILATION The most difficult thing about BVM ventilation is to get an adequate seal between the mask and face to ensure that the air is delivered

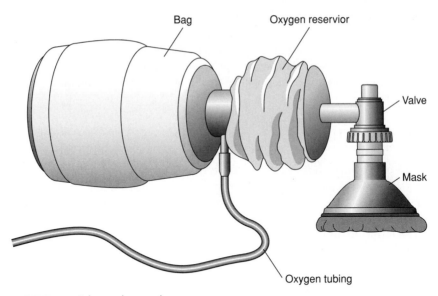

Bag   Oxygen reservior

Valve

Mask

Oxygen tubing

FIGURE 6-6 A bag-valve-mask setup.

to the lungs, not the cheeks. This is difficult for one person because one hand is needed to hold the mask and the other to squeeze the bag. When possible, use two people to "bag": one uses both hands to ensure a tight mask-face fit, and the other squeezes the bag (Fig. 6-7) The bag should always be connected to 100% oxygen when it is available. As you are bagging, watch the chest rise and listen to both lungs for breath sounds ensure adequate ventilation.

TIPS AND TRICKS:

Unfortunately, the tongue may still fall back and obstruct the airway, so proper head position is needed. Artificial airways, such as oral or nasal airways, are also used in conjunction with the BVM ventilation.

For specific respiratory illnesses, see Chapter 7.

CIRCULATION: EVALUATION AND TREATMENT

CRITICAL ACTION:

Stop bleeding first with direct pressure, then find the cause.

ASSESSING CIRCULATION PROBLEMS

Take the pulse (see Table 6-1 for normal ranges) and blood pressure. Note the regularity or type of irregularity of the pulse (irregularly irregular or regularly irregular).

FIXING CIRCULATION PROBLEMS (GENERAL TREATMENT OF SHOCK)

Circulatory problems present as either pulselessness or "shock" (hypotension, tachycardia, tachypnea). If the patient is pulseless, check the airway and begin rescue breathing and chest compressions immediately. If they still have a pulse, continue a rapid evaluation while starting IV access. Fluid resuscitation is the initial treatment of essentially all causes of shock. Other basic care includes the following:

■ Stop all bleeding immediately. Direct pressure against the bleeding source is the best method. Once the pressure is applied, don't let up. After 5 to 10 minutes

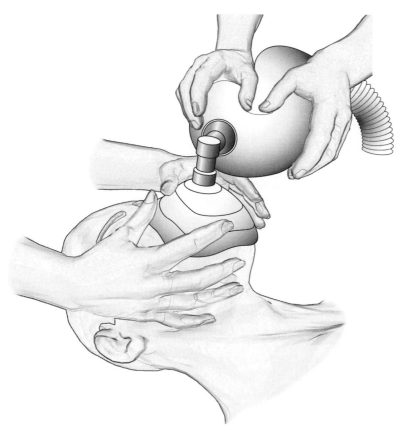

FIGURE 6-7 Hand positioning with two-person bagging.

without significant bleeding, a pressure dressing can be applied. Tourniquet use should be avoided if possible.

■ Elevate the patient's feet (lift the end of the bed).

■ Keep the patient warm and covered as much as possible.

INTRAVENOUS ACCESS Intravenous access is essential to treat shock. However, IV fluid is probably used too often to treat dehydration from diarrhea, when oral rehydration solution (ORS) is sufficient. In case of shock, IV access should be established as soon as possible. This is best done by an assistant who can begin the procedure while the team leader completes the ABC survey and treatment.

PERIPHERAL ACCESS Generally, peripheral access is the first choice. The most common site is the antecubital vein of either arm. Other sites include the forearm, back of the hand, and external jugular (neck veins).

CENTRAL ACCESS Central IV access is needed when the patient has poor peripheral access, when rapid resuscitation is necessary, and when a more reliable delivery of cardiac resuscitation drugs is needed. It is also useful because central venous pressure (CVP) readings can be taken to monitor therapy.

The most common sites for central venous access are the femoral, subclavian, and internal jugular (IJ) veins. There are advantages and disadvantages to each. In general, the femoral approach is easier and has fewer complications, but the subclavian and IJ routes deliver drugs to the heart more reliably in a cardiac resuscitation. The specific methods for peripheral and central access are discussed in Chapter 14, Trauma Management.

SURGICAL ACCESS Surgical venous access is an open technique in which the skin is incised and the vein isolated and then cannulated. This technique is the most difficult and time consuming and so is usually reserved as the final attempt when other methods have failed. The most common site for open access is the saphenous vein just anterior to the medial malleolus at the ankle.

FLUID RESUSCITATION For the initial treatment of shock, normal saline (NS) or lactated Ringer solution (LR) should be given through a large-bore (18-gauge or greater) IV catheter. LR and NS are more effective for volume resuscitation (not D_5W) because they include more electrolytes and less free water. Use two IV lines for patients with advanced signs of shock. To facilitate rapid fluid infusion, use a large drip chamber and IV tubing. Use pressure on the IV fluid bag (squeeze it or apply an inflated blood pressure cuff around it) for even more rapid delivery.

Give fluid boluses of 20 mL/kg, then reassess the patient's vital signs and condition. These boluses may be repeated up to two additional times as needed before turning to alternative therapies such as blood transfusions and pressors.

BLOOD TRANSFUSION Emergent blood transfusion may be required for patients with continued hypotension despite the fluid, or if the bleeding cannot be controlled. In many settings blood transfusions are not available and the patient must be transferred. When transfusions are possible the only blood available may be whole blood from a cross-matched donor. Ideally, fully cross-matched blood should be used, but this generally takes 45 to 60 minutes. For severe or rapidly progressive shock, type O-negative blood should be used. Transfuse 10 mL/kg of packed red blood cells (if available), or whole blood for patients with blood loss.

PRESSORS (SYMPATHOMIMETICS) These drugs have little effect if the cause of shock is continued blood loss. However, they can be very useful for other causes of shock. Potential vasoconstrictors include the following:

■ Norepinephrine is an almost pure vasoconstrictor (alpha-1) that can increase blood pressure and maintain perfusion to vital organs.
■ Epinephrine has both alpha- (vasoconstriction) and beta- (cardiac output, etc.) adrenergic effects. It increases both blood pressure and cardiac output.
■ Dopamine has dose-dependent effects. At low dose, it is a vasodilator that increases cardiac output. At higher doses, it has more pure alpha (vasoconstrictor) effect.
■ Dobutamine increases cardiac output with some vasodilatory activity and is often used with high-dose dopamine.

MONITORING TREATMENT A patient in shock must be reevaluated frequently to determine if the therapy is working. The patient's mental status, speech, pulse, blood pressure, respiratory rate, skin perfusion, and urine output should be followed. If the patient does not show correction of the shock state or respond sufficiently, then more aggressive treatment may be indicated.

When available, CVP is a useful parameter for assessing and monitoring shock and guiding treatment. It is most useful to manage acute circulatory failure, large-volume fluid or blood replacement, and to diagnose pericardial tamponade. CVP is usually best read from the subclavian or internal jugular vein. Besides the supplies for venous access, the only supplies needed are a three-way stopcock and graduated manometer tube.

OBTAINING CENTRAL VENOUS PRESSURE READING

■ The three-way stopcock is placed in the IV tubing between the patient and the IV fluid bag.
■ The manometer tube is attached and held vertically at the level of the heart.
■ The stopcock is turned so that the IV solution fills the manometer to 25 cm of H_2O.
■ The position of the stopcock is then reversed so that the manometer is open to the patient, but not to the IV bag.
■ The fluid will equilibrate to the pressure; take the reading at the end of inspiration.
■ Between readings the stopcock is turned off to the manometer so that the IV fluid can flow freely to the patient.

A normal CVP can range from 0 to 7 cm H_2O. To interpret the results, see Table 6-2.

TABLE 6-2 CENTRAL VENOUS PRESSURE INTERPRETATION AND CAUSES

READING	INTERPRETATION	CAUSE
<6 cm H_2O	Low	Hypovolemia or poor vascular tone (sepsis, anaphylaxis)
6–12 cm H_2O	Medium	Could be normal or pathologic, consider the clinical situation
>12 cm H_2O	High	Poor heart function (CHF), fluid overload, tamponade, pulmonary embolism

Serial CVP measurements are useful for assessing the response to therapy, but care must be taken to ensure that the CVP manometer is always held at the same level in relation to the patient's body (make a mark on the patient). A fluid challenge also can be used in patients with potential heart failure to assess their ability to accept more fluid.

1. Take a preliminary reading.
2. Give 200 mL of NS or LR over 10 minutes.
3. Wait 10 minutes.
4. Take a second reading.

If the reading has increased by more than 5 cm H_2O, then stop giving fluid. If the increase is less than 2 cm H_2O, then more fluid may be given.

SHOCK

Shock occurs when the tissues and organs don't get enough oxygen, usually from lack of blood reaching the tissues. It is important to recognize a patient in shock and to begin treatment immediately. Identifying the cause of shock comes after the primary resuscitation. Initial treatment is IV access and fluid resuscitation for all patients.

KEY POINTS:

Symptoms of shock:
- Weakness
- Lightheadedness (dizziness)
- Nausea
- Sense of impending doom

Signs of shock:
- Tachycardia
- Cool, clammy skin
- Hypotension (a late finding, particularly in children)
- Decreased mental status or confusion
- Decreased urine output (very late finding)

> **KEY POINT:**
>
> Performing laboratory tests in the shock patient is much less important than administering treatment.

DIAGNOSIS When there is time, the most useful blood test is a type and crossmatch for blood, especially if bleeding is a potential cause of the shock. Other tests, such as hematocrit and white blood cell count, and analysis of blood sugar and electrolytes, are secondary.

> **TIPS AND TRICKS:**
>
> The initial hematocrit may be normal despite severe acute blood loss, and the white blood cell count may be normal, high, or low, even with septic shock.

TREATMENT OF COMMON CAUSES OF SHOCK

- Dehydration
  - Fluid resuscitation

- Bleeding (hemorrhagic)
  - Stop all external bleeding immediately with direct pressure.
  - Fluid resuscitation. Give 3 mL of LR or NS for every 1 mL of estimated blood loss. For example, a patient with an estimated blood loss of 1,000 mL should be resuscitated with 3 L of crystalloid.
  - The patient may require a blood transfusion. Vasoconstrictors are not effective.

- Septic
  - IV fluid boluses
  - IV antibiotics as soon as possible
  - Drain any infected fluid accumulation present.
  - IV vasopressors if no response to loading IV fluids

- Anaphylactic
  - IV fluid boluses
  - Epinephrine 0.01 mg/kg (1:1,000) solution subcutaneously up to 0.3 mg in adults. Repeat as necessary every 3 to 5 minutes.
  - For severe patients use IV epinephrine. Dilute 0.1 mg of epinephrine in at least 10 mL of NS or D5W. Then give slowly IV to maintain blood pressure.
  - IV diphenhydramine 1 mg/kg (50 mg in adults)
  - Corticosteroids either 100 mg of hydrocortisone or methylprednisone IV or prednisone 1 to 2 mg/kg orally or IV. Remember to give this dose of IV corticosteroids in any patient suspected of having shock due to adrenal insufficiency.
  - Consider the use of a histamine blocker (cimetidine 300 mg IV).

- Neurogenic shock
  - Fluid bolus up to 30 mL/kg
  - If hypotension continues, give a continuous IV alpha vasoconstrictor drip such as epinephrine or dopamine.
  - Consider high-dose IV steroids (30 mg/kg methylprednisone) for treatment of spinal cord injury.

- Cardiogenic
  - Treat dysrhythmias (see list of specific cardiac problems below)
  - Congenital heart defects are difficult to treat without advanced capabilities, so transfer if possible. Stabilizing treatment includes the following:
  - Oxygen
  - Fluid bolus
  - Knee-chest position
  - May be able to maintain blood pressure with either IV epinephrine or dopamine.

- Obstructive shock
  - Tension pneumothorax
    - Immediate needle decompression of the affected lung by piercing the pleural space with a 14-gauge needle at the second intracostal space in the mid-clavicular line. If a rush of air is obtained, then a thoracostomy tube should be placed in the same side (see Chapter 14 for details).
  - Cardiac tamponade
    - Initial IV fluid boluses
    - Then (if available) emergent echocardiography to confirm diagnosis.
    - If hypotension continues, consider an emergent pericardiocentesis.
    - Transfer as needed.
  - Carbon monoxide poisoning (see Chapter 19)
    - Oxygen by nonrebreather mask

ADVANCED CIRCULATION TREATMENT

A common cause of cardiogenic shock is dysrhythmia. Specific dysrhythmias should be treated based on the electrocardiographic (ECG) findings. If you don't have an ECG, or even a cardiac monitor, it is difficult to diagnose specific dysrhythmias. Therefore, the treatment may be based on the blood pressure and the rate and regularity of the pulse. In general, do not treat someone with an adequate blood pressure unless you are sure of the specific dysrhythmia and its treatment. For patients with decreased blood pressure thought to be due to a cardiac problem, there are three basic pulse patterns to treat: pulseless, slow pulse (bradycardia), and fast (irregular or regular) pulse (tachycardia).

Patients should not be treated for any irregular pulse unless they have unstable signs or symptoms:

- Unstable symptoms: light-headed, syncope, chest pain, shortness of breath
- Unstable signs: heart rate greater than 150 or less than 40 beats/min, hypotension, CHF, myocardial infarction, altered level of consciousness

PULSELESS Differential diagnosis for pulseless patients should include the following:

- Ventricular fibrillation (VF)
- Ventricular tachycardia (VT)
- Asystole
- Pulseless electrical activity
- Severe hypotension (make sure you check the carotid pulses)

Empiric treatment for the pulseless patient should include the following:

- Give a firm chest thump with a closed fist to the mid-sternum (for possible VT or VF).
- Begin with the emergency assessment and ABCs, including bag ventilation, or intubate the patient and begin chest compressions.
- Start an IV and give 1 mg of epinephrine (0.01 mg/kg) every 3 to 5 minutes (consider increasing up to 0.1 mg/kg for the repeat doses), or vasopressin 40 units IV. It also may be given through the ETT, but mixed with 5 mL of NS; start the dose at 0.1 mg/kg.
- Give 1 mg of atropine (0.02–0.03 mg/kg) every 5 minutes for three doses.
- Give a fluid bolus of 20 mL/kg of NS or LR. Repeat two more times, then consider blood products or pressors.
- Sodium bicarbonate 1 amp (50 meq) may be given in prolonged arrest.

While giving the above series of medications, evaluate the patient for other causes, such as pericardial tamponade, tension pneumothorax, and drug toxicity. If pulselessness continues, then give lidocaine 1 to 1.5 mg/kg IV or amiodarone 150 mg over 10 minutes to treat VF or VT.

SLOW PULSE (BRADYCARDIA)

DIFFERENTIAL DIAGNOSIS

- Normal heart rate in a healthy patient
- Hypoxemia
- Sinus bradycardia
- Vagal stimulation
- Ventricular escape beats
- Third-degree heart block

EMPIRIC TREATMENT If the patient has bradycardia and a normal blood pressure, do not intervene; rather, monitor the patient's heart rate and blood pressure. Start an IV if the patient has been symptomatic (lightheaded, syncope).

TABLE 6-3 TREATMENTS OF COMMON CAUSES OF SHOCK

CAUSE	SYMPTOMS	FINDINGS	TESTING
HYPOVOLEMIA			
Dehydration (diarrhea)	History of diarrhea or poor fluid intake; may have heat exposure	Sunken eyes, dry lips, skin tenting	None necessary. May have concentrated urine, or poor urine output.
Bleeding	History of trauma, or GI bleeding	With trauma external bleeding is obvious, internal (spleen or liver) may have abdominal pain and tenderness. Blood or black stool for GI bleed	Hematocrit (Hct) Guiac testing for occult blood in stools
Severe anemia	History suggestive of malaria or other process	Pale, white conjunctiva Splenic enlargement	Hct Malaria smear
VASOGENIC			
Sepsis	History of fever (usually) History of an infection (requires a complete review of systems, especially GU, lung, GI, and ENT	Usually febrile (but not always) May have an obvious source, especially the urine or lungs	Urine for WBCs CXR for pneumonia WBC is not specific
Anaphylaxis	May have a history of exposure (drug, insect sting, etc.) The only symptom may be light-headedness or near syncope	May be hypotensive, or only have orthostatic hypotension May have associated rash, wheezing, or GI symptoms	None indicated
Toxic ingestions	Various	See Chapter 19	

TABLE 6-3 TREATMENTS OF COMMON CAUSES OF SHOCK *(continued)*

CAUSE	SYMPTOMS	FINDINGS	TESTING
NEUROGENIC	History of trauma (spinal cord injury), usually with pain at the injury site	Hypotension without tachycardia. May have a spinal cord level of neurologic findings, indicating the fracture level; flaccid paralysis and loss of sensation	X-rays of the entire spine
CARDIOGENIC			
Dysrhythmias	Symptoms of an irregular or rapid heartbeat. Light-headedness or near syncope	Rapid, irregular, weak, or slow pulse	Check ECG/cardiac rhythm
Congenital	Various presentations	Poor feeding, respiratory distress	CXR may show an enlarged heart. Cardiac ultrasound is diagnostic
Obstructive Periocardial tamponade	History of trauma, cancer, renal failure, etc.	Tachycardia, muffled heart sounds, dilated neck veins	CXR may show an enlarged heart. Cardiac ultrasonography is diagnostic
Tension pneumothorax	Usually a history of trauma. Short of breath, may have chest pain	Tachypnea and tachycardia. Unilateral absent breath sounds, tracheal shift, tympanic chest	Chest radiography is diagnostic, but treat with needle decompression first for unstable patients
TOXIC Carbon monoxide poisoning (prevents blood from carrying O$_2$)	History of stove or fire exposure. Normal BP; headaches, nausea, mental status changes	Mental status may vary from mild confusion to coma. Assess advanced mental functions such as short-term memory, addition; may be subjectively short of breath	Carbon monoxide level, only available in advanced laboratories

If the patient has unstable signs such as lethargy or confusion, the following measures may be taken:

■ Oxygen 100% by BVM or intubation as needed
■ Fluid resuscitation with 20 mL/kg boluses of LR or NS (may repeat)
■ Stop any vagal stimulation that is present (nausea, vomiting, etc.)
■ Atropine 1 mg every 5 minutes for three doses
■ Epinephrine 1 mg IV, repeated every 3 to 5 minutes
■ Consider pacing, or a continuous infusion of IV epinephrine or dopamine (see later section on bradycardia)

FAST PULSE (TACHYCARDIA)

DIFFERENTIAL DIAGNOSIS Pulses can be either regularly irregular (there is a regular, repetitive change, such as a missed beat) or irregularly irregular (the pulse has no repeating rhythm, but is completely inconsistent).

REGULAR PULSE

■ Shock from noncardiac causes, including sepsis and blood loss (Table 6-3)
■ Sinus tachycardia
■ Atrial flutter
■ Paroxysmal supraventricular tachycardia (PSVT)
■ Nonparoxysmal atrial tachycardia (digitalis toxicity)
■ VT

REGULARLY IRREGULAR PULSES

■ Second-degree type I or type II AV block (heart rate usually (<70 beats/min)
■ Regular interval premature ventricular contractions (PVCs; trigeminy, quadrageminy, etc.)

IRREGULARLY IRREGULAR PULSES

■ Shock from noncardiac causes, including sepsis and blood loss (Table 6-3)
■ Atrial fibrillation: completely irregular
■ PVCs: intermittent missed beats with a normal underlying pulse
■ Sinus arrhythmia: pulse rate slows with inspiration
■ VT with a poorly transmitted pulse: variable
■ Nonparoxysmal atrial tachycardia (digitalis toxicity, usually regular): variable, usually regular

EMPIRIC TREATMENT If the patient does not have unstable signs or symptoms, then start an IV at a maintenance rate and monitor the blood pressure to ensure it does not decrease. If the patient is asymptomatic and there is no blood pressure change after 6 hours, he or she can be referred for a more detailed evaluation. For unstable patients

- Give oxygen 100% by BVM or intubate as needed.
- Start fluid resuscitation with 20 mL/kg boluses (may be repeated up to a total of 60–80 mg/kg).
- Evaluate for underlying causes of shock.

If a cardiac cause is considered for the shock or the tachycardia remains greater than 150 beats/min despite fluids, then take the following measures:

- Adenosine 0.05 mg/kg by rapid IV push (push 5–10 mL of fluid immediately after the adenosine for best effect). The subsequent doses are 0.10 mg/kg and finally 0.15 mg/kg for a total of three doses (6, 12, and 18 mg for the average adult). If this is unsuccessful, then give
- Amiodarone 150 mg in 20 mL of DS/NS over 10 minutes
- Consider a calcium channel blocker (diltiazem or verapamil), particularly if there is a sustained irregularly irregular pulse (atrial fibrillation) of greater than 150 beats/min.
- Consider a beta blocker (propranolol, metoprolol), particularly if there is a sustained regular or irregular pulse (atrial fibrillation vs. VT) of greater than 150 beats/min.

PULSELESS RHYTHMS

VENTRICULAR FIBRILLATION OR PULSELESS VENTRICULAR TACHYCARDIA

Ventricular fibrillation is a deadly dysrhythmia that you can treat. But you must intervene (defibrillate) within minutes to be successful. Pulseless VT is treated the same way.

The ECG reveals a disorganized, wide, irregular rhythm, with no specific waves (Fig. 6-8).

TREATMENT

CRITICAL ACTION:

VF = immediate defibrillation

This is the only variation from the usual ABCs. The goal is to defibrillate as fast as possible. Therefore, as soon as a monitor or ECG identifies VF or pulseless VT, defibrillate—do not wait for an airway or IV line to be placed. Take the following steps for a pulseless patient when a defibrillator is present:

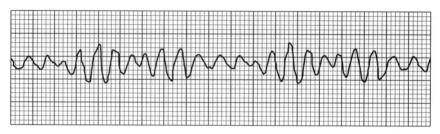

FIGURE 6-8 Ventricular fibrillation.

- Begin with the ABCs.
- Perform CPR until a defibrillator is available (it is best to check the rhythm with the defibrillator first so that you can shock immediately, rather than hook up a monitor and then reach for the defibrillator).
- Confirm that VF or VT is present, and confirm that there is no pulse.
- Defibrillate immediately, up to three times until normal sinus rhythm is reestablished: 200, 300, and 360 J.

If VF or VT persists or recurs after three shocks, continue CPR, intubate, and obtain IV access. Then take the following measures:

- Epinephrine 1 mg IV push (or Vasopressin 40 units IV-one dose)
- Defibrillate at 360 J within 30 to 60 seconds.
- Administer medications that may help with persistent or recurrent VF, then defibrillate at 360 J within 30 to 60 seconds after each dose given:
  - Lidocaine 1 to 1.5 mg/kg IV push (or may be repeated every 5 minutes to a total dose of 3 mg/kg)
  - Amiodarone 150 mg IV push after epinephrine and defibrillation. May repeat 150 mg IV drip.
  - Magnesium 1 to 2 mg IV
  - Procainamide 30 mg/min to a total dose of 17 mg/kg
  - Sodium bicarbonate 1 mEq/kg IV can be considered for a prolonged arrest.

ASYSTOLE

The patient will have no pulse and the ECG will be a flatline. Always confirm asystole in more than one lead. It is very difficult to resuscitate someone from asystole even under the best circumstances.

TREATMENT Begin with the ABCs. Start the following drug therapy:

- Epinephrine 1 mg IV push, repeated every 3 to 5 minutes (may increase to high dose of up to 10 mg IV push)

■   Atropine 1 mg IV push, repeated every 3 to 5 minutes, up to 0.04 mg/kg

Consider and treat possible causes:

■   Hypoxia: ventilate and give oxygen, intubate if possible.
■   Hyperkalemia: calcium chloride, sodium bicarbonate, furosemide, insulin, glucose
■   Acidosis: Intubate, ventilate, and give sodium bicarbonate 1 mEq/kg IV.
■   Drug overdose: see Chapter 19
■   Hypothermia: Begin rewarming.

If still unsuccessful, consider termination of resuscitative efforts.

PULSELESS ELECTRICAL ACTIVITY (PEA) ALGORITHM

The ECG or heart monitor will demonstrate electrical activity (usually wide QRS complexes or ventricular escape beats), but there is no palpable pulse. The treatment is essentially the same as for asystole.

Consider possible causes and then treat the underlying cause:

■   Hypovolemia: fluid resuscitation
■   Hypoxia: ventilate and give oxygen, intubate if possible.
■   Cardiac tamponade: pericardiocentesis
■   Tension pneumothorax: needle thoracostomy
■   Hypothermia: begin active rewarming.
■   Massive pulmonary embolism: thrombolytics (streptokinase) or emergency surgery
■   Drug toxicity
    ■   Tricyclic antidepressants
    ■   Digitalis
    ■   Beta blockers
    ■   Calcium channel blockers
■   Hyperkalemia: calcium chloride, sodium bicarbonate, furosemide, insulin, glucose
■   Acidosis: intubate, ventilate, and give sodium bicarbonate 1 mEq/kg IV.
■   Massive acute myocardial infarction: thrombolytics (streptokinase)

If the cause is not obvious, or if pulselessness continues, take the following measures:

■   Epinephrine 1 mg IV push, repeated every 3 to 5 minutes
■   If bradycardia (<60 beats/min), give atropine 1 mg IV push, repeated every 3 to 5 minutes up to 0.04 mg/kg.

BRADYCARDIAS

Bradycardia is defined as a heart rate of less than 60 beats/min. This rate can be normal in young, athletic individuals, so the rate must be taken in context with the patient and their blood pressure. Pathologic causes of bradycardia include sinus bradycardia and atrioventricular blocks.

Decide if the bradycardia is unstable:

- Unstable symptoms: lightheaded, syncope, chest pain, shortness of breath
- Unstable signs: hypotension, CHF, myocardial infarction, altered level of consciousness

SINUS BRADYCARDIA

DIAGNOSIS Sinus bradycardia usually has a regular pulse and rhythm, with a rate of less than 60 beats/min. It should not be treated in patients without unstable signs or symptoms. However, the patient should be monitored or undergo ECG evaluation to determine if the cause is an atrioventricular (AV) block.

TREATMENT If unstable, take the following measures:

- Atropine 0.5 to 1 mg IV, repeated every 3 to 5 minutes to a total dose of 0.03 to 0.04 mg/kg (atropine could be harmful for patients with a third-degree or type II second-degree heart block, so use it cautiously, if at all)
- Transcutaneous pacing, if available
- Dopamine infusion of 5 to 20 µg/kg IV per minute for hypotension
- Epinephrine infusion of 2 to 10 µg/min for refractory hypotension
- Prepare for transvenous pacing.

ATRIOVENTRICULAR BLOCKS

An AV block is a delay in the conduction between the atria and ventricles. There are three types of AV block: first, second, and third degree.

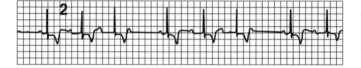

FIGURE 6-9 Type I second-degree atrioventricular block.

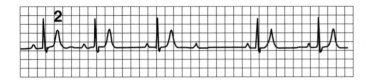

FIGURE 6-10 Type II second-degree atrioventricular block.

FIRST-DEGREE BLOCK A first-degree AV block has little clinical significance unless the patient is unstable. It has a regular pulse and rhythm with a P-R interval longer than 0.20 seconds and a normal ECG.

SECOND-DEGREE BLOCK There are two types of second-degree block: type I and type II. The latter has significant association with mortality and usually requires long-term treatment with an implanted pacemaker.

A type I second-degree (Wenckebach) block usually involves a regularly irregular pulse. The ECG demonstrates gradually lengthening P-R intervals until a beat (QRS complex) is "dropped" (does not occur). The QRS complex is normal (Fig. 6-9). This can cause a pulse with a continuous series of two to four regular beats and then a pause. Treatment is not needed unless the patient is unstable. Then treat like any bradycardia.

A type II second-degree block usually involves a regularly irregular pulse. The ECG reveals a dropped QRS complex with no change in the P-R interval. The complex may be normal or wide (Fig. 6-10). Treatment is not needed unless the patient is unstable. Then treat like any bradycardia, but be cautious with atropine and use pacing earlier.

THIRD-DEGREE BLOCK This block is also known as AV dissociation because the atrial pulses are completely blocked from the ventricles. Long-term pacing is almost always required.

The pulse is usually regular, but slow (40-60 beats/min). On the ECG the atrium is firing at a rate that is either equal to, but usually faster than, the ventricular rate. The QRS complex can be normal or wide. Treatment is not needed unless the patient is unstable, but patients should always be admitted for a more complete cardiac evaluation. Then treat like any bradycardia, but be cautious with atropine and use pacing earlier.

TACHYCARDIAS

There are many types of supraventricular tachycardias, but the basic approach is the same:

- PSVT
- Junctional tachycardia
- Nonparoxysmal atrial tachycardia
- Atrial fibrillation
- Atrial flutter
- Sinus tachycardia

GENERAL APPROACH

As always start with the ABCs, oxygen, etc. Decide if the tachycardia is serious (unstable):

- Serious symptoms: lightheaded, syncope, chest pain, shortness of breath
- Serious signs: heart rate greater than 150 beats/min, hypotension, CHF, myocardial infarction, altered level of consciousness

If the patient is unstable, use immediate synchronized cardioversion (you may quickly attempt medications if their symptoms and vital signs are borderline). Make sure you use the synchronized setting on the defibrillator (you must reset after each shock). Be prepared for advanced cardiac life support and possible intubation.

- Provide sedation if possible (ketamine, midazolam).
- For atrial flutter and PSVT, start at 50 J, then 100, 200, 300, and 360 J.
- For VT or atrial fibrillation, start with 100 J, then 200, 300, and 360 J.

For stable patients, adenosine is now the first drug of choice for all narrow QRS tachycardias (where available). But while you're starting the IV, try the following measures:

- Vagal maneuvers: if patient has normal (or borderline) vital signs, then attempt vagal maneuvers while starting an IV:
  - Carotid massage: Listen for carotid bruits first. Never push on both carotids at the same time. Make sure that the carotid is directly under your fingers and not under the sternocleidomastoid muscle.
  - Diver's reflex: Immerse the patient's face in a pan of ice water (messy). Avoid if patient has a history of coronary artery disease.
  - Valsalva maneuver: Push on the patient's abdomen while asking him or her to push back.
  - Don't attempt eyeball pressure because of the possibility of retinal detachment.
- Adenosine 6-mg rapid IV push, then 12-mg rapid IV push (may be repeated with 12–18 mg). Adenosine works best with very rapid administration into the most central line available and with a 10- to 20-mL fluid bolus pushed behind it.

The adenosine should unveil the underlying rhythm even if it does not restore a sinus rhythm. Further treatment is determined by the width of the QRS complex.

WIDE COMPLEX TACHYCARDIA (>0.12 SECONDS)

- Lidocaine 1.0 to 1.5 mg/kg IV push and magnesium 2–4g IVP.
- If unstable: synchronized cardioversion starting at 100 J

NARROW COMPLEX TACHYCARDIA (<0.12 SECONDS) If the blood pressure is normal, take the following measures:

- Calcium channel blocker (choose one):
    - Diltiazem 0.25 mg/kg IV over 2 minutes (about 20 mg in an adult). May be repeated at 0.35 mg/kg (25 mg) if no effect in 15 minutes, or
    - Verapamil 2.5 to 5 mg IV over 2 minutes (beware of hypotension). May be repeated at 5 to 10 mg if no effect in 15 to 30 minutes.
- Consider digoxin or beta blockers (be cautious after a calcium channel blocker).

If the blood pressure is low, attempt synchronized cardioversion starting at 100 J.

PAROXYSMAL SUPRAVENTRICULAR TACHYCARDIA

Patients experience repetitive episodes of tachycardia that start abruptly and may or may not cause symptoms. The pulse is usually regular.

TREATMENT Paroxysmal supraventricular tachycardia can often be stopped with vagal maneuvers, but adenosine or other narrow complex tachycardia interventions are also useful.

JUNCTIONAL TACHYCARDIA

The pulse is regular. The ECG reveals a rapid, narrow ventricular rate, but no P waves. Treat the same as PSVT.

NONPAROXYSMAL ATRIAL TACHYCARDIA

Nonparoxysmal atrial tachycardia (NAT) is usually caused by digitalis toxicity (previously called multifocal atrial tachycardia). The pulse and rhythm may be regular or irregular. NAT is usually associated with an AV block on the ECG. Review the ECG carefully to look for an AV block and question the patient about exposure to digitalis.

TREATMENT Treat for digitalis toxicity.

ATRIAL FIBRILLATION

DIAGNOSIS Atrial fibrillation produces an irregularly irregular pulse and rhythm (Fig. 6-11). There are no distinct P waves in an irregularly irregular rhythm, usually with a rate of 130 to 170 beats/min. When the rate is fast, the baseline is hard to see, so look for P waves in the slowest portions of the monitor tracing.

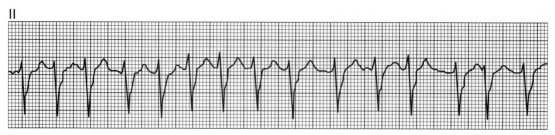

FIGURE 6-11 Atrial fibrillation.

TREATMENT Synchronized cardioversion should be considered for unstable patients. For stable patients there is usually no treatment immediately needed. Consider possible underlying causes:

- Acute myocardial infarction: thrombolytics (streptokinase), aspirin, heparin
- Hypoxia: ventilate and give oxygen, intubate if possible.
- Hypothermia: begin active rewarming.
- Pulmonary embolism: aspirin, heparin, thrombolytics (streptokinase)
- Drug toxicity, especially digoxin and quinidine
- Electrolyte abnormalities
- Thyrotoxicosis

If treatment is indicated (heart rate >150 beats/min, or mild symptoms) then consider using the following options:

- Calcium channel blocker (diltiazem or verapamil)
    - Diltiazem 0.25 mg/kg IV over 2 minutes (about 20 mg in an adult). May be repeated at 0.35 mg/kg (25 mg) if no effect in 15 minutes, or
    - Verapamil 2.5 to 5 mg IV over 2 minutes (beware of hypotension). May be repeated at 5 to 10 mg if no effect in 15 to 30 minutes.
- Beta blockers (propranolol, atenolol, metoprolol)
- Digoxin
- Procainamide 30 mg/min IV up to a total dose of 17 mg/kg

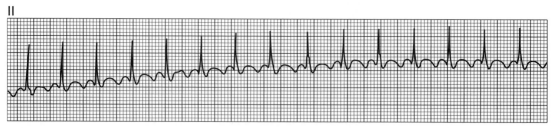

FIGURE 6-12 Atrial flutter.

■ Quinidine
■ Anticoagulants

Beta blockers are useful and effects are additive to those of digoxin.

There is a risk of arterial embolization if a patient with chronic atrial fibrillation or flutter is converted and clots have formed in the left atrium.

ATRIAL FLUTTER

DIAGNOSIS Atrial flutter usually produces a regular pulse and rhythm. The atrium beats 150 to 350 times per minute. On the ECG this usually appears as a sawtooth flutter wave (Fig. 6-12). Flutter is easy to miss when the ventricular response is at a rate of 150 beats/min with a 2:1 conduction.

SINUS TACHYCARDIA

DIAGNOSIS Sinus tachycardia is characterized by a heart rate of 100 to 150 beats/min with normal P waves. Rates can be higher with exercise or acute blood loss.

TREATMENT Treat the underlying cause, including volume loss, exercise, fever, thyrotoxicosis, drugs, pulmonary embolus, etc.

PREMATURE VENTRICULAR CONTRACTIONS

DIAGNOSIS Premature ventricular contractions cause an irregular (usually irregularly irregular) pulse because the pulse is usually not felt with the disorganized contraction of a PVC (Fig. 6-13). On ECG a PVC appears as an intermittent beat with a widened QRS complex (>0.12 seconds) and a compensatory pause (no change in the

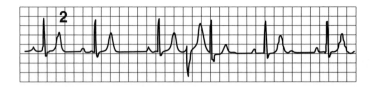

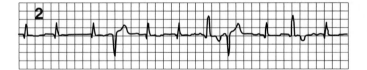

FIGURE 6-13
Premature ventricular contractions.

overall P-P interval between beats). ST segments and T waves are inverted because of the abnormal repolarization.

TREATMENT Generally PVCs do not require treatment. For patients with an acute myocardial infarction, PVCs indicate the need for aggressive treatment of cardiac ischemia. In any circumstance PVCs may indicate the presence of hypoxia and the need for oxygen and ventilation. Consider treating PVCs if more than six occur per minute, if they are multifocal, or if they occur in couplets.

Treat frequent or atypical PVCs with

- Lidocaine
- Procainamide: initial dose of 100-mg slow IV push, can be repeated up to 1 g total dose
- Dilantin (drug of choice for PVCs caused by digitalis toxicity if lidocaine fails)

VENTRICULAR TACHYCARDIA

DIAGNOSIS Patients with VT may be completely pulseless, particularly if they have any underlying cardiac dysfunction (Fig. 6-14). If they do have a pulse, it is usually regular, but may be irregularly irregular. When three or more PVCs occur in a row, the rhythm is considered VT. The rate is always greater than 100 beats/min and usually 160 to 250 beats/min. The rate (R-R interval) is usually regular, varying by no more than 0.04 seconds. If the VT is irregular, it is more likely atrial fibrillation.

TREATMENT For unstable symptoms or vital signs, defibrillate starting at 200 J, then 300 J, then 360 J.

For patients with a good blood pressure and no unstable symptoms, the rhythm can be converted first chemically and then electrically:

- Amiodarone 150 mg over 10 minutes

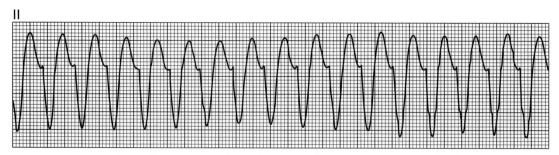

FIGURE 6-14 Ventricular tachycardia.

- Lidocaine 1 to 1.5 mg/kg IV push, repeat doses of 0.5 to 0.75 mg/kg IV every 5 to 10 minutes up to a total of 3 mg/kg. Then start a continuous infusion of 2 to 4 mg/min, or
- Synchronized cardioversion starting at 100 J is usually effective. Then 200 J, 300 J, and 360 J until the rhythm converts.

APPENDIX 6.1. ADVANCED AIRWAY TECHNIQUES

The capability for advanced airway management depends on the proper equipment and the expertise of trained health-care workers. Decisions must be made in advance as to whether these techniques should even be attempted. This book describes oral and nasotracheal intubation and simple open techniques (surgical airways).

ENDOTRACHEAL INTUBATION

In almost all circumstances, orotracheal intubation with paralysis (rapid sequence intubation or RSI) is the optimum method for advanced airway control. But only experienced practitioners should attempt it. Nasotracheal and orotracheal intubation without paralysis is less likely to be successful and more likely to have complications. It is usually best to attempt the technique that you are most experienced with first.

STEPS FOR RAPID SEQUENCE INTUBATION There are many combinations of medications used for RSI, with some better than others depending on the circumstances (Table 6-4). This section will outline the steps of RSI using the most commonly available drugs with the fewest side effects (Table 6-5).

Steps for RSI are as follows:

1. Preparation
2. Pretreatment
3. Paralysis
4. Intubation
5. Protect/confirm

STEP 1. PREPARATION: Good preparation is the key to successful intubation. First prepare yourself by studying the drugs, equipment, and methods in advance. Then practice mock codes and intubations with the entire health-care team. Always prepare for the worst. Have ACLS drugs and cricothyrotomy equipment nearby.

Prepare the patient. All patients need preoxygenation, IV access, proper positioning, and monitoring.

Preoxygenate. If the patient is adequately preoxygenated, you have 3 to 5 minutes to complete the intubation. There are several ways:

TABLE 6-4 COMMON DRUGS FOR RAPID SEQUENCE INTUBATION

Sedatives/induction agents

Midazolam hydrochloride (Versed)

Dose: 0.2–0.3 mg/kg IV over 30 seconds (lower doses if premedicated)
Onset: 3–5 min
Duration: 15–45 min
Effects:
  Sedation, unconsciousness
  Antero- and retrograde amnesia
Negative side effects
  Respiratory depression, apnea
  Cardiovascular depression: slightly decreased, BP, CO, SVR (these effects are potentiated by the
  addition of narcotics)
Contraindications
  Glaucoma
  Hemodynamically unstable patients

Thiopental sodium (Pentothal)

Dose: 4 mg/kg
Onset: 1 circulation time (about 40 seconds)
Duration: About 10 min
Effects:
  Sedation, unconsciousness
  Decreased ICP
Negative side effects
  No analgesia
  May cause apnea
  Cardiovascular suppresion leading to hypotension, especially in hypovolemic patients
  May increase airway secretions and cause bronchospasm
Contraindications
  Asthma, especially status asthmaticus; significant hypovolemia; porphyria

Ketamine hydrochloride (Ketalar)

Dose: 1–2 mg/kg
Onset: 1 min
Duration: 10–20 min
Effects:
  Dissociative anesthesia
  Simulates the cardiovascular system, leading to increased BP and HR
  Bronchodilatation
Negative side effects
  Increased ICP and IOP
  Increased myocardial oxygen demand
  Increased airway secretions
  Hallucinations (rarely)
Contraindications
  Hypertension
  Head injury
  Penetrating eye injury

TABLE 6-4 COMMON DRUGS FOR RAPID SEQUENCE INTUBATION *(continued)*

Analgesics/narcotics

Fentanyl citrate (Sublimaze; usually used in conjunction with midazolam)

Dose: Titrate 25–50 μg at a time

Onset: 4–5 min (peak 10–15 min)

Duration: Dose dependent (about 1 h for a 100-mg dose)

Effects:

  Sedative

  Analgesic

  Reduces the tachycardia associated with intubation (blunts the sympathetic response)

  Cardiovascular stability is maintained

Negative side effects

  Respiratory depression (dose dependent)

  May get hypotension secondary to lack of reflex tachycardia

Contraindications

  Concurrent use of MAO inhibitors

Paralytic agents

 Depolarizing

  Succinylcholine chloride (Anectine)

  Dose:

    Adults: 1mg/kg without pretreatment, 1.5–2 mg/kg with pretreatment

    Children: 1–2 mg/kg

    Infants: 2 mg/kg

  Onset: 15–60 seconds

  Duration: 5–10 min

  Effects: Rapid paralysis

  Negative side effects

    Fasciculations: increased ICP, increased intraocular pressure and intraabdominal pressure, leading to regurgitation

    Hyperkalemia (increased 0.5 mEq/L for 15 min). This may be exaggerated in patients with burns, massive trauma (but usually a week later, not in the acute phase), intraabdominal sepsis, tetanus, or upper and lower neuron lesions.

    Can cause malignant hyperthermia

    May cause bradycardia, salivation, etc. (muscarinic), especially in children

  Contraindications

    Hyperkalemia (patients with renal failure or extensive burns, massive trauma)

    History of significant neuromuscular disease, malignant hyperthermia, glaucoma, or pseudocholinesterase deficiency

    Penetrating eye injuries

    There is no documentation that CRF is a contraindication.

 Nondepolarizing

  Pancuronium (Pavulon; usually used for pretreating prior to succinylcholine)

  Dose: Pretreating: 0.01 mg/kg

      Intubating: 0.05–0.2 mg/kg

  Onset: 2–3 min

  Duration: Average 78 min at 0.1 mg/kg dose

  Effects:

    Nondepolarizing paralysis

    Less cardiovascular and histamine effects

TABLE 6-4 COMMON DRUGS FOR RAPID SEQUENCE INTUBATION *(continued)*

Negative side effects
   Long acting
   Increased HR and BP (vagolytic effect and sympathetic stimulation)
   Rare ventricular tachycardia and severe hypertension
   May cause histamine release: bronchospasm and hypotension
Contraindications
   Myasthenia gravis

Atracurium bresylate
Dose: 0.4–0.5 mg/kg
Onset: 1–5 min (dose dependent)
Duration: 20–30 min
Effects:
   Nonfasciculating paralysis
   Fewer cardiovascular effects than Pavulon
Negative side effects
   Relatively long-term paralysis
   Not always reliable rapid paralysis
   Hypotension from vasodilatation secondary to histamine release (especially with rapid injection of large doses)
Contraindications
   Myasthenia gravis

Vecuronium bromide
Dose: 0.1–0.2 mg/kg
Onset: 1–5 min (dose dependent: higher doses, more rapid onset)
Duration: 30–40 min at 0.1 mg/kg.
Effects:
   Paralysis
   No cardiovascular effects
Negative side effects
   Relatively long-term paralysis
   Not always reliable rapid paralysis
Contraindications
   Myasthenia gravis

- If the patient is spontaneously breathing give him or her 5 minutes of 100% oxygen by tight nonrebreathing face mask, or (if time is limited)
- Have the patient take three deep breaths of 100% oxygen.
- If the patient isn't breathing, bag him or her with cricoid pressure on 100% oxygen for 3 to 5 minutes or to 100% saturation by pulse oximetry.

KEY POINT:

   Do not bag a breathing patient. This forces air into the stomach and may lead to vomiting and aspiration.

TABLE 6-5 RAPID SEQUENCE INTUBATION STEPS

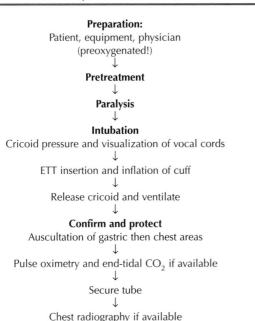

Preparation:
Patient, equipment, physician
(preoxygenated!)
↓
Pretreatment
↓
Paralysis
↓
Intubation
Cricoid pressure and visualization of vocal cords
↓
ETT insertion and inflation of cuff
↓
Release cricoid and ventilate
↓
Confirm and protect
Auscultation of gastric then chest areas
↓
Pulse oximetry and end-tidal CO_2 if available
↓
Secure tube
↓
Chest radiography if available

Position: Proper head position is essential (for a nontraumatized patient). Use the "sniffing" position:

- Place a small (1- to 2-cm) pad below the patient's occiput.
- Tilt the head back and extend the chin.

Monitor the patient. A pulse oximeter is more important than a cardiac monitor, but use what is available.

Prepare the equipment and setting:

- Test all equipment in advance. If possible, have two of everything and extra quantities of each drug. See Table 6-6 for a list of important equipment.
- Use the mnemonic "SOAP ME" to help remember the preparation needed: suction, oxygen, airway, pharmacology, and monitoring equipment (Table 6-7).
- The ETT should have a lubricated stylette inserted into its center and then be bent at a 45-degree angle about one third from the balloon end.
- Use an assistant (or ideally two) who know what they are doing to
    - Prepare the drugs and IVs
    - Give the drugs when ordered

TABLE 6-6 EQUIPMENT FOR INTUBATION

Anesthesia bag (ambu bag)
Assorted masks (pediatric to adult)
Assorted airways (nasal and oral)
Laryngoscope handle
Laryngoscope blades
   Straight (Miller 2 or 3)
   Curved (MacIntosh 3 or 4)
Assorted endotracheal tubes
Syringe (10-mL)
Stylet
Suction with rigid tip
Viscous lidocaine or lube
Anesthetic spray
Magill's forceps
Cricothyrotomy tray

- Apply proper cricoid pressure
- Provide in-line cervical stabilization for trauma patients

TABLE 6-7 THE SOAP ME PREPARATION FOR INTUBATION

S	Suction (*This is critical*)
O$_2$	An O$_2$ delivery system A mask that fits
Airway	Oral or nasal airway
Pharmacology	IV line Sedatives: midazolam or valium Paralytics: Succinylcholine Analgesic: Fentanyl or morphine Code drugs: Epinephrine, atropine, etc.
Monitoring	Cardiac Rhythm Pulse oximeter (To assess oxygenation) Blood pressure cuff (To assess circulation) End-Tidal CO$_2$ (To assess ventilation)
Equipment	(see complete list below) Endotracheal tube (ETT) with stylette Check the ETT cuff with a 10 cc syringe Laryngoscope (Check the light)

STEP 2. PRETREATMENT The goal of pretreating with drugs is to prepare the patient mentally (sedation) and physiologically for intubation. This step can be skipped in the completely unresponsive patient. The sequence of drugs administration is as follows:

- First, give a defasciculating dose of a nondepolarizing paralytic agent such as pancuronium (Pavulon) 0.01 mg/kg IV push (or 1–1.5 mg in an average adult), or use vecuronium.
- Second, give a sedating agent:
  - Ketamine (Ketalar) 1 to 2 mg/kg IV push (100 mg in an average adult), or
  - Midazolam (Versed) 0.1 to 0.2 mg/kg IV push (7–15 mg in an average adult) Less with hypotension/hypovolemia, or
  - Sodium thiopental (Pentothal) 3 to 5 mg/kg IV push (200–300 mg in an average adult), less with hypotension/hypovolemia
- Wait for 2 to 3 minutes to allow the sedation to take effect, then paralysis.

STEP 3. PARALYSIS Succinylcholine, vecuronium, and pancuronium are the most common paralytic agents. Succinylcholine is the most reliable and has the fastest onset and shortest half-life. Succinylcholine 1.5 to 2 mg/kg IV push (100–150 mg) is usually used in an average adult.

The assistant must be ready to apply cricoid pressure. Wait for 30 to 60 seconds for the patient to become paralyzed.

STEP 4. INTUBATION When the patient begins to fasciculate (fine tremors may be most noticeable in the face and eyelids) or spontaneous respirations cease (in about 45 seconds),

- Brush the eyelash to see if it twitches, or assess the laxity of jaw to see if the patient is paralyzed. If not paralyzed, wait and check every 15 seconds.
- Have the assistant begin cricoid pressure (Fig. 6-15).

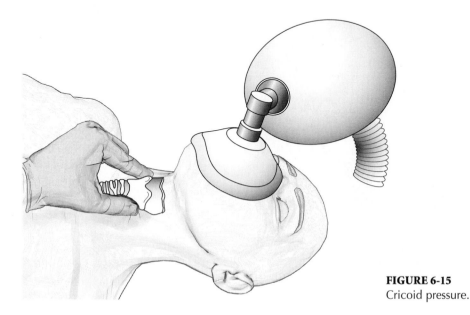

FIGURE 6-15
Cricoid pressure.

■ Apply direct, firm posterior pressure on the cricoid cartilage. This occludes the esophagus and prevents passive aspiration of gastric contents (but is not effective against active emesis).

■ Pressure should not be released until the ETT cuff is inflated and tube placement is confirmed.

■ If active emesis occurs, release cricoid pressure, place the patient in the head-down position, suction, and, if possible, turn the head and body to the side.

■ If no paralysis at 2 minutes, repeat the dose of succinylcholine.

Once the patient is paralyzed and cricoid pressure has been applied, use the laryngoscope to begin intubation. There are two basic types of laryngoscope blades (Fig. 6-16): the Macintosh, or curved blade and the Miller, or straight blade. With the Macintosh the tip enters the vellecula above the epiglottis and indirectly lifts it. The Miller tip directly lifts the epiglottis to view the vocal chords.

Take your time to find the accurate landmarks (the gray-white vertical stripes of the vocal cords). If a patient has been adequately preoxygenated, then you have more than 3 minutes to secure the airway. Have the suction in your hand to clear any secretions. Hold the laryngoscope in the left hand and insert it into the right side of the mouth and

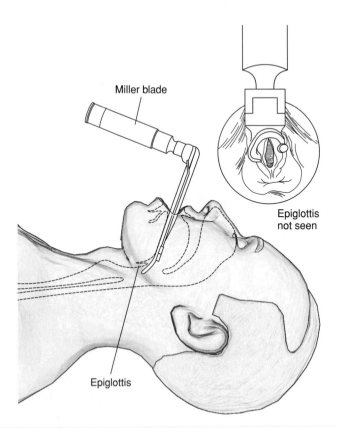

Miller blade

Epiglottis
not seen

Epiglottis

FIGURE 6-16
Intubation with the Macintosh versus Miller blades.

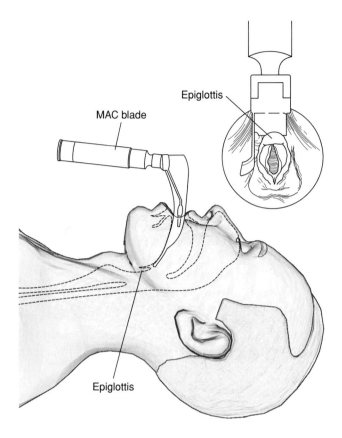

Epiglottis

MAC blade

Epiglottis

FIGURE 6-17 View of the vocal cords through a laryngoscope.

sweep the tongue to the left to allow more space for visualization and introduction of the ETT (Fig. 6-17):

- Slowly slide the blade deeper along the tongue to locate the epiglottis.
- Suction as necessary.
- Once the vocal cords are visualized, the ETT is passed through the cords and into the trachea.
- Inflate the ETT balloon and attach the BVM.

> **CRITICAL ACTION:**
>
>   Do not insert the ETT until you can see the vocal cords, and can observe the ETT passing through them. It is better to pull out, bag the patient, and look again than it is to intubate the esophagus.

STEP 5. PROTECT AND CONFIRM Confirm: Use multiple methods to confirm that the ETT is in the mainstem bronchus.

Listen:

■ Listen over the stomach first. If you hear gurgling and the stomach expands, stop bagging immediately and reintubate.

■ Listen on both sides of the chest, preferably deep in the axilla because there is less transmission of stomach sounds there.

■ If the breath sounds are greater on one side, deflate the balloon and withdraw the tube 2 to 3 cm and relisten.

Look:

■ Look for symmetrical chest expansion (especially important in children).

■ If available, use the pulse-oximeter. Follow the trend, not a single reading.

■ If available, use an end-tidal CO_2 monitor for a minimum of three breaths.

■ If in doubt, look down the throat again with the endoscope to ensure that the tube passes through the cords.

■ Check a chest radiograph for final confirmation.

■ Other modalities to confirm placement: condensation in ETT, bag compliance, palpation of chest rise

PROTECT THE ETT FROM BEING DISLODGED Secure the tube to the patient by wrapping the tape completely around his or her neck and around the ETT from both sides of the face. Then place an oral airway so the patient will not bite on the ETT if the paralysis wears off. Consider providing long-term paralysis with pancuronium (and sedation if possible).

NASOTRACHEAL INTUBATION

To perform the nasal intubation technique, the patient must be breathing. Nasotracheal intubation has a higher complication rate and lower success rate than oral intubation, but it may be useful when

■ Physicians are more familiar with the nasal technique.

■ Patients have facial or neck injuries, cancer, or infection that distorts the oral anatomy.

Nasotracheal intubation is similar to placing a nasopharyngeal airway. The critical actions for nasotracheal intubation include the following:

■ Ensure patient has no signs of facial fractures.

■ Provide anesthesia to the patient's nasal passages. Squirt liquid or gel lidocaine or other topical anesthetic into the nose.

■ Hold the lubricated ETT with the beveled end facing the nose. Insert the tube into the nose and gently push it past the nasal turbinates.

- Advance the ETT while listening to the end until the tip is just above the cords (the breath sounds become loud; if they decrease or stop, you have gone too far). The patient's breath is heard and felt through the tube.
- Listen for the timing of the breathing, when the patient inspires, the vocal cords open. Quickly advance the ETT into the trachea.
- Continue listening to see if the breath sounds are still present. If not, withdraw and try again.
- Confirm and protect the same as with orotracheal intubation.

SURGICAL AIRWAY: CRICOTHYROIDOTOMY

This surgical technique of introducing the ETT into the trachea through the cricothyroid membrane is used when you cannot intubate the trachea orally or nasally. The cricothyroid membrane is avascular and easy to find. To locate the membrane, stabilize the thyroid cartilage with the thumb and middle finger. Then slide your other index finger along the midline of the neck up from the sternal notch until you palpate a slight depression between the thyroid cartilage and the cricoid cartilage. This space is the cricothyroid membrane (Fig. 6-18).

- Use a needle to pierce through the cricothyroid membrane and into the trachea.
- Aspirate air to confirm that you have found the trachea.
- Use a scalpel to make a small (about 2.5 cm) lateral incision through the membrane.

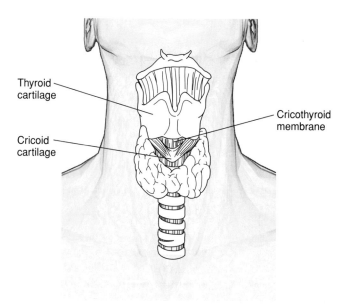

Thyroid cartilage

Cricoid cartilage

Cricothyroid membrane

FIGURE 6-18
The location of the cricothyroid membrane.

- A skin hook can be used to hold the edge of the cartilage from above (rest your hand on the patient's chin to steady it).
- Insert the ETT (size 5 or 6 for adults) through the incision and into the trachea.
- Confirm and protect as described above.
- Control bleeding if needed.

The procedure is relatively contraindicated in children under 8 years of age.

CHAPTER 7

Adult Emergencies and Illnesses

Thomas D. Kirsch and C. James Holliman

As a health provider in remote or developing settings, you will encounter a wide variety of adult medical emergencies. Your challenge is to recognize and treat these conditions with limited resources and to know when to refer a patient to a higher level of care.

AIRWAY PROBLEMS

Airway emergencies are discussed in Chapter 6.

BREATHING PROBLEMS

SHORTNESS OF BREATH (DYSPNEA)

Dyspnea is a symptom, not an illness. You must identify the cause of the patient's shortness of breath. There are some common actions in the evaluation and treatment of these patients. The most important first step is to stabilize the ABCs (airway, breathing, and circulation).

CRITICAL ACTIONS:

- ABCs
- Always consider the possibility of upper airway obstruction in every patient with dyspnea.
- Treat the acute symptoms prior to making the final diagnosis.
- Start high-flow oxygen in patients with respiratory distress and where hypoxia is suspected or confirmed.
- Decide if diagnostic tests or simply empiric treatment will be necessary.

CLINICAL PRESENTATION Shortness of breath can be caused by a number of serious medical problems:

- An exacerbation of asthma or chronic obstructive lung disease
- Acute congestive heart failure (CHF)
- Acute coronary syndrome [myocardial infarction (MI) or angina]
- Pneumonia
- Pulmonary embolism
- Pneumothorax
- Pulmonary effusion
- Sepsis
- Severe anemia

HISTORY

- Question the patient and the family about the time course, rapidity of onset, progression, if continuous versus episodic, exertional versus resting, positional effects.
- Associated symptoms: chest pain/discomfort, edema, fever, chills, neurologic symptoms
- Past history of pulmonary [asthma, chronic obstructive pulmonary disease (COPD)] or cardiac disease (MI, angina, dysrhythmias)
- Current medications

PHYSICAL EXAMINATION For acute coronary syndrome, the examination is notoriously inaccurate. For respiratory disease it is more reliable. The following should be assessed:

- General appearance: Level of distress, obvious signs of respiratory distress (wheezing, stridor)
- Vital signs: The respiratory rate is critical and often misestimated. Count for at least 1 minute in a quiet patient. An elevated temperature may indicate an infection. If available, a pulse oximetry reading can direct the need for oxygen. Assess for pulsus paradoxus in severe asthma and COPD.

- Head and neck: Look for jugular venous distention (JVD), hepatojugular reflux (HJR), and tracheal deviation.
- Chest: Look for retractions. Auscultate for rales, wheezes, and rhonchi. Percuss for dullness.
- Abdomen: Check for tenderness and ascites.
- Extremities: Assess for pretibial (ankle) edema.

DIAGNOSIS

   LABORATORY TESTS Routine laboratory tests are not usually indicated. An arterial blood gas (ABG) reading can provide valuable information in assessing overall ventilatory function (CO_2), oxygenation, and acid/base status. An ABG is useful in acutely ill patients, but it is not necessary in most patients presenting with dyspnea.

   RADIOLOGY Chest radiography (CXR) should be performed on essentially all patients with dyspnea. Radiographs can be used to help differentiate between pneumonia, CHF, pneumothorax, and pleural effusion.

OTHER DIAGNOSTIC STUDIES

- Pulse oximetry is a valuable screening tool for oxygenation when it is available. The information it provides is even more useful with repeated or continuous readings.
- Electrocardiography (ECG) should be performed with acute CHF or significant chest pain to look for signs of myocardial ischemia.
- Expiratory flow rates (peak expiratory flow rate and forced expiratory volume in 1 second) are helpful in patients with wheezing and bronchospastic disorders (asthma, COPD). Peak flow rates can help gauge the severity of the attack and to monitor therapeutic response.

   TREATMENT Treatment should be directed at the specific cause of the dyspnea. However, some actions are useful for most patients. Make patients comfortable. Loosen tight clothing; let them assume the position that is most comfortable for them.

   If myocardial ischemia is even a slight possibility, then the patient should be given a single aspirin immediately. The only contraindication to this is a known severe allergic reaction to aspirin or an active gastrointestinal (GI) bleed.

   Oxygen, when it is available, should be given to all patients. Because oxygen is usually a limited resource, only the minimum needed for patient comfort (and to reach an SaO_2 of >94%) should be used. The various delivery sources include the following:

- A nasal cannula can deliver up to 6 L of oxygen per minute and is sufficient for most mild to moderate dyspnea.
- Face masks can be used to deliver up to 100% oxygen (with a well-fitting nonrebreather mask). Some face masks deliver a specific percentage of oxygen based on Venturi valves.

■ Bagging and intubation are invasive and should be used only if absolutely necessary.

PLEURAL EFFUSION

Pleural effusion is an accumulation of fluid within the pleural space. This is caused by either transudates or exudates. Transudates are from CHF, nephrosis, and myxedema. Exudates occur with infections, neoplasm, and some connective tissue disorders.

CLINICAL PRESENTATION Many pleural effusions are entirely asymptomatic, but patients generally have gradually increasing shortness of breath and exercise intolerance. Some may also have pleuritic chest pain.

PHYSICAL EXAMINATION On the side with the effusion

■ Chest auscultation reveals decreased or absent breath sounds
■ Dullness on percussion
■ Decreased tactile fremitus

DIAGNOSIS

■ A CXR is diagnostic and helps to direct therapy. There must be more than 200 mL of fluid to be evident on CXR.
■ Blood tests are generally not indicated except to evaluate for associated diseases.
■ Pleural fluid should be tested for signs of an infection, including a Gram stain, cell count, differential cell count, culture, protein, glucose, and pH.

TREATMENT

■ For a patient with respiratory distress, thoracentesis rapidly improves symptoms, but may work only temporarily, until the fluid reaccumulates.
■ An indwelling chest tube may be needed in a complicated effusion with pus, bacteria, or a pH less than 7.
■ The underlying cause for the effusion, such as cancer or an infection, must be identified. Repeat chest radiography should be performed after the tap to look for this cause, or the patient should be referred for a complete evaluation.

PULMONARY EMBOLUS

Patient risk factors for a pulmonary embolus (PE; blood clot to a pulmonary artery) include the presence of cancer, injuries (especially to the lower limbs), immobility of the lower limbs (extended seated travel, hospitalization), use of birth control pills in smokers, and previous deep venous thrombosis (DVTs) or PEs.

CLINICAL PRESENTATION Symptoms vary from minor symptoms to sudden death. Patients often have sudden onset of symptoms, including

- Shortness of breath
- Pleuritic chest pain
- Tachypnea
- Tachycardia

PHYSICAL EXAMINATION There are no specific physical findings. Patients are often tachycardic and may be tachypneic. With large PEs a murmur may be heard, and the patient may present in shock. Always check the lower extremities for signs of a DVT: swelling, tenderness, erythema, and palpable veins.

DIAGNOSIS Few tests are commonly available that diagnose a PE. A chest radiograph and ECG are usually performed to rule out the presence of other diseases.

> **TIPS AND TRICKS:**
>
> Patients with signs of a DVT and symptoms of a PE should be treated for a PE with IV heparin even before diagnostic studies are undertaken.

Screening tests include the following:

- Pulse oximetry is a poor screening test unless the patient is found to be hypoxemic (a normal or near normal reading tells you nothing about the presence of a PE).
- If ABG testing can be performed, it can yield valuable clues, particularly based on the alveolar-arterial (A-a) gradient. For normal patients breathing room air at sea level, the A-a gradient can be estimated using the following equation: $150 - 1.2(PaCO_2) - PaO_2$. A gradient greater than 15 may indicate the presence of a PE.
- CXR is useful to rule out other causes, but usually has minimal changes (particularly with small PEs, which are the most difficult to diagnose). With large PEs you will occasionally see a triangular infiltrate with its apex pointed toward the hilum on the pleural border (Hamptom's hump) or dilated pulmonary vessels that end suddenly at the embolism (Westermark's sign).

Advanced diagnostic studies include the following:

- Pulmonary angiography is considered the gold standard, but is rarely available and has significant complications.
- Ventilation-perfusion (VQ) scanning can be diagnostic, but the necessary equipment is rarely available. Interpretation of these studies is based on a combination of the physician's suspicion and the probability of the scan (low, medium, high,

indeterminate). Spiral computed tomography (CT) scans may be useful if the equipment is available.

■ Venography or Doppler ultrasonography of the lower extremities: These tests are not specifically diagnostic of a PE, but are useful for identifying DVT, the most common cause of a PE.

TREATMENT Without advanced diagnostic equipment (VQ scan, etc.), the diagnosis of a PE must be based on clinical suspicion. However, the therapy (heparin) is difficult to manage and has frequent, severe complications. The decision to treat is complicated.

For serious cases (sudden onset of severe shortness of breath, hypotensive) treat the patient aggressively, particularly a patient with signs of DVT:

■ High-flow oxygen by facemask
■ Intravenous (IV) fluid bolus
■ Give heparin 5,000 to 10,000 U IV bolus (or 80 U/kg), then start a continuous infusion of 800 to 1,000 U (or 18 U/kg) per hour.
■ Consider an IV thrombolytic agent [streptokinase or tissue plasminogen activator (tPA)] if the diagnosis is strongly suspected and the patient is unstable.
■ Transfer for further care.

For less serious cases where you suspect a PE as the cause of dyspnea:

■ Give an aspirin (80–325 g)
■ Consider heparin 5,000 to 10,000 U IV bolus, then start a continuous infusion of 800 to 1,000 U/h.
■ Transfer the patient for a definitive study.

PNEUMOTHORAX

Pneumothorax is the entry of air into the pleural space. This can occur spontaneously from a ruptured pleural bleb, or more commonly occurs as a result of chest trauma or procedure-induced complications.

The risk factors for pneumothorax include the following:

■ Recent injury (blunt or penetrating)
■ History of asthma or COPD
■ Use of mechanical ventilators
■ Spontaneous pneumothorax can occur in patients with underlying lung infections, asthma, emphysema, and cancers. This is most common in tall, thin men 20 to 40 years of age.
■ Penetrating medical procedures to the chest area (subclavian central line, etc.)

CLINICAL PRESENTATION A patient with a simple pneumothorax may present with mild respiratory distress and minimal chest pain. A tension pneumothorax can rapidly progress to respiratory arrest.

Symptoms are similar to those of a PE:

- Chest pain, usually on the affected side and pleuritic
- Shortness of breath
- Tachypnea
- Tachycardia
- Unilateral decreased or absent breath sounds

PHYSICAL EXAMINATION Physical findings of a simple pneumothorax are often subtle, usually with only decreased breath sounds on the affected side.

Physical findings of a tension pneumothorax progress to include the following:

- Unilateral hyperresonance of the chest
- Distended neck veins
- Hypotension and tracheal deviation occur late and are ominous findings.

DIAGNOSIS The definitive diagnostic study is CXR. Laboratory tests are not indicated.

If a patient is in acute distress with signs of a tension pneumothorax, decompress the chest with a needle; don't wait for the CXR.

TREATMENT See Chapter 14 for details on the procedure.

For a tension pneumothorax

- Perform immediate needle decompression even prior to CXR.
- Then place a tube thoracostomy (chest tube).

For a simple pneumothorax, the treatment depends on the size of the lung collapse, its cause, the patient's health, the presence of underlying pulmonary disease, and the availability of resources. Options include

- Observation: If the pneumothorax is less than 20% of the hemithorax, the patient can be observed with repeated radiography over 24 to 48 hours. Increasing symptoms dictate the need for another CXR or a chest tube.
- Needle aspiration (see Chapter 14)
- Tube thoracostomy (see Chapter 14)

ACUTE ASTHMA

Asthma is a chronic inflammatory lung condition, with acute exacerbations that cause attacks of wheezing and shortness of breath. Precipitating factors include respiratory tract infections, allergens (pollen, dust, animals, etc.), smoke, changes in the weather, and exercise. The evaluation of patients with known asthma is very different from those in whom you are trying to make the first diagnosis.

CLINICAL PRESENTATION Asthma presentation can range from a mild, chronic cough to respiratory arrest. Patients generally have previous symptoms or a history of asthma. Symptoms include

- Wheezing
- Shortness of breath
- Coughing (A chronic or frequent cough may be the only sign of asthma.)

> When a patient presents with respiratory distress and wheezing without a history of asthma, the evaluation must be much more detailed. The differential diagnosis should include the following:
>
> - Pneumonia
> - Foreign body aspiration (especially in young children and the elderly)
> - Croup (children)
> - Tracheitis
> - Allergic reaction
> - Cardiac (CHF)
> - Toxic inhalations

Ask the patient about fevers and sputum production (infections), possible toxic or allergic exposures, history of smoking, rapidity of onset (weeks or months may mean a cancer or mass), presence of prior symptoms (asthma, allergic), and other associated symptoms in the review of systems.

The following are risk factors for severe disease and death in asthma patients:

- History of intubation for asthma
- Hospitalized more than twice in the prior 12 months (especially if any intensive care) for asthma
- More than three health center, hospital, or emergency department visits in the prior 12 months for asthma exacerbations
- A visit for asthma to a health center, hospital, or emergency department in the past month
- Current or recent use of oral steroids for asthma
- Other health problems such as CHF and COPD

PHYSICAL EXAMINATION The first priority of the examination is to identify patients at immediate risk for respiratory failure. These patients may be sitting upright, arms pushed straight against the bed, and may be sweating with obvious signs of labored breathing. Other signs include the following:

- Confusion, lethargy, or other mental status changes are ominous findings.
- Vital signs are important; look especially for a fever, which helps to identify an infectious source.
- A lung examination shows wheezes (inspiratory, expiratory or both).
  - Decreased or absent breath sounds occur in severe cases.
  - An asymmetric lung examination usually indicates a cause other than asthma.
- Retractions or the use of accessory muscles (especially in children)

DIAGNOSIS

- Peak expiratory flow (PEF) meters are a useful measure of severity, and can be used repetitively during extended treatments to assess improvement. Normal PEF levels are based on the patent's age, sex, and height.
- Pulse oximetry (when available) is useful to identify patients who have significant respiratory compromise. A single reading is not a good predictor of outcome, except that a low reading (<92%) generally requires admission.
- CXRs are not indicated for routine exacerbations, except for new-onset asthma, an asymmetric lung examination, or suspicion of a pneumothorax, pneumonia, or other diagnoses such as CHF or PE.
- Complete blood counts (CBCs) and other blood tests are not indicated even if pneumonia is suspected (check the CXR).
- ABGs should rarely be used but can be considered when the patient deteriorates despite therapy and when intubation is being considered.

TREATMENT For the known asthmatic, the severity of the attack directs the treatment. Beta agonists (inhaled or injected) are the mainstay of emergency treatment, whereas steroids are used for long-term treatment and prevention.

1. Start with aerosol therapy in acute asthma exacerbation.
2. Then use injected therapies.
3. Oral steroids are inexpensive and readily available. They should be used for all but the most minor attacks.
4. For severe cases use multiple medicines and delivery methods. Give oral or IV steroids as soon as possible.

> **TIPS AND TRICKS:**
>
> Steroids (prednisone) are cheap, safe, and the most effective therapy for asthma.

AEROSOL THERAPY This form of therapy requires a high-flow air or oxygen source and nebulizer equipment.

- Albuterol nebulized (0.5% = 5 mg/mL)
    - For adults give 5 mg in 2 to 3 mL of normal saline (NS) every 20 minutes, or continuously in severe cases.
    - For children give 0.05 to 0.10 mg/kg diluted with 1 to 2 mL NS.
- As a backup, terbutaline in the same doses diluted with 2 to 3 mL of saline can be delivered by a nebulizer.
- Nebulized atropine 0.01 to 0.03 mL/kg (0.01 mg/mL) in 1 to 2 mL NS also may help, especially for COPD and emphysema. Beware of the cardiac effects.

As an alternative to nebulized therapy, an albuterol (or other beta-agonist) inhaler (puffer) works as well as nebulized solution for moderate cases. Patients may have difficulty coordinating the delivery of the puff with their inspiration. The use of a spacer delivers more drug to the lung.

TIPS AND TRICKS:

Many plastic tubes, such as a 1-L soda bottle, can be used as a spacer (do not use paper or wood, which may absorb the drug).

INJECTED THERAPY When nebulizers or inhalers are unavailable, use the following:

- Epinephrine (adrenaline) 0.3 to 0.5 mL of the 1:1,000 solution subcutaneously (SC) every 20 minutes as needed (for children, 0.01 mL/kg of the 1:1,000 solution SC every 20 minutes to a maximum dose of 0.3 mL), or
- Terbutaline 0.25 mg SC every 20 minutes as needed (for children, 0.01 mL/kg SC to a maximum of 0.25 mL)

INTRAVENOUS THERAPY IV therapy should be reserved for severe attacks:

- IV terbutaline: Give a 10 µg/kg loading dose followed by an infusion of 0.4 µg/kg/min. Titrate up to 6 µg/kg/min as needed.
- IV epinephrine
- There is little evidence that IV aminophylline is useful in an acute asthma exacerbation, and the risk of toxicity is great (but it could be the only drug available). If it is to be used, give a 6 mg/kg IV bolus, then start an infusion at 1 mg/kg/h. However, aminophylline levels should be checked to prevent toxicity.

ORAL THERAPY Ultimately it is the use of steroids (glucocorticoids) that reduces the airway inflammation, stops the symptoms, and lessens the chance of further attacks.

- Give a bolus of prednisone 1 mg/kg orally or IV.

■   A short course of 3–5 days of prednisone 0.5 to 1.0 mg/kg orally is usually suffi-
    cient for mild to moderate cases. Severe asthmatics that require steroids fre-
    quently need longer courses, or even continuous daily oral prednisone. Patients
    with no access to other asthma medications may require longer courses also.

OTHER THERAPY In patients with severe acute asthma not responding to treatment, consider intubation after sedation with ketamine. Other medicines to consider if
the aerosols do not seem to be effective include magnesium (3–4 g IV) and ketamine
(1–2 mg/kg IV).

PREVENTION

MEDICATIONS Outpatient therapy in developing countries is difficult because the
medications are either expensive (inhalers), difficult to manage (theophylline), or have
significant long-term complications (oral steroids). Local factors and the severity of the
patient's asthma will determine the treatment methods.

■   Steroid and cromolyn sodium inhalers can reduce the number of exacerbations.
    Steroid inhalers should be used twice a day, every day to prevent attacks.
■   Patients with severe asthma may require chronic oral steroids. They should be
    weaned to the lowest dose and put on an every-other-day regimen if possible.

Patients (or their parents) should be instructed to avoid situations or materials that
worsen asthma: smoking in the home, air pollution (smoky fires, heavy traffic, etc.),
animals in the house, and dust and animal hairs.

CHRONIC OBSTRUCTIVE PULMONARY DISEASE

The presentation, evaluation, and treatment of COPD and asthma are similar. COPD
patients are generally long-term smokers and may respond better to atropine-like
agents. Therefore, this section focuses on the treatment of patients with COPD.

TREATMENT The therapy is similar to that for asthma. These patients, however,
also may respond to inhaled agents:

■   Nebulized atropine 0.01 to 0.03 mL/kg (0.01 mg/mL) in 1 to 2 mL NS. Beware of
    the cardiac effects.
■   Glycopyroliate (0.5 mg) in 1 to 3 mL NS
■   Ipratropium (if available)

These inhaled agents can be added to the beta 2 aerosols in patients during the
treatment of an acute exacerbation.

> **KEY POINT:**
>
> Beware of the use of high-flow oxygen in COPD patients. Many patients may be CO_2 retainers, and high-flow oxygen can reduce the respiratory drive in these individuals and cause them to become apnic.

SPECIFIC CARDIAC PROBLEMS

CHEST PAIN

> **CRITICAL ACTIONS:**
>
> ■ Assume all chest pain is serious until proven otherwise.
> ■ Give an aspirin to essentially everyone with chest pain.
> ■ Give sublingual nitroglycerin (NTG) for any suspicion of cardiac chest pain.

For patients with chest pain, the goal is to identify and stabilize the most serious problems (MIs, pulmonary embolisms); to diagnose, treat, and refer other serious problems (pneumonias, pneumothorax, etc.); and to treat the simplest problems (Table 7-1). The most serious patients may need to be transferred.

> **KEY POINT:**
>
> The diagnosis of chest pain is based primarily on the history, not the results of laboratory tests or ECGs. Spend time to elicit an accurate history. If interpreters are used, make sure that they are very careful in their presentation and translation.

CLINICAL PRESENTATION

HISTORY Cover the following areas:

■ Type/quality of pain (be aware that cardiac pain can include any of these):
  ■ Sharp, piercing, precisely localized pain exacerbated by palpation is usually from the superficial chest wall.
  ■ Pain that increases with breathing is usually pleuritic: consider PE, pneumonia, costochondritis (see section on Breathing Problems above).
  ■ Poorly localized, dull, or aching pain is often visceral: consider an abdominal source.
  ■ Pressurelike pain with or without radiation, sweating, or nausea: cardiac
■ Rapidity of onset: sudden or progressive over several minutes or hours

TABLE 7-1 THE GENERAL DIFFERENTIAL DIAGNOSIS OF CHEST PAIN

	SYMPTOMS	FINDINGS	TESTING
Emergent causes			
Acute MI	Chest pain or pressure >15 min with radiation to the arms or neck. SOB is common and may be only symptom. Diaphoresis and nausea	Few reliable physical findings. Severe myocardial infarction present with congestive heart failure, hypotension, and altered heart sounds.	Classic ECG with 2 mm ST segment elevations, but may have nonspecific changes.
Unstable angina	Similar to the symptoms of an MI, but no cardiac damage	Usually none	ECGs usually normal, or with small ST elevations or depressions
Aortic dissection	80% are hypertensive men between the ages of 50 and 70. Abrupt onset of tearing chest or back pain	May have new heart murmur or thoracic bruit. May be hypotensive.	CXR with classic findings of wide mediastinum, obscure aortic arch, pleural effusion, etc.
Pulmonary embolus	Most patients have predisposing factors to venous thrombosis (trauma, immobility, BCPs). Symptoms: pleuritic chest pain, dyspnea, tachypnea, and tachycardia, but may have nonpleuritic musculoskeletal chest pain.	Rare physical findings. May have a low pulse oximetry with large embolisms.	CXR is usually normal, may see wedge-shaped infarct. ABG shows an A-a gradient >15.
Esophageal rupture	Associated with vomiting or trauma. Severe throat and chest pain, usually without respiratory symptoms	May have neck tenderness and crepitis from subcutaneous air.	CXR may demonstrate mediastinal air.
Tension pneumothorax	Severe dyspnea with pleuritic chest pain	Unilateral decreased or absent breath sounds and tympanic. Distended neck veins	CXR diagnostic, but don't wait: needle decompression first.
Cardiac tamponade	Increasing SOB with or without chest pain	Distended neck veins. Decreased heart sounds. Sometimes a cardiac rub	ECG with decreased voltage, and possible electrical alterans
Urgent causes			
Pneumonia	History of fever and cough with progressive dyspnea. May have pleuritic chest pain.	Febrile. Tachypnea. May have rales or wheezes on auscultation.	CXR with an infiltrate. Pulse oximetry with hypoxia
Angina pectoris	Episodic pain, lasts 5–15 min; caused by exertion, relieved by rest or NTG. Usually retrosternal (over 90%) and 70% radiate.	Pain relief with NTG	No ECG changes
Pericarditis	Severe retrosternal pain with radiation, may increase with each heartbeat, chest motion, or respiration	May have a pericardial friction rub and decreased heart sounds.	Evolutionary ST and T changes on ECG, small pericardial effusion on echocardiogram

TABLE 7-1 THE GENERAL DIFFERENTIAL DIAGNOSIS OF CHEST PAIN *(continued)*

	SYMPTOMS	FINDINGS	TESTING
Esophageal disorders (reflux, hiatal hernia, achalasia, spasm, etc.)	Achy chest pain may begin several minutes after exercise, eating, or reclining and persist for hours. Usually does not radiate. May have heartburn, acid regurgitation, odynophagia, globus sensation.	Rare physical findings	CXR rarely useful, may see a hiatal hernia if air filled. Diagnose by endoscopy or swallowing x-ray with contrast.
Spontaneous pneumothorax	Usually in 20–40-year-old males. Pleuritic chest pain with dyspnea that increases with the size of the lung collapse	Decreased breath sounds on affected side	CXR with lucent lung border
Cardiac valve diseases	Various presentations depending on the affected valve and lesion. CP, SOB, synope, CHF, etc.	Heart murmur usually present, other physical findings vary with the affected valve.	CXR may demonstrate an enlarged heart of abnormal border. Echocardiogram is diagnostic.
Non–life-threatening			
Chest wall pain/costochondritis	Usually sharp, pleuritic chest pain and may be short of breath (mild).	May have palpable chest tenderness.	No studies useful. ECG may help to rule out MI.
Pleuritis	Sharp, pleuritic chest pain, not present when holding breath. May have mild shortness of breath. May be febrile if caused by an infection.	No physical findings	No labs or x-rays ECG normal

Other causes include anxiety, thoracic spine disease, thoracic shingles, fibrositis.

MI, myocardial infarction; SOB, shortness of breath; CHF, congestive heart failure; ECG, electrocardiogram; CXR, chest x-ray; ABG, arterial blood gases; NTG, nitroglycerin; CP, chest pain.

- Duration: seconds, minutes, hours, days (cardiac pain lasts at least 5 minutes but usually much more without treatment)
- Temporal pattern of the pain: Is the pain present now? If so, is it better, worse, or unchanged? Has the pain come and gone?
- Location and radiation: Is the pain localized to a single point or is it more diffuse? Pain from myocardial ischemia and aortic dissection typically radiates to the left arm, neck, or back.
- Provocation of symptoms: Exact activity of patient when pain first noted (e.g., resting, sitting, standing, etc.). Does anything the patient do make the pain worse? Cardiac pain usually comes on with stress or exercise. Pain relief with sublingual NTG should occur within 3 minutes.
- Assess for risk factors for specific causes of chest pain.

PHYSICIAN EXAMINATION

- General appearance and level of distress
- Vital signs, including pulse oximetry, if available; blood pressure (BP) should be taken in both arms if an aortic dissection is considered.
- Chest wall palpation (however, chest wall tenderness is found in up to 50% of patients with coronary artery disease (CAD) and 15% of patients with an MI.)
- Chest auscultation: rales, wheezes, decreased or absent breath sounds
- Cardiac palpation and auscultation: S_3, murmurs, displaced PMI
- Abdominal examination to assess for referred tenderness
- Assess peripheral pulses, including the carotids and femorals for strength and symmetry.
- Neck: tenderness, carotid pulses/bruits
- Limbs: peripheral pulses, edema

DIAGNOSIS

ELECTROCARDIOGRAPHY All patients with chest pain and cardiac risks should undergo ECG to screen for an acute myocardial infarction (AMI). If the characteristic changes of AMI are found, it is helpful, but does not rule out other causes of chest pain (only about half of patients with angina have ECG changes).

CHEST RADIOGRAPHY Chest radiography is a useful tool to diagnose pulmonary causes of chest pain, but the results are usually normal for patients with cardiac chest pain. It is useful for diagnosing lung pathology (PE, pneumothorax, pneumonia, effusions).

BLOOD TESTS Except for cardiac enzymes to assess for an MI, blood tests are rarely indicated. In addition, there are many settings where tests are unavailable. The goal is to stabilize the patient, to begin treatment for the most severe suspected cause, and to transfer to a facility with more resources. See the specific problems for recommended testing.

TREATMENT

CRITICAL ACTION:

Treat all patients with chest pain as having a potentially emergent condition—"Assume the worst, hope for the best."

On any patient, be sure to address the ABCs first. You can then take the following steps to address possible serious threats:

- Give all patients with a possible MI an aspirin (80–325 mg) orally.
- Start an IV or heparin lock (do not give much fluid unless hypotensive).

■ Start 3 L of oxygen by nasal cannula, or more if the patient is potentially hypoxic.
■ Place the patient on a monitor in an easily observed bed.

See the specific causes of pain for the specific treatments.

DISPOSITION If you work in a situation with limited resources, you may consider admitting the patient when you cannot prove that no serious disease exists and when the patient's risk of severe disease is low to moderate. Transfer seriously ill patients and those with a high probability of serious disease. Some patients have trivial pain and can be safely discharged.

CORONARY ARTERY DISEASE

The presentation of acute chest pain from CAD ranges from angina, to unstable angina, to non–Q-wave MIs, to Q-wave MIs. Chest pain may be a result of tissue ischemia or the possibility of infarction.

ANGINA

Angina is self-limited cardiac pain that is brought on by stress or exercise, lasts less than 15 minutes, and is relieved by rest or sublingual NTG.

DIAGNOSIS ECG shows changes in less than 50% of patients, and these are generally small ST depressions or nonspecific ST changes.

TREATMENT Acute anginal attacks are treated with sublingual NTG 0.3 to 0.6 mg every 3 to 5 minutes for three doses. If patients do not get relief after three doses of NTG, they need evaluation for acute MI.
Chronic outpatient treatment can include the following:

■ Aspirin (acetylsalicylic acid; ASA) 80 to 325 mg each day helps prevent MIs (for all patients without known allergic reaction to ASA).
■ Nitrates: either with the use of intermittent doses of sublingual NTG to relieve symptoms or the use of longer acting nitrates to help prevent them.
   ■ NTG 2% ointment (or patch) 1.5 to 4.5 cm two to three times daily.
   ■ Isosorbide dinitrate 5 to 40 mg orally two to four times daily (there is also a sustained-release version using 40 mg twice daily).
■ Beta blockers
   ■ Atenolol: Start with 50 to 200 mg every day up to 200 mg total daily.
   ■ Metoprolol: Start with 50 to 100 mg twice daily up to 400 mg total daily.
   ■ Propranolol: Start with 10 to 60 mg four times daily up to 320 mg total daily.
■ Calcium channel blockers

- Diltiazem: Start with 30 to 60 mg four times daily, or 60 to 120 mg twice daily or 180 mg every day up to a total dose of 360 mg daily.
- Nicardipine 20 mg three times daily or 30 mg twice daily.
- Nifedipine: Start with 10 to 20 mg three times daily or 30 to 60 mg every day up to a total dose of 120 mg daily.
- Verapamil: Start with 80 to 120 mg three times daily or 180 to 240 mg every day up to a total dose of 480 mg daily.

PREVENTION See section on Myocardial Infarction below.

UNSTABLE ANGINA

Unstable angina is a more unpredictable and dangerous form of angina. It may precede an MI. Unstable angina is defined as follows:

- Angina that started less than 4 to 8 weeks ago
- Increasingly severe angina that is brought on by less exercise, lasts longer, or takes more NTG to relieve (Remember that NTG loses its potency gradually over 6 months.)
- Angina that occurs at rest

DIAGNOSIS ECG may demonstrate initial changes similar to an AMI (ST elevations) that may persist for several hours, but Q waves do not develop.

TREATMENT The treatment of unstable angina needs to be almost as aggressive as that for AMI. Start with the simplest interventions and add more if the symptoms are not relieved (progressive treatment).
   All patients should receive the following:

- Oxygen: Start with 2 to 4 L by nasal cannula (more if hypoxemic)
- Aspirin: 80 to 325 mg orally
- Sublingual NTG every 5 minutes for three doses

If symptoms continue, add the following:

- IV NTG infusion
- Heparin, IV bolus and infusion, then
- Beta blocker IV, preferably a continuous esmolol infusion (500 mg/kg IV over 1 minute then 50 mg/kg/min titrated to a maximum dose of 200 mg/kg/min), but you can use boluses of
    - Metoprolol (preferably) or
    - Propranolol

Increasing anginal symptoms indicate worsening CAD and increased risk of mortality. Therefore, all of these patients should be admitted and referred for further evaluation and treatment.

MYOCARDIAL INFARCTION

An MI is diagnosed from the history (with help from an ECG). It is one of the most difficult diagnoses to make, even in the best of circumstances. MIs occur most often between 6 a.m. and noon. There is a second peak in the late afternoon.

RISK FACTORS

- Male gender
- Family history of an MI before age 50
- Age over 45 years
- Cigarette smoking
- Diabetes mellitus
- Hypertension
- Hypercholesterolemia

CLINICAL PRESENTATION The following symptoms are considered to be more common with cardiac pain, but patients can be completely asymptomatic during their MI, particularly diabetics:

- Chest discomfort can be described as pain, pressure, heaviness, or constriction that lasts more than 30 minutes, but can be any kind of pain.
- The pain often radiates to the left arm, neck, or back.
- Shortness of breath
- Diaphoresis (sweating)
- Nausea
- Palpitations

TIPS AND TRICKS:

"Atypical" symptoms and vague pain are common presenting complaints in the elderly and in diabetics.

PHYSICAL EXAMINATION Results of the physical examination are usually normal. Potential (but usually nonspecific) findings include soft S4 and S3 heart sounds, a paradoxically split S2, pericardial rubs, and CHF.

DIAGNOSIS

ELECTROCARDIOGRAPHY The ECG can be diagnostic of AMI, but only half the patients with an AMI have diagnostic changes on their ECG. Serial readings can be helpful.

- The most specific finding of an AMI is a greater than 2 mm ST segment elevation in two leads.
- More patients have ST depressions, which is far less specific.
- T-wave inversion may be seen.
- After several hours, Q waves develop.

LABORATORY TESTS Many blood tests are used to diagnose AMI. They are often not available in areas with limited resources. Some tests, such as troponin, are now available on simple cards that only require a drop of the patient's serum. Specific tests include the following:

- Myoglobin is the earliest serum marker of myocardial injury/infarction, but it is not very sensitive or accurate.
- Total creatinine kinase (CK) is not usually useful because of its low sensitivity and specificity.
- CK-MB isoenzyme is more specific (accurate) for identifying AMI. This test is helpful in patients with nondiagnostic ECGs. Its accuracy is increased by three serial samples taken every 3 to 6 hours (peaks at 18 to 36 hours). The test is not helpful for patients with unstable angina.
- Troponin is another useful marker for AMI, and has increased sensitivity with serial samples.

The timing of these tests depends on their availability and cost, but the ability to detect an AMI increases with serial tests every 3 to 6 hours for 9 to 18 hours.

Other potential tests include an echocardiogram and radionuclide studies to detect cardiac muscle abnormalities, but these are not always available.

TREATMENT

- Oxygen 2 to 4 L/min by nasal cannula (more if needed for CHF or hypoxia)
- Aspirin (ASA) alone is effective for revascularizing a thrombosed coronary artery. Give 160 to 325 mg orally (chewed ASA may act faster).
- Nitrates: Give 0.4 mg sublingual NTG every 3 to 5 minutes as long as the systolic BP remains above 100 mm Hg and the patient has continued symptoms (pain or shortness of breath).
- Start an IV, preferably with D5W at a "keep vein open" (KVO) rate only.
- Morphine 2 to 5 mg IV
- Thrombolysis: tPA or streptokinase when available. Should be given no later than 12 hours after the onset of symptoms (preferably less than 6 hours). (See Table 7-2 for contraindications and doses.)

TABLE 7-2 CONTRAINDICATIONS AND DOSES FOR THROMBOLYTIC THERAPY

Contraindications
Absolute contraindications
  Any previous hemorrhagic stroke
  A nonhemorrhagic CVA within 1 year
  Known intracranial neoplasm
  Active internal bleeding (not menses)
  Suspected aortic dissection by symptoms, history, or CXR

Relative contraindications
  Uncontrolled blood pressure >180/110 mm Hg
  Known bleeding disorder or current anticoagulant use
  Major surgery within the previous 3 weeks
  Serious injury or internal bleeding within 2–4 weeks
  Active peptic ulcer
  Pregnancy
  Noncompressible vascular punctures (e.g., subclavian access attempts)
  CPR (chest compressions) more than 10 minutes, or with possible injuries
  History of chronic, severe HTN

Streptokinase is also relatively contraindicated in patients who have already received it because of possible anaphylaxis, especially with a prior allergic reaction.

Doses
tPA
  15 mg IV bolus, then
  0.75 mg/kg IV over the first 30 min (up to 50 mg), then
  0.50 mg/kg IV over the following 60 min (up to 35 mg)

Begin heparin therapy prior to the end of the tPA infusion.

Streptokinase
  1.5 million IU over 1 hour (no heparin needed)

CVA, cerebrovascular accident; CXR, chest x-ray; CPR, cardiopulmonary resuscitation; HTN, hypertension; tPA, tissue plasminogen activator.

■ Beta blockers reduce myocardial damage (started within 12 hours): metoprolol, propranolol, atenolol, esmolol.

If thrombolytics are not available, then start the patient on the following:

■ Heparin 5,000 U bolus then 700 to 1,000 U/h IV
■ IV NTG titrated to pain-free or a systolic BP of over >100 mm Hg. Should be continued for 24 to 48 hours.

- Angiotensin-converting enzyme (ACE) inhibitors within the first 12 to 24 hours
- Lidocaine is not needed for premature ventricular contractions (PVCs) unless they are more frequent than six per minute or are coupled.

CHEST WALL PAIN

Chest wall pain is probably the most common cause of chest pain, but it is the last diagnosis considered, only after the more serious causes (including lung disease) are ruled out. If there is clearly chest wall tenderness, no risk factors, and a normal ECG, the patient can probably be discharged.

Treatment consists of administration of nonsteroidal antiinflammatory drugs (NSAIDs) or acetaminophen for the pain.

HEART FAILURE/PULMONARY EDEMA

CRITICAL ACTION:

Vasodilatation with NTG is the primary therapy for acute pulmonary edema, then turn to a diuretic and morphine.

Heart failure has many causes and presentations, but it is most commonly CHF due to poor cardiac output (usually left ventricular). CHF is caused by CAD, hypertension, cardiomyopathies, and valvular heart disease, but also by more easily correctable causes such as arrhythmias, infections, and metabolic disorders such as anemia, hyperthyroidism, and beriberi.

CLINICAL PRESENTATION Heart failure can affect either the left ventricle or right ventricle.

- Right ventricular failure is manifested by peripheral edema (lower extremity) and evidence of increased venous pressure (JVD or HJR).
- Left ventricular failure is manifested by progressively increasing dyspnea that occurs while lying horizontally. Lung auscultation shows rales. Left-sided CHF usually progresses to include the right-sided symptoms of ankle edema and JVD.

The difference between CHF and pulmonary edema is that CHF worsens slowly over days, whereas pulmonary edema has a rapid onset, commonly in the early morning hours, and the BP of patients with pulmonary edema is often extremely high (systolic 200–260 mm Hg). AMI is often the cause of pulmonary edema.

DIAGNOSIS

■ CXR is useful to diagnose heart failure, but may be normal in patients with early or sudden heart failure. The CXR often shows increased vascular markings and a large heart (greater than half the width of the chest cavity).
■ ECG can help identify AMI.
■ Laboratory tests are not often useful, except to look for underlying causes such as an MI or infection.

TREATMENT Fix any correctable cause of heart failure such as an infection or arrhythmia.

PULMONARY EDEMA TREATMENT

■ Oxygen 100% by nonrebreather mask. Intubate if necessary.
■ Give 0.4 mg sublingual NTG immediately and every 2 to 5 minutes to maintain a systolic BP of over 120 mm Hg. A continuous NTG infusion may be needed to reduce BP and congestion.
■ Start an IV at a KVO rate.
■ Furosemide 60 to 120 mg IV or orally if necessary) as soon as possible. Monitor the urine output.
■ Consider IV morphine (2–4 mg) to help reduce the patient's anxiety.
■ Give an aspirin if an MI may be the cause of the pulmonary edema.

If a patient is hypo- or normotensive with pulmonary edema, start the following:

■ Dopamine 1 to 10 μg/kg/min IV, and
■ Dobutamine 2 to 20 mg/kg/min
■ A central venous pressure (CVP) monitor may be useful.

Other potential therapies include the following:

■ Aminophylline (200 mg IV per 20 minutes) may reduce the bronchospasm of cardiac asthma.
■ Phlebotomy can reduce blood volume, especially for patients with renal failure.
■ Rotating limb tourniquets are an unconventional treatment to reduce the return of blood to the heart and pulmonary congestion.

TREATMENT FOR EXACERBATION OF CONGESTIVE HEART FAILURE

■ Oxygen at least 2 L by nasal cannula. Titrate to relieve symptoms.
■ Furosemide: Start with 20 to 40 mg IV or orally during an acute exacerbation (more if already on diuretics). Double the dose every 30 to 60 minutes, depending on the urine output.

- Vasodilators
- Nitrates (NTG) are also useful for exacerbations of CHF. Sublingual administration usually is sufficient.

CHRONIC CONGESTIVE HEART FAILURE TREATMENT Restriction of salt intake and vasodilators are the mainstay of therapy. Vasodilators include the following:

- Calcium channel blockers such as diltiazem and nifedipine
- ACE inhibitors such as captopril
- Venous dilators include NTG and isosorbide dinitrate.
- Other agents include hydralazine and minoxidil.

Diuretics are secondary agents, but may be the only type available. Use them in combination with vasodilators for patients with signs of fluid retention. There are two main classes of diuretics: thiazide diuretics and loop diuretics. The combination of loop and thiazide diuretics may be synergistic.

- Loop diuretics (furosemide) are generally more useful in the acute phase, but can be used for chronic therapy. The difficulty is that they cause a significant loss of potassium. Use furosemide 20 to 40 mg orally once or twice a day.
- Thiazide diuretic: HCTZ (and others) 25 to 50 mg orally once or twice a day for maintenance.

The final medication for treating CHF is an inotropic agent. Start digitalis (digoxin), with a loading dose of 10 to 15 µg/kg (lean body mass). Care must be taken and levels monitored to prevent toxic levels (be especially cautious in patients with renal failure).

PREVENTION Hypertension and MIs are the most common causes of CHF, so preventive measures must be directed toward them.

CARDIAC TAMPONADE

CRITICAL ACTIONS:

- If patients present with shock (hypotension) and dilated jugular veins, think tamponade.
- Fluid bolus is the first line of therapy.
- Pericardiocentesis can be life saving.

Cardiac tamponade is caused by the accumulation of fluid in the pericardial space surrounding the heart that leads to decreased cardiac output. Causes include blunt and penetrating injuries (including iatrogenic), infections, neoplasms, uremia, collagen-vascular diseases, and post-MI myocardial rupture.

CLINICAL PRESENTATION

- The classic symptoms of tamponade are described as Beck's triad: hypotension, JVD, and muffled heart sounds. Hypotension is a late finding.
- Kussmaul's sign is an increase in JVD with inspiration.
- Other evidence of high venous pressures may be present, such as hepatojugular reflux and peripheral edema.
- Tamponade may present as pulseless electrical activity in a cardiac arrest. Consider a pericardiocentesis in a cardiac arrest.

DIAGNOSIS

- Pulsus paradoxus of greater than 10 mm Hg systolic BP with inspiration occurs when checking the BP.
- ECG may demonstrate low-voltage and nonspecific ST–T changes. Occasionally you will see electrical alternans (beat-to-beat changes in the axis of the QRS complex on the ECG).
- Ultrasonography of the heart is the most useful test to identify tamponade.

TREATMENT Initial therapy is the same as for any patient in shock:

- Oxygen
- IV resuscitation with NS or lactated Ringer's (LR) solution. Start with a 500-mL bolus.

The optimum treatment is to open the pericardial sac sterilely in the operating room. When this is not available, a simple, needle pericardiocentesis can be attempted (see Table 7-3 and Fig. 7-1). Simple pericardiocentesis may be sufficient for patients with nontraumatic tamponade. Pericardiocentesis may be used to determine the cause of the effusion or for treatment of tamponade.

THORACIC ANEURYSM (AORTIC DISSECTION)

Aortic dissection is the tearing and disruption of the thoracic aorta. In areas with limited resources, there are only a few temporizing measures that can be taken for patients with an acute dissection. The definitive treatment is surgical.

CLINICAL PRESENTATION Symptoms include

- Severe, sharp pain from the anterior chest, often radiating straight through to the back. The pain also may radiate to the neck and jaw, or into the belly.

TABLE 7-3 PERICARDIOCENTESIS

Pericardiocentesis is indicated for any patient with an acute tamponade and signs of shock or respiratory distress.

There are two approaches for a simple needle pericardiocentesis: subxiphoid and fifth intercostal approaches. It can be done blindly or more accurately with ECG guidance.

Equipment
> Sterile drapes and preparation solution
> Local anesthetic
> Needle: at least 9 cm long and 16 gauge. Ideally it will be a needle/plastic catheter combination to allow the catheter to remain indwelling.
> 30–50 mL syringe
> Sterile alligator clip (or clamp) to connect the ECG to the needle
> ECG

General technique
> The patient should be lying supine with the head elevated 20–30 degrees.
> Prepare and drape the patient for all procedures.
> Inject local anesthetic (1%–2% lidocaine without epinephrine) to the area.
> Connect the ECG V lead with the sterile clip to the needle.
> Gradually introduce the needle while gentle aspirating and watching the ECG monitor.
>> A pop may be felt as you pierce the pericardium.
>> Fluid and/or blood should be seen immediately.
> You've gone too far (stop immediately and withdraw slightly) if
>> ST elevations are seen, then you've hit the ventricle myocardium.
>> PR elevation then the atrial myocardium
>> Arrhythmias are noted.
>> A scratching sensation is felt against the needle
> Blood from the pericardial space should not clot when squirted into a container.
> The patient's blood pressure should improve rapidly if the pericardial fluid is removed.
> If the needle includes a catheter and the patient reaccumulates fluid, then withdraw the needle, but leave the catheter in place and seal it with a three-way stopcock.
> Pericardial fluid can be analyzed for cell count/differential, cytology, protein, glucose, and cultures including bacterial, acid-fast, and fungal cultures.

Fifth intercostal approach
> This is the preferred site for pericardiocentesis.
>> The needle is introduced straight down through the left fifth intercostal space 1 cm lateral to the sternum.

Subxiphoid approach
> The needle is introduced 1–2 cm below the costal margin, just left of the xiphoid process. Aim toward the middle of the clavicle toward the back at a 30–45 degree angle.

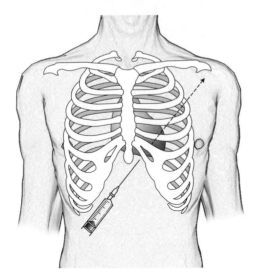

FIGURE 7-1 Pericardiocentesis.

- Syncope may occur.
- 20% of patients will have a neurologic deficit.

Physical findings can be diagnostic of aortic dissection.

- Patients may present in shock.
- The patient may not have a pulse on one side of the body, or in a single upper limb.
- There may be differences in the BPs between limbs.
- Acute aortic regurgitation may occur.
- Pericardial tamponade may occur.
- The combination of severe chest pain and neurologic findings is extremely suggestive of aortic dissection (tracking into the carotid artery). Patients have an altered mental status or hemiplegia.

TIPS AND TRICKS:

- Diagnose by presentation (tearing chest pain, altered pulse, neurologic findings).
- Treat by lowering the BP and shearing forces of blood flow.

DIAGNOSIS

- ECGs do not diagnose a dissection, but can rule out an AMI as the cause of the chest pain.
- The CXR is abnormal in the majority of cases:

- Mediastinal widening
- Pleural effusions
- Bulging of the aortic contour
- Separation of a calcified inner aortic wall from the outer most portion of the aortic contour
- Echocardiography is relatively sensitive for detecting a dissection, and transesophageal cardiography is more sensitive.
- CT scan can be helpful but is not as sensitive.
- Aortography is the most helpful in making the diagnosis and providing preoperative information for repair.

TREATMENT Definitive treatment is surgical: transfer patients as soon as possible.

KEY POINT:

The initial treatment of most forms of shock is a fluid bolus of 250 to 500 mL.

To stabilize, treat either the shock or hypertension. When the patient is hypertensive, the goal is to reduce the BP and the shear forces on the wall of the aorta. A combination of drugs is often needed.

- Labetalol is a suitable single-agent choice (it has both beta- and alpha-blocking effects).
- Trimethaphan is also a good single agent, but can cause tachycardia. It is a ganglionic blocking agent and produces a wide array of autonomic symptoms such as orthostasis, pupil area abnormalities, diplopia, urinary retention, and ileus.
- Beta blockers work in combination with vasodilating agents like nitroprusside by preventing reflexive tachycardia and increased shear forces. Perhaps the best combination is esmolol and nitroprusside because both can be quickly titrated by continuous IV infusion, but other beta blockers can be used.

HYPERTENSION

The presentation of hypertension is generally divided into emergent, urgent, and chronic varieties based on their clinical presentation. The approach to each is different. In addition, chronic hypertension can be considered mild to severe depending on the BP:

- Mild hypertension is considered a diastolic BP of 90 to 99 mm Hg and a systolic BP of 140 to 159 mm Hg.
- Moderate hypertension is diastolic BP of 100 to 109 mm Hg and systolic BP of 160 to 179 mm Hg.
- Severe hypertension is diastolic BP of 110 to 119 mm Hg and systolic BP of 180 to 209 mm Hg.

> **KEY POINTS:**
>
> Patients with hypertension can be grouped into the following categories:
>
> - Emergency: presents with hypertension and end-organ damage (chest pain, mental status changes, renal failure)
> - Urgency: diastolic BP over 130 mm Hg
> - Chronic: diastolic BP under 130 mm Hg with no specific symptoms (as above)

Hypertension should not be diagnosed on the basis of a single measurement. If the initial reading is elevated, it should be repeated after the patient has been resting quietly on his or her back for 5 minutes, and should be checked in both arms.

HYPERTENSIVE EMERGENCIES A hypertensive emergency is diagnosed not by a specific BP, but is defined as an increased BP that causes acute end-organ (brain, heart, kidneys, and eyes) damage.

CLINICAL PRESENTATION The presentation depends on the specific hypertensive emergency that occurs:

- AMI/chest pain
- Cerebrovascular accident (CVA)/subarachnoid hemorrhage (SAH)
- Hypertensive encephalopathy (Patient presents with a severe headache, vomiting, blurred vision or double vision, altered mental status, seizures, focal neurologic deficits, coma.)
- CHF/pulmonary edema
- Aortic dissection

DIAGNOSIS Laboratory tests may be useful to check for evidence of end-organ damage:

- Electrolytes may be helpful to assess for kidney damage [blood urea nitrogen (BUN) and creatinine], or associated electrolyte abnormalities (especially hypokalemia with diuretic therapy).
- Urinalysis to look for kidney damage (the presence of protein and red cells)

RADIOLOGY

- Chest radiography can be used to assess for cardiomegaly. It is particularly useful if CHF or pulmonary edema are possible sequelae.
- A head CT is useful for hypertensive patients with altered mental status.

ELECTROCARDIOGRAHY The ECG is essential to check for myocardial damage (AMI, unstable angina).

TREATMENT The BP must be reduced rapidly to slightly above normal to limit or prevent life-threatening complications. The amount and rapidity that the BP should be reduced depends on the particular hypertensive emergency. In general, avoid sublingual nifedipine to treat hypertension urgently.

DID YOU KNOW?

In treating hypertension, reducing the BP in stroke patients or those with cerebral vascular disease too quickly may cause worsening of symptoms (stroke).

Treatments for specific hypertensive emergencies include the following:

- Hypertensive encephalopathy: Decrease the BP by less than 20% in the first hour (or to a diastolic BP of 110 mm Hg). Do not decrease the BP by more than 30% over the next 48 to 72 hours. IV nitroprusside infusion is a great method, but requires frequent, accurate BP checks (do not lower the BP too much).
- CVA, SAH, or intracerebral hemorrhage: The need to reduce the BP is controversial. If the diastolic BP is persistently over 140 mm Hg, then slowly reduce the BP by 20% to 30% over 12 to 24 hours. Nitroprusside or labetalol can be used.
- AMI/chest pain (See the section on Myocardial Infarctions.)
  - Sublingual (or preferably IV) NTG is the best drug because it increases coronary blood flow. Titrate the infusion to reduce the BP to normal levels.
  - Beta blockers are also indicated in patients with cardiac ischemia.
- CHF/pulmonary edema
  - Use an IV NTG infusion to reduce the BP to normal or near-normal levels.
  - Do not use beta blockers with CHF.

HYPERTENSIVE URGENCIES

Hypertensive urgency is defined as a diastolic BP over 130 mm Hg. Patients may have chronic end-organ damage, but no evidence of acute, life-threatening dysfunction.

TREATMENT The goal is to lower the BP slowly over 24 to 72 hours, usually by starting with a single oral agent (Tables 7-4 and 7-5).

CHRONIC HYPERTENSION

TREATMENT The most important treatment for chronic hypertension is to educate the patient about the importance of weight loss, exercise, salt restriction, and the need for chronic therapy and ongoing care. Unless continued medical therapy is available, there is little reason to start drugs.

TABLE 7-4 RECOMMENDED HYPERTENSIVE MEDICATIONS BASED ON PATIENT VARIABLES

	DIURETIC	BETA BLOCKER	CALCIUM CHANNEL BLOCKER	ACE INHIBITOR	ALPHA BLOCKER
Patient demographics					
Elderly	++	+/–	+	+	+
Black race	++	+/–	+	+	+/–
Patient medical condition					
Angina	+/–	++	+	++	+
Post AMI	+	++	+	+/–	++
CHF	++	?	+	–	++
CVA	+	+	+/–	++	+
Renal insufficiency	++	+/–	+	++	++
Diabetes	–	–	++	+	++
Dyslipidemia	–	–	++	+	+

ACE inhibitor, angiotensin-converting enzyme inhibitor; AMI, acute myocardial infarction; CHF, congestive heart failure; CVA, cerebrovascular accident.

TABLE 7-5 COMMON ANTIHYPERTENSION MEDICATIONS

DRUG	STARTING DOSE	USUAL DOSE
Diuretics		
Furosemide	20 mg daily	20–320 mg
Hydrochlorothiazide	25 mg daily	12.5–50 mg
Beta blockers		
Atenolol	50 mg daily	25–100 mg
Metoprolol	50 mg b.i.d.	50–450 mg
Propranolol	40 mg b.i.d.	40–240 mg
Proponolol LA	80 mg daily	60–240 mg
Labetalol	100 mg b.i.d.	200–1,200 mg
Calcium channel blockers		
Diltiazem	5 mg daily	2.5–10 mg
Diltiazem SR	60–120 mg b.i.d.	120–360 mg
Diltiazem CD	180 mg b.i.d.	180–360 mg
Nicardipine	20 mg t.i.d.	60–120 mg
Nicardipine SR	30 mg b.i.d.	60–120 mg
Nifedipine XL	30 mg daily	30–90 mg
Verapamil SR	120–140 mg daily	120–480 mg
ACE inhibitors		
Captopril	25 mg b.i.d.	50–450 mg
Enalapril	5 mg daily	2.5–40 mg

b.i.d., twice daily; ACE inhibitors, angiotensin-converting enzyme inhibitors.

First-line drugs to treat hypertension include diuretics, beta blockers, calcium channel antagonists, ACE inhibitors, and alpha-adrenergic antagonists. The drug choice is affected by coexistent patient factors such as age, race, and associated medical problems (e.g., angina, CHF, renal insufficiency, left ventricular hypertrophy, obesity, hyperlipidemia, gout, and bronchospastic disease) (Table 7-4).

GASTROINTESTINAL PROBLEMS

ACUTE ABDOMINAL PAIN

Like chest pain, abdominal pain is a common and complicated complaint. Even in well-equipped outpatient departments, 40% to 60% of patients with abdominal pain are discharged without a specific diagnosis. Abdominal pain can originate in the abdomen, can be referred from another site (lung, kidney, back), or can result from metabolic (diabetic ketoacidosis (DKA), sickle cell) or neurogenic (herpes zoster) causes.

CLINICAL PRESENTATION

The history provides the most information when diagnosing abdominal pain (Table 7-6). The key areas to cover in the history are as follows:

- Onset and time course: sudden (mechanical obstruction or perforation) versus gradual
- Character and severity (dull, sharp, burning, crampy)
- Intermittent versus constant
- Location, change in location, radiation
- Provoking factors, relieving factors
- Associated symptoms: fever, chills, anorexia, nausea, vomiting and diarrhea, genitourinary symptoms
- Gynecologic and menstrual history in women
- Recent medication (especially aspirin, NSAIDs, steroids, coumadin) and alcohol use
- Previous abdominal illness and surgery

PHYSICAL EXAMINATION

Multiple, repeated physical examinations over a number of hours is the best method to evaluate significant abdominal problems when the initial history and physical is inconclusive. Examine for the following:

- Vital signs: Look for signs of shock or dehydration.
- Abdomen: Appearance, distention, auscultation, palpation to localize the pain, signs of peritonitis such as
    - Guarding
    - Rebound (pain with the rapid lifting of the examining hand)

TABLE 7-6 COMMON CAUSES AND FINDINGS OF ABDOMINAL PAIN

	SYMPTOMS	FINDINGS	TESTING
GI causes			
Esophagitis	History of hiatal hernia, heartburn, no radiation to back, pain may increase with eating, not relieved by bowel movement.	Abdomen usually nontender.	Labs: Usually normal x-rays: CXR normal or may see hiatal hernia.
Peptic ulcer	Nighttime or postprandial pain, relief with antacids or food, age >40, history of PUD, smoking, NSAIDs	Epigastric tenderness, but no peritoneal signs. May have guaiac + stools.	Labs not needed. Chronic ulcers may cause anemia. Upright abdominal x-ray only if perforation suspected.
Gastroenteritis	Nausea, vomiting, diarrhea, cramping pain	Usually non- or mildly tender abdomen. Bowel sounds may be hyperactive.	Microscopic stool for O&P. Guaiac for blood in stool.
Cholecystitis and cholelithiasis (gallstones)	RUQ or epigastric pain for 1–24 hours starting >1 hour after eating, steady in quality, pain may radiate to the upper back. Nausea and vomiting	Localized RUQ tenderness, no peritoneal signs (unless ruptured)	Slight increase LFTs. US for stones. If increased WBCs, consider infection.
Cholangitis	Abdominal pain (RUQ or diffuse) with fever, chills, and vomiting	High fever, severe tenderness or peritonitis, often with jaundice. Severe cases can have shock.	Labs: Elevated WBCs, bilirubin, and LFTs. X-rays: US is most useful, plain x-rays may show air in the biliary tree.
Pancreatitis	Severe, constant, boring epigastric or diffuse pain that usually radiates to the back. Usually with anorexia and vomiting. Most common causes are gallstones, alcohol abuse and medications.	Marked epigastric tenderness with guarding but rebound is uncommon. Bowel sounds are reduced or absent.	Labs: Increased amylase or lipase. Serious if high WBCs, sugar, LDH and GOT, and low calcium. X-rays. May see pancreatic calcifications if chronic. US may find an abscess.
Small bowel obstruction (SBO)	Crampy abdominal pain leading to severe nausea and vomiting with or without abdominal distention	Most commonly a previous history of abdominal surgery. Mild to moderate tenderness, often tympanitc. Rushing, high-pitched bowel sounds	Labs: Usually normal, may show dehydration. Elevated amylase can means strangulation and bowel death. X-rays: Dilated loops of small bowel, air-fluid levels
Mesenteric ischemia	Elderly patient with vague but severe pain out of proportion to physical findings	Minimal abdominal tenderness compared with discomfort. Unexplained shock or acidosis	Labs: Leukocytosis, elevated LDH, phosphate, lactate. X-rays. Ischemic changes such as ileus, thumb printing, bowel wall thickening, gas in bowel wall
Appendicitis	RLQ that was initially diffuse or migrated from the midline, anorexia, nausea, and fever	RLQ tenderness, low-grade fever. Maybe tenderness on rectal and with flexion/rotation at hip joint. If the appendix ruptures, then the patient will have signs of peritonitis.	Labs: Leukocytosis with a left shift. X-rays. <20% have a visible stone in RLQ.

TABLE 7-6 COMMON CAUSES AND FINDINGS OF ABDOMINAL PAIN *(continued)*

	SYMPTOMS	FINDINGS	TESTING
Diverticulitis	Localized LLQ pain which may worsen with bowel movements	LLQ tenderness, often febrile Usually older than 45 years	Labs: Leukocytosis
Large bowel obstruction	Diffuse crampy of colicky pain with vomiting	Usually elderly Abdominal distention, tympanitic Absent bowel sounds or rushes	X-rays: Markedly distended loops of bowel
Non-GI causes			
Ectopic pregnancy	Pelvic or lower abdominal pain with vaginal bleeding. May be dizzy (shock). Patient may not be aware of pregnancy (LMP <10 weeks ago).	Mild to severe abdominal tenderness Vaginal bleeding May be hypotensive if large bleed.	Labs: Positive pregnancy test, anemia (unreliable) X-rays: Plain films useless US to identify ectopic vs. normal pregnancy Culdocentesis for blood
Salpingitis (PID)	Severe lower abdominal pain with a vaginal discharge in a sexually active female (multiple partners = high risk)	Fever, marked LQ tenderness Cervical motion tenderness on pelvic exam	Labs: Leukocytosis, check hCG. X-rays: Plain films useless US to rule out tubal abcess or ectopic. Culdocentesis for blood
Abruption placenta Placenta previa	Painful, severe vaginal bleeding in a pregnant woman Painless, variable bleeding in a pregnant woman	Marked abdominal tenderness, more mild with previa May present in shock Bright blood on vaginal exam	Positive pregnancy test (but usually palpable uterus and amenorrhea)
Cystitis/ Pyelonephritis (UTI)	Suprapubic or flank pain associated with urinary frequency, pain and urgency Pyelonephritis includes fever.	Mild to moderate suprapubic tenderness (cystitis) CVA tenderness and fever (pyelonephritis)	Leukocyte esterase and nitrites on urine dipstick WBCs on urine microscopy Blood test not indicated
Nephrolithiasis (kidney stone)	Mild to severe flank pain radiating to the groin May have nausea and vomiting.	CVA tenderness, minimal abdominal tender	RBCs on urine dipstick and microscopic exam X-ray with stone <25%
Testicular torsion	Usually rapid onset of testicle pain in adolescents, but younger present with nonspecific abdominal pain.	Abdomen nontender. Unilateral testicular tender with swelling and abnormal rotation	Ultrasound if available

There are also chest sources of abdominal pain: myocardial ischemia or acute myocardial infarction, pneumonia, pneumonia, pneumothorax, pulmonary embolus, pericarditis.

Labs, laboratory studies; CXR, chest x-ray; PUD, peptic ulcer disease; NSAIDs, nonsteroidal antiinflammatory drugs; RUQ, right upper quadrant; LFT, liver function tests (aspartate transaminase, ALT, bilirubin, alkaline phosphate, etc.); US, ultrasonography; WBCs, white blood cells; RLQ, right lower quadrant; LLQ, left lower quadrant; LMP, last menstrual period; PID, pelvic inflammatory disease; hCG, human chorionic gonadotropin; UTI, urinary tract infection; CVA, costovertebral angle (flank); RBCs, red blood cells.

- Pain worse with movement, coughing, sneezing, jostling (bed movement, heel percussion, etc.)
- Pain with light percussion of the abdomen
- Referred pain (palpation of one area with pain in another)
- Rectal: Signs of bleeding, hemorrhoids, fissures. Point tenderness (especially right side appendicitis)
- Male genital examination: Infections (urethral discharge, lesions), testicular tenderness from torsion or epididymitis
- Pelvic examination: Signs of abnormal bleeding (ectopic, fibroids), discharges or cervical motion tenderness (infections, pelvic inflammatory disease), masses
- Lung examination to assess for pneumonia, PE, or pneumothorax

---

TIPS AND TRICKS:

The general appearance of a patient with abdominal pain may provide a clue to the diagnosis. Anxious patients who move around and are unable to get comfortable may have visceral pain, such as with a kidney stone. Patients who are very still may have somatic pain, such as with peritonitis.

Signs of inflammation of the peritoneum (peritonitis) are ominous; these include the following:

- Severe abdominal pain
- Abdominal wall rigidity
- Rebound tenderness (Even bumping the bed may cause severe pain.)
- Fever (late)
- Decreased or absent bowel sounds
- Abdominal distention (late)

DIAGNOSIS

LABORATORY TESTS

- A pregnancy test is essential for all women of reproductive age.
- CBC: Although a common test, it has a limited role in decision-making. It is nonspecific and usually unnecessary.
- Urinalysis: To look for hematuria, pyuria, and bacteriuria. Even urine dipsticks are useful to assess for many important functions: blood, nitrites, sugar, ketones, specific gravity.
- Amylase/lipase (to evaluate for pancreatitis)
- Other laboratory tests such as liver function tests (AST, ALT, bilirubin, alkaline phosphatase) and kidney tests (BUN/creatinine) are rarely available and only useful if clinically indicated.

RADIOLOGY

- Abdominal radiographs have little utility for generalized abdominal pain. They are useful (with an upright film) for patients with vomiting or peritoneal signs to identify
  - Small bowel obstruction (SBO)
  - Pneumoperitoneum (perforated viscus)
  - Foreign body ingestion
  - Renal or biliary calculi (sometimes)
  - Aortic vascular calcifications [abdominal aortic aneurysm (AAA)]
  - Air in biliary tree (ascending cholangitis)
- Ultrasonography is useful for diagnosing biliary colic, abdominal aorta aneurysms, renal colic, ectopic pregnancy, and even appendicitis.
- Abdominal CT could be used to diagnose suspected ureterolithiasis, diverticulitis, tumor, intraperitoneal hemorrhage (if hemodynamically stable).

OTHER STUDIES Electrocardiography should be performed in patients over 40 years of age with upper abdominal symptoms, particularly if they are short of breath or have any other cardiac or respiratory symptoms.

DIFFERENTIAL DIAGNOSIS The life-threatening causes of abdominal pain include the following:

- Appendicitis
- Bowel obstruction
- Bowel infarction
- Ruptured ectopic (tubal) pregnancy
- Ruptured AAA
- Ruptured liver or spleen (usually traumatic but can be caused by malaria, mononucleosis, or hematologic disease)
- Ruptured viscus (leading to peritonitis)

GENERAL TREATMENT OF ABDOMINAL PAIN For patients in severe pain or with signs or symptoms of shock or hypotension, immediately start the following:

- IV fluids (LR or NS) and give boluses of 20 mL/kg.
- If an intraabdominal infection is suspected (peritonitis, appendicitis, cholecystitis, ruptured viscus), start IV antibiotics immediately (penicillin or cephalosporin with gentamicin and metronidazole).

For all patients consider the following:

- Antiemetics such as hydroxyzine [50 mg intramuscularly (IM)] or prochlorperazine (10 mg IV or IM)

- Decide if parenteral pain medications are needed (morphine 2–8 mg IV or meperidine 10–25 mg IV repeated as needed).
- If an SBO is suspected, then a nasogastric (NG) tube is needed to decompress the stomach and bowel. Ideally the NG tube is connected to low, intermediate suction.
- Emergent transfer if surgery may be needed

DISPOSITION

- Patients with a potential surgical cause for their pain should be referred to a surgeon immediately.
- Patients with an unexplained source of their abdominal pain should be admitted for observation and serial examinations for 12 to 48 hours.
- High-risk patients (the elderly, immunocompromised, diabetics, those with significant chronic diseases) should be admitted.
- Patients with intermittent or colicky pain or pain that has been relieved can often be discharged.

Discharged patients should return within 24 hours if the pain is worse, vomiting is persistent, or fever is maintained (better yet, admit them for observation and serial examinations).

TREATMENT OF SPECIFIC ABDOMINAL PROBLEMS See Table 7-6 for recommendations on the symptoms, findings, and testing of patients with abdominal pain.

ESOPHAGITIS Esophagitis and reflux are not life threatening, but perforations are.

- Elevate the head of the patient's bed.
- Prohibit fatty foods.
- Prohibit alcohol, caffeine, and cigarettes.
- Give antacids 1 hour after each meal and at bedtime.
- Severe cases may require H_2 blockers (cimetidine, ranitidine, etc).

PEPTIC ULCER Untreated ulcers can lead to perforation, peritonitis, and death. Treatment is as follows:

- Bland diets (no spicy foods) and more frequent feedings are often used, but there is no proof that they work.
- Prohibit alcohol, caffeine, and cigarettes.
- Give antacids 1 hour after each meal and at bedtime.
- Severe cases may require the use of H_2 blockers:
    - Cimetidine 400 mg orally twice daily or 800 mg at bedtime
    - Ranitidine 150 mg orally twice daily or 300 mg at bedtime
    - Sucralfate 2 g twice a day before meals

CHOLECYSTITIS/CHOLELITHIASIS Gall bladder disease ranges from simple stones (cholelithiasis), to stones causing obstruction and inflammation (cholecystitis) to severe infections (acute cholangitis). Surgery is the definitive treatment, but episodes of pain can be treated temporarily. Treatment consists of the following:

■ IV fluid rehydration with nothing by mouth (or only clear fluids if necessary)
■ Antiemetics for the control of vomiting
■ Severe vomiting may require NG suctioning.
■ Antispasmodics such as glycopyrrolate can be used.
■ IV pain medications may be needed (morphine).

CHOLANGITIS Treatment is as follows:

■ IV resuscitation and vasopressors if necessary for shock
■ IV antibiotics (ampicillin, gentamicin, and metronidazole)
■ The gallbladder must be drained either by open surgery or with drains placed directly or with ultrasonographic or laparoscopic guidance.

PANCREATITIS Pancreatitis can usually be managed with fluids and pain medications. Hemorrhagic pancreatitis is often fatal. Complications include pleural effusions, infiltrates, and acute respiratory distress syndrome. Treatment consists of the following:

■ Fluid resuscitation with NS or LR
■ Antiemetics for the control of vomiting
■ Severe vomiting may require NG suctioning.
■ IV pain medications may be needed (morphine).

SMALL BOWEL OBSTRUCTION The most common cause of SBO is adhesions from previous surgery. Other causes include tumors, intestinal parasites, stenosis, and hernias.

■ Patients are often significantly dehydrated and require fluid resuscitation with 1 to 3 L of NS.
■ Patients in shock should receive blood products when available.
■ IV potassium is often needed.
■ NG suction is used for all patients and may be curative by itself.
■ Operative intervention is needed for patients whose symptoms don't resolve with suction, their pain worsens, or they develop signs of peritonitis.

APPENDICITIS Appendicitis is particularly difficult to diagnose in children, the elderly, and pregnant patients. Untreated appendicitis often progresses to a rupture with a resulting peritonitis and high mortality.

■ The treatment is surgical. Transfer if needed.
■ Antibiotics are indicated for all patients, particularly if a rupture is suspected (ampicillin, gentamicin, and metronidazole, or clindamycin).

DIVERTICULITIS Diverticulitis is relatively rare in non-Western countries. It can lead to severe, painless hemorrhage, rupture with peritonitis, or a large bowel obstruction (LBO). Treatment is as follows:

■ IV fluid with nothing by mouth, or only clear liquids
■ IV antibiotics (ampicillin, gentamicin, and metronidazole)
■ IV pain medications (morphine, etc.)
■ Frequent reexamination for worsening findings (peritonitis consistent with perforation)

LARGE BOWEL OBSTRUCTION Large bowel obstructions are caused by cancer, volvulus, and diverticuli. A volvulus occurs when (generally) the sigmoid colon twists upon itself. It is most common in elderly patients with other debilitating diseases and in patients with severe psychiatric or neurologic disorders. Treatment consists of the following:

■ IV fluid resuscitation
■ IV antibiotics
■ The bowel can often be decompressed with a barium enema, or more likely with a colonoscopy or even sigmoidoscopy.

BOWEL INFARCTION Patients are usually elderly and present with severe abdominal pain, but with little tenderness. The mortality rate is 80% to 90% despite therapy:

■ IV fluids
■ IV antibiotics
■ Heparin IV may help to revascularize.
■ Emergent surgical intervention

RUPTURED ECTOPIC (TUBAL) PREGNANCY See Chapter 12 for discussion of ectopic pregnancy.

RUPTURED ABDOMINAL AORTIC ANEURYSM Patients are usually elderly with underlying vascular disease. There is usually severe abdominal pain followed by shock and signs of peritonitis from the free blood in the abdomen. Treatment consists of the following:

■ IV fluid resuscitation for shock
■ Blood transfusions are usually needed.
■ Operative repair is usually needed immediately, but some patients can be stabilized and transferred for surgery.

RUPTURED LIVER OR SPLEEN The cause is usually traumatic in nature, but can result from malaria, mononucleosis, or hematologic disease. Patients present with peritonitis and hypotension. Treatment is as follows:

- IV fluid resuscitation
- Emergent surgical intervention

RUPTURED VISCUS (LEADING TO PERITONITIS) Usually there is abdominal pain prior to the perforation. It may be temporarily relieved after the perforation occurs, but then returns as the peritonitis develops. It is treated as follows:

- IV fluid resuscitation
- IV antibiotics
- Emergent surgery

GASTROINTESTINAL BLEEDING

> **CRITICAL ACTION:**
>
> Always assume that a GI bleed is serious and evaluate quickly.

GI bleeding may be acute or chronic, trivial or life threatening. The good news is that approximately 85% of GI bleeding stops spontaneously. GI bleeding may be rapid and apparent (hematemesis, hematochezia, or melena) or slow and occult, presenting with such symptoms as shock, angina, syncope, weakness, or confusion. The bleeding can come from the stomach or esophagus (upper) or from the small and large bowels (lower).

The causes of upper GI bleeding include peptic ulcer, gastritis, esophagitis, esophageal varices, Mallory-Weiss tear (from forceful vomiting), and swallowed blood (from bleeding of the nose or mouth).

The causes of lower GI bleeding include diverticulosis, ulcerative colitis, colon cancer, polyps, Crohn's disease, parasites, hemorrhoids, and rapid transit of upper GI blood.

HISTORY It is important to differentiate between vomiting blood (hematemesis) and coughing up blood (hemoptysis). Differentiating between upper and lower GI bleeding is also useful.

- Attempt to estimate the amount of blood loss (number of episodes, volume of each).
- Associated symptoms: painful or not, location of pain (esophagus vs. stomach)
- Upper (vomiting blood) versus lower (bloody, maroon stools)
- Any prior history of GI bleeding (although the current bleeding may not be from the same site)
- History of alcohol abuse or liver disease (Cirrhosis leads to esophageal varices, a frequent cause of bleeding.)
- Prior surgery, especially for ulcers and abdominal aortic grafts (May bleed massively from a fistula.)
- Current medications: Antiinflammatories (aspirin, NSAIDs), anticoagulants, and steroids all lead to ulcers.

PHYSICAL EXAMINATION The clinical presentation identifies the bleeding site only 40% to 60% of the time, and the severity of bleeding is a poor predictor of the site.

- The ABCs: Tachycardia and hypotension are emergencies.
- Physical evidence of blood loss: Hematemesis and grossly bloody stool indicate a potentially serious hemorrhage.
- General physical examination: Examine for abdominal tenderness, signs of peritonitis. Look for evidence of abdominal disease. Palpable spleen and visible abdominal veins mean portal hypertension.
- Rectal examination to test stool for occult blood. Twenty mL of blood will give a positive result; 100 to 200 mL of blood will turn the stool maroon or black (melena).

DIAGNOSIS

LABORATORY TESTS

- Type and cross-match is the most important blood test (when possible).
- A hematocrit is an indicator of blood loss, but in rapid blood loss the decrease in the hematocrit may lag by up to 24 hours. A platelet count and prothrombin time/partial thromboplastin time are useful if available.
- Liver function studies can indicate liver disease and the possibility of cirrhosis, but are not very sensitive or specific.

RADIOLOGY

- CXR may help differentiate bleeding from the lungs (abscess, TB, etc.) versus the GI tract when uncertain of the source.
- Abdominal films are generally useless unless a perforated ulcer is suspected as the source of the bleeding (accompanied by signs of peritonitis).

NASOGASTRIC TUBE An NG tube can help to identify upper versus lower GI bleeding (Table 7-7; Fig. 7-2). An NG tube is indicated for the treatment of bowel obstruction, pancreatitis, and toxic ingestions, as well as to evaluate for upper GI bleeding and to decompress the stomach during anesthesia or CPR. Contraindications include possible basilar skull fracture, severe nasal/facial fracture, coagulopathy, sinusitis, and a caustic ingestion (such as lye).

The following specific diagnostic tests are useful, but usually are available only at tertiary hospitals:

- Endoscopy: The most precise diagnostic tool, but it does not necessarily improve the outcome.
- Radiology: GI arteriography (bleeding rate of 0.5–2.9 mL/min) and radionuclide scanning are useful in selected patients.

TABLE 7-7 INSERTING A NASOGASTRIC TUBE AND EVALUATING THE RESULTS

1. Tilt the patient's head forward slightly.
2. Gently push the NG tube straight backward into the nares (see Fig. 7-2).
3. As the tube passes through the turbinates, it gets easier to push and can be seen in the back of the throat.
4. Give the patient sips of water to swallow while gently sliding the tube farther down.
5. If the patient begins coughing or cannot speak, the tube is probably in the trachea and should be withdrawn partially and repositioned.
6. Confirm that the tube is in the stomach by squirting 10–20 cc of air into the tube while listening for a gurgle over the stomach.

To assess for bleeding gently instill 200 mL (10 ml/kg in children) of water into the stomach and then either suction it out or allow it to drain to gravity (place the end of the NG tube in a bowl on the floor). NG tube aspirate is diagnostic of UGI bleed if it consists of

   10 mL of gross blood, or
   30 mL of pink fluid with flecks of blood, or
   30 mL of dark usually brown fluid strongly positive for occult blood

NG, nasogastric; UGI, upper gastrointestinal.

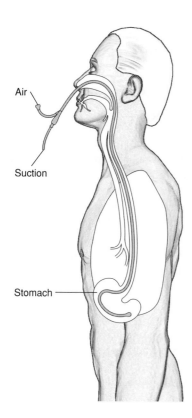

Air

Suction

Stomach

FIGURE 7-2 Inserting a nasogastric tube.

TREATMENT

> **TIPS AND TRICKS:**
>
> When in doubt about the severity of a GI bleed, admit the patient for observation.

Most bleeding stops without intervention. For more serious bleeding, the goals are to stabilize the patient and to transfer him or her for definitive diagnosis and therapy.

- Fluid resuscitation is the first priority (the ABCs) for treatment of shock.
- Supplemental oxygen, cardiac monitor
- Gastric lavage: There is little evidence that lavage reduces bleeding (don't bother to pour in and draw out large volumes of fluid through the NG tube). Its most useful function is to monitor bleeding and prepare patients for endoscopy.
- Antacids and H_2 blockers are probably effective for bleeding due to ulcers but ineffective for other causes. Oral antacids include
    - Aluminum hydroxide
    - Magnesium hydroxide
- H_2 blockers include
    - Cimetidine 300 mg IV over 15 to 20 minutes
    - Ranitidine 50 mg IV over 5 to 10 minutes
    - Famotidine 20 mg IV over 5 minutes

Advanced treatments include the following:

- Balloon tamponade may be useful for bleeding esophageal varices (from cirrhosis). But these tubes (such as the Sengstakken-Blakemore tube) have a high incidence of significant complications and should be used only as a last resort for patients with continued bleeding despite other therapy.
- Endoscopic guided sclerotherapy, laser coagulation, or electrocoagulation
- Surgery: actively bleeding, hemodynamically unstable, refractory to volume resuscitation

DISPOSITION The overall mortality rate is 10%, but most deaths occur in patients over 60 years of age. Admit high-risk patients such as the elderly or any patient with hemodynamic changes or signs of continued bleeding.

- Intensive care monitoring is indicated for those with continued hemodynamic instability or continued bleeding and high-risk patients such as those with abdominal aortic grafts, those over 60 years of age, and those with significant other illnesses, especially heart and lung disease.
- Admit to the regular floor if they are hemodynamically stable and have no active bleeding; also admit patients with coagulopathies.

■ Short observation is recommended for those who report "vomiting blood" but there is no evidence of blood loss.

NEUROLOGIC PROBLEMS

HEADACHE

CRITICAL ACTIONS:

■ Identify life-threatening causes of headache (meningitis is the most treatable).
■ Treat suspected meningitis immediately with antibiotics (do not wait for test results).
■ Decide if lumbar puncture and cerebrospinal fluid (CSF) examination are needed.
■ Decide early if a higher level for care is needed (head CT, neurosurgery).

The majority of patients with a complaint of headache do not have a life-threatening problem, but it is important to identify the few that do. Potentially life-threatening headaches may be caused by the following:

■ Infections: meningitis, encephalitis, abscess
■ Brain injury with intracranial hemorrhage: subdural or epidural hematoma
■ Spontaneous subarachnoid or parenchymal hemorrhage
■ Increased intracranial pressure from trauma or brain lesions (tumors) or abscesses

Other causes of headache are as follows:

■ Vascular (migraines)
■ Tension (musculoskeletal)
■ Infections, such as otitis media, sinusitis, malaria, etc.

CLINICAL PRESENTATION Key historical features to elicit are as follows:

■ Recent head trauma (concussion, subdural hematoma)
■ Rapidity of onset (a SAH occurs suddenly, particularly while straining such as lifting, sexual activity, etc.)
■ Fever (meningitis, malaria, sinusitis, etc.)
■ Syncope (SAH)
■ Vision changes (vascular, mass, temporal arteritis)
■ Nausea or vomiting (many causes)
■ Neck stiffness (meningitis for infection or intracranial bleeding)
■ Possible exposure to carbon monoxide or other toxins
■ Associated seizures (subdural or epidural hematomas, SAH, infections)

PHYSICAL EXAMINATION

GENERAL

- Changes in mental status (confusion, lethargy, combativeness, unconsciousness) are serious and require more rapid evaluation and treatment.
- Look for petechiae and purpura due to meningitis from *Neisseria* (especially hands and feet).

VITAL SIGNS

- Temperature: Most patients with meningitis are febrile, but not all, particularly children and the elderly.
- Blood Pressure (BP): Headaches can be caused by elevated BP. Treat for malignant hypertension for patients with a headache, abnormal mental status, and increased BP (see earlier section on Hypertensive Emergencies).

HEAD

- Palpate the scalp for tenderness, specifically temporal artery tenderness (temporal arteritis). With head trauma, a tender skull outside the area of impact may indicate a fracture.
- Tympanic membrane: Look for hemotympanum (basilar skull fracture) and otitis media (a frequent cause of meningitis in developing countries).
- Eyes: Check visual acuity, extraocular motions, and the fundi for signs of increased intracranial pressure, such as papilledema and small retinal hemorrhages.
- Nose and throat: Signs of infection including sinusitis.

NECK Assess for meningeal signs (if there is no possibility of cervical spine injury). Pain or stiffness with flexion could be due to meningeal irritation, infection, or SAH. Other signs include the following:

- Kernig sign (pain or resistance to passive extension of the lower leg when the patient is supine with the hip flexed)
- Brudzynski sign (involuntary hip flexion when the neck is flexed)

NEUROLOGIC

- Assess all cranial nerves.
- Check the strength, sensation, and deep tendon reflexes of all extremities.
- Coordination tests such as walking the patient and finger to nose are sensitive methods of picking up lesions affecting the cerebellum.

DIAGNOSIS

LABORATORY TESTS Few laboratory studies are useful for patients with headaches. The major exceptions are lumbar puncture and sedimentation rate:

- Lumbar puncture is useful when the potential diagnosis is meningitis or SAH (see Chapter 8 for details on performing lumbar puncture and interpreting the results).
    - SAH: The CSF will show red blood cells or xanthrochromia (yellow discoloration if the blood is more than 24 hours old).
    - Meningitis: White blood cells, and maybe low glucose, high protein, and bacteria on Gram stain.
- An elevated sedimentation rate (usually >20 mm/hr) helps diagnose temporal arteritis.

RADIOLOGY

- When available, CT is useful to diagnose spontaneous subarachnoid hemorrhage, traumatic injuries, masses, and abscesses.
- Plain radiographs of the skull are not useful if CT is available. If only radiography is available, they can be used to diagnose a skull fracture. If a fracture is present, the patient has a higher likelihood of more severe intracranial injury and should be referred for a CT, or at least observed for a minimum of 24 hours.

TREATMENT

KEY POINT:

In developing countries, particularly in the "meningitis belt" of sub-Saharan Africa, always rule out meningitis (and malaria) as the cause of a headache.

The treatment is determined by the cause of the headache. Once life-threatening causes have been excluded, the major goal of treatment is to reduce the patient's pain. General treatment for headache (pain control) is instituted. Start simply and increase the strength and doses of medications as needed:

- Acetaminophen 650 to 1,000 mg every 4 hours. May be used in combination with
- Ibuprofen 400 to 800 mg every 4 to 8 hours (or other NSAID).

Narcotic analgesics include codeine, oxycodone, hydrocodone orally. Morphine, meperidine (Demerol), and others may be given IV, IM, or subcutaneously.

Treatments for specific causes of headaches are described in the following sections:

INCREASED INTRACRANIAL PRESSURE Patients with suspected intracranial pathology (brain tumor, abscess, injury) whose mental status deteriorates should be treated for increased intracranial pressure (ICP). However, in areas with limited resources and no neurosurgical capabilities, there are few definitive treatments, and patients rarely survive. Methods to reduce ICP include the following:

- Mannitol 0.25 to 2.0 g/kg IV, then repeat doses at 0.25 g/kg as needed.
- Steroids, preferably dexamethasone (Decadron) 0.15 mg/kg IV
- Diuretics (furosemide 0.5–1 mg/kg)
- If a brain abscess is suspected, start IV antibiotics.
- If available, intubate with paralysis and hyperventilation.

MENINGITIS See Chapter 8 for a discussion on meningitis.

SUBARACHNOID HEMORRHAGE Patients present with sudden onset of pain, and may have mental status changes (including coma). Some die immediately. The definitive treatment is neurosurgery; therefore, transfer is usually necessary.

- Keep the patient in a quiet room with little stimulation to attempt to prevent rebleeding.
- If possible, prevent hypertension by gently titrating IV NTG to a systolic BP of 100 to 120 mm Hg (see earlier section on Hypertension), but do not lower the BP too much.
- The calcium channel blocker nimodipine is ideal to treat SAH in patients who are not comatose, but it is rarely available (60 mg orally every 4 hours for 21 days). Consider other calcium channel blockers.

TEMPORAL ARTERITIS Persistent or point temporal artery tenderness should be treated empirically, particularly if the patient's vision is affected. Failure to treat can lead to blindness.

- Start prednisone 60 to 100 mg orally per day.
- Refer the patient for temporal artery biopsy.

VASCULAR (MIGRAINES) Classic symptoms of migraine headaches include unilateral headache associated with nausea, vomiting, and even mental status changes or cranial nerve palsies. There also may be an aura that precedes the pain. Patients usually present in severe discomfort.

- Place the patient in a quiet, dark room to rest.
- Start with acetaminophen and NSAIDs.
- Caffeine and antiemetics (prochlorperazine) may improve pain control.
- Narcotic analgesics such as morphine are often needed.

Advanced therapies include the following:

- Dihydroergotamine mesylate (DHE-45) 1 mg IV or IM every 1 hour, up to two or three doses, respectively
- Sumatriptan (Imitrex), 6 mg subcutaneously, may be repeated once after 1 hour, but it is unlikely to work if not initially effective.

CHANGES IN MENTAL STATUS

CRITICAL ACTIONS:

- ABCs first
- Identify life-threatening causes of altered mental status:
  - Hypoxia
  - Metabolic, especially hypoglycemia
  - Infectious: meningitis, sepsis, malaria, etc.
  - Intracranial: brain injury, SAH, mass, etc.
  - Toxic (all kinds of drugs and toxins)
- Rapidly assess for hypoxia and hypoglycemia. Treat empirically with oxygen and glucose if diagnostic studies are not available.
- If there is a possibility of trauma, immobilize the cervical spine in a collar or with sandbags on each side of the head.

Altered mental status can vary from mild confusion to total unresponsiveness (coma). Altered mental status can be caused by the following:

- Intracranial: bleeding due to SAH or trauma; masses such as cancer, abscesses, or hematomas
- Infectious: meningitis, abscess, malaria, sepsis, etc.
- Metabolic
  - Hypoglycemia or hyperglycemia
  - Brain ischemia or anoxia
  - Severe acidosis
  - Hyponatremia or hypernatremia
  - Hypothermia or hyperthermia
  - Hepatic or uremic encephalopathy
  - Endocrine disorders such as adrenal insufficiency or myxedema
- Toxic
  - Alcohol
  - Sedatives (barbiturates, benzodiazepines, phencyclidine)
  - Narcotics
  - Carbon monoxide

■ Other medications such as tricyclics, anticholinergics, or phenothiazines.
■ Heavy metals
■ Psychiatric, such as hysterical or psychogenic coma. Clues to a psychogenic coma include unusual posturing, resisting opening the eyelids, and a change in the patient's position when they think they are not observed.

CLINICAL PRESENTATION Key components of the physical examination are described in the following sections:

GENERAL

■ ABCs to check for hypoxia as a cause
■ Check the vital signs to assess for hypotension or fever.

HEAD, EARS, EYES, NOSE, AND THROAT

■ Look first for signs of head or facial trauma as a possible cause.
■ Eyes: Look for pupil size and reaction (toxins, brain injury), and extraocular movements (brain injury, stroke).
■ Ears: Otitis media (meningitis, abscess) or perforation or hemotympanum (injury)
■ Throat: Infection, tongue movements (stroke)

NEUROLOGIC Neurologic examination is usually the key to identify the cause of altered mental status.

■ The best method to assess and describe alertness is AVPU:
   ■ A = alert
   ■ V = responds to voice commands
   ■ P = responds to painful stimulus
   ■ U = unresponsive to any stimulus
■ Strength, sensory, and reflexes to assess for symmetry or abnormal responses
■ Gait (normal, toe and heel walking, and line walking are important indicators of cerebellar and fine motor functioning).
■ Other important findings:
   ■ Assess the patient's orientation to self, place, and time to look for confusion.
   ■ Focal neurologic findings usually indicate a structural intracranial problem (although hypoglycemia also can be a cause).
   ■ If there are no lateralizing signs, altered pupil response and normal "doll's eyes" (oculocephalic reflex), then a toxic or metabolic cause is more likely.

DIAGNOSIS Because there are many potential causes of altered mental status, diagnosing the cause can be difficult. Oxygenation should be checked by pulse oximetry or an ABG if they can be performed.

> **TIPS AND TRICKS:**
>
> ■ Hypoglycemia is a common cause of mental status changes; check the glucose level.
> ■ Infections are another common cause, especially for children.

LABORATORY TESTS

■ Rapid glucose on all patients
■ Lumbar puncture if an infection or bleed (SAH) is considered
■ Other important tests include electrolytes, blood urea nitrogen, calcium, CBC, and carboxyhemoglobin when available.
■ Optional tests include alcohol and drug or toxin levels, cortisol level, thyroid function studies, liver function tests, and blood cultures.

RADIOLOGY

■ CT is the most useful test, but is often unavailable.
■ A skull radiograph that demonstrates a fracture can help indicate a brain injury.
■ Cervical spine films are needed if trauma is suspected.

TREATMENT

■ Oxygen for potentially hypoxic patients
■ Glucose 25 g IV, particularly if the patient has a history of insulin or hypoglycemic use (1 mL/kg of 25% glucose for pediatric patients)
■ Start an IV for fluid resuscitation if shock is a possible cause (if the patient might have increased ICP, then limit the fluid to a KVO rate).
■ Administer 0.4 to 2 mg of naloxone IV if narcotic overdose is suspected.
■ IV antibiotics if an infection is considered (see Chapter 8)
■ If a possible drug overdose is identified as the cause for coma, then placement of an NG tube with lavage and administration of activated charcoal should be considered.
■ If the patient is found to be either hypo- or hyperthermic, then aggressive management of temperature by cooling or warming methods is indicated (see Chapter 20).

SEIZURES

> **CRITICAL ACTIONS:**
>
> ■ ABCs: Determine if there is any respiratory compromise caused by the seizure.
> ■ Differentiate intermittent seizures from status epilepticus.
> ■ Determine if a structural (brain injury) or metabolic (hypoglycemia, hypoxia) cause is present.

Intermittent seizures (convulsions) in a patient with previously diagnosed epilepsy are common and do not require emergency intervention. Continuous or repetitive seizures (status epilepticus) are true emergencies that require rapid management. The causes and evaluation of seizures are similar to that of altered mental status.

Causes of seizures include the following:

- Hypoxemia should be excluded as a cause first.
- Discontinuation of antiepileptic medications is the most common cause.
- Infections such as meningitis, encephalitis, and brain abscesses
- Alcohol or sedative (especially benzodiazepines) withdrawal
- Drug intoxication or drug interaction, such as anticholinergics, aminophylline, cocaine, or amphetamines
- Structural abnormalities such as hemorrhagic stroke, head trauma with intracranial bleed, tumor, or degenerative central nervous system (CNS) diseases
- Metabolic causes
    - Hypoglycemia: Always check for this early.
    - Hyponatremia
    - Hypocalcemia
    - Hypomagnesemia
- Uremia
- Inflammatory diseases and collagen vascular diseases such as systemic lupus erythematosus
- Congenital brain disorders

CLINICAL PRESENTATION Seizures can present as the classic grand mal (tonic-clonic), as a coma or altered mental status (postictal), or as petit mal (absence) seizures.

Grand mal seizures are usually tonic-clonic in nature. That is, the patient has a period with a loss of consciousness with convulsions and rigidity in posture. This is usually followed by a postictal phase where the patient goes from being unresponsive to awake, but confused, then returns to the normal state. The postictal phase can last 1 to 24 or more hours, but usually lasts less than 2 hours.

Petit mal seizures are subtler in their presentation and may just appear to be brief periods of a loss of attention. They are not usually associated with a postictal phase.

DIAGNOSIS The classic tools for evaluating seizures [CT, magnetic resonance imaging (MRI), and electroencephalography (EEG)] are often not available in areas with limited resources. Therefore, the physical examination and simple blood tests become very important. The evaluation is similar to that for altered mental status:

- See earlier section on Changes in Mental Status for the key steps in the evaluation.
- Patients with a known seizure disorder who return to their normal level of consciousness after a seizure should have a complete physical examination and determination of anticonvulsant levels (if the patient is taking anticonvulsants).
- See Chapter 11 for the evaluation and treatment of children who had a simple febrile seizure.

TREATMENT Treat first based on the underlying cause of the seizure (injury, infection, etc.). A single idiopathic seizure (those with no specific identifiable cause) should probably not be treated with anticonvulsants without further referral and evaluation. Managing the levels of anticonvulsants is difficult without advanced laboratory services.

The decision to treat recurring idiopathic seizures should be based on your ability to follow the patient and to regulate his or her medication levels. Where levels cannot be determined, phenytoin doses can be slowly increased to the point where the seizures stop but the symptoms of toxicity have not yet started. Symptoms of toxicity include the following:

1. Nystagmus
2. Tremors
3. Nausea and vomiting, then
4. Ataxia, and finally
5. Changes in mental status, including seizures and coma

See Table 7-8 for general medications used to treat seizures.

PREVENTION Idiopathic seizures cannot be prevented, but all of those with identifiable causes can be. The most common of these are infections and brain injuries. Identify infections early and treat them with appropriate antibiotics and teach patients of the importance of helmet and seatbelt use (and other ways of preventing brain injuries).

STATUS EPILEPTICUS

> ### CRITICAL ACTIONS:
>
> - Status epilepticus is a true emergency; continuous seizures can directly and indirectly cause cerebral hypoxia. Rapid intervention is essential.
> - ABCs first; paralysis and intubation may be necessary.
> - Paralysis alone is not sufficient; seizure activity must be stopped with medications. Sometimes continuous IV infusions of benzodiazepines or barbiturates are needed.
> - Use a benzodiazepine (diazepam) first.

CLINICAL PRESENTATION Status epilepticus is either a seizure lasting more than 30 minutes or a series of seizures where the patient does not return to the normal level of consciousness between seizures. The mortality rate can be as high as 30%, depending on the cause.

DIAGNOSIS Diagnosis is determined as for regular seizures, but additional focus should be placed on the following:

TABLE 7-8 COMMON MEDICATIONS FOR SEIZURES

Phenytoin (Dilantin)

Indications: The primary drug for long-term control for all seizure types except absence.

Dose:
    Adults 3–5 mg/kg/day (usually 300 mg/day in a single dose)
    Children 4–7 mg/kg/day daily in 2–3 divided doses
    The ideal therapeutic range is between a total plasma concentration of 10–20 µg/mL.
    Toxicity usually occurs above 30 µg/mL.

Toxicity:
    If given too rapidly IV, it can cause cardiac arrhythmias, with or without hypotension and CNS depression.
    An acute oral overdose causes nystagmus, ataxia, diplopia, and vertigo.
    Chronic therapy can cause gingival hyperplasia.
    Hypersensitivity reactions (morbilliform rash) can oocur in 2%–5% of patients.

Drug interactions:
    The phenytoin level is increased by chloramphenicol, coumadin, disulfiram, isoniazid, cimetidine, sulfonamides, phenylbutazone, salicylates.
    The phenytoin level is decreased by carbamazepine.
    The use of phenytoin increases clearance of (decreases the level of) theophylline, steroids and oral contraceptives.

Barbiturates (phenobarbital and others)

Indications: A primary (or secondary to phenytoin) drug for all seizure types except absence. Often used in combination with phenytoin.

Dose:
    Adults: 1–5 mg/kg/day (60–250 mg/day)
    Children: 3–6 mg/kg/day
    Therapeutic level 10–30 µg/mL

Toxicity: Sedation, irritability, and hyperactivity in children; agitation and confusion in the elderly.

Drug interactions: Potent activator of the P-450 microsome enzyme system.

Carbamazepine (Tegretol)

Chemically related to the tricyclic antidepressants.

Indications: Useful for all seizure types except absence.

Dose: 200–1,200 mg orally each day

Toxicity:
    Acute intoxication can result in stupor, coma, hyperirritability, seizures, respiratory depression.
    Chronic toxic effects include drowsiness, ataxia, diplopia, and serious hematologic toxicity.

Drug interactions:
    Drug levels are decreased by phenytoin and phenobarbital (metabolism increased).
    Drug levels are increased by erythromycin and propoxyphene (metabolism inhibited).

TABLE 7-8 COMMON MEDICATIONS FOR SEIZURES *(continued)*

Benzodiazepines

Indications: These are used mostly for the emergent treatment of status epilepticus. Only clonazepam (Klonopin) and clorazepate (Tranxene) have been approved for the chronic treatment of seizures.

Toxicity: Minimal: lethargy, drowsiness. Status epilepticus may be precipitated if these drugs are withdrawn suddenly.

Dose:
Diazepam (Valium) is primary drug of choice for the treatment of status epilepticus.
Midazolam (Versed) may be given IM, IV, or rectally.
Lorazepam (Ativan) is also effective.

Valproic Acid (Depakene)

Indication: More useful for absence seizures

Dose:
15–60 mg/kg/day, therapeutic level 50–100 µg/mL

Toxicity:
GI irritation
Elevation of hepatic enzymes in 15%–30% of patients
Fulminant hepatitis (rare)

Drug interactions: Can raise phenobarbital levels by much as 40% when given concurrently.

Ethosuximide (Zarontin)

Indications: A primary agent for absence seizures

Dose: 250–500 mg orally daily, therapeutic level 40–100 µg/mL

Toxicity: Blood dyscrasias and hepatic and renal impairment are rare. Sedation is common.

Drug interactions:
May increase phenytoin levels.
Effect of valproate is variable.

- Hypoxia: Check pulse oximetry if possible.
- Hyperthermia: Check the rectal temperature early.
- Hypoglycemia: Perform a fingerstick glucose test as soon as possible.
- Blood can be drawn with the IV stick, and the tests to consider include glucose, electrolytes, blood urea nitrogen, calcium, magnesium, CBC, anticonvulsant levels, and blood alcohol or other drug or toxin levels.
- Lumbar puncture if an infection or bleed (SAH) is considered

TREATMENT

- ABCs: Oxygen is needed for essentially all patients who have a low threshold for intubation.

- Start an IV with NS.
- Start rapid cooling measures if the patient is hyperthermic.
- Glucose 25 g IV, particularly if the patient has a history of insulin or other hypoglycemic use; 1 mL/kg of 25% glucose for pediatric patients
- Naloxone 0.4 to 2.0 mg IV if narcotic overdose is suspected
- IV antibiotics if an infection is considered (See Chapter 8.)
- If a possible drug overdose is identified as the cause for coma, then placement of an NG tube with lavage and administration of activated charcoal should be considered.

The medication sequence for status epilepticus is as follows:

- Benzodiazepines first (diazepam is 80%–90% effective in terminating the status):
  - Diazepam, 2.5 to 5 mg IV for adults or 0.05 to 0.1 mg/kg IV for children (not IM)
  - Midazolam 2.5 to 5 mg IV for adults or 0.05 to 0.1 mg/kg IV for children (Can be given IM or rectally.)
  - Lorazepam (longest duration of action) 2.5 to 5 mg IV for adults or 0.05 to 0.1 mg/kg IV for children (Can be given IM.)
  - The initial dose can be repeated up to total dose of 0.3 to 0.4 mg/kg if the seizure activity continues.
- The next medication is phenytoin (Dilantin).
  - Give a loading dose of 18 mg/kg at an IV rate of 1 mg/kg/min in children to a maximum of 50 mg/min in adults. In stable patients with isolated seizures, this dose of phenytoin can be given as a loading dose orally.
  - If the seizures persist, then give phenobarbital 10 to 20 mg/kg IV loading dose at a rate of 60 mg/min. This often causes significant respiratory depression, and the patient will require intubation and assisted ventilation.

If the patient is still having persistent seizures after loading with phenobarbital, then the mortality rate is very high and additional treatments are often unsuccessful. Additional medications to consider include the following:

- Lidocaine may be useful in instances of acute CNS lesions, but may increase seizures in chronic epilepticus. Give 2 mg/kg IV then a continuous infusion of 3 to 10 mg/kg/h.
- Paraldehyde 0.1 to 0.15 mL/kg IM, using only glass equipment. IV use is indicated only in extreme situations. The drug must be diluted in NS and infused over 1 hour.
- Clonazepam or carbamazepine administered via NG tube
- General anesthesia may be tried as a last resort: neuromuscular blockade to stop muscular hyperactivity, mechanical ventilation to support respirations, and inhalation anesthetic to quell seizure activity in the brain. But EEG monitoring is required, because the patient may still be having seizure activity, even though it will not be manifest because of the muscle relaxation from the general anesthetic.

DIZZINESS

CRITICAL ACTIONS:

■ First differentiate lightheadedness due to vertigo from other causes of dizziness.
■ Treat with fluid rehydration if orthostatic hypotension or shock is identified.
■ Differentiate peripheral from central vertigo.
■ Treat or refer appropriately.

Dizziness is an imprecise term that is better described as lightheadedness or vertigo or even weakness. The differential diagnoses and evaluation for these complaints are very different.

■ Lightheadedness/orthostasis: This is the symptom of nearly passing out due to poor blood supply to the brain, usually on rapid standing. This is one of the primary symptoms of dehydration or blood loss (shock).
■ Vertigo: This is a sensation that the environment is spinning or that the patient's body is spinning, or a sensation of involuntary compulsion for a particular movement of the body.
■ Weakness is a vague symptom with a large number of potential causes that are listed in Tables 7-9 and 7-10.

General evaluation of the dizzy patient should proceed as follows:

■ First try to differentiate lightheadedness from vertigo by the history:
  ■ The spinning sensations of vertigo often worsen with head movements, even when reclining.

TABLE 7-9 COMMON CAUSES OF GENERALIZED WEAKNESS

Adrenal crisis	Hysteria and malingering
AIDS (SIDA)	Lyme disease
Alcohol intoxication	Myasthenia gravis
Anemia	Myotonic (and other) dystrophy
Brain mass or tumor	Myxedema (hypothyroidism)
Botulism	Neurosyphilis
Cancer	Parkinson's disease
Cervical myelopathies	Periodic paralysis
Cervical spinal cord injury	Poliomyelitis
Chronic fatigue syndrome	Postical states
Collagen vascular disease	Radiation myelopathies
Congenital disorders, including meningomyelocele	Sepsis
Diabetes	Tick paralysis
Diphtheria	Toxic myopathies
Drug overdoses	(lead, arsenic, mercury)
Guillain-Barré syndrome	Transverse myelitis (rule out polio first)

TABLE 7-10 CASES OF FOCAL OR ASYMMETRIC WEAKNESS

Systemic	Spinal cord
Arthritis	Spinal cord injury or radiculopathies
Diabetes	Intervertebral disc disorders
Multiple myeloma	Motor neuron disease
Multiple sclerosis	Spinal vascular disease
Poliomyelitis	(ischemic, hemorrhagic)
Polyarteritis	**Peripheral nerves**
Rabies	Peripheral nerve injury or entrapment
Intracranial	
Brain tumors	
Cerebral palsies	
Cerebrovascular disease	
(ischemic, hemorrhagic)	

- ■ Vertigo is often associated with nausea and vomiting.
- ■ Check orthostatic vital signs. They are positive for orthostatic symptoms if
  - ■ the patient becomes lightheaded with standing.
  - ■ the pulse increases by greater than 20 beats/min or systolic blood pressure drops by over 20 mm Hg after 3 to 5 minutes.
- ■ Careful physical examination should include
  - ■ Vital signs to assess for signs of hemodynamic instability and infection
  - ■ Complete neurologic examination
  - ■ Eyes: Check visual acuity and look for nystagmus at rest and with lateral gaze. Check discs for signs of increased intracranial pressure.
  - ■ Ears: Look for a foreign body (including earwax), infection, and mastoiditis. Clear canals completely. Grossly assess hearing.
  - ■ Look for possible sources of infection.
- ■ Consider ECG.
- ■ Consider laboratory tests if etiology not clear from examination. In order of usefulness:
  - ■ Hemoglobin or hematocrit to evaluate for anemia
  - ■ Glucose (diabetes can cause either lightheadedness or vertigo)
  - ■ White blood cell count for signs of an infection
  - ■ Blood urea nitrogen and creatinine
  - ■ Electrolytes
  - ■ Medication levels (elevated serum levels of medications can cause dizziness). See Table 7-11.

TABLE 7-11 COMMON DRUGS THAT CAUSE DIZZINESS

Phenytoin (Dilatin)	Alcohol
Salicylates (aspirin)	Aminoglycosides
Quinine	Erythromycin

VERTIGO The evaluation should attempt to differentiate central from peripheral causes of vertigo. Causes of central (intracranial) causes of vertigo include the following:

- Intracranial infection (encephalitis, meningitis, abscess)
- Posttraumatic injury/postconcussive syndrome
- SAH
- Brain tumor (especially of the posterior fossa)
- Cerebellar hemorrhage
- Vertebral basilar insufficiency
- Rare causes include basilar artery migraine, acoustic neuroma, multiple sclerosis, and temporal lobe seizures.

Causes of peripheral vertigo are related to the inner ear and include the following:

- Otitis media or other ear infection
- Foreign body in the ear canal
- Vestibular neuronitis
- Benign peripheral vertigo
- Ménière disease

CLINICAL PRESENTATIONS

TIPS AND TRICKS:

The key areas to differentiate central from peripheral vertigo are

- The rapidity of onset and duration of the symptoms
- The presence of other neurologic findings (central)
- Changes in hearing (peripheral)
- The type and duration of nystagmus

Central vertigo is usually characterized by gradual onset, nystagmus that does not stop after a few beats with lateral gaze, and other neurologic findings (cranial nerves, gait, fine motor, weakness). See Table 7-12.

Peripheral vertigo is characterized by sudden onset, with fatigable nystagmus and hearing changes. The ear canals must be completely cleaned to fully assess for peripheral vertigo (this often cures the vertigo). Specific syndromes include the following:

- Vestibular neuronitis: Patients present with vertigo but normal hearing in both ears. There should be no associated headache, and neurologic examination should be normal.
- Ménière's disease is characterized by episodic attacks of vertigo associated with temporary deafness, sensation of ear fullness, and tinnitus. Patients often have intractable nausea and vomiting.

TABLE 7-12 DIFFERENCES IN CENTRAL AND PERIPHERAL VERTIGO

	CENTRAL	**PERIPHERAL**
Symptoms		
Onset	Gradual (SAH are sudden)	Rapid or even sudden
Duration	Weeks to months, usually steadily progressive	Hours to days, varies in severity
Severity	Mild, but gradually increasing	Often associated with vomiting, severe vertigo
Physical findings		
Nystagmus	Persistent nystagmus may occur without lateral gaze. Rotary and vertical nystagmus occurs.	Nystagmus for only 5–10 beats Almost always horizontal
Neurologic findings	Gait disturbance and other neurologic deficits	No other neurologic findings
Hearing findings	Normal hearing	May have decreased hearing acuity or tinnitus

SAH, subarachnoid hemorrhage.

■ Labyrinthitis: Symptoms include vertigo, decreased hearing on the affected side, and pain in the mastoid area. If suspected to be bacterial in origin, this would require admission for parenteral antibiotics because of the risk of progression to meningitis.

■ Benign positional vertigo: This diagnosis can be made if the patient's symptoms are exactly reproduced only with the head in certain positions.

DIAGNOSIS The diagnosis is based mostly on the history, and then on the physical examination. Additional testing is rarely needed, except for a head CT scan if a central cause is suspected.

PHYSICAL EXAMINATION Besides the examinations listed in the general diagnosis of dizziness, the key to the physical examination is the neurologic system, including a good ear examination, eye examination for nystagmus, and positional testing. Nystagmus or nausea that develops with positional testing implies a peripheral cause of the vertigo.

POSITIONAL TESTING:

If there is no nystagmus at rest (and the patient isn't severely nauseated or vomiting), then positional testing may be attempted:

- Sit the patient upright.
- Tilt the head back and rotate it 30 degrees to one side.
- Rapidly lower the patient to a supine (reclining) position.
- Observe for nystagmus.
- Repeat with the extended head rotated in the other direction.

NEUROLOGIC EXAMINATION

- Cranial nerves (including corneal reflex)
- Cerebellar testing: finger-nose, gait, dysdiadochokinesia

TREATMENT The symptoms of central vertigo can be treated (vertigo, nausea, vomiting), but the patient requires referral for further evaluation and treatment. The primary advanced test is a CT scan of the head.

Peripheral vertigo is usually self-limited. If an underlying condition such as otitis media or mastoiditis is identified, treat it with the appropriate medications. Acute bacterial labyrinthitis requires IV antibiotics.

Nausea and vomiting may require treatment with a parenteral antiemetic:

- Hydroxizine 50 mg IM, or
- Prochlorperazine 5 to 10 mg IV or IM

The vertiginous symptoms can be treated as follows:

- Meclizine (Antivert) 12.5 to 25 mg orally every 8 hours as needed, or
- Diphenhydramine 25 to 50 mg IV or orally every 6 to 8 hours, and/or
- Benzodiazepines such as diazepam 2 to 10 mg IV, orally, or rectally are also effective.

WEAKNESS Weakness is a vague term that requires a more detailed explanation. Focus on the history to rule out the various causes listed in Tables 7-9 and 7-10. The physical examination can help determine if the weakness is generalized or isolated to specific muscles. Generalized weakness might be the only presenting symptom of AMI in the elderly, and an ECG should be considered. Clues to the diagnosis of weakness are given in Table 7-13.

PARALYSIS

The most common cause of paralysis is injury. If an injured patient has paralysis and any possibility of spine trauma, then spine immobilization should be performed imme-

TABLE 7-13 CLUES TO THE DIAGNOSIS OF WEAKNESS

SIGNS AND SYMPTOMS	PROBABLE CAUSE
Upper motor neuron dysfunction	Brain or spinal cord lesion
Lower motor neuron dysfunction	Peripheral nerve or muscular disorder
Upper and lower motor neuron dysfunction	Amyotrophic lateral sclerosis
Hemiparesis	Cerebral lesion
Paresis	Spinal or peripheral lesion
Cervical weakness	Amyotrophic lateral sclerosis
	Myasthenia gravis
Cranial nerve weakness	Bulbar palsy
	Pseudobulbar palsy
	Amyotrophic lateral sclerosis
	Myasthenia gravis
	Botulism
Sensory level and pain present	Spinal cord compression
No sensory level or pain present	Guillain-Barré syndrome
Flaccid paralysis (no reflex)	Poliomyelitis

diately. You must determine if a central nervous system versus peripheral nervous system lesion is the cause. A rapid, complete neurologic examination is the key to differentiating the two. Non-neurologic toxic causes also should be determinable from the history. Toxic causes of generalized paralysis include the following:

- Botulism
- Late phase of organophosphate insecticide poisoning
- Tic paralysis
- Paralytic or neurotoxic shellfish poisoning

Patients with weakness or paralysis possibly due to spinal cord compression require emergent radiographic imaging (plain radiographs, then CT or MRI) of the spine with rapid neurosurgical consultation. These patients may require emergent decompressive surgery to prevent permanent spinal cord damage. Nontraumatic causes of spinal cord compression include the following:

- Pathologic vertebral body fractures and tumors
- Spontaneous epidural hemorrhage
- Epidural abscesses

SYNCOPE

Syncope is a transient loss of consciousness due to the following:

- Cardiac arrhythmias
  - Ventricular tachycardia

- - Second- or third-degree atrioventricular block
  - Sick sinus syndrome
- Cardiac outflow obstruction
  - Aortic stenosis
  - Hypertrophic cardiomyopathy
  - PE
- Central nervous system (seizures, migraine, CVA, vertebrobasilar transient ischemic attack, normal pressure hydrocephalus)
- Other
  - Reflex syncope (vasovagal, orthostatic hypotension, carotid sinus syncope, etc.)
  - Situational (micturition, defecation, coughing)
  - Drugs (see Table 7-14)
  - Metabolic (hypoglycemia, hyperventilation)
  - Psychogenic

The most common cause of syncope is vasovagal or fainting, particularly in young patients (<60 years) with no other symptoms. Predisposing factors include hunger, exhaustion, alcohol, vasodilating drugs, stress, and even postprandial (after eating) hypotension in elderly.

The goal is to stabilize the emergent patients and to identify the high-risk patients who need transfer or rapid referral for evaluation and treatment. The cause of 40% to 50% of all syncopal episodes will never be found even after an extensive evaluation.

PRESENTATION The history of the event is critical for the diagnosis. Attempt to determine the exact course of the event: the body position, sudden body movements, the presence of a prodrome, fall, and the postevent course.

Cardiac arrhythmias should be considered as the cause of syncope in anyone over 60 years of age. Symptoms of cardiac-caused syncope include the following:

- Sudden onset syncope with no or brief prodrome symptoms
- Syncope with exertion
- Occurs in any position (Vasovagal syncope does not occur when the patient is horizontal.)

TABLE 7-14 COMMON DRUGS
CAUSING SYNCOPE

Alcohol	Calcium channel blockers
ACE inhibitors	Diuretics
Antiarrhythmics	Lithium
Antidepressants	Nitrates
Antihypertensives	Phenothiazines

ACE inhibitors, angiotensin-converting enzyme inhibitors.

Symptoms of vasovagal syncope include the following:

- There is usually a prodrome that lasts 10 to 20 seconds that includes nervousness, pallor, diaphoresis, nausea, lightheadedness, weakness, and decreasing visual acuity (tunnel vision), and finally decreasing auditory acuity.
- Loss of consciousness occurs before a fall to the ground. This can lead to significant injuries. However, the prodrome that patients feel often leads them to sit or lie down.
- If loss of consciousness occurs, there may be a brief period (5–10 seconds) of muscle twitching and myoclonic jerks that can be confused with seizure activity. Occasionally there is urinary incontinence.
- Once the patient is horizontal, he or she becomes conscious within seconds to minutes and is alert and oriented almost immediately.
- If a pulse is taken during the event, the patient will have a paradoxic bradycardia with hypotension.

DIAGNOSIS Past medical history is the basis for diagnosis:

- Medications (see Table 7-14)
- Past history of cardiac disease, especially CAD, MI, CVA, dysrhythmias, a pacemaker, or prosthetic valve are significant for high-risk patients.

PHYSICIAN EXAMINATION

GENERAL

- Check orthostatic vital signs. Check the BP and pulse first while the patient is lying flat, then immediately upon standing and again after 3 minutes.
    - Symptoms of lightheadedness are the most sensitive finding.
    - A heart rate increase of over 30 beats/min is significant.
    - A systolic BP decrease of 20 mm Hg is significant, but not sensitive.

NECK

- Bruits for carotid stenosis
- Radiated murmurs of aortic stenosis

CARDIAC Cardiac examination for murmurs, especially aortic stenosis.

GASTROINTESTINAL Rectal examination is indicated to check for occult blood loss.

NEUROLOGIC

- Look for findings of a CVA.
- Meningismus from an acute SAH

LABORATORY TESTS

- Hematocrit: Severe anemia may lead to vasovagal syncope.
- Glucose: Hypoglycemia is an uncommon cause (for those not taking diabetes medications), but always check in an unconscious or confused patient.
- Electrolytes are rarely needed.
- Urine pregnancy test in women of reproductive age

RADIOLOGY A CXR is rarely useful.

OTHER STUDIES

- ECG: Arrhythmias are a common cause. Look for ventricular tachycardia, bradycardia or pauses, superventricular tachycardia, and AMI.
- Cardiac rhythm monitoring is usually not very helpful, but may identify a dysrhythmia.

ADVANCED DIAGNOSTIC STUDIES

- An echocardiogram is diagnostic for myocardial or valvular causes.
- For CNS causes: a head CT, MRI, and EEG
- A VQ lung scan (if pulmonary embolism suspected)

TREATMENT Treat the underlying cause of the syncope.

DISPOSITION

- Discharge:
    - Patients up to 30 years of age with typical vasovagal syncope
    - Low-risk group includes patients under 60 with vasovagal, psychogenic, or unknown causes for syncope. Poor outcome is seen in about 1% at 1 year.
- Refer urgently for further evaluation:
    - Patients over 30 with CNS or metabolic/toxic causes of syncope.
    - Patients over 60 with vasovagal, psychogenic, or unknown causes of syncope.
- Transfer:
    - High-risk patients are those with cardiac causes by history or examination.
- If you are unsure of the cause and have the capabilities, then monitor the cardiac rhythm for 24 hours.

CHAPTER 8

Adult Infectious Diseases

Thomas D. Kirsch

GENERAL CONSIDERATIONS

Infectious diseases are the leading cause of health problems in many developing countries. Health workers practicing in rural or refugee settings will encounter a wide range of infectious illnesses. Appendix 3 contains World Health Organization (WHO) treatment guidelines for a range of common infectious diseases in adults and children. This chapter describes a more detailed approach to the evaluation of infectious diseases in adults.

RISKS FOR SIGNIFICANT INFECTIONS

When evaluating patients with an acute infectious process, first assess the possibility of a life-threatening infection (check the ABCs). Patients with an infectious disease also should be categorized as either high-risk (those more likely to develop systemic infections and sepsis) or low-risk patients (those who are immunocompetent and less likely to develop sepsis). High-risk patients should be treated more aggressively, and may require hospitalization to start therapy. If patients have one or more of the following characteristics, they can be considered at high risk for developing serious infections or sepsis:

High-Risk Patients
1. Under 1 year or over 60 years of age
2. Any immunocompromised state, such as
   - diabetes

219

- AIDS
- substance abuse [alcoholism or intravenous (IV) drug use]
- cancer and chemotherapy
- severe malnutrition
3. Unable to comply with treatment or follow-up

The following symptoms indicate the presence of sepsis or a serious complication in a patient with an infectious disease:

High-Risk Signs and Symptoms
1. Toxic- or "shocky"-appearing patient:
   - lethargic
   - altered mental status
   - diaphoretic
   - pale, cool, clammy
2. Hypotension (orthostatic hypotension), tachycardia, delayed capillary refill
3. Persistent fever greater than 39.5 to 40.0 (C)
4. Oliguria, anuria

See Table 8-1.

> **KEY POINT:**
>
> Always look for high-risk patients and high-risk signs and symptoms in anyone with an infection.

Patients with these characteristics or symptoms require emergent, aggressive intervention (especially if they have both or more than one). This includes fluid resuscitation, IV antibiotics, hospitalization, and even the use of vasopressors to support blood pressure.

TABLE 8-1 RISK FACTORS FOR SEPSIS

Gram-negative sepsis
   Diabetes mellitus
   Severe burns
   Liver cirrhosis
   Intravenous drug use (IVDU)
   Invasive procedures or indwelling devices
   Treatment with immunosuppressant drugs (neutropenia)
Gram-positive sepsis
   Intravascular catheters
   Indwelling mechanical devices
   Severe burns
   IVDU

ANTIBIOTIC USE AND ABUSE

Not all infections are treated with antibiotics. Antibiotics are effective against most bacterial and parasitic infections but not against viral illnesses. Many health workers prescribe antibiotics for minor viral infections because the patient expects them. Unfortunately, this encourages a cycle of expectation, inappropriate use of resources, and dependence that is good for neither the patient nor the health of the community. Such inappropriate use of antibiotics is also costly and contributes to drug resistance.

Antibiotic resistance is a universal problem of increasing importance. The widespread availability of antibiotics without prescription in many developing countries contributes to the problem. In many regions *Escherichia coli*, gonorrhea, tuberculosis (TB), malaria, *Staphylococcus aureus*, pneumococci, *Shigella*, and many types of *Streptococcus* are now widely resistant to common antibiotics. The WHO recognizes antibiotic resistance as one of the most serious threats to health.

Antibiotics must be chosen carefully and used only when bacterial infections are suspected. An awareness of the resistance patterns in your location is important to properly tailor antibiotic therapy. Patients must understand the importance of sticking to the schedule and completing the course of therapy.

EMERGING DISEASES

New infectious threats and "old" diseases once thought controlled are increasing problems. Examples of emerging infectious agents include the Ebola virus and the human immunodeficiency virus (HIV-AIDS-SIDA). The reemergence of infectious diseases (such as TB, cholera, and malaria) is also a major problem. The emergence of multidrug-resistant tuberculosis (MDRTB) has been called one of the greatest health threats of the twenty-first century. Dengue and cholera have returned to the Americas, where there had not been a case of cholera in over 100 years. Diphtheria has become a significant problem in the countries of the former Soviet Union. The reasons for these changing disease patterns are complex, but include the overuse of antibiotics and insecticides, poor sanitary conditions, increasing crowding of cities, and increased international travel.

PREVENTION

IMMUNIZATIONS

One of the greatest successes in the history of health care was the eradication of smallpox from the earth in 1979. The World Health Organization's Expanded Programme on Immunization (EPI) developed from that effort and now leads the fight against vaccine-preventable diseases. With the assistance of UNICEF and national governments, approximately 80% of the world's children are now immunized against TB, poliomyelitis, diphtheria, tetanus, pertussis, and measles. This translates to the preservation

TABLE 8-2 RECOMMENDED IMMUNIZATION
SCHEDULE

BCG	At birth
DTP	At 6, 10, and 14 weeks, and at 18 months of age
OPV	At birth, 6, 10, and 14 weeks of age
Measles	At 9 months of age
TT	All women of childbearing age, and with each pregnancy

of at least 2.7 million lives from measles, neonatal tetanus, and pertussis and the prevention of 200,000 cases of paralytic polio. Unfortunately, the coverage is not 100%, and vaccine-preventable diseases continue to kill millions of children, accounting for 20% to 35% of all deaths in children under 5 years of age. Measles alone still kills 1.5 million children annually.

It is important that all health workers promote childhood immunizations and be familiar with the recommendations and delivery of EPI vaccines (Table 8-2). It is likewise important to use routine patient encounters to screen for compliance with routine immunizations. Immunization schedules vary considerably between countries, so individual schedules must be reviewed. Some regions and countries use additional vaccines depending on their local disease epidemiology. These include hepatitis A and B, Japanese B encephalitis, yellow fever, group A meningococcus, mumps, and rubella. Prior to embarking on any international work, health-care workers should familiarize themselves with local immunization schedules (see International Travel References at the end of this chapter).

INFECTIONS BY SYSTEM

SYSTEMIC INFECTIONS/SEPSIS

SEPSIS

DEFINITION Sepsis can be caused by any type of microorganism, but is most commonly due to gram-negative and gram-positive bacteria (80%–90% of all cases), particularly *Staphylococcus* and Group A *Streptococcus*. Even with advanced care, the mortality rate is over 25%. The release of bacterial toxins and the body's own immune response can lead to septic shock, particularly in high-risk patients (Table 8-1). Septic shock results from a marked decrease in systemic vascular resistance, hypovolemia from capillary leakage, and the resultant poor tissue perfusion. If shock is not corrected, multiple organ systems are damaged, which leads to death.

CLINICAL PRESENTATION Symptoms can vary (with atypical presentations in the extremes of age) but include

- Hyperventilation
- Fever
- Chills
- Tachypnea
- Tachycardia
- Altered mental status
- Hypotension

Hyperventilation is often an early sign, whereas hypotension may not occur until late (particularly in children). Findings such as disorientation and confusion also may develop, particularly in the elderly.

DIAGNOSIS The diagnosis must be made on clinical findings to prevent mortality. No specific laboratory analyses are readily available to diagnose sepsis.

- The white blood cell (WBC) count is usually elevated, but may be normal or suppressed.
- Lactate levels may be elevated.
- Blood cultures are useful to identify the organism, but treatment cannot await these results.

TREATMENT

KEY POINT:

If sepsis is a possibility, treat first, then make the diagnosis.

Start broad-spectrum antibiotics immediately on suspicion of sepsis. *Staphylococcus*, *Streptococcus*, and gram-negative organisms must be covered.

- A third-generation cephalosporin (cefotaxime 2 g every 4 to 8 hours or ceftriaxone 2 g every 12 hours) plus
- Aminoglycoside (gentamycin or tobramycin 2 mg/kg IV loading dose then 1.7 mg/kg every 8 hours) plus
- Metronidazole (500 mg IV every 6 hours) or clindamycin (600 mg IV every 6 hours) to cover for an intraabdominal source
- If *Staphylococcus* infection is suspected (history of injecting drugs, or indwelling IV line), add vancomycin (1 g IV every 12 hours) or nafcillin (3 g IV every 6 hours)

Other recommended antibiotic regimens (when available) include combining metronidazole or clindamycin with either

- Fluoroquinolone (ciprofloxacin or ofloxacin 400 mg every 12 hours or levofloxacin 500 mg daily) or
- Ticarcillin/clavulanate 3.1 g IV every 4 hours or
- Imipenem 500 mg IV every 6 hours or
- Maintain the blood pressure

See Chapter 6 for further details on the treatment of shock. Initial fluid resuscitation should be rapid.

- For adults, start with 1 to 2 L of normal saline or lactated Ringer solution (>5 L may be needed).
- For children, begin with a bolus of 20 mL/kg of the same fluid and repeat twice more if needed (check vital signs and capillary refill to assess perfusion).
- Vasopressor agents such as dopamine 5 to 10 µg/kg/min, epinephrine, or norepinephrine may be needed if volume resuscitation fails.

Remove the source of infection. Search carefully for the source of the infection and remove it: incise and drain abscesses, remove catheters, and clean wounds. Examine the entire patient, including all orifices.

Monitoring
- Monitoring of the patient should include frequent blood pressure assessment.
- Urine output is the best indicator of good tissue perfusion, so a Foley catheter is helpful. Minimum urine output should be 0.5 mL/h.
- A central venous pressure (CVP) monitor is very useful, but is not always available. CVP should be maintained between 10 and 12 cm H_2O. CVP can be estimated by the jugular venous pressure.

PREVENTION Early recognition is the key to preventing death. Extreme care must be taken to ensure the cleanliness and sterility of hospitals, and the number of invasive procedures performed and indwelling catheters placed must be kept to a minimum.

TOXIC SHOCK SYNDROME

DEFINITION Toxic shock syndrome (TSS) is caused by an entrapped bacterial source. It may occur with tampon use, postpartum infections, septic abortions, surgical wound infections, nasal packing, cutaneous and subcutaneous abscesses, osteomyelitis, and peritonsillar abscess. TSS is caused by strains of *Staphylococcus aureus* that produce a toxin that leads to massive vasodilatation and fluid redistribution.

CLINICAL PRESENTATION By definition, TSS affects multiple organ systems, so the presentation may vary. Symptoms usually develop rapidly and include

- Fever
- Chills
- Headache
- Lightheadedness
- Skin erythema
- Nausea
- Watery diarrhea

Additional complaints include sore throat (50%), photophobia, abdominal pain, and cough. Physical findings include

- Hypotension, tachycardia, tachypnea, etc.
- Erythematous rash (initially a diffuse blanching erythema that then fades within 3 days and is followed by desquamation, especially of the palms and soles)
- Mucous membrane hyperemia (pharyngitis with strawberry red tongue, vaginitis)
- Conjunctival hyperemia, abdominal tenderness
- Altered states of consciousness
- Renal and hepatic insufficiency

DIAGNOSIS The diagnosis of TSS is based on the multisystem symptom pattern. Laboratory tests are generally not helpful.

TREATMENT

- First, assess the ABCs for shock.
- Start broad-spectrum antibiotics (see earlier section on Sepsis) and include an antistaphylococcal penicillin.
    - nafcillin or oxacillin 2 g IV every 4 hours or
    - cephalosporin with β-lactamase stability is needed (cefazolin 1 to 2 g IV every 6 hours)
- Find the source of the infection and treat or remove it (drain abscesses, remove tampons, etc.).

PREVENTION

- Some studies suggest avoiding the use of tampons.
- Use antistaphylococcal antibiotics whenever packing a patient's nose.
- Recurrences can occur within 60 days, but antibiotics reduce their frequency and severity.

RICKETTSIAL INFECTIONS

TYPHUS

DEFINITION Typhus is caused by the *Rickettsia* organisms, which have characteristics of both bacteria and viruses. There are two major vectors for epidemic typhus: louse-borne (*Rickettsia prowazekii*) and rat/flea-borne (*Rickettsia mooseri*). Both cause similar symptoms (although the rat-borne variety is milder) and are treated the same. They occur most often in Africa and Asia and occasionally in Europe. Another typhus infection, Tsutsugamushi fever (scrub typhus) is transmitted by chiggers. It occurs in the southwest Pacific and Southeast Asia in an area bordered by Pakistan, Japan, and the Solomon Islands. It has the same presentation and treatment as the others, but a chronic necrotic eschar develops at the site of the bite.

CLINICAL PRESENTATION After an incubation period of 7 to 14 days, rapid onset of the following symptoms may be observed:

- Fever may fluctuate irregularly over a week and is associated with a significant headache.
- After the fever starts, a rash quickly spreads peripherally into scattered, firm macules/papules and then petechially from the trunk to the extremities.
- Other symptoms include cough, abdominal pain, nausea, and vomiting.
- Untreated patients progress with decreasing mental status, and ultimately heart and renal failure.

DIAGNOSIS Diagnosis is primarily clinical; look for the fever and peripherally spreading rash. The Weil-Felix test result is positive.

TREATMENT

- Doxycycline 100 mg twice daily orally (PO) or IV for 7 days (or 2 days after afebrile)
- Chloramphenicol 500 mg every 6 hours PO or IV for 7 days (or 2 days after afebrile)

PREVENTION

Vaccination with the typhoid vaccine (Typhim Vi) 25 μg intramuscularly (IM) (single dose)
Louse/flea control

Additional Rickettsial Diseases
- Q fever: Similar in presentation and treatment as the above, except that a rash rarely develops and pneumonia develops in 50% of cases. It is transmitted from

animals (particularly cattle and sheep) to people, and so is most common around slaughterhouses.

■ Rocky Mountain spotted fever: Occurs most often in the eastern United States.

SOFT TISSUE INFECTIONS: SKIN, MUSCLE, AND BONE

CELLULITIS

DEFINITION Cellulitis is an infection of the subcutaneous tissues. In adults the most common causes are staphylococci and/or streptococci, and in young children *Hemophilus.*

CLINICAL PRESENTATION Patients usually complain of pain at the site of the cellulites, and there is often a preceding injury. Findings depend on the severity of the infection and progress from

■ Local erythema, warmth, and tenderness (without fluctuance), to
■ Lymphangitis and regional lymphadenopathy, to
■ Fever with leukocytosis (uncommon in healthy patients)

DIAGNOSIS Diagnosis is by physical examination; laboratory tests are not indicated. If an abscess is suspected, then incision and drainage or needle exploration can be performed to look for pus.

TREATMENT

■ Admit high-risk patients (see earlier definition of high-risk patients) or those with facial cellulitis for IV antibiotic therapy.
  ■ penicillinase-resistant penicillin (nafcillin or oxacillin 2 g IV every 4 hours) or
  ■ cephalosporin (such as cefazolin 1 g every 8 hours) or
  ■ vancomycin
■ For less severe infections (extremities, healthy patients):
  ■ dicloxacillin 500 mg PO every 6 hours or
  ■ ampicillin/clavulanate 875/125 mg twice daily or 500/125 mg every 8 hours PO

PREVENTION Teach patients the need for cleanliness in caring for their wounds— even minor skin trauma can lead to infection/cellulitis/abscess in high-risk patients. Clean all wounds immediately with soap and water, or at least copious amounts of the cleanest water available.

ABSCESSES

DEFINITION Abscesses (boils) are caused by minor trauma, ingrown hairs (pilonidal abscesses), obstructed sebaceous or apocrine glands, anal cysts (perirectal abscesses), or obstructed Bartholin glands (vulvovaginal abscesses). The most common aerobic organisms are *Staphylococcus aureus*, *Proteus mirabilis*, and *Escherichia coli* (most common in intraabdominal abscesses). Anaerobes are common in abscesses in the perineal area and are usually mixed infections. If it stinks, think anaerobic infection.

Recurrent perianal abscesses suggest inflammatory bowel disease, and recurrent axillary or inguinal abscesses suggest hidradenitis suppurativa.

CLINICAL PRESENTATION Patients complain of severe local pain and swelling. Physical findings include

- Local tenderness with fluctuance
- Erythema and swelling
- Warmth

A fever may indicate a systemic infection or may be evidence of immunocompromise. Nonhealing or recurring abscesses may be related to diminished immunity.

DIAGNOSIS Diagnosis is based on the clinical examination; laboratory tests are not useful.

TIPS AND TRICKS:

If you are uncertain of the location of the abscess or if the presence of pus is in doubt, attempt a needle aspiration to localize the pus.

TREATMENT

- Incision and drainage is the primary treatment in healthy, nontoxic patients (Fig. 8-1).
- If the abscess is not fluctuant, have the patient apply warm compresses four to five times daily and return for a follow-up visit in 24 to 48 hours.

TIPS: ABSCESS INCISION AND DRAINAGE

Narcotic premedication may be necessary prior to incision and drainage, and local anesthesia may be useful as a ring block infiltration or into the abscess roof. Larger abscesses and those in difficult areas (neck, perirectal) may require general anesthesia.

- Antibiotics are usually not indicated, but may be considered for
  - high-risk patients or those with
  - fever
  - signs of sepsis
  - an abscess in the mastoid area or central triangle of the face

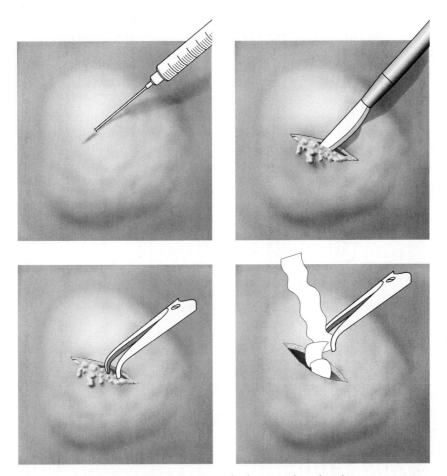

FIGURE 8-1 Abscess incision and drainage. The key: quick and wide.

1. Inject local anesthetic (if possible)
2. Incise with #11 scalpel blade along the length of fluctuant area, attempt to follow the natural skin folds.
3. Explore bluntly with forceps (or the opposite end of the scalpel) to break up loculations. Squeeze out the pus. Irrigate (with sterile water or saline if available).
4. Loose packing, or better yet just a gauze wick (do not pack tightly unless you intend to personally repack two to three times daily).

  ■ patients at risk for endocarditis (artificial valve or cardiac murmur)
 ■ The patient should be instructed to return for follow-up in 24 to 48 hours (sooner for complicated infections and facial abscess).
 ■ Have the patient remove the packing in 24 to 48 hours if they cannot present for follow-up.

PREVENTION Teaching patients about cleaning all wounds, even the most minor, can prevent the formation of many abscesses. This is particularly important for high-risk patients.

GAS GANGRENE

DEFINITION Gas gangrene is a soft tissue infection that leads to muscle necrosis, gas production, and significant systemic toxicity. It usually is the result of contaminated wounds with poor care. It is caused by *Clostridia.*

CLINICAL PRESENTATION The clostridial infection is rapidly progressive.

■ The patient initially complains of muscle heaviness and dull pain.
■ Pain may rapidly increase and shock can develop.
■ Systemic symptoms include fever and then signs of shock.

Physical findings include the following:

■ Local discoloration with a dark, malodorous exudate may be observed.
■ There may be cutaneous bullae.
■ Crepitance from the gas is a key clinical finding.

DIAGNOSIS An infected wound with crepitance should be considered gangrene. An x-ray may reveal subcutaneous and intramuscular air.

KEY POINT:

Any wound with crepitance (crackling feeling under the skin when palpating) should be considered gangrene and treated aggressively.

TREATMENT Rapid and aggressive therapy is needed to save the patient's life.

■ Admit all patients.
■ Start IV antibiotic therapy immediately:
  ■ penicillin 4 to 6 million units IV every 6 hours with
  ■ clindamycin 900 mg IV every 8 hours or
  ■ ceftriaxone 2 g IV every 12 hours

In penicillin-allergic patients, use

■ Erythromycin 1 g IV every 6 hours or
■ Chloramphenicol 4 g/day or
■ Clindamycin alone

Prompt surgical exploration with extensive debridement under general anesthesia is needed. Localized incision, drainage, and debridement can be performed if general anesthesia is not immediately available. Always give the patient tetanus prophylaxis.

PREVENTION Early wound care and cleanliness should be practiced, particularly in high-risk patients.

IMPETIGO

DEFINITION A superficial infection of the skin caused by *Streptococcus*, with *Staphylococcus* as a secondary invader. If untreated, spreading continues and a deeper infection results. It is very infectious, and the bullae and pustules can spread quickly. It most commonly affects young children.

CLINICAL PRESENTATION

- Impetigo usually occurs under the nose and perioral area.
- There is a weeping yellow crust covering an erythematous area with irregular margins and sometimes vesicles.
- Bullae (large blisters) also may form.
- Patients may become febrile.

DIAGNOSIS Physical examination only.

TREATMENT

- Wash the area with warm, soapy water three to four times daily and remove the crusts.
- Topical antibiotics containing bacitracin or gentian violet can be used on isolated areas after each washing.
- Oral antibiotics are indicated for advanced cases and febrile patients.
    - For nonbullous (honey-crust) lesions, use penicillin VK 500 to 1,000 mg every 6 hours or a first-generation cephalosporin (cefalexin)
    - For bullous lesions, use antistaphylococcal drugs (dicloxacillin, oxacillin, azithromycin, or ampicillin/clavulanate).

PREVENTION Cleanliness is the key. Teach parents to keep the perinasal area clean and to treat early infections with soap and water and warm compresses.

ERYSIPELAS

DEFINITION Erysipelas are a distinctive variety of cellulitis caused by group A *Streptococcus*, usually occurring on the face or scalp of infants, or sometimes in the elderly and patients with skin ulcers. If untreated, the mortality rate reaches 40%.

CLINICAL PRESENTATION

- Small raised, red, and painful plaques have a distinct advancing edge.
- The rash desquamates during convalescence.
- In children the infection is usually periorbital.
- Occasionally patients present with a high fever and sepsis.

DIAGNOSIS Physical examination only.

TREATMENT

- Admit all patients for IV antibiotics.
- Clean the wound with warm, soapy water and elevate the infected area, if possible.
- Antibiotic therapy is the same as for in-patient cellulitis.

PREVENTION Cleanliness and early wound care.

TINEA CORPORIS (RINGWORM), PEDIS, CRURIS, AND CAPITAS

DEFINITION Tinea corporis is a superficial fungal infection of the epidermis caused by *Trichophyton* and *Microsporum* fungi.

CLINICAL PRESENTATION The presentation depends on the location of the infection.

- Intense pruritus is common to all forms.
- The classic presentation is a raised, scaly, erythematous ring with a clear center that gradually expands.
- Atypical presentations are common from local erythema or vesicles.
- Tinea capitas on the scalp often presents with hair loss.

TREATMENT

- Local treatment with antifungal creams (clotrimazole, miconazole, haloprogin) twice daily for 2 to 4 weeks
- Oral griseofulvin 10 to 15 mg/kg/day for 6 weeks for severe cases and those involving the hair

---

TIPS AND TRICKS:

Make sure the patient uses topical therapy for a full 2 weeks (the lesion may be gone before this time), or the infection can return.

CANDIDA

DEFINITION Candida fungal infection affects many body parts: oral (thrush), esophageal, vaginal, and skin. Oral and skin (diaper rash) candidiasis is common in infants under 6 months of age. If oral thrush is seen in an adult, consider AIDS or another underlying immunocompromising disease.

CLINICAL PRESENTATION The presentation depends on the affected area.

- Skin: Monilial dermatitis presents with sharply demarcated erythematous areas in skin creases, particularly of the thighs. Satellite papules and pustules are often seen.
- Mouth: Thrush appears as white, "cheesy" patches on the mucous membranes in the mouth. These pseudomembranes leave a tender erythematous base when removed.
- Vagina: "Yeast" infection with a "cheesy" vaginal discharge, usually with vaginal and labial erythema (see Chapter 12 for details).

DIAGNOSIS

- Examine a scraping of the lesion (or discharge) under the microscope after adding a few drops of 10% potassium hydroxide (KOH). Budding yeast and pseudohyphae can be found.
- No laboratory tests are needed (unless you suspect an underlying immunosuppressing disease).

TREATMENT

- Skin: Instruct the patient to dry the area, and to wear loose-fitting clothing, take off shoes and socks every day.
  - Local treatment with antifungal creams (lotrimin, others) for 2 to 4 weeks may be indicated.
  - Oral griseofulvin with a dose of 10 to 15 mg/kg for 6 weeks may be used for severe cases and those involving the hair.
- For thrush, use oral nystatin 200,000 to 500,000 units swish and swallow every 6 hours for 10 to 14 days or fluconazole 200 mg PO in a single dose or 100 mg daily for 14 days.
  - Don't allow children to constantly suck on a bottle.
- Vaginal candidiasis responds to antifungal creams or suppositories intravaginally every night for 1 week or a single oral dose of fluconazole (150 mg).

SCABIES

DEFINITION Infection is caused by infestation of the insect *Sarcoptes scabiei*, which burrows into the skin and deposits eggs and feces. Symptoms may not develop for 4 to

6 weeks after the initial infestation. Infestations occur commonly below the neck and particularly in the interdigital area in older children and adults. Younger children are affected on the palms and soles or even the face and scalp.

CLINICAL PRESENTATION The primary symptom is unremitting intense pruritus that is worse at night. Patients also may develop papules and tiny vesicles. The linear burrows are rarely seen in children.

DIAGNOSIS

- The history and physical examination may be sufficient.
- A microscopic examination of skin scrapings may identify mites or eggs to confirm the diagnosis.
  - Place a drop of oil over a fresh vesicle and scrape it with a knife blade or the edge of a slide.

TREATMENT

- Apply either permethrin 5% or lindane 1% to the entire body (chin to toes) for 8 to 10 hours, then wash it off (do not use on children <2 months of age or on pregnant women).
  - Repeat after 1 week if symptoms persist.
- Gentian violet also may be applied topically to the affected area, but is less effective.
- Trim fingernails.
- Family members also should be treated, and bedding and clothing sterilized.

PEDICULOSIS (LICE)

DEFINITION The human head louse only infects people. It is 1 to 4 mm long and white, and is hard to see.

CLINICAL PRESENTATION

- The primary symptom is intense pruritus.
- The only physical finding is that the nits (eggs) can resemble dandruff.

DIAGNOSIS

- Careful examination of hair from the affected area (scalp or groin) may reveal small oval nits or the small crab-like lice attached to hair shafts. A microscope or magnifying glass helps.
- Nits may appear as dandruff on gross examination, but are not easily removed.

TREATMENT

- Vigorous cleaning of the infested areas is important.
- Wash the hair with permethrin 5%, leave on for 10 minutes, then rinse out (no shampoo or soap) and comb. Repeat in 7 to 10 days.
- If the entire body needs treating, then use lindane (gamma benzene hydrochloride) or permethrin, as above.
- Family members will often be infected and need treatment also.
- All clothing and bedding must be washed with hot (boiling if possible) soapy water and treated with either
  - 1% malathion powder or
  - 10% DDT powder

TETANUS

DEFINITION Tetanus is a highly fatal neuroparalytic disease. Even with optimum treatment the mortality rate is over 40%. The disease is caused by *Clostridium tetani*, a gram-positive anaerobic rod that is everywhere, particularly in the feces of animals and people. The bacteria produce a toxin that ascends peripheral nerves to the spinal cord and brain; thus, symptoms may develop weeks after the original inoculation. There are two major types of tetanus infections: neonatal tetanus (NNT) and adult tetanus. In adults, dirty wounds lead to the infection. NNT is caused by unclean birth practices, particularly regarding the care of the cord. See Chapter 11 for details on NNT.

CLINICAL PRESENTATION

Neonatal Tetanus See Chapter 11. Symptoms develop 3 to 14 days after birth.

- Poor feeding and then continuous crying are the first symptoms.
- The umbilical cord may show signs of infection.

Adult Tetanus

- Half of adults present with trismus (pain) and difficulty with swallowing.
- Increasing rigidity of the neck and jaw then develops.
- Patients then begin having difficulty walking.
- Finally tetanic spasms develop:
  - The patient arches the back and retracts the arms with flexion at the elbow.
  - The spasms are brought on by even slight stimuli (such as a touch, or bright lights).
- Often no wound can be found.

Depending on how late the symptoms develop, cases are considered mild, moderate, or severe:

- Mild cases (incubation period longer than 10 days) develop stiffness in an isolated muscle group (localized tetanus) and have a lower mortality.
- Moderate cases present with dysphagia and paroxysmal spasms but no respiratory difficulty.
- Severe cases present with severe spasms, respiratory difficulty, gluteal spasm, and respiratory arrest.

DIAGNOSIS

- Classic tetanic spasms are diagnostic.
- Hyperreflexia is a prominent early finding, including in the newborn.
- No laboratory tests are indicated.

TREATMENT

- Maintain the airway; endotracheal intubation may be needed in severe cases.
- Neutralize the unbound toxin with 3,000 to 10,000 units IM of human tetanus immunoglobulin (TIG, Hypertet), if available.
- Control muscle spasms with IV diazepam or phenobarbital. Very large doses may be required.
  - Neuromuscular blockade may be required.
- IV antibiotics
  - Penicillin G, 4 to 6 million units IV every 6 hours or
  - Metronidazole 500 mg IV every 6 hours or 1 g every 12 hours or
  - Doxycycline 100 mg IV every 12 hours
- Irrigate and debride all wounds (check the entire body carefully).
- Avoid stimulating patients—keep them in a quiet environment.
- Maintain hydration with nasogastric or IV fluids (formula or breast milk can be used for infants).
- Begin immunizations if necessary.

PREVENTION Immunization is the key. The target groups are all children under 2 years of age and all women of childbearing years.

- Pregnant women should receive Td toxoid.
- Children should receive at least four doses of the diphtheria-tetanus-pertussis (DTP) vaccine (follow your country's immunization schedule). For those over 7 years of age, use boosters of Td toxoid every 5 to 10 years.
- Neonatal tetanus is also prevented by proper birth practices.

EAR, NOSE, AND THROAT INFECTIONS

OTITIS MEDIA

DEFINITION Most (60%–80%) ear infections in children are viral. When bacterial in origin the three most common organisms are *Streptococcus pneumoniae, Hemophilus influenzae,* and *Branhamella catarrhalis.* It most commonly affects children under 5 years of age. Complications include meningitis and mastoiditis.

CLINICAL PRESENTATION Symptoms include

- Fever
- Localized ear pain
- Headache
- Decreased hearing acuity
- Crying and/or fever in infants

Physical findings include the following:

- The external ear and canal should be normal.
- The tympanic membrane should be erythematous, bulging, and dull. Look especially at the posterior, superior quadrant of the tympanic membrane.
- Pneumatic otoscopy demonstrates fluid behind the ear if the tympanic membrane does not move.
- There may be palpable anterior cervical nodes.

DIAGNOSIS Physical examination only; clean the canal to be sure of the diagnosis.

TREATMENT Most cases do not require antibiotic therapy. In patients with obvious findings and high-risk factors, treat with amoxicillin 250 mg every 8 hours for 10 days. Double the first dose of any antibiotic. Compliance with therapy is important. Don't overcall it just to satisfy parents; it is the leading cause of partially treated meningitis.

OTITIS EXTERNA

DEFINITION Otitis externa is caused by trauma to the ear canal or by a foreign body or water in the canal. It can occur at any age, but in children beware of the possibility of a foreign body.

CLINICAL PRESENTATION Symptoms include local pain with or without discharge from the ear.

Physical Examination
- Pain with manipulation of the pinna
- An edematous, erythematous ear canal
- Often with purulent discharge.
- Try to visualize the tympanic membrane to ensure that the discharge is not coming from a foreign body (in children) or from a tympanic membrane perforated by otitis media.

DIAGNOSIS Based on the history and physical.

TREATMENT

- Remove debris by irrigation with normal saline (which is slightly acidic).
- Lower the pH in the canal with mild acid drops, such as 2% acetic acid (vinegar) solution every 6 hours for 7 days.
- Use antibiotic drops if needed: polymyxin B/neomycin/hydrocortisone drops every 6 hours for 10 days.
- Oral antibiotics are only indicated in patients with fever or surrounding cellulitis [trimethoprim/sulfamethoxazole (TMP/SMX) PO twice daily or dicloxacillin 500 mg PO every 6 hours for 7 to 10 days].
- Admit diabetic patients for IV antibiotics (must cover for *Pseudomonas*):
    - ciprofloxacin 400 mg IV every 12 hours or 750 mg PO every 12 hours or
    - ceftazidime 2 g IV every 8 hours or
    - ampicillin and an aminoglycoside (gentamycin, tobramycin, etc.) may be used, but are generally less effective

PREVENTION The canal should be dried thoroughly, and no objects should be inserted in the canal.

SINUSITIS

DEFINITION Infection of the perinasal sinuses (usually maxillary) is a common complication of an upper respiratory infection and allergic rhinitis. The infection occurs because the sinus ostia becomes obstructed. The most common bacteria are *Streptococcus*, *Branhamella*, and *Hemophilus influenzae*. Untreated infections can lead to orbital infections and meningitis by direct extension, or cavernous sinus thrombosis. Symptoms usually resolve rapidly with antibiotic treatment.

CLINICAL PRESENTATION Sinusitis initially presents as a chronic "cold" that lasts more than 10 days. There also may be a chronic cough. The nasal discharge varies from clear to purulent or bloody. Symptoms then progress to

- Facial pain
- Upper tooth pain
- Malodorous breath with increasing severity

Findings of the physical examination are often normal but may include

- Low-grade fever
- Tenderness to percussion of the anterior face and forehead

DIAGNOSIS The diagnosis should be based on the history of a prolonged "cold" with local pain and fever. Facial x-rays may reveal an air-fluid level, particularly the occipitomental view for the maxillary sinuses.

TREATMENT

- Local heat (warm water–soaked cloths) applied across the bridge of the nose and cheeks may provide some symptomatic relief and help to soften the mucus.
- Decongestant nasal spray (such as oxyphentolamine) may help the sinuses to drain.
- Do not use antihistamines—they may dry the mucus and further obstruct the ostia. Antibiotics should be considered if the patient's temperature is over 39°C, the symptoms have lasted more than 14 days, or there is significant facial swelling. Therapy includes
    - TMP/SMX double strength (DS) 1 tablet PO twice daily or
    - ampicillin or amoxicillin 500 mg PO every 8 hours for 10 days or
    - amoxicillin/clavulanate 875/125 mg PO twice daily or 500/125 mg every 8 hours; very effective, but expensive
- Aspiration and irrigation of the sinus intranasally through the lateral sinus wall below the inferior turbinate may be needed for complicated or chronic cases.

PHARYNGITIS

DEFINITION Most cases of pharyngitis (60%–80%) are caused by viral, not bacterial, infections. The most common bacterial cause is Group A β-hemolytic *Streptococcus* (GABHS). GABHS pharyngitis is rare before age 3 and peaks in early school years. In developing countries diphtheria also must be considered. Don't forget gonorrhea in sexually active adolescents.

CLINICAL PRESENTATION Symptoms vary widely and usually resolve untreated in 3 to 5 days. They include

- Sore throat, fever, chills, and malaise
- Abdominal pain, nausea, and vomiting, especially in children

Physical findings include

- Mucosal erythema of the pharynx
- Exudate on tonsils and posterior pharynx
- Enlarged and tender anterior cervical lymph nodes

DIAGNOSIS There is no way to distinguish bacterial from viral pharyngitis by the history and physical examination alone. Consider viral pharyngitis in patients with accompanying cough and rhinorrhea. Testing is generally not needed.

- A culture for *Streptococcus* is the gold standard but difficult to perform and to follow up.
- The results of some rapid *Streptococcus* tests are available instantly. They are very specific (>95%), but less sensitive (55%–90%) (i.e., they may miss a lot of streptococcal infections).

> **KEY POINT:**
>
> Diphtheria (see Chapter 11)
>   Pharyngitis is also commonly caused by *Corynebacterium diphtheriae* in develop-
> ing countries. The distinguishing clinical feature is the pseudomembrane found in the
> throat, which occurs in 50% to 90% of patients. Unlike streptococcal exudates, pharyn-
> gitis can spread far beyond the tonsillar pillars, and dislodging the membrane leads to
> bleeding. The onset of pain and fever is usually gradual over days, and nausea and vom-
> iting may be common with children. Diphtheria produces a systemic toxin that causes
> multiple effects such as neuritis, myocarditis, and focal damage to kidneys, adrenal
> glands, and the liver. It can lead to cardiovascular collapse and shock. In tropical cli-
> mates cutaneous infections are more common than respiratory diphtheria. These infec-
> tions are usually secondary to scabies, impetigo, or other forms of dermatitis.

TREATMENT Antibiotics are not usually needed for simple pharyngitis. But be
aware of the incidence of *Streptococcus* A and associated rheumatic fever in your geographic area. If rheumatic fever is common, be more liberal with antibiotic treatment.
If antibiotics are to be used, then long-acting IM penicillin is the most effective method
and guarantees compliance.

- Benzathine penicillin G 1.2 million units IM (600,000 units IM in children weigh-
  ing >27 kg) or
- Penicillin V 250 mg PO every 6 hours for 10 days or
- Erythromycin 250 mg (10 mg/kg) PO every 6 hours for 10 days

COMPLICATIONS Serious complications include rheumatic fever, meningitis, and
pharyngeal abscesses. Others include scarlet fever.
   Scarlet fever is caused by *Streptococcus*, most commonly pharyngitis. It presents with

- "Sandpaper" rash (fine papules and erythema) that starts on the upper trunk and
  spreads outward, sparing the soles and palms, and more prominent in the folds of
  the skin
- "Strawberry" tongue (enlarged papillae and a coated tongue)
- Desquamation of the soles and palms as the rash resolves in 6 to 9 days

RHEUMATIC FEVER Rheumatic fever is a late sequela of a *Streptococcus* A infection,
resulting in damage to heart valves (most commonly), joints, skin, subcutaneous tissue,
and the central nervous system (CNS). Rheumatic fever remains an important cause of
childhood deaths in developing countries. The principal causes of death are endo-,
myo-, and pericarditis (acutely); death also results from the long-term complications
of valvular damage. Infections most commonly occur in individuals 5 to 15 years of age
and are more common with outbreaks of streptococcal pharyngitis. Recurrences are
common, and the effects on the heart and valves accumulate. Therefore, antibiotic prophylaxis for patients with previous rheumatic fever is needed.

TABLE 8-3 THE JONES CRITERIA FOR
DIAGNOSING RHEUMATIC FEVER

If the patient has two major or one major and two minor
  manifestations, rheumatic fever is highly probable.

Major manifestations
   Carditis
   Polyarthritis
   Chorea
   Erythema marinatum
   Subcutaneous nodules

Minor manifestations
   Fever
   Arthralgias
   Prolonged PR interval on electrocardiogram
   Elevated sedimentation rate or C-reactive protein

CLINICAL PRESENTATION AND DIAGNOSIS The diagnosis is based on major and
minor findings in the Jones criteria (Table 8-3). The most common findings include

- Fever
- Migratory polyarthritis
- Carditis

  Less common features include

- Subcutaneous nodules
- Sydenham chorea
- Erythema marginatum

TREATMENT

- Treat acute infections with benzathine penicillin 1.2 million units IM in adults or
  600,000 U in children daily for 10 days.
- Treat any future infection or fever in patients with a history of rheumatic fever
  with antistreptococcal antibiotics to prevent recurrence and further valve damage.

PREVENTION

- Antibiotic treatment with anti-*Streptococcus* for other streptococcal infections
  (especially pharyngitis) prevents rheumatic fever.
- Antibiotics are particularly indicated in patients with pharyngitis when streptococcal outbreaks occur.
- Prophylactic antibiotics can be provided to exposed family members, especially
  children.

■ To prevent recurrent rheumatic fever, antibiotic prophylaxis with monthly doses of IM penicillin is indicated, but extremely difficult to deliver. This should be maintained until the child reaches 18 years of age, or for 5 years in adults.

COMPLICATED PHARYNGITIS: ABSCESSES

DEFINITION Peritonsillar, retropharyngeal, and parapharyngeal abscesses occur most often in adolescents and young adults. Group A *Streptococcus* is the leading cause.

CLINICAL PRESENTATION Patients present with 1 to 2 days of pharyngitis with fever and severe posterior pharyngeal pain (often unilateral). As the infection progresses they develop

■ Drooling (it is too painful to even swallow their own saliva)
■ Trismus (pain with opening, or inability to open the mouth)
■ Moderate dehydration due to difficulty swallowing

The physical examination may just show mild posterior pharyngeal erythema, but usually reveals

■ Marked erythema and swelling
■ Asymmetric soft palate
■ The uvula shifted from the midline
■ The swollen area may be fluctuant

TIPS AND TRICKS:

When examining a patient with suspected peritonsillar abscess, have the patient pant rapidly while you attempt to palpate the posterior pharynx; this helps to prevent them from gagging.

DIAGNOSIS The history and physical examination usually determines the diagnosis. If an abscess is not certain, a needle aspiration of the area may help to find the purulent fluid (see Chapter 21 for details).

TREATMENT

■ Incision and drainage (or at least aspiration) of the mass are the mainstays of therapy.
■ Simple abscesses can be needle drained with little difficulty.
■ More complex, deep abscesses require operative drainage under sedation or general anesthesia (Fig. 8-1).
■ IV antibiotics are often used initially and the patients are usually dehydrated and require fluid resuscitation (normal saline or lactated Ringer solution).

- Use IM or PO medicine for simple presentations.
- Antibiotic therapy with penicillin or ampicillin may be sufficient, but there are often anaerobic bacteria present, so broader coverage may be needed, such as
  - penicillin 4 mg IV every 6 hours with metronidazole 1 g load then 500 mg every 6 hours or
  - clindamycin 150 to 450 mg PO every 6 hours or
  - amoxicillin/clavulanate 500 mg PO every 6 hours for 7 to 10 days
- Most patients in developing countries should be hospitalized for at least 24 hours.

CARDIAC INFECTIONS

ENDOCARDITIS

BACKGROUND Endocarditis, myocarditis, and other infections of the heart are difficult to diagnose and treat, usually requiring advanced services. Endocarditis is an infection, with resulting destruction of the heart valves. Endocarditis is usually caused by bacteria, but can be caused by any infective agent. Predisposing factors include rheumatic heart disease, IV drug use, congenital abnormalities, and prosthetic valves.

CLINICAL PRESENTATION The presentation of endocarditis can range from subtle, nonspecific symptoms to strokes and cardiovascular collapse. The most common early symptoms are

- Intermittent fever
- Malaise
- Other symptoms may or may not occur: chest pain, dyspnea, myalgias, headache, cough, and anorexia

As the infection worsens, the valve may begin to release septic emboli, causing strokes that lead to hemiparesis, personality changes, and alterations in consciousness.

DIAGNOSIS The most common physical examination finding is a regurgitant heart murmur (except for IV drug users). Other findings include

- Fever
- Vascular lesions such as petechiae, splinter hemorrhages (under the fingernails), Janeway lesions (nontender red lesions of the fingertips), or Osler nodes (painful red nodes of the palms and soles) (seen in 50%)
- Splenomegaly
- Retinal flame hemorrhages with pale centers (Roth spots) (rare, seen in <10%)

Laboratory tests may reveal

- Increased WBC count with a shift in polymorphonuclear cells (PMNs)
- Elevated erythrocyte sedimentation rate

- Microscopic hematuria (from emboli to the kidneys)
- Results of blood cultures usually will determine the diagnosis, but such analyses may not be available. Ideally draw two to four cultures from different sites prior to starting antibiotics.

Electrocardiography may demonstrate conduction abnormalities, but results are usually normal. Echocardiography (ultrasonography) is useful (80% sensitive) to demonstrate valvular damage on natural valves. The clinical diagnosis is based on the finding of a new or changing murmur combined with evidence of emboli.

TREATMENT Most infections are by streptococcal organisms. If the disease course has been rapid and the patient appears toxic, treat immediately for *Staphylococcus* also. Cultures are essential to direct long-term therapy. Empiric treatment regimens for patients with native (nonprosthetic) valves include

- Penicillin G 3.5 million units IV every 4 hours (or ampicillin 2 g every 4 hours) with
- Oxacillin or nafcillin 2 g IV every 4 hours (to cover for *Staphylococcus*) and
- Gentamicin 1 mg/kg IV or IM every 8 hours

For penicillin-allergic patients

- Vancomycin 15 mg/kg IV every 12 hours (no more than 2 g/day) and
- Gentamicin 1g/kg IV or IM every 8 hours

Therapy must be continued for 4 to 12 weeks, depending on the organism. Specific antibiotic therapy must be directed by blood culture results.

PREVENTION Patients with known valve anomalies, significant heart murmurs, artificial valves, or a history of rheumatic heart disease should receive prophylactic antibiotics whenever an invasive dental, gastrointestinal, genitourinary, or skin (incision and drainage) procedure is performed. Recommended regimens include

- Dental procedures
    - amoxicillin 2 g PO 1 hour before the procedure or
    - clindamycin 600 mg PO or cephalexin 2 g PO if patient is penicillin allergic
- Gastrointestinal or genitourinary procedures
    - ampicillin 2 g IV or IM 30 minutes prior to the procedure then 1 g 6 hours later and
    - gentamicin 1.5 mg/kg IV
    - If patient is penicillin allergic, use vancomycin 1 g IV over 1 to 2 hours and gentamicin
- Incision and drainage of an abscess
    - Cephalexin 2 g PO 1 hour before the procedure and 500 mg PO 6 hours after the procedure

RESPIRATORY INFECTIONS

PNEUMONIA

GENERAL DEFINITION Pneumonia is an infection of the lower respiratory tract. For the most part, in developing countries you will not have the resources to identify the specific infectious agent. Therefore, you must treat pneumonia with broad-spectrum antibiotics. Patients with underlying medical problems (see earlier definition of high-risk patients), pregnancy, or sickle cell disease, and postsplenectomy patients are at risk for complications and require even more aggressive therapy. You must familiarize yourself with the etiologies and recommended therapies for pneumonia in your geographic area.

GENERAL CLINICAL PRESENTATION The most common presentation is

- Cough with sputum (green, brown, or bloody)
- Fever
- Shortness of breath

Symptoms and findings that indicate a serious infection include

- Toxic (sick) appearance
- Hypoxemia (pulse oximetry <90%–92%)
- Increased respiratory rate (>26–30 breaths/min in adults)
- Multilobar pneumonia
- Virulent organisms (i.e., *Staphylococcus, Klebsiella, Varicella*)

GENERAL DIAGNOSIS The diagnosis of pneumonia in a low-risk, otherwise healthy adult can almost always be made based on a careful history and physical examination. A chest x-ray is not always necessary.

- Pulse oximetry is useful to confirm the need for admission.
- Chest x-rays are indicated when the diagnosis is uncertain or the patient is at high risk for complications.
- A sputum Gram stain and microscopic examination are useful to determine the specific etiology. It is difficult to get a good sample.
    - An adequate specimen has greater than 10 squamous cells per high-power field (HPF) and greater than 25 WBCs/HPF.
    - Visually examine the sputum for blood, color, thickness, or foul smell.

TIPS AND TRICKS:

   When collecting a sputum sample, coach the patient to produce sputum from the lungs, not spit from the mouth.

- When available, sputum cultures can be useful for high-risk patients or those with severe disease.
- Other potential (but rarely useful) studies:
  - Arterial blood gases: rarely available or needed. A-a gradient can be used if pulmonary embolism is suspected.
  - WBC count is nonspecific and is rarely needed.
  - Blood cultures: not indicated, rarely useful.

GENERAL TREATMENT Given the lack of available follow-up and available health resources, most patients should be hospitalized when diagnosed with pneumonia, especially high-risk patients. If the patient is to be treated as an outpatient, antibiotic therapy is generally indicated, even if you are suspicious that the cause is viral. General antibiotic recommendations are described as follows (see also specific organism-specific therapies below):

Outpatient/Oral Therapy

- Erythromycin is usually the most available and appropriate drug for commonly-acquired peneumonia.
- Clarithromycin (Biaxin) 500 mg PO twice daily or azithromycin 500 mg PO load then 250 mg every day for 10 days are better choices if available.
- Second- and third-generation cephalosporins (cefuroxime 250–500 mg PO twice daily, cefprozil 250 mg PO twice daily)
- Levofloxacin 500 mg PO twice daily is very useful in areas with high *S. pneumoniae* resistance to penicillin.

For hospitalized patients give

- Oxygen if hypoxic or respiratory rate is greater than 24 to 30 breaths/min in an adult.
- Antibiotics:
  - third-generation cephalosporin (cefotaxime 2 g IV every 4–8 hours, or ceftriaxone 2 g IV daily, or ceftazidime 2 g IV every 8 hours) or
  - azithromycin 500 mg IV daily
  - add erythromycin (to the cephalosporins) 4 to 5 mg/kg IV every 6 hours if the patient is very ill
- Fluids may be required if dehydrated.
- Treat fever, pain, and cough (acetaminophen and codeine are useful to treat all of these at once).
- All patients should be followed up in 1 to 3 days.

SPECIFIC PNEUMONIA ETIOLOGIES

STREPTOCOCCUS PNEUMONIAE

DEFINITION S. pneumoniae is a gram-positive diplococci and is the most common cause of community-acquired bacterial pneumonia.

CLINICAL PRESENTATION The classic presentation is the rapid onset of a high fever with a single rigor associated with a productive cough with rusty sputum and pleuritic chest pain.

DIAGNOSIS

- A Gram stain of the sputum demonstrates the gram-positive organism.
- If a chest x-ray is taken, it usually shows a single lobe infiltrate.
- Sputum culture is positive in only 50%, blood culture in 30%.

TREATMENT Penicillin resistance is increasing, but it is generally the drug of choice.

- Outpatient therapy
    - penicillin VK 500 mg every 6 hours for 10 to 14 days or
    - amoxicillin 250 to 500 mg PO every 8 hours
- Other therapies
    - erythromycin 500 mg every 6 hours or
    - clarithromycin 500 mg twice daily, or
    - cefuroxime axetil (Ceftin)
- Inpatient therapy
    - penicillin G 1.2 to 2.4 million units every 4 to 6 hours IV until afebrile, then penicillin 500 mg PO every 6 hours for 5 days

PREVENTION Pneumococcal vaccine is about 80% effective. It is recommended for elderly and postsplenectomy patients, as well as those with sickle cell anemia, cardiac disease, or chronic lung disease. It is contraindicated in pregnancy or for patients under 2 years of age.

STAPHYLOCOCCAL PNEUMONIA

DEFINITION This variety accounts for less than 1% of community-acquired pneumonia in the United States. It occurs after influenza or measles, as well as in debilitated patients and IV drug users.

CLINICAL PRESENTATION This infection is generally an acute disease but can be insidious in the elderly and debilitated. Symptoms include cough, rigors, shortness of breath, pleurisy, and fever.

DIAGNOSIS The sputum is often bloody and/or purulent.

- Gram stain of sputum shows gram-positive cocci in clumps.
- Chest x-ray shows patchy infiltrate progressing to necrotizing pneumonitis.

TREATMENT All patients require hospitalization. Antibiotics include

- Nafcillin/methicillin 2 g IV every 4 hours for 2 weeks (6 weeks if bacteremia is present)
- Vancomycin 500 mg every 6 hours as an alternative

HEMOPHILUS INFLUENZAE

DEFINITION This infection is common in patients with chronic obstructive pulmonary disease (COPD), as well as in smokers and debilitated, hospitalized, and nursing home patients.

CLINICAL PRESENTATION Little to differentiate it from other etiologies: fever, dyspnea, occasionally pleurisy, and rales.

DIAGNOSIS

- Gram stain often misses the gram-negative pleomorphic rod.
- Chest x-ray shows patchy alveolar infiltrate that is sometimes lobar.

TREATMENT

- Outpatient
    - Amoxicillin/ampicillin 500 mg PO every 6 hours for 10 to 14 days
    - Other therapies
        - ciprofloxacin 500 mg twice daily for 10 days or
        - TMP/SMX DS 1 tablet PO twice daily or
        - amoxicillin clavulanate, Ceclor
- Inpatient
    - Chloramphenicol 50 mg/kg/day divided every 6 hours IV
    - Cephalosporins
        - cefotaxime 1 g IV every 8 hours
        - ceftriaxone 1 to 2 g IV twice daily
        - cefuroxime 1 g IV every 8 hours

KLEBSIELLA PNEUMONIAE *AND OTHER GRAM-NEGATIVE PNEUMONIAS*

DEFINITION Klebsiella is an encapsulated gram-negative bacillus that occurs in pairs and is the most common gram-negative community-acquired pneumonia. It is common in patients with COPD, as well as in alcoholics, diabetics, and residents of hospitals and nursing homes. *E. coli, Pseudomonas, Enterobacter, Serratia,* and other gram-negative bacteria cause 10% of community-acquired pneumonia and 50% of all nosocomial pneumonia. The mortality rate from gram-negative pneumonia is 50%.

CLINICAL PRESENTATION The classic symptom for *Klebsiella pneumoniae* is "currant jelly" sputum (thick and bloody). Otherwise the symptoms are similar to those of other pneumonias.

DIAGNOSIS

■ The Gram stain results can be confused with those of *Pneumococcus* because the bacilli are short and fat.
■ The chest x-ray may demonstrate a necrotizing labor pneumonia with a bulging fissure sign.

TREATMENT Admit all patients because they are high risk. Antibiotics include the following:

■ Gentamicin 1 mg/kg IV every 8 hours with cefazolin 1 to 2 g IV every 6 hours.
■ Alternative drugs include second- or third-generation cephalosporins with gentamicin.
■ Alternative therapy includes a third-generation cephalosporin such as ceftazidime 1 g IV every 8 hours and an antipseudomonal, β-lactamase–susceptible penicillin such as carbenicillin, ticarcillin, or piperacillin.

LEGIONELLA

DEFINITION *Legionella* infection occurs in clusters of cases, has an unclear transmission mechanism, and may account for as much as 5% to 15% of community-acquired pneumonia. Individuals at risk include those with COPD, as well as debilitated patients, diabetics, the elderly, smokers, and alcoholics.

CLINICAL PRESENTATION In addition to symptoms of pneumonia, the patient often has

■ Nausea, vomiting, and diarrhea
■ Myalgias, malaise
■ Persistent fever
■ Hematuria
■ Progression to confusion and coma
■ Relative bradycardia

DIAGNOSIS

■ The sputum Gram stain does not demonstrate organisms.
■ The chest x-ray shows unilateral or bilateral patchy infiltrates progressing to frank consolidation.

TREATMENT All patients must be hospitalized.

Antibiotics

■ Erythromycin 1 g IV every 6 hours for 3 to 4 weeks.
■ Alternative drugs include rifampin 600 mg/day or azithromycin of levofloxacin IV.

MYCOPLASMAL PNEUMONIA

DEFINITION A common cause of community-acquired pneumonia, mycoplasmal pneumonia usually occurs in the young (3–30 years). Extrapulmonary disease such as myocarditis, pericarditis, hepatitis, hemolytic anemia, and meningitis or encephalitis can occur.

CLINICAL PRESENTATION The disease presents with a "viral" pattern including upper respiratory infection (rhinitis), cough, headache, fever, earache, and diarrhea. It also may present with wheezing. The generalized symptoms (fever, myalgias) resolve within 3 weeks, but cough may persist longer. The classic finding in the ear examination is bullous myringitis.

DIAGNOSIS

■ Results of the sputum Gram stain are negative.
■ The chest x-ray shows a diffuse reticulonodular pattern in both lower lobes. Chest x-ray findings are more impressive than physical examination findings. Effusions occur in 20%.

TREATMENT

Antibiotics

■ Erythromycin or tetracycline 500 mg PO every 6 hours
■ Alternative therapy: TMP/SMX DS 1 tablet PO twice daily, ciprofloxacin 500 mg PO every 6 hours, clarithromycin 500 mg twice daily, azithromycin 250 mg daily

TUBERCULOSIS

DEFINITION Tuberculosis is caused by *Mycobacterium tuberculosis*, an aerobic, acid-fast rod, transmitted by respiratory exposure. It causes the formation of granulomas in affected tissues. It most commonly presents as pulmonary, but as the organism spreads rapidly from the lung throughout most organs, a third of cases can have extrapulmonary findings, affecting any organ system.

Tuberculosis has made a tremendous comeback in developing and developed countries in the past decade, and the emergence of MDRTB is a major health threat worldwide. The onset of the AIDS epidemic has played a major role in this. Despite therapy, the mortality rate remains as high as 15%, and there is a 60% mortality rate with untreated TB, usually within 3 years. Patients with AIDS have a much more rapid and virulent course, and more than half present with extrapulmonary TB.

CLINICAL PRESENTATION The classic symptoms of TB include

- Cough lasting more than 3 weeks
- Weight loss
- Persistent fever
- Pleuritic chest pain
- Hemotysis as the infection progresses

Children may present with weight loss and intermittent fevers initially. TB presents in one of four ways:

1. Primary: The initial pulmonary infection with TB is usually asymptomatic, but may present with nonspecific pneumonia/bronchitis symptoms of cough and fever. The chest x-ray classically shows an apical infiltrate with hilar nodes.
2. Reactivation: The most classic presentation of low-grade fever, malaise, weight loss, and a chronic cough with hemoptysis. PPD is positive in 80%. The chest x-ray demonstrates an upper lobe scar or cavity with hilar nodes.
3. Miliary: A generalized TB infection characterized by a diffuse fine nodular pattern on chest x-ray. Many organ systems involved. The symptoms vary widely depending on the affected system. Some of the classic extrapulmonary presentations include
   - Scrofula: chronic lymphadenitis and swelling of the cervical nodes
   - Potts disease: TB of the mid-thoracic spine leading to collapse of the vertebral body and sharply angled kyphosis
   - Meningitis, particularly in children
4. Extrapulmonary: Occurs in 20% to 30% of cases. Common sites include joints, pericardium, peritoneum, meninges, kidney, and bone. Look for masses and prominent adenopathy.

DIAGNOSIS Tuberculosis bacilli can be found in the urine and other body fluids or tissues, but is most often found in the sputum. The Board of Health or Ministry of Health will often provide the staining and microscopic evaluation. There are many stains for TB, the most common being carbolfuchsin. The organism is a small, slender rod that is often curved and may be seen in pairs or clumps.

- Sputum. Proper sputum collection is essential because there are relatively few organisms. Collect at least three, but not more than five, specimens on different days. Alternative methods include early morning gastric aspiration and bronchoscopy. All specimens should be collected in a safe environment or outdoors away from other people.
- Specimens for microscopic examination also can be collected from granulomas located anywhere on the body.

- A chest x-ray is an important diagnostic tool. There are various presentations seen from pneumonia to signs of old infections. The healed primary lesion often leaves a calcified apical scar. If there is an associated calcified hilar node, it is call a Ghon complex. Active pulmonary TB often presents with upper lobe infiltrates, frequently with cavities. As the acute infection resolves, scarring and fibrotic changes occur, sometimes with calcifications and loss of volume in the upper lobes.
- The tuberculin skin test (PPD) is a useful screening tool in areas of low incidence, but it is more difficult to interpret the results in high-incidence areas and in tropical areas and where the bacillus Calmette-Guerin (BCG) vaccine is used. Consult with the local TB control program for recommendations of its use.
- Cultures are difficult and should be performed by a reference laboratory.

TREATMENT The key to treating TB is to ensure compliance with therapy. Directly observed therapy is recommended for all TB patients. This means working closely with the government's TB control program. Therapy usually include at least two drugs, generally these will be

- Isoniazid (INH) 300 mg PO daily with rifampin 600 mg PO daily for 6 to 12 months. Other combinations include INH with ethambutol (15 mg/kg daily) or INH and thioacetazone (150 mg daily). Streptomycin, ethambutol, or pyrazinamide (PZA) also may be used.
- For immunocompromised patients or if drug resistance is suspected, three to four drugs are used (INH, PZA, ethambutol, streptomycin) for 18 to 24 months.

> **KEY POINT:**
>
> Compliance with TB therapy is essential; use directly observed therapy whenever possible.

PREVENTION Tuberculosis is highly infectious.

- Respiratory isolation of the patient is mandatory. Patients and staff should wear well-fitting high-efficiency particulate filter (HEPA) masks.
- BCG vaccine given in infancy is moderately effective in preventing some forms of TB and may improve the immune response.
- Chemoprophylaxis with INH for 12 months is usually recommended for immunocompromised patients exposed to TB, family members of TB patients, and those under 35 years of age with a newly positive PPD reaction. Referral to a TB control program is essential.

INFLUENZA

DEFINITION Influenza is an acute respiratory illness caused by influenza viruses A and B. It is the most common cause of viral pneumonia in adults. It occurs seasonally in the winter, with worldwide epidemics every 10 years as major changes in the viral antigens occur. *Staphylococcus* is a common cause of postinfluenza pneumonia.

CLINICAL PRESENTATION Influenza, the "flu," is not a cold or diarrhea. Symptoms include

- Rapid onset of a high fever
- Myalgias
- Low-grade cough

DIAGNOSIS Diagnosis is usually made on the classic symptoms that occur in a number of cases during the flu season. The laboratory diagnosis of influenza is difficult and expensive.

TREATMENT The current therapies are generally too expensive for most persons. They are also not curative, but reduce the length and severity of the infection. The antivirals must be started within 48 hours of the onset of symptoms (amantadine or rimantadine 100 mg PO twice daily).

PREVENTION Prevention is the key. The vaccine is indicated for the elderly, those with chronic, particularly pulmonary diseases, and medical care personnel.

PNEUMOCYSTIS CARINII

DEFINITION *Pneumocystis carinii* is a protozoan parasite that infects only immuno-compromised patients (i.e., organ transplant recipients and those with AIDS). Person-to-person spread does not occur.

CLINICAL PRESENTATION Symptoms include the gradual onset of fever and cough with progressive dyspnea.

DIAGNOSIS Consider the diagnosis with any immunocompromised patient, particularly those with AIDS.

- Chest x-ray shows diffuse bilateral and symmetric hilar interstitial infiltrates, but may be normal initially.
- The definitive diagnosis is made by bronchoscopy or open lung biopsy.

TREATMENT

- Inpatient therapy
    - IV TMP/SMX is preferable, but PO is effective.
    - TMP 25 mg/kg/day with SMX 75 to 100 mg/kg/day or
    - pentamidine 4 mg/kg every day IV for 14 to 21 days or

- dapsone 100 mg/day and TMP 15 to 20 mg/kg/day divided every 6 hours also may be used
- Outpatient therapy
  - TMP/SMX DS 2 tablets PO twice daily is useful for mild cases
  - prednisone 40 mg twice daily tapered over a 21-day period in severe cases to decrease the inflammatory effects of *Pneumocystis carinii* pneumonia (PCP)
  - TMP/SMX DS 1 PO daily is useful for prophylaxis

GASTROINTESTINAL INFECTIONS

HEPATITIS There are literally dozens of causes of hepatitis, from infections, to toxins, to idiopathic causes. The difficulty for a clinician in an area with limited laboratory resources is to distinguish between the various causes. For infectious hepatitis the lengthy incubation period makes intervention during an outbreak difficult, so maintenance of sanitation is important. The elevations in aminotransferases and bilirubin are not predictive of disease severity or outcome and so are not needed when resources are scarce. Prothrombin time (PT) elevation is a better predictor of liver dysfunction and is a more appropriate test for severe cases.

HEPATITIS A

DEFINITION Hepatitis A is spread by fecal-oral transmission. It has a relatively low morbidity rate and rare mortality. It is ubiquitous throughout the developing world, with infection rates that approach 100% by 5 years of age in some areas.

CLINICAL PRESENTATION It is generally a mild disease, with the majority of patients essentially asymptomatic. Symptomatic patients have nausea and vomiting with icterus from hyperbilirubinemia.

DIAGNOSIS

Laboratory Diagnosis

- Aminotransferases (AST, ALT) are elevated, starting late in the incubation period. They will always be elevated if symptomatic.
- Elevated bilirubin; direct and indirect bilirubin will be approximately equal.
- The PT is the best indicator of liver dysfunction and prognosis.
- Serology will determine viral etiology; other causes also may need to be sought out.

TREATMENT Treatment is supportive. Patients are rarely admitted for IV hydration from gastrointestinal loss.

PREVENTION Prevention is primarily centered around maintaining adequate sanitation and clean water supplies, and avoiding close contact with carriers. For the health worker in the field, most water sterilization techniques do not prevent transmission of hepatitis A, but some viral water filters do. See the recommendations of the Centers for Disease Control and Prevention for hepatitis A vaccination.

HEPATITIS B

DEFINITION Hepatitis B is a major problem worldwide, with more than 2 billion people infected at some time in their lives, of which 350 million are chronic carriers. Hepatitis B causes over 1 million deaths annually from fulminant liver disease, cirrhosis of the liver, or primary hepatocellular cancer.

Countries are considered to have high, intermediate, or low hepatitis B virus (HBV) endemicity. Highly endemic areas are those where as much as 95% of the population has serologic evidence of previous HBV infection. In these countries infections usually occur during the perinatal period or childhood, and chronic carriers make up 5% to 20% of the population. High endemicity areas include Africa, eastern Asia, the Pacific Basin, the Amazon Basin, the Arctic Rim, the Asian Republics of the former Soviet Union, and portions of the Middle East, Asia Minor, and the Caribbean.

In intermediate and low countries, most infections occur in adults through sexual contact, injecting drug use, or occupational exposure to blood.

Hepatitis B virus is transmitted by human body fluids such as blood and serum. The incubation period for HBV is 30 to 180 days (mean 75). HBV infection leads to one of three outcomes: death from fulminant hepatitis acutely, recovery after the infection with lifelong immunity, or development of a persistent infection, the chronic carrier state. About one third of adults develop symptoms of hepatitis B with jaundice, and 6% to 10% become chronic HBV carriers. In highly endemic areas, infected newborns rarely develop symptoms of acute hepatitis, but almost all become HBV carriers. Young children rarely develop symptomatic HBV infection with jaundice, but are more likely to become carriers, with the chronic carrier state occurring in about 25% of those infected under the age of 7.

CLINICAL PRESENTATION The stages of a hepatitis infection are incubation, preicteric, icteric, convalescent, and chronic. Most cases are asymptomatic and do not involve jaundice. Initial symptoms include the following:

- A serum sickness–like prodrome develops, with myalgias and low-grade fevers during the preicteric phase.
- Gastrointestinal complaints include malaise, anorexia, nausea and vomiting, and right upper quadrant pain.
- During the icteric phase (1–4 weeks), dark urine and jaundice may develop.

The physical examination varies with the severity of the infection.

- Patients may be afebrile or have a low-grade fever.
- There may be a urticarial or macular/papular rash during the prodrome.

- Jaundice occurs 1 to 2 weeks after flulike illness (in blacks check the mucous membranes and conjunctiva).
- Hepatomegaly and/or splenomegaly develops with a right upper quadrant tenderness.
- Fulminant cases can present with encephalopathy.

DIAGNOSIS The diagnosis requires advanced laboratory capabilities that may not be readily available.

- PT is the best measure of the degree of liver dysfunction.
- Transaminases and bilirubin will be elevated.
- Hepatitis B surface antigen (HBsAg) increases before and during clinical hepatitis.
- Hepatitis B surface antibody (Anti-HBs) appears and HgsAg clears.
- Hepatitis B core antibody (Anti-HBc) is the antibody found during the "window" between HgsAg and anti-HBs.
- Hepatitis B e antigen (HBeAg) is indicative of a high degree of infectivity or chronic infection.

TREATMENT Supportive care and IV hydration if necessary for dehydration.

PREVENTION Vaccination with hepatitis B vaccine can prevent the disease and carrier state from developing. Given the increased severity of the disease in childhood, the vaccine has been incorporated into the routine infant immunization schedule in almost 100 countries. There is significant variation in the immunization recommendations for most countries, so it is important to understand the indications and schedule for your geographic area. The vaccines are highly protective in 90% to 97% of healthy individuals, including infants. Hepatitis B vaccines are extremely safe, with mild, transient local reactions the most common side effect.

> **KEY POINT:**
>
> All health-care workers must be fully immunized against HBV prior to working internationally.

Hepatitis B immune globulin (HBIG) also can be given to newborns of HBeAg-positive mothers to increase the efficacy of hepatitis B vaccine. But it is extremely expensive because of the cost of the vaccine ($25–$50 per child) and its use requires serologic testing of mothers to determine their HBsAg status.

HEPATITIS C

DEFINITION Hepatitis C virus (HCV) was previously commonly called non-A, non-B hepatitis and is the most common cause of posttransfusion hepatitis. A chronic infection state develops in 80% of those infected.

The WHO estimates that up to 3% of the world's population has been infected with HCV, and there may be more than 170 million chronic carriers. About 20% of patients with chronic infections develop cirrhosis, and 1%–5% of these develop primary hepatocellular carcinoma. Most patients with primary hepatocellular carcinoma have either hepatitis B or hepatitis C infection.

Hepatitis C is not as infectious as hepatitis B or HIV. Transmission occurs through blood transfusions, through the use of inadequately sterilized equipment, or through injecting drug use with shared needles. Sexual and perinatal transmission also may occur, although less frequently.

CLINICAL PRESENTATION The incubation period is 15 to 150 days. The vast majority of cases (up to 90%) are asymptomatic, but when symptoms are present they include fatigue and jaundice.

DIAGNOSIS Differentiating the various types of hepatitis requires advanced serologic testing, often not available. The presence of HCV-RNA indicates an active infection and a potential for the development of chronic liver disease.

TREATMENT There is little practical treatment available in developing countries because of the high cost and limited efficacy. Treatment with interferon is effective in only about 20% of patients.

PREVENTION Measures to prevent HCV infection include the screening of blood products, universal precautions, destroying disposable needles, and adequate sterilization of reusable surgical and dental instruments. There is no effective vaccine against HCV.

DIARRHEA

DEFINITION Diarrhea is a ubiquitous disease and one of the leading causes of death in children globally. Diarrhea is a symptom, not a disease, and has many causes, from infectious, to metabolic, to toxic. Diarrhea can be described as being invasive, infectious, or toxigenic.

CLINICAL PRESENTATION Symptoms include loose or watery stools more than three to five times daily. Dysentery (invasive diarrhea) usually presents with bloody stools, fever, and abdominal cramping.

The purpose of the physical examination is to determine if the patient requires hospitalization, antibiotics, fluids, or other therapy. The rectal examination is a simple study that provides important information for diagnosing and treating diarrheal disease, such as the presence of blood, mucus, and WBCs.

DIAGNOSIS Determining the cause of diarrheal illnesses may be aided by microscopic stool examination for fecal WBCs, which correlates with positive stool cultures in 85% to 90% of cases. Examination for ova and parasites is also helpful. Stool cultures, if available, are useful for determining the etiology of resistant forms of diarrhea.

TREATMENT The WHO offers excellent treatment guidelines that are generally readily available in most countries (Table 8-4). Most treatment is focused on the prevention of dehydration.

- For most diarrheas oral rehydration is sufficient. The key is small amounts frequently. In young children this means 5 to 10 mL every few minutes. Use fluids that contain sugar and salts (oral rehydration fluids, oral rehydration salts (ORS) etc). Homemade soup (sugar, fluid, salt) or other sugar-containing fluids work well, but avoid fluids with a high osmolality such as soda pop. Use D5W-0.9 Normal Saline (D5/0.9NS) for IV fluids.
- Specific treatment may include antiemetics for those unable to tolerate PO fluids (prochlorperazine).
- Antidiarrheal agents such as kaolin-pectin or bismuth subsalicylate (Pepto-Bismol) are not effective even at high doses.
- Antimotility agents such as loperamide (Imodium) and diphenoxylate HCl-atropine (Lomotil) may be used in toxigenic diarrheas but should generally be avoided in most infectious diarrheas.
- Empirical use of antibiotics is not indicated in toxigenic diarrhea; only infectious diarrhea should be treated empirically with antibiotics.
  - TMP\SMX DS 1 tablet PO twice daily; 5 to 7 days of treatment is usually sufficient.
  - Alternatives include ciprofloxacin 500 mg PO or norfloxacin 400 mg PO or ofloxacin 300 mg PO twice daily for 3 days.

The specific etiologies vary between region and country, but include the following:

CHOLERA (VIBRIO CHOLERAE) Cholera reestablished itself throughout the world in the late 1980s and is now endemic in most tropical regions. It is associated with profuse "rice water" diarrhea and massive fluid losses.

TABLE 8-4 GUIDELINES FOR PRESUMPTIVE TREATMENT OF DIARRHEA

Treat mild to moderate dehydration with oral rehydration solution (ORS).

Treat severe dehydration with intravenous (IV) fluid (0.9 NS or LR) or nasogastric tube (if trained).

After initial treatment
  Assess for ability to take ORS.
  Reassess after 6 hours of therapy the need for continued IV fluid vs ORS.

Antibiotics should only be used for dysentery and for suspected cholera with severe dehydration.

Antiparasitic drugs should only be used for Amoeabiasis, giardiasis or resistant shigella (with bloody stool).

Treatment Fluid replacement (IV or PO) is the mainstay of therapy. Measure the stool output and replace the same amount. Use IV normal saline (NS) or lactated Ringer's solution (LR).

Antibiotics shorten the course of the illness and reduce fluid losses:

- Ciprofloxacin 1 g PO single dose or
- Norfloxacin 400 mg PO twice daily for 3 days or
- Doxycycline 300 mg PO single dose or
- TMP/SMX or erythromycin

CAMPYLOBACTER *Campylobacter* is a common cause of infectious diarrhea, especially in those exposed to animals, birds, and poultry.

SALMONELLA *Salmonella* is associated with eggs, turkeys, unpasteurized milk, and animals, especially dogs and cats.

SHIGELLA *Shigella* is a common cause of bloody diarrhea, and is spread easily. *Shigella* should be treated with antibiotics even if the patient is asymptomatic when cultures return.

ENTEROHEMORRHAGIC ESCHERICHIA COLI *0157:H7* Enterohemorrhagic *Escherichia coli* 0157:H7 is a common cause of diarrhea in developing countries, and is associated with nursing homes, travel to Mexico, and food poisoning. It causes bloody diarrhea. Hemolytic-uremic syndrome and thrombotic thrombocytopenic purpura (TTP) are serious complications.

ROTAVIRUS Rotavirus is the most common cause of diarrhea in children, and leads to protracted watery diarrhea. There is now a vaccine for rotavirus for children, although it is generally too expensive for developing countries.

YERSINIA ENTEROCOLITICA *Yersinia enterocolitica* can produce an appendicitis-like picture, with focal abdominal pain and fever.

GIARDIASIS Symptoms vary widely from none to intermittent malodorous diarrhea to acute diarrhea with abdominal pain and fever. Treat with metronidazole 250 mg PO every 8 hours for 5 days or a similar agent.

AMEBIASIS Amebiasis occurs commonly in travelers and is transmitted by contaminated water. Acute illness includes malodorous diarrhea associated with abdominal pain and fever. The course may be prolonged, with intermittent symptoms. There is also a carrier state, especially in immunocompromised patients. Treat with metronidazole 750 mg PO every 8 hours for 10 days followed by iodoquinol 650 mg PO every 8 hours for 20 days or paromomycin 500 mg PO every 8 hours for 7 days.

ANTIBIOTIC-ASSOCIATED COLITIS (PSEUDOMEMBRANOUS COLITIS) This colitis is caused by *Clostridium difficile* overgrowth in the gut after antibiotic use. It is most common after broad-spectrum antibiotic use, particularly those active against anaerobes, such as clindamycin, ampicillin, or cephalosporins. Treat with oral metronidazole 500 mg PO for 10 to 14 days or vancomycin 125 mg PO every 6 hours (IV antibiotics do not work).

"TRAVELERS' DIARRHEA" Diarrhea affects 25% to 50% of travelers to developing countries. It is caused by ingesting fecally contaminated food or beverages, even transmitted by ice. Enterotoxic strains of *Escherichia coli* are the most common cause. For short trips where a diarrheal illness cannot be tolerated, prophylaxis with short-course ciprofloxacin (500 mg PO every day) is advised.

Prevention

- Cleanliness: Wash your hands, and teach patients to wash theirs.
- "Peel it, boil it, cook it, or forget it" (doesn't always work).
- Prophylactic non–antimicrobial agents such as bismuth subsalicylate (Pepto-Bismol): Requires very high continuous doses.
- Prophylactic use of antibiotics (begin the day before travel and continue until 2 days after returning home):
  - Ciprofloxacin 250 to 500 mg PO daily
  - Doxycycline 100 mg PO daily
  - TMP/SMX DS 160 mg/800 mg PO daily

The antiperistaltic agents diphenoxylate and loperamide are not effective and may actually increase the incidence of diarrhea.

GENITOURINARY INFECTIONS

URINARY TRACT INFECTIONS

DEFINITION There are two major types of urinary tract infections: lower (cystitis or bladder) and upper (pyelonephritis or kidney). Urinary tract infections are usually caused by local (rectal/gastrointestinal) bacteria, most commonly *E. coli* (80%–90%). Females are anatomically at risk due to a short urethra in proximity to the anus.

Risks for developing a urinary tract infection include

- Sexual activity
- Pregnancy
- Urethral instrumentation or catheterization (a single catheterization = 1%–3% infection rate, up to 15% in pregnant and debilitated patients)
- Persons with urinary tract abnormalities (prostate hypertrophy)

Patients at high risk for complications are similar for any infection:

- Demographic groups include pregnant women, children, and the poor
- Hospitalized patients
- History of urethral catheterization

- History of neurogenic bladder
- Immunocompromised (diabetes, sickle cell disease, chronic renal failure, cancer, etc.)
- Anatomic abnormality or kidney stone
- A complicated urinary history, including
    - History of previous urinary tract infection
    - History of pyelonephritis
    - Three urinary tract infections in preceding 12 months
    - Recent (<30 days) antibiotics
    - History of relapsing urinary tract infections
    - History of urinary tract infection before 12 years of age
    - Urinary tract infection symptoms for more than 7 days

Pregnant women are at extreme risk for complications with a urinary tract infection and should all be hospitalized for treatment.

CLINICAL PRESENTATION Classic symptoms for cystitis are

- Dysuria
- Urgency
- Frequency of urination
- Blood in the urine (hemorrhagic cystitis)

Pyelonephritis (kidney infection) may result from an asymptomatic urinary tract infection. Common symptoms include

- Fever
- Flank, back, and/or abdominal pain
- Dysuria
- Frequency
- Urgency

The physical examination is important to rule out other intraabdominal processes [appendicitis, pelvic inflammatory disease (PID), others].

- Costovertebral angle tenderness is typical with pyelonephritis.
- A palpable kidney implies an anatomic abnormality or abscess and mandates admission.
- A palpable bladder (must be >150 cm³ in adults) is significant for urinary retention and the need for admission.
- A genital examination is especially needed for males to assess for sexually transmitted diseases (STDs) and urethritis.
- A rectal examination is also indicated for all males to assess for prostatitis.

DIAGNOSIS The most useful laboratory study is a microscopic urinalysis. The first void of the day is the most accurate—collect in mid-stream, clean catch. It must be examined within 1 hour, or the test will be inaccurate. Optimally the sample is centrifuged for 5 minutes at 2,000 rpm, but it also may be examined directly. The sediment is examined, then stained.

- If pyuria is noted (5–10 WBCs/HPF) or any WBCs are present in a symptomatic patient, treat for urinary tract infection.
- Dipstick urinalysis: Blood in the urine (a nonmenstruating female or male) is highly suggestive of a urinary tract infection.
- If the pH is above 8.0, think proteus.
- Nitrite is not very sensitive (urine needs to be in the bladder for 6 hours), but the leukocyte esterase has a sensitivity of 74% to 96% and a specificity 94% to 98%. If either are positive, then treat.
- Urine cultures are rarely indicated, except in the most complicated cases. The classic definition of a positive culture was greater than 100,000 colony-forming units (CFU)/mL. Now with urinary tract infection symptoms in females, a culture with greater than 100 CFU/mL for a known uropathogen is considered positive.

TREATMENT

Acute Cystitis A 3- or 7-day course of antibiotics can be used. Three days is sufficient for the most simple cases in a patient with no risk factors, but in the developing world 7 days may be safer. For sexually active males it is more likely that the symptoms of a urinary tract infection are actually an STD. Examine and question men carefully and consider empiric treatment for gonorrhea and chlamydia.

- Antibiotics: TMP/SMX DS 1 tablet PO twice daily for 7 days (a 3-day course may be used for the most simple infections and reliable patients.
- Alternatives include nitrofurantoin and quinolones. There is significant resistance to ampicillin, but it is still an acceptable preliminary choice for pregnant women.

Acute Pyelonephritis Most patients should be hospitalized for at least the first day for IV therapy, unless they are otherwise healthy and have readily available follow-up. Antibiotics are generally the same as those for cystitis, but the total course should be 10 to 14 days.

Initial IV antibiotics include aminoglycosides combined with penicillin [gentamicin 100 mg (1–1.5 mg/kg)] IV every 8 hours and ampicillin 1 g IV every 6 hours. Patients can be started on oral therapy when they are afebrile.

Admission criteria for acute pyelonephritis:

- High risk for a complicated infection (see above)
- Clinical toxicity
- Inability to take oral antibiotics

- All children under 6 months of age
- Inability to follow up

SEXUALLY TRANSMITTED DISEASES

Sexually transmitted diseases are a major problem globally, particularly in the Americas, Southeast and South Asia, and Africa. With the international devastation caused by AIDS, the prevention of all STDs has become increasingly important. Patients should be taught to use condoms or to abstain from sex. Partners should always be empirically treated.

> **KEY POINT:**
>
> Definitive diagnostic studies are often not available. Treat sexually transmitted diseases based on symptoms and suspicions.

GONORRHEA

DEFINITION Gonococcal infections are caused by the gram-negative diplococci *Neisseria gonorrhoeae* and affect the genitals, rectum, pharynx, and eyes. If untreated, the infection may cause PID (salpingitis) in women, or become disseminated, leading to perihepatitis (Fitz-Hugh Curtis syndrome), bacteremia, meningitis, or endocarditis. Transmission is usually by genital contact, but is is also transmitted congenitally or even from hands to eyes. The incubation period is 2 to 7 days. The incidence of gonorrhea is highest in young adults, especially men, and peaks at 20 to 24 years in men and 18 to 24 in women.

CLINICAL PRESENTATION

- Males are almost always symptomatic with gonorrhea urethritis, presenting with urethral discharge and dysuria.
- Females with gonorrhea cervicitis are often asymptomatic or may have nonspecific vaginal and/or urethral irritation or dysuria.
- Gonorrhea pharyngitis is usually asymptomatic and has a spontaneous remission after 10 to 12 weeks. Consider this with resistant pharyngitis infections.
- Gonorrhea conjunctivitis usually occurs with a current urethral infection and is spread by the hand to the eyes. Symptoms are typical for conjunctivitis, with mucopurulent discharge, tearing, and a foreign body sensation. If gonorrhea is suspected, the best diagnostic technique is the Gram stain of the exudate (gram-negative diplococci).

DIAGNOSIS

- In a male the penis can be "milked" to express the discharge for a Gram stain. The Gram stain will demonstrate gram-negative intracellular diplococci.
- There are also many rapid tests available.

■ The gold standard is a culture (especially for females because the normal vaginal flora make a Gram stain less accurate).

TREATMENT In areas of high endemicity, treat for gonorrhea and chlamydia on suspicion or history. The key is to prevent the complications in females and to reduce transmission. To ensure compliance and reduce resistance, use single-dose therapy when possible. In general, gonorrhea is resistant to penicillin globally.

For genital, throat, rectal, and ocular infections, use single-dose therapy with either

■ Ciprofloxacin 500 mg PO or
■ Ceftriaxone (Rocephin) 250 mg IM or
■ Cefixime (Suprax) 400 mg PO or
■ Spectinomycin 2 g IM

KEY POINT:

When treating for suspected gonorrhea, treat for chlamydia also (azithromycin, doxycycline).

Hospitalize all patients with a suspected disseminated gonococcal infection (DGI). With a purulent arthritis/synovitis, elevate and immobilize the affected joint. Antibiotic therapy includes

■ Ceftriaxone 1 g IM or IV every 24 hours for 7 days or
■ Ceftizoxime 1 g IV every 8 hours for 7 days or
■ Cefotaxime 1 g IV every 8 hours for 7 days
■ If allergic, then spectinomycin 2 g IM every 12 hours for 7 days

Reliable patients can be discharged after 24 to 48 hours and treated with PO ciprofloxacin 250 mg twice daily or cefuroxime 250 to 500 twice daily.

DISSEMINATED GONOCOCCAL INFECTIONS Untreated genital gonorrhea can lead to a DGI. Women, especially pregnant women, are more commonly affected than men, probably because their initial infection is asymptomatic (and untreated). A coinfection with chlamydia is very common (treat for both).

CLINICAL PRESENTATION Arthritis and rash are the most common symptoms of DGI and occur 3 weeks after the genital symptoms (only 50%–85% of males and 30%–50% of females will recall any genitourinary symptoms). The arthritis begins as a migratory polyarthritis and/or tenosynovitis and then the inflammation settles into a single joint in about 70% of patients. The wrist, knees, and hands are most commonly affected.

> **KEY POINT:**
>
> Most cases of septic arthritis in young, sexually active adults are due to gonorrhea, especially if the wrists, knees, or hands are affected.

- About 40% of patient with DGI develop a painful, usually petechial, rash. The rash also may present as papular or even necrotic. There are usually 10 to 15 widely scattered lesions on the distal limbs, including the palms and soles.
- Meningitis and endocarditis are uncommon, but the endocarditis causes a rapid destruction of valves and should be suspected in patients with a new murmur with the associated symptoms of DGI.

PELVIC INFLAMMATORY DISEASE Approximately 15% of women with untreated gonorrhea cervicitis progress to PID. Chlamydia and other flora are also causes. Symptoms range from chronic pelvic pain to an acutely tender "surgical" abdomen and fever. Onset is often during or immediately after menstruation. Findings usually include marked cervical motion tenderness, a fever greater than 38°C, and a leukocytosis greater than 20,000/mL. Treatment is usually IV antibiotics except for the most simple cases.

SYPHILIS

DEFINITION Syphilis is caused by the spirochete *Treponema pallidum*. Transmission is usually by sexual contact through mucous membranes, but it also can be passed from mother to child congenitally. The incubation period is 10 days to 10 weeks (average 3 weeks). Syphilis chancres are associated with an increased risk of contracting HIV infection. There are other forms of syphilis infections, including a nonsexually transmitted *T. pallidum* infection among infants in Africa called endemic syphilis as well as pinta, yaws, and bejel.

CLINICAL PRESENTATION The signs and symptoms vary by the three clinical phases of syphilis infections:

- Primary: At about 3 weeks after exposure, a painless ulcer with serous exudate and an erythematous, raised margin appears. The chancre occurs at the site of the initial infection but is often intravaginal and hard to find in females.
- Secondary (approximately 6 weeks): The lesions of this stage affect many systems and present in many forms, including a rash and condyloma lata.
    - The rash is usually a diffuse, symmetrical, nonpruritic erythema associated with painless lymphadenopathy. It occurs on the trunk and limbs but its presence on the palms, soles, and face is highly suspicious for syphilis.
    - Condyloma lata are large gray or pinkish plaques that occur in warm, moist areas of the body (perineum, perianal area, axillae). They are highly contagious.

- Patients also may develop alopecia, mucous patches, laryngitis, uveitis, hepatitis, and nephrotic syndromes.
- Tertiary (months to years after exposure): Tertiary syphilis is a result of inflammation of many different organs. Patients may have recurrent rashes with progressive CNS and cerebrovascular damage.
  - The most benign form of tertiary syphilis is composed of skin lesions called gummas. They are usually single granulomatous/ulcerative lesions with necrotic centers. They then develop a hypopigmented central atrophic area surrounded by hyperpigmentation. Lesions occur on the face, legs, buttocks, trunk, and scalp, but also may occur on the mucous membranes, preferentially on the palate, nose, and pharynx.
  - Visceral syphilis results from gummas on internal organs, including the liver, eyes, lungs, stomach, and testes.
  - Neurosyphilis is initially asymptomatic, with an elevated cell count and protein in the cerebrospinal fluid (CSF). When symptoms develop, they range from peripheral neurologic symptoms such as tabes dorsalis (sensory changes, ataxia, muscle hypotonia, etc.), to encephalopathy.
  - Cardiovascular syphilis: The ascending aorta is most often affected. The chronic vasculitis leads to aortitis, aortic regurgitation, coronary ostial stenosis, and eventually an aortic aneurysm. Patients present with symptoms related to this pathology from heart failure, to myocardial infarction, to a dissection. Antibiotic treatment arrests the progress of the disease but cannot repair existing aortic damage.

DIAGNOSIS

- Primary syphilis is diagnosed by dark-field or phase microscopy of discharge from the base of the chancres.
- Serologic studies include the rapid plasma reagin (RPR) and Venereal Disease Research Laboratory (VDRL) tests. There are many causes of false-positive results. The RPR is a good screening test but cannot distinguish an acute from chronic infection. The VDRL can estimate infection acuity. The fluorescent treponemal antibody-absorption (FTA-ABS) test is more specific (so decreases false-positive results) and the most sensitive test available.

TREATMENT

- Primary: Benzathine penicillin 2.4 million units IM (single dose) or doxycycline or erythromycin PO.
- Secondary and tertiary: Benzathine penicillin G 2.4 million units IM each week for 3 weeks, or 250 mg tetracycline or erythromycin PO every 6 hours for 30 days.

PREVENTION Condom use or abstinence is advised. Screening pregnant females with a VDRL test is important to prevent the devastating sequelae of congenital syphilis. At the least, a careful prenatal vaginal examination is important.

CHLAMYDIA Chlamydia trachomatis is an obligate intracellular parasite/bacteria. There are two different types of genital infections caused by *Chlamydia trachomatis:* urethritis/vaginitis and lymphogranuloma venereum (LGV). Additional infections include ophthalmologic and systemic infections such as Reiter disease and perihepatitis.

CHLAMYDIAL URETHRITIS/VAGINITIS

DEFINITION Sexually transmitted chlamydia infections are more common than previously thought. They are often asymptomatic, and chlamydia may be the leading cause of PID and perihepatitis.

CLINICAL FINDINGS Patients are usually asymptomatic and have no physical findings. Even males may experience only a mild dysuria without discharge (think chlamydia or other STD when sexually active males complain of dysuria). There are rare physical findings in males. On examination, women usually have a mild cervicitis with mucopurulent discharge, erythema, and hypertrophic lesions.

DIAGNOSIS Culture or rapid enzyme tests

TREATMENT Because diagnostic studies are usually unavailable, treat on suspicion. Treat all cases of gonorrhea for chlamydia also.

- Azithromycin 2 g PO once (single dose = higher compliance) or
- Tetracycline 500 mg PO every 6 hours for 10 days or
- Doxycycline 100 mg PO twice daily for 10 days or
- Erythromycin 500 mg PO every 6 hours for 10 days

LYMPHOGRANULOMA VENEREUM

DEFINITION Lymphogranuloma venereum is an STD that occurs throughout the world, but it is most common in subtropical Africa and Southeast Asia. It occurs more often in males (80%), especially homosexuals. Transmission is by contact with the infectious lesions. The incubation period is 1 to 3 weeks.

CLINICAL PRESENTATION Lymphogranuloma venereum causes a slow-growing lesion that starts as a painless genital ulcer or papule. The traditional findings include the following:

- Fluctuant, draining, painful, usually unilateral lymphadenopathy (buboes) is featured, associated with fever, chills, and malaise.
- About 25% of patients have a transient primary vesicle or ulcer at the site of the inoculation (genitalia).
- The lymph nodes eventually become matted (buboes), fluctuant, and finally necrotic, with 75% forming draining sinus tracts.

■ In women the affected lymph nodes may be internal (iliac and sacral), so that there are fewer external signs of the disease. Lesions may be present in the vaginal vault, or there may just be a mild cervicitis with purulent discharge from the os. Backache and adnexal tenderness may develop from the pressure of the retro-peritoneal nodes.

DIAGNOSIS Careful history taking for possible exposures is important, especially for women.

■ A Gram stain of a sample from the lesion will demonstrate lymphocytes with intracellular inclusion bodies.
■ Serologic studies exist, but they may not be available.
■ Culture is difficult and not commonly used.

TREATMENT

■ Tetracycline 500 mg PO every 6 hours for 10 to 14 days or
■ Erythromycin 500 mg PO every 6 hours for 10 to 14 days (or longer if lesions do not resolve)
■ Needle aspiration of fluctuant buboes to prevent the formation of sinus tracts (incision and drainage are not necessary)

NEONATAL CHLAMYDIA OPHTHALMIA

DEFINITION Neonatal chlamydia ophthalmia is a congenitally transmitted infection secondary to maternal genital chlamydia infection. The incubation period is 1 to 40 days (usually 5–14).

CLINICAL PRESENTATION Newborns present with acute papillary conjunctivitis with swollen and erythematous eyelids with profuse mucopurulent discharge. If the infection remains untreated, a pseudomembrane, follicles, and scarring may develop.

DIAGNOSIS The diagnosis is made by visualizing chlamydial inclusion bodies in microscopic examination of conjunctival scrapings.

TREATMENT Treatment can be with topical or oral antibiotics.

■ Tetracycline or erythromycin eye ointment every 8 hours for 5 to 6 weeks—there is a high incidence of treatment failures due to the difficulty of applying ointment to the eyes of neonates.
■ Systemic therapy with PO erythromycin for 3 weeks is highly effective.

The infection often can be prevented with topical ocular antibiotics and silver nitrate solution applied at birth.

ADULT CHLAMYDIAL OPHTHALMIA

DEFINITION Adult chlamydial ophthalmia occurs in adults with active genital infections and is transmitted from the genitals by hand. It may present as an acute or subacute infection with an incubation period of 1 to 2 weeks.

CLINICAL PRESENTATION Patients present with watery or mucopurulent discharge with lid edema and erythema. The patient may experience slight photophobia and a foreign body sensation.

The conjunctiva is most severely infected, particularly the fornices and lower lid. Clinical diagnosis is based on the numerous large follicles found subtarsally and in the fornices. The cornea is occasionally affected, and a fluorescein stain may reveal a fine punctate keratitis. If untreated, a punctate keratoconjunctivitis can lead to opaque corneal infiltrates.

DIAGNOSIS Laboratory diagnosis involves advanced studies often not available in rural areas of developing countries.

TREATMENT The treatment is the same as for neonatal infections and can be either:

- Topical erythromycin or tetracycline ointment every 8 hours for 5 weeks or
- Tetracycline or doxycycline PO for 7 to 14 days, which should always be used because the eye infection is associated with a genital infection

CHANCROID

DEFINITION Chancroid is caused by *Hemophilus ducreyi,* a pleomorphic, gram-negative rod. It causes a localized infection with no systemic complications. Most common in Southeast Asia and sub-Saharan Africa, it also occurs in the Americas, Europe, and Australia. Transmission is by direct contact with infectious lesions. The organism invades through disrupted dermis. The incubation period is 3 to 14 days.

CLINICAL PRESENTATION Chancroid initially develops as a pustule that ruptures and becomes a painful necrotic ulcer or suppurative inguinal adenopathy. The ulcer edges are usually soft, in contrast to the firm edges of a syphilitic ulcer. In women the lesion commonly involves the labia minora and may occur on the thighs, but cervical lesions are rare. Painful inguinal adenopathy occurs in 50% to 70% of cases, and about 30% to 50% develop into buboes. Also unlike syphilis, secondary infections at the ulcer site are common, but systemic symptoms do not occur.

DIAGNOSIS

- Gram stain: The bacteria can be identified in 50% of smears from edges of the lesion, but suprainfective bacteria of similar morphology lowers the specificity of the test.

■ Culture is the definitive diagnostic test, but very difficult to do, requiring special medium.

TREATMENT Treat until the lesions are gone.

■ Single-dose ceftriaxone (250 mg IM) or
■ Azithromycin (1 g PO) or
■ Erythromycin 250 to 500 mg PO every 6 hours for 7 to 10 days or
■ TMP/SMX (Bactrim) DS twice daily for 7 to 10 days or
■ Ciprofloxacin PO for 3 days

TRICHOMONIASIS

DEFINITION The causative organism is *Trichomonas vaginalis,* a protozoan. It causes a localized, usually symptomatic infection of the vagina. It most commonly infects sexually active females, but it is also found in elderly women, nonsexually active women, and even neonates. Males are rarely symptomatic. The incubation period is 4 to 20 days.

CLINICAL PRESENTATION Many women are asymptomatic carriers. Symptoms include

■ A characteristic yellow, foamy, malodorous vaginal discharge
■ Vaginal pain and pruritus
■ Dysuria
■ Dyspareunia

Physical findings may include multiple small erythematous areas on the cervix and vagina (strawberry patches) as well as local vulvular edema. The vaginal pH is more alkaline (pH 5–8) than the normal pH of 4 to 5.

DIAGNOSIS The best diagnostic method is the immediate wet (normal saline) prep examination of the discharge. Vaginal secretions are mixed with a drop of NS and immediately observed under light microscopy (or preferably dark-field microscopy). This demonstrates the motile organisms moving through the solution. Cultures are also available but require a special medium.

TREATMENT

■ Metronidazole (Flagyl) 2 g PO single dose or
■ Metronidazole 500 mg PO per day for 7 days

Sexual partners also should be treated. If the treatment is unsuccessful, a second 7-day course should be used. During pregnancy metronidazole is contraindicated during the first trimester; its safety is unknown later in pregnancy. Mildly symptomatic infections should not be treated or only with betadine douches.

HERPES PROGENITALIS (HERPES SIMPLEX VIRUS TYPE 2)

DEFINITION Genital herpes is caused by herpes simplex virus (HSV) type 2 and occasionally HSV type 1 (usually causes oral lesions). Transmission is by direct contact with lesions (sexual) or is congenital. The incubation period is 2 to 12 days.

CLINICAL PRESENTATION The primary infection with herpes is often accompanied by systemic symptoms such as fever and malaise. Primary infection occasionally presents with diffuse skin lesions and even encephalitis. Patients can continue to have recurrent, intermittent (secondary) infections.

PHYSICAL FINDINGS

- Multiple painful, clustered vesicles that lead to shallow ulcers occur at the site of the original inoculation.
- Inguinal adenopathy.

In males the lesions usually occur on the glans, coronal sulcus, or penile shaft. In females the lesions are usually labial and intravaginal.

Encephalitis usually occurs with the primary infection and is particularly serious in the neonate. The patient presents with headaches and fevers of 40° to 41°C, which are resistant to antipyretics. Personality changes may precede changes in mental status, seizure, and coma. The mortality rate is greater than 60%, with the survivors often suffering from severe neurologic sequelae.

DIAGNOSIS The physical finding of multiple, painful genital ulcers/vesicles is the key.

- A Tzank smear of lesions demonstrating multinucleated (giant) ballooning epithelial cells also may be used.
- Encephalitis is diagnosed by lumbar puncture, which demonstrates a leukocytosis, increased protein, and a normal glucose.

TREATMENT There is no known cure for herpes infection, but some treatments are effective for suppressing the recurrence of the virus. However, the therapies are very expensive.

- Genital: acyclovir 200 mg PO five times daily for 7 to 10 days or vidarabine
- Rectal: acyclovir 400 mg PO five times daily for 10 days or until lesions are resolved
- Severe infections and encephalitis: acyclovir 5 mg/kg IV every 8 hours for 5 to 7 days

GRANULOMA INGUINALE (DONOVANOSIS)

DEFINITION The causative organism is *Calymmatobacterium granulomatis.* Granuloma inguinale is a slowly progressing granulomatous disease of the inguinal and anal-genital region that can cause massive local tissue destruction and may predispose to cancer. It is endemic in areas of the South Pacific, the Caribbean, and southern India, but rare elsewhere.

Males are more commonly affected than females and it is increased in dark-skinned races and in people of lower socioeconomic status. It is difficult to transmit, but it is thought to be conveyed by repeated direct contact.

CLINICAL PRESENTATION Initially small nodules or papules slowly spread by direct invasion into large ulcerative or granulomatous lesions on the genitalia and into the moist inguinal folds. There are no systemic symptoms unless a secondary infection develops. Patients may present with huge lesions with much local tissue destruction.

DIAGNOSIS

- Stained preparations of the lesions reveal intracellular organisms, particularly in the cytoplasm of histocytes (Donovan bodies).
- No cultures or serologic studies are available.

TREATMENT

- Tetracycline 500 mg PO every 6 hours for 15 days or
- Streptomycin or
- Chloramphenicol or
- TMP-SMX DS 1 tablet PO twice daily

Longer treatment is necessary for slowly healing lesions. Relapses are common due to inadequate therapy. Treatment of secondary infections also may be necessary (cephalexin or erythromycin).

NEUROLOGIC INFECTIONS

MENINGITIS

KEY POINT:

Treat immediately on suspicion of meningitis—never delay for definitive studies. Treatment must cover *Streptococcus, Hemophilus,* and *Neisseria.*

DEFINITION Meningitis occurs globally, but its infection pattern varies greatly. In temperate regions the disease is endemic, with a continuous but small number of cases. In the "meningitis belt" of sub-Saharan Africa, however, there is a seasonal pattern, with increasing incidence from the end of the dry season to the onset of the rains as well as an epidemic pattern with large 2- to 3-year outbreaks occurring every 8 to 12 years. These epidemics increased dramatically in the 1990s. The countries most commonly affected include Burkina Faso, Mali, Niger, and Nigeria. Other affected countries include Cameroon and Chad. Epidemic meningitis also occurs in South America and China.

Meningitis is most commonly caused by *Streptococcus, Hemophilus influenzae,* and *Meningococcus.* In temperate countries the most common cause is *Streptococcus pneumoniae* in adults and *H. influenzae* in newborns, infants, and children. In sub-Saharan Africa, *Neisseria meningitidis* is the most common cause. *N. meningitidis* is a gram-negative diplococcus that lives in the nasopharynx of humans. Infections are most common in children 6 months to 3 years of age.

The mortality rate of untreated bacterial meningitis is greater than 90%, but if promptly treated it is less than 20%. Of the survivors, 15% to 20% will suffer with neurologic sequelae such as deafness and mental retardation. The focus of this discussion will be on *N. meningitidis,* but all treatment for meningitis should include coverage for the other common organisms.

Transmission is by direct contact, most commonly from droplets from the noses and throats of infected persons. Colonization of the nasopharynx leads to local invasion and bacteremia (meningococcemia), and then the bacteria seed the meninges (meningitis). Most infections are subclinical, with up to 40% of patients having meningococcemia without meningitis. The incubation period ranges from 2 to 10 days, most commonly 3 to 4 days.

CLINICAL PRESENTATION Initial symptoms are similar to those of an upper respiratory infection and pharyngitis. This is followed by more specific symptoms:

- Headache
- Fever and chills
- Myalgia, arthralgia
- Nausea and vomiting

With *N. meningitidis* meningitis, 75% of patients develop a rash that can be petechial, ecchymotic, or maculopapular. As the infection worsens, the headache and vomiting increase and the patient may become confused and lethargic, eventually comatose. In the elderly and infants (particularly those under 6 months of age) symptoms can be very nonspecific, such as poor feeding and decreased activity.

DIAGNOSIS Physical findings may be nonexistent, except for rare petechiae or a bulging fontanelle in infants. Key findings include the following:

- Neurologic evaluation: Focal neurologic deficit indicates the need for a CT scan before lumbar puncture.
- Eye examination: Papilledema indicates increased intracranial pressure, suggesting other possible causes for altered mental status. Do not perform a lumbar puncture without a head CT.
- Evidence of meningeal irritation and nuchal rigidity
  - Brudzinski's sign: When the patient's neck is flexed, the patient flexes the hips and knees.
  - Kernig's sign: With the hips flexed, there is pain with passive extension of the knee past 120 degrees.
- Skin examination: Look carefully for very small peripheral petechiae or purpura or a more general ecchymotic rash.

The only essential laboratory study is the examination of the CSF obtained by a lumbar puncture. However, treatment should be started as soon as the diagnosis is considered and should never be delayed by the lumbar puncture.

Important components of a lumbar puncture include

- Opening pressure: normal 150 $\pm$ 33 mm H_2O, but it tends to be higher in patients with bacterial meningitis. Remove less fluid with a marked elevation and treat for increased intracranial pressure by elevating the head of the bed and administering mannitol if necessary.
- CSF cell count: Normal adult CSF cell count is 0 to 5 mononucleated cells/μL and no PMNs or red blood cells. In bacterial meningitis there are 500 to 10,000 WBCs/μL, with a predominance of PMNs. In traumatic tap or after subarachnoid hemorrhage, one WBC may be subtracted from the total WBC count in the CSF for each 1,000 red blood cells. In viral meningitis there are usually fewer than 100 WBCs with mononuclear predominance.
- CSF Gram stain is extremely useful and finds the organism in 70% to 90% of bacterial cases.
- CSF glucose: Glucose decreases with bacterial meningitis. The normal CSF to serum glucose ratio is 0.6. The absolute level is often less than 40 mg/dL in bacterial, fungal, and tubercular meningitis. Assessment can be made by glucose dipstick, but it is not very accurate.
- CSF protein: The protein increases markedly in meningitis. Normal CSF protein is 38 $\pm$ 10 mg/dL. In bacterial meningitis it is usually 100 to 500 and less than 100 in viral meningitis.
- Xanthochromia (pink or yellow color of the CSF supernatant): This does not come from a traumatic tap but rather from old bleeding, such as a subarachnoid hemorrhage.
- Countercurrent immunoelectrophoresis (CIE) and latex agglutination can rapidly detect antigens for *H. influenzae*, *S. pneumoniae*, *N. meningitidis*, and group B streptococci, but they are rarely available.
- India Ink may to used to identify *Cryptococcus* in immunocompromised patients.

TREATMENT Meningitis is a medical emergency. All patients should be admitted to a hospital or health center. Antibiotics should be administered within 30 minutes. Base antibiotic therapy on Gram stain results or likely etiologies of meningitis. Empiric treatment for adults should cover for *Streptococcus pneumoniae* that is resistant to penicillin and chloramphenicol (use vancomycin) and can include any of the following:

- Penicillin 4 million units IV every 4 hours or
- Ampicillin 3 to 4 g IV every 4 hours with
- Vancomycin 1,000 mg IV every 6 hours (give over 1 hour)

For patients with a history of anaphylaxis to penicillin, administer chloramphenicol 1.5 g every 6 hours (but give with vancomycin). Chloramphenicol may be the drug of choice in limited circumstances due to its long duration and good coverage.
Other choices include

- Third-generation cephalosporin, cefotaxime (Claforan) 2 g IV every 4 to 6 hours or ceftriaxone (Rocephin) 2 g IV every 12 hours. Third-generation cephalosporins are not effective against enterococci, methicillin-resistant staphylococci, or *Listeria.*
- If *Pseudomonas aeruginosa* infection is suspected (immunocompromised patients), then give ampicillin with ceftazidime 2 to 4 g every 8 hours.
- In patients over 50, give ampicillin and a third-generation cephalosporin (ceftriaxone or cefotaxime).

ADJUNCTIVE THERAPY Also give dexamethasone 0.4 mg/kg IV every 12 hours for two doses. It must be given in conjunction with or just before the antibiotics.

PREVENTION Chemoprophylaxis should be considered for people in close contact with patients (family) in the endemic situation, but it is ineffective during an epidemic. Potential chemoprophylaxis antimicrobial agents include rifampin, ceftriaxone, mynocycline, spiramycin, and ciprofloxacin. In some countries, vaccination is used against meningococcal disease to prevent secondary cases.

HIV INFECTION AND AIDS

BACKGROUND Acquired immunodeficiency syndrome (AIDS) is a viral disease with a latency period of several years. As the virus propagates, the immune system of the body is diminished, leading to death from opportunistic illnesses and infections.

An estimated 60 million people are infected with the AIDS virus worldwide. There are an estimated 10 million orphaned children as a result of HIV. Several countries report a seroprevalence of over 30% of urban populations. AIDS has various names in other regions, including SIDA in French-speaking countries, slim disease in Uganda,

VIGS in South Africa, and others. It is essential that any health worker in the international setting be aware of the risk factors, clinical signs of infection, treatment options, and preventive measures to address the profound health threat of AIDS.

TRANSMISSION The most common route of transmission of the HIV virus is sexual intercourse, either heterosexual or homosexual. Other routes of transmission include blood transfusion, contaminated needles, accidental exposure to blood (doctors, dentists, midwives), and maternal-newborn transmission before or during birth.

CLINICAL PRESENTATION AIDS has many presentations because the body's crippled immune system allows various infections to occur. Health workers must be familiar with the array of illnesses related to AIDS and the risk factors leading to HIV infection. The risk factors for HIV include those listed in Table 8-5.

The clinical stages of HIV infection range from acute viral infection to end-stage disease. The initial presenting complaint is typically a viral syndrome with flu-like symptoms. This typically goes unrecognized, but may include fever, rash, sore throat, and myalgias. Four to 12 weeks after HIV exposure, antibodies to the virus are detectable in the blood (seroconversion). This is followed by an asymptomatic phase that may last 1 to 10 years. During this time, HIV replicates and kills CD4 immune cells until the CD4 count decreases to the point that opportunistic infections occur. The earliest infections may include non–AIDS-defining illnesses, such as oral thrush, severe vaginal candidiasis, and recurrent herpes zoster infection. Once the CD4 count drops below $200/mm^3$, more serious AIDS-defining opportunistic infections occur.

GENERAL SYSTEMIC SYMPTOMS Many HIV-infected patients seek medical care for complaints of

■ Weight loss
■ Chronic fever
■ Generalized weakness
■ Cough
■ Headaches

TABLE 8-5 RISK FACTORS OF HIV INFECTIONS

Male homosexual contact
Injection drug use
Repeat use of needles in health centers
Multiple heterosexual contacts and prostitution
Blood transfusion
Maternal-neonatal transmission
Inadequate precautions among health workers

Because patients with AIDS have difficulty mounting an adequate response to infection, they may have serious infections without the typical clinical picture. Fever, for example, may be caused by undiagnosed pneumonia, TB, lymphoma, or other opportunistic infections. The clinician must then search for the cause of infection and begin appropriate treatment.

DIAGNOSIS Essentially all patients should be screened on behavioral issues and exposures to determine their risk of being HIV positive. This helps to educate the patient about the AIDS risk factors and give you valuable information for your evaluation.

TIPS AND TRICKS:

Here is a 1-minute survey for determining if a patient has risk factors for HIV infection:
1. Do you think you may have been exposed to HIV infection?
2. Have you ever used any kind of injected drug (outside of the hospital)?
3. Have you ever received a blood transfusion outside the United States, or in the United States between 1978 and 1985?
4. For men: Have you ever had unprotected sex with a prostitute or someone who has used injected drugs? Have you ever had sex with another man?
5. For women: Have you ever had sex with a bisexual man or someone that has used injected drugs?

The diagnosis of AIDS is most commonly made with laboratory tests and the presence of one or more AIDS-defining illnesses, also called indicator conditions. These include those conditions listed in Table 8-6.

LABORATORY There are several laboratory methods used to diagnosis HIV infection, including

■ Detection of the virus-specific antigen
■ Assays for HIV antibodies
■ Isolation of the virus by culture

The most common assay used to detect viral antibody is an enzyme-linked immunoassay (EIA). This is 99% specific and 98.5% sensitive. A positive EIA result is then confirmed by a Western blot test, which is nearly 100% sensitive. Assessing the CD4 counts and viral load is helpful to characterize clinical presentation and the risk of opportunistic infections.

AIDS-RELATED ILLNESSES

PULMONARY Pulmonary complications are some of the most common and life-threatening illnesses faced by HIV patients. Patients may present with classic complaints

TABLE 8-6 CONDITIONS FOR THE DEFINITION OF AIDS

Candidiasis of upper airway, lower airway, or esophagus
Cytomegalovirus retinitis
Cryptococcus
Cryptosporidiosis
Cerebral toxoplasmosis
Herpes simplex virus
Kaposi's sarcoma
Lymphoma (brain, Burkitt, or immunoblastic)
Mycobacterium avium complex
Pneumocystis carinii pneumonia
Progressive multifocal leukoencephalopathy
Disseminated histoplasmosis
Salmonella septicemia
Isosporiasis
HIV encephalopathy
HIV wasting syndrome
Disseminated *Mycobacterium tuberculosis*
Pulmonary tuberculosis
CD4 cell count <200 cells/μL
Recurrent bacterial pneumonia
Invasive cervical cancer

of pneumonia, with shortness of breath, pleuritic chest pain, fever, and sputum production. They frequently, however, have nonspecific complaints of myalgias, general weakness, and fever. The most common cause of HIV-related pulmonary complications are community-acquired bacterial (nonopportunistic) infections. Other infections include PCP, TB, histoplasmosis, and cytomegalovirus (CMV).

Like any pulmonary illnesses, the diagnosis depends on the clinical examination and a chest x-ray. Chest x-ray findings can include

- Diffuse interstitial infiltrates (PCP, CMV, histoplasmosis)
- Focal consolidation (bacterial pneumonia, *Mycobacterium* infection, PCP)
- Cavitary lesions (PCP, bacterial infections, fungal infections, *Mycobacterium tuberculosis*)

Diagnosis of the specific organism usually depends on sputum Gram stain, culture or AFB, or possibly bronchoscopy.

GASTROINTESTINAL Gastrointestinal complications of HIV are also common. The most common presenting gastrointestinal complaint is abdominal pain and diarrhea. Diarrhea occurs in the majority of patients with AIDS, and may be caused by a number of pathogens (Table 8-7).

TABLE 8-7 CAUSES OF DIARRHEA IN
HIV-INFECTED PATIENTS

Shigella
Salmonella
Escherichia coli
Campylobacter
Cryptosporidium
Cytomegalovirus
Antibiotic-induced *(Clostridium difficile)*
Amoeabiasis
Giardiasis
Other parasitic infections

Like all cases of diarrhea, initial treatment includes ensuring adequate hydration. Empiric treatment for severe diarrhea is recommended if a bacterial etiology is suspected, although a number of patients with AIDS have watery diarrhea with no identifiable organism. The best initial antibiotic is ciprofloxacin 500 mg twice daily until an organism can be identified. Avoid unnecessary antibiotics, because repeated dosing may lead to antibiotic-induced *Clostridium difficile* infection.

In addition to gastrointestinal causes, there are a number of illnesses that target the esophagus and oral cavity. The most common of these lesions is oral candidiasis (thrush). Oral thrush occurs in over 80% of patients with AIDS, and is a source of significant discomfort. Clotrimazole, nystatin, or other antifungal liquids can be used to treat oral candidiasis. Esophageal involvement may be caused by candidiasis, HSV, or CMV and can lead to dysphagia and odynophagia.

NEUROLOGIC Central nervous system complications eventually occur in almost all patients with AIDS. Symptoms range from a mild headache to confusion, lethargy, or seizures.

Computed tomography scan (if available) and lumbar puncture aid in the diagnosis of a specific organism and detect other neurologic causes, such as masses, bleeding, or CNS infection.

Neurologic illnesses are caused by a variety of opportunistic infections, including toxoplasmosis and *Cryptosporidium* infection.

■ Toxoplasmosis is the most common cause of focal encephalitis in HIV patients. CT is typically required to confirm the diagnosis.
■ Cryptococcal CNS infection can present with a fever, headaches, and focal neurologic deficits. The use of cryptocooccal antigen is virtually 100% sensitive, but may be unavailable in many field settings.

Other AIDS-related illnesses include those listed in Table 8-8.

TABLE 8-8 OTHER HIV-RELATED MANIFESTATIONS

ORGAN SYSTEM	MANIFESTATION
Ophthalmologic	CMV retinitis, herpes zoster
Cutaneous	Kaposi's sarcoma, seborrheic dermatitis, herpes simplex, varicella zoster
Renal	Renal insufficiency from dehydration or drug toxicity
Psychiatric	AIDS psychosis, mood disorder, and depression

TREATMENT Treatment of HIV patients in the field setting presents a major problem. Most antiretrovirals and many antibiotics are not available in countries with limited resources. If medications are available, Table 8-9 describes current recommendations for treatment of HIV and HIV-related infections.

Vaccinations can reduce the risk of vaccine-preventable illnesses, including diphtheria, tetanus, pertussis, and pneumococcal infection. Do not immunize HIV-infected patients with live vaccines, including the oral polio vaccine and the measles, mumps, rubella (MMR) vaccine.

PREVENTION One of the most important contributions that a field health worker can make is to screen for high-risk patients and support prevention efforts and AIDS education programs. Although limited success has been noted in slowing the explosive epidemic of AIDS in some countries (Uganda), there is a desperate need for aggressive, community-integrated AIDS education programs all over the world.

Patients who enter a hospital or clinic also must be protected from exposure. It is important to adequately sterilize equipment, even in a remote setting with limited access to state-of-the-art sterilization methods. This means autoclaving or boiling any reusable equipment and cleaning surfaces with a diluted bleach solution.

Another important component of prevention is the protection of health workers who may be exposed to HIV through patient contact. The observation of universal precautions is essential, and must be supported and practiced in the clinical setting, no matter how remote.

KEY POINT:

Observe universal precautions when working with any blood product or body fluid where there is a potential for injection, spray, or splash, even in remote settings. These include the use of gloves and eye protection when working with fluids. Also use sharps containers for disposing needles and contaminated sharp instruments.

The majority of work-related exposures are from needle sticks. High-risk needle-stick exposures include those from hollow (blood draw) needles, deep intradermal sticks, and those from a known HIV-positive patient. Depending on the type of

TABLE 8-9 TREATMENT RECOMMENDATIONS FOR HIV AND COMMON HIV-RELATED INFECTIONS

ORGAN SYSTEM	INFECTION	THERAPY
Antiretroviral therapy	HIV infection (recommendations based on CD4 count; patients should be followed closely after initiating treatment)	One of the following: Efavirenz, indinavir, nelfinavir, ritonavir/saquinavir plus Stavudine or zidovudine plus Lamivudine or didanosine
Systemic	*Mycobacterium avium-intracellulare*	Clarithromycin 500 mg PO b.i.d. plus Ethambutol 15 mg/kg/day PO plus Rifabutin 300 mg/kg/day PO
	CMV	Gancyclovir 5 mg/kg IV b.i.d. or Foscarnet 60 mg/kg IV every 8 h
Pulmonary	PCP	15–20 TMP/kg/day and 75–100 mg SMZ/kg/day PO or IV for 3 weeks Pentamidine 4 mg/kg/day IV or IM for 3 weeks
	Tuberculosis	Isoniazid 5 mg/kg/day PO plus Rifampin 10 mg/kg/day PO plus Streptomycin 15 mg/kg/day IM
Central nervous system	Toxoplasmosis	Pyrimethamine 50–100 mg/day PO plus Sulfadiazine 4–8 mg/kg/day plus Folinic acid 10 mg/day PO
	Cryptococcosis	Amphotericin B 0.7 mg/kg/day IV with or without Flucytosine; maintenance therapy required
Ophthalmologic	CMV	Ganciclovir 5 mg/kg b.i.d. for 2 weeks; maintenance therapy required
Gastrointestinal	Candidiasis: thrush	Clotrimazole 10 mg 5 time a day, troches or Nystatin lozenges 5 times a day, gargle
	Esophagitis	Fluconazole 100 mg/day PO
	Salmonellosis	Ciprofloxacin 500 mg b.i.d. for 2–4 weeks; maintenance therapy required
	Cryptosporidiosis	No known effective cure
Cutaneous	Herpes simplex	Acyclovir 1,000 mg/day PO or Acyclovir 5–10 mg/kg/day IV
	Herpes zoster	Acyclovir 4,000 mg/day PO; IV therapy required for ocular involvement or dissemination
	Candida, Tricophyton	Clotrimazole, miconazole, or ketoconazole

CMV, cytomegalovirus; PCP Pneumcystis carinii pneumonia.

exposure, there are a number of recommendations for antiretroviral therapy for post-exposure prophylaxis. For high-risk exposures treat with

■ Zidovudine (AZT)
■ Lamivudine (3TC)
■ Crixivan

Postexposure prophylaxis is usually continued for 4 weeks. Refer to the CDC recommendations for determining when to start postexposure prophylaxis.

CHAPTER SUMMARY

Infectious diseases are the most common cause of illness throughout the world. As noted in this chapter, most of these diseases can be diagnosed without the assistance of complex laboratory or diagnostic testing. It is therefore important to learn distinguishing historical and clinical findings to treat the broad spectrum of infectious diseases you will encounter.

INTERNATIONAL TRAVEL REFERENCES

Health Information for International Travel (published yearly) and Advisory Memoranda on
    Travel (published periodically), Centers for Disease Control and Prevention
The CDC international travelers' hotline is available 24 hours a day, 7 days a week, at (404) 332-
    4559. Information on acute disease outbreaks such as cholera, specific destination advisement,
    food and water precautions, travelers' diarrhea, vaccines, AIDS, etc., is available on tape-
    recorded messages. During normal business hours you also can speak with a travel expert.

REFERENCES

American College of Physicians Task Force on Adult Immunization/Infectious Diseases Society
    of America. Guide for adult immunization. 3rd ed. Philadelphia: American College of
    Physicians; 1994.
Centers for Disease Control. Update on adult immunization: recommendations of the
    Immunization Practices Advisory Committee (ACIP). MMWR 1991:40(RR-12), 1.
Peter G, ed. 1994 Red Book: Report of the Committee on Infectious Diseases. 23rd ed. Elk Grove
    Village, IL: American Academy of Pediatrics; 1994:371, 375.

CHAPTER 9

Tropical Infectious Diseases

Jon Mark Hirshon and Michael J. VanRooyen

The purpose of this chapter is to review the diagnosis and treatment of tropical diseases. Helminth and protozoa causing illnesses are found around the world, but the frequency and severity of parasitic diseases is greatly increased in the tropics and subtropics. Some of these organisms, especially malaria, are the dominant cause of morbidity and mortality in many countries. It is important to recognize when someone is sick due to a tropical infection, determine the specific agent causing the disease, and treat them appropriately.

The following subjects are covered in this chapter:

- Brief review of critical actions when someone is severely ill
- Discussion on how to differentiate between types of tropical diseases
- Review of specific common tropical diseases: malaria, schistosomiasis, onchocerciasis, dracunculiasis, intestinal parasites

CRITICAL ACTIONS

EVALUATION OF THE ILL PATIENT

One of the most important first steps in evaluating people who are sick is to determine if they have a problem that could threaten their life. Evaluation of any acutely ill individual requires attention to the ABCs of resuscitation (airway, breathing, and circulation; see Chapter 6).

RECOGNITION OF MEDICAL EMERGENCIES

After making sure that the patient has an open airway, is breathing, and has a pulse, be sure to look for signs and symptoms of serious illnesses and life-threatening conditions that may be related to tropical diseases. Some of these signs and symptoms include the following:

■ Coma and decreased level of consciousness (not talking or acting normally): Consider cerebral malaria, meningitis, or opportunistic central nervous system infections in an immunocompromised patient.
■ Seizures or status epilepticus (convulsions): Consider cerebral malaria, meningitis, or cysticercosis.
■ Shortness of breath: Consider pneumonia.
■ Severe vomiting, diarrhea, or abdominal pain: Consider cholera, bacterial diarrhea, or intestinal parasites.

Other potentially serious problems related to infection can include high, persistent fever; rapid heart rate; blood in vomit, urine, or stool; skin lesions; jaundice; blindness; and marked weight loss.

WHEN TO SEEK HELP OR TRANSFER A PATIENT (KNOW YOUR LIMITS)

Many rural clinics and hospitals do not have the ability or resources to treat very sick or critically ill people. The first thing to do is to stabilize the patient (give oxygen, protect the airway, give intravenous fluids) as much as local circumstances allow. Consider transporting the patient to a bigger or better equipped hospital if the local resources are not good enough and more intensive medical care is likely to help the individual. This may be necessary for either someone who is very ill, not getting better despite therapy or is getting progressively worse.

DIFFERENTIATING TYPES OF TROPICAL DISEASES

DIFFERENCES BETWEEN VIRAL, BACTERIAL, AND PARASITIC DISEASES

Infectious diseases can be caused by many different organisms. It is important to perform a complete history and physical to help determine the cause of a disease. In many areas of the world, there are very limited modern medical resources; laboratory testing may not be available. The health-care worker will need to depend on what he or she uncovers on history and physical examination as well as sound clinical judgment to develop an appropriate list of possible diseases. Although there are effective medications for many bacterial and parasitic diseases, there are few treatment options for viral infections. If the patient has a viral illness, such as an upper respiratory tract infection (a cold) or viral hepatitis, it is important to provide supportive care and avoid the misuse of antibiotics. Antibiotics may be difficult to obtain locally and do not work against viruses. Antibiotic misuse can lead to the development of bacteria that are resistant to antibiotic treatment.

AVAILABILITY AND USE OF LABORATORIES

Information from a laboratory can greatly help a health-care worker in discovering the cause of an illness and deciding on the proper treatment. Although laboratory testing may or may not be readily available, it is important to use what is available wisely. Efficient and effective use of a laboratory will not waste precious resources that may be needed at a later time.

Try not to order unnecessary laboratory tests, but only the tests that are likely to affect how the patient will be treated. This means obtaining only appropriate, focused laboratory tests based on a short list of potential diagnoses after a thorough history and physical has been completed (see Chapter 23 for details on field laboratories).

THE NEED TO DISTINGUISH BETWEEN ILLNESSES

It is important to avoid using medications indiscriminately, especially the use of antibiotics without a good indication. Treating a patient who has multiple complaints with multiple antibiotics indicates that the health-care provider doesn't know what illness the patient has. This can lead to antibiotic misuse and overuse. Such treatment may or may not make the patient better, and there are always risks to taking any medication (e.g., severe allergic reactions). Ask more questions and examine more thoroughly; order fewer tests and use fewer antibiotics.

KNOW THE DISEASES THAT ARE COMMON IN THE LOCAL AREA

Speak with other health-care providers and local residents to find out what diseases are commonly seen, and think twice before treating an illness that is not typically found in the local region. For example, if you are treating a patient in the Americas for Guinea worm (dracunculiasis), which is not normally found in the Western Hemisphere, think about other causes for the patient's symptoms.

SPECIFIC COMMON TROPICAL DISEASES

This section describes the major findings in common tropical illnesses. For a detailed description of tropical illnesses, refer to Appendix 9.1 to 9.9.

MALARIA

Malaria is the disease caused by infection of humans with a protozoan parasite of the *Plasmodium* species, primarily *P. falciparum, P. vivax, P. ovale,* and *P. malariae.* It is transmitted from person to person through the bite of an infected female *Anopheles* mosquito, which usually bites at night from dusk until dawn. Malaria is widespread throughout most tropical and subtropical areas of the world, infecting approximately 300 million people and causing more than 1 million deaths each year. Disease can occur within 6 to 8 days after being bitten by an infected mosquito or several months later, after antimalarial drugs are stopped.

CLINICAL PRESENTATION The severity of malaria can range from mild to life threatening, depending on the infecting species and the amount of parasites. The classic triad is fever, spleen enlargement, and anemia. A typical malarial attack has three stages:

Stage 1. It often begins with shaking chills, headache, malaise, muscle aches, and a rising fever, but also may include nausea, vomiting, and diarrhea.
Stage 2. Then a high fever of 40°C or higher develops, and the patient may be weak, flushed, and delirious.
Stage 3. Sweats and decreasing temperature ensue as the patient begins to improve.

Usually the patient has continuous symptoms at first, and then fevers every 2 or 3 days, depending on the infecting species. Serious malarial attacks occur primarily in young children (<5 years old), pregnant women, individuals not previously infected with malaria, and debilitated patients with other medical problems. Signs of a life-threatening malarial attack (typically *P. falciparum*) can include the following:

- Cerebral malaria: confusion, delirium, coma, or repeat seizures
- Pulmonary edema: shortness of breath, frothy sputum
- Renal failure: blood in the urine (hemoglobinuria) or decreased urine output (oliguria), leading to confusion and coma
- Hemolysis: hemorrhagic syndrome (destruction of red blood cells) usually leads to profound anemia and jaundice

Recrudescence or relapse can lead to splenomegaly, severe anemia, generalized weakness, and wasting.

DIAGNOSIS The diagnosis of malaria is based on clinical suspicion combined with laboratory evidence of protozoa in the blood. Every individual who lives in an endemic area or has recently traveled to an endemic area who has a fever of over 38.5°C (101.4°F) of unclear cause should get a malarial (thick and thin) blood smear (see Chapter 23). Repeated smears may be needed in chronic cases because the number of parasites may be less. In highly endemic areas, presumptive treatment may be indicated (Appendix 9.1).

TREATMENT The treatment for malaria depends on the area where the infection was acquired (Fig. 9-1). Common drugs used in the treatment of malaria include chloroquine, mefloquine, pyrimethamine-sulfadoxine, quinine, tetracyline, and halofantrine (Table 9-1).

PREVENTION The risk of getting malaria can be markedly decreased by taking preventive measures, both on a personal and on a community level. Extra efforts should be made for at-risk individuals—young children, pregnant women, and debilitated patients.

- Mosquito netting: The use of bed netting, especially impregnated (soaked) with an insecticide such as permethrin, can decrease the likelihood of getting bitten by mosquitoes at night.
- Insect repellants: The use of insect repellents, especially those containing diethyltoluamide (DEET), on bare skin can help prevent the bite of mosquitoes.
- Avoidance behavior: Long-sleeve shirts and pants should be worn from dusk to dawn to decrease the likelihood of getting bitten by an *Anopheles* mosquito.
- Help with mosquito control efforts: A number of efforts can be taken on a local or community level, including draining areas of standing water where mosquitoes can breed; using of larvicides and biological controls in standing water to eat the larva of mosquitoes; and spraying residual insecticides where appropriate.
- Chemoprophylaxis, usually for expatriates and pregnant women (Table 9-2):
  - Regimen A. For areas where chloroquine-resistant *P. falciparum* has not been reported, chloroquine alone is recommended.

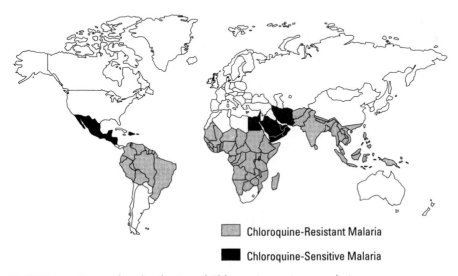

Chloroquine-Resistant Malaria

Chloroquine-Sensitive Malaria

FIGURE 9-1 Geographic distribution of Chloroquine-resistant malaria

TABLE 9-1 MALARIA TREATMENT REGIMENS

USAGE	DRUG	ADULT DOSAGE	CHILD DOSAGE	COMMENTS & PRECAUTIONS
Chloroquine sensitive: *P. falciparum,* and most infections with *P. malariae, P. ovale,* and *P. vivax*	Chloroquine phosphate	25 mg of chloroquine base/kg administered over a three-day period: Day 1: 10 mg/kg initially (~600 mg), then 5 mg/kg (~300 mg) 6 hours later Day 2: 5 mg/kg (~300 mg) Day 3: 5 mg/kg (~300 mg)	See adult dosage	Organism drug sensitivity varies area to area. Every effort should be made to find out what is the best treatment for malaria in the area where the infection was acquired.
Chloroquine resistant: *P. falciparum,* or *P. vivax* acquired in Oceania	Mefloquine	15 mg/kg, single dose	See adult dosage	Not recommended for individuals with seizure disorders, severe psychiatric disorders, cardiac conduction abnormalities or known allergy to mefloquine
Chloroquine resistant and mefloquine resistant (or patient unable to take mefloquine) *P. falciparum*	Pyrimethamine-sulfadoxine	3 tablets as a single oral dose (75 mg pyrimethamine + 1,500 mg sulfadoxine)	5–10 kg: ½ tablet 11–20 kg: 1 tablet 21–30 kg: 1½ tablet 31–45 kg: 2 tablets >45 kg: 3 tablets	Should not be used if allergic to sulfa drugs
	Quinine + doxycycline or tetracycline	Quinine: 30 mg/kg/day divided in 3 doses for 3–7 days depending on where infection was acquired Doxycycline: 100 mg twice a day for 7 days Tetracycline: 250 mg four times a day for 7 days		Doxycycline and tetracycline should not be used in pregnant or nursing women and children under 8 years; can cause photosensitivity.
	Halofantrine			Sudden death has occurred with use; see package insert for precautions and dosage
Severe malaria infections	Quinine dihydrochloride	20 mg/kg base, diluted in 500 mL normal saline or glucose, administered over 2–4 hours. May repeat in 8 hours at 10 mg/kg.	See adult dosage	If used >48 hours, and unable to monitor drug levels, reduce by 30%. Hypoglycemia is a common side effect. Quinine is not available in the United States. Convert to oral medications as soon as able to tolerate.
P. vivax or *P. ovale* infections	Primaquine	0.3 mg base/kg/day (~15 mg base) for 14 days	See adult dosage	The use of primaquine is decided on a case-by-case basis. Consider after prolonged exposure. Use after initial therapy due to risk of intrahepatic infection. Do not use in pregnancy (consider chloroquine until postpartum). Check for G-6-PD enzyme deficiency.

■ Regimen B. For areas where chloroquine-resistant *P. falciparum* has been reported, mefloquine alone is recommended. Alternative drug regimens include doxycycline or chloroquine plus proguanil.

Overdose of antimalarial drugs can be fatal. Medication should be stored in child-proof containers and out of reach of children.

TABLE 9-2 MALARIA PREVENTION REGIMEN

DRUG	USAGE	ADULT DOSAGE	CHILD DOSAGE	COMMENTS & PRECAUTIONS
Mefloquine	In areas with chloroquine-resistant *P. falciparum*	228 mg base (250 mg salt) orally, once/week	<15 kg: 4.6 mg/kg (base), 5 mg/kg (salt) 15–19 kg: ¼ tablet/wk 20–30 kg: ½ tablet/wk 31–45 kg: ¾ tablet/wk >45 kg: 1 tablet/wk	Start 1 week before and continue until 4 weeks after visit to malaria-risk area. Not recommended for individuals with seizure disorders, severe psychiatric disorders, cardiac conduction abnormalities, or known allergy to mefloquine.
Doxycycline	An alternative to mefloquine	100 mg orally, once/day	>8 years of age: 2 mg/kg orally/day up to maximum adult dose	Start 1 or 2 days before and continue until 4 weeks after visit to malaria-risk area. Should not be used in pregnant or nursing women and children under 8 years. Can cause photosensitivity.
Chloroquine phosphate	In areas with chloroquine-sensitive *P. falciparum*	300 mg base (500 mg salt) orally, once/wk	5 mg/kg base (8.3 mg/kg salt) orally, once/wk up to maximum adult dose	Start 1 week before and continue until 4 weeks after visit to malaria-risk area.
Hydroxy-chloroquine sulfate	As an alternative to chloroquine	310 mg base (400 mg salt) orally, once/wk	5 mg/kg base (6.5 mg/kg salt) orally, once/wk up to maximum adult dose	Start 1 week before and continue until 4 weeks after visit to malaria-risk area.
Chloroquine + proguanil	A less effective alternative for use in Africa, only if mefloquine or doxycycline cannot be used	Weekly chloroquine dose (as above) + proguanil dose of 200 mg orally, once/day	Weekly chloroquine dose (as above) + proguanil dose <2 years: 50 mg/day 2–6 years: 100 mg/day 7–10 years: 150 mg/day >10 years: 200 mg/day	Seek medical care immediately after treatment if individual develops fever or flulike symptoms.
Pyrimethamine-sulfadoxine	Self-treatment drug to be used if medical care is not available within 24 hours	3 tablets orally as a single oral dose (75 mg pyrimethamine + 1,500 mg sulfadoxine)	5–10 kg: ½ tablet 11–20 kg: 1 tablet 21–30 kg: 1½ tablet 31–45 kg: 2 tablets >45 kg: 3 tablets	Seek medical care immediately after treatment. Should not be used if allergic to sulfa drugs.

RELAPSING FEVER

Relapsing fever is a bacterial infectious disease caused by the *Borrelia* species, transmitted by either lice or ticks. The borreliae reproduce in body fluids, and produce endotoxins, which affect the liver, spleen, and capillary endothelial, cells.

■ In louse-borne relapsing fever (*Borrelia recurrentis*), the disease occurs in overcrowded conditions, particularly in refugee settings, where people may harbor lice in clothing or in their hair.
■ Tick-borne relapsing fever (*Borrelia duttoni*) is transmitted by ticks, and is clinically significant in children and pregnant women.

CLINICAL PRESENTATION As the name of the disease implies, the most characteristic presentation is that of a fever that relapses a week after its initial presentation. Initially, after an incubation period of 3 to 10 days, patients may present with:

■ fever
■ chills
■ headache
■ myalgias
■ abdominal pain and jaundice may also occur.

After 5 to 7 days, the temperature may return to normal, then near day 14 the patient may again become febrile. The patient may develop mental status changes, meningitis, myocarditis and hepatic failure.

DIAGNOSIS The diagnosis is made by clinical suspicion and confirmation by performing a thick and thin blood smear and identifying spirochetes. Malaria should also be considered in the differential diagnosis of relapsing fever.

TREATMENT Both louse-borne and tick-borne relapsing fever can be treated with:

■ single oral dose of 500 mg tetracycline or
■ doxycycline 100 mg PO BID for 10 days
■ erythromycin 500 mg PO single dose

PREVENTION Patients with relapsing fever are considered contagious until they have been deloused and clothing and bedding have been washed.

DENGUE FEVER

Dengue fever occurs in tropical Central and South America, East and West Africa, the Caribbean, and in South East Asia. It is mosquito borne, and is most often found in urban environments. Many health authorities use increasing rates of dengue as a marker for urban decay and lack of sanitary practices. A more serious form of the disease, Dengue hemorrhagic fever, occurs with re-infection.

CLINICAL PRESENTATION Dengue fever presents after an incubation period of 4 to 7 days. Patients present with:

- sudden high fever
- headaches
- nausea
- vomiting
- myalgias

Patients may develop red eyes, painful eye movement, and a puffy face. There may also be a fine pale maculo-papular or morbilliform rash. Small children my present with symptoms of an upper respiratory tract infection. Spleen enlargement is unusual, and more indicative of malaria.

Dengue hemorrhagic fever can cause petechial hemorrhages that can be initially indistinguishable from meningococcemia. Hemorrhagic fever occurs in tropical America, the Caribbean, and Southeast Asia in infants of immune mothers. It is more common in children, especially those over 1 year of age and those with recurrent infections, especially if the virus strain is new to the individual. Symptoms of dengue hemorrhagic fever can include the following:

- shock
- hemorrhagic pleural effusions
- bleeding diathesis
- thrombocytopenia

DIAGNOSIS The diagnosis is based on clinical findings, as laboratory tests are often unavailable.

TREATMENT

- Treatment is supportive in uncomplicated dengue fever and consists of oral fluids and analgesics.
- Dengue hemorrhagic fever requires intensive IV supportive treatment with lactated Ringer's or normal saline, plasma, and/or whole blood. Supplemental oxygen and sedation may be required.

PREVENTION Prevention of dengue depends on the reduction of mosquito breeding by insecticide spraying and repellants. Sleeping nets are not as effective, since the vector bites by day.

YELLOW FEVER

Yellow fever is an acute infectious disease caused by a flavivirus and is found in jungle monkeys. It is transmitted by the Aedes mosquito. Yellow fever ranges in severity from an undifferentiated self-limited flu-like illness to a hemorrhagic fever that is fatal in 50% of cases.

CLINICAL PRESENTATION After an incubation period of 3 to 6 days, the patient develops:

- fever
- headache
- myalgias
- conjunctival injection
- facial flushing
- relative bradycardia

In most cases, the patients recover from this initial period of infection. In others, the fever resolves for a few hours to several days, and is followed by renewed symptoms, with high fever, headache, back pain, and bleeding diathesis. In severe cases, the following can occur:

- hypotension
- shock
- metabolic acidosis
- myocardial dysfunction and arrhythmias (late stages)
- confusion, seizures, and coma (late stages)

Death usually occurs within 7 to 10 days after onset. If the patient survives the critical period of illness, secondary bacterial infections may complicate the course.

DIAGNOSIS The diagnosis is primarily clinical. Leukopenia and albuminuria may be seen on laboratory tests. Direct bilirubin levels rise and liver function tests may also rise for several days during the time that azotemia and oliguria ensue.

TREATMENT Treatment is supportive with fluid replacement and treatment of complications.

PREVENTION A live virus vaccine is effective and should be administered every 10 years. It is important to obtain this immunization prior to travel in and between endemic countries, as yellow fever vaccination is still required for entry in many countries, and officials may mandate immunization prior to border crossing.

BACTERIAL INFECTIONS

TYPHOID FEVER

Enteric fever is caused by the gram-negative bacteria *Salmonella typhi* and *S. paratyphi A and B*. The bacteria are transmitted by ingestion of food or water contaminated by feces or urine from active cases of disease or healthy carriers of the infection. The bacteria invade the liver, spleen and lymphoid tissue and are disseminated by blood. Untreated mortality is 10–15%, mostly in small children.

CLINICAL PRESENTATION Typhoid classically begins with:

- progressive onset of fever with chills
- headache
- abdominal distention and nausea, vomiting, diarrhea
- *Relative bradycardia* is a classic feature, but may be absent.

After several days of fever a pale red macular rash may appear on the trunk ('rose spots"). As the disease progresses, splenomegaly may be appreciated. In 10% of cases there is evidence of CNS involvement with acute psychosis, delirium, and seizures.

DIAGNOSIS Diagnosis is made clinically and by culture of the organism from blood, urine, or stool (during the second week), or by "rose spot" biopsy or bone marrow aspirate. Proven cases almost always have a significant leukopenia. The differential diagnosis includes malaria, typhus, viral hepatitis, amoebic liver abscess, and other infective causes of enteritis.

TREATMENT Enteric fever can be treated with several different drugs:

- Chloramphenicol 500 mg 4 times a day IV or PO for 14 days is used in most developing countries.
- Fluoroquinolones—(i.e., ciprofloxin 500 mg PO twice a day for 10 days) are used when available and where antibiotic resistance is a problem.
- Azithromycin oral 1 g the first day then 500 mg per day for 6 days is effective.
- Ampicillin 25 mg/kg every 6 hours for 7–10 (PO or IV).

PREVENTION Typhoid vaccine is recommended for travelers to areas where it is difficult to follow good hygienic practices with water and food. Two vaccines are recommended in the United States, and both provide only about 70% protection. An oral, live-attenuated vaccine is given in capsule form, one capsule PO every other day for four doses; a booster series is required every 5 years. An injectable capsular polysaccharide vaccine given in a single dose provides protection for 2 years. Control in communities depends on improved sanitation and water treatment and control of restaurants and food handlers.

CHOLERA

Cholera is an acute, diarrheal illness caused by the bacterium *Vibrio cholerae*. The infection may be mild, but can also be severe and life threatening, particularly in malnourished or vulnerable populations. Cholera is transmitted by contaminated drinking water or food, and has an incubation period of 2 to 3 days. In an epidemic, the source of the contamination is typically fecal contamination of the water supply. Although it takes a significant ingestion of bacteria to produce a clinical infection, the disease can spread rapidly in areas with inadequate treatment of sewage and drinking water.

CLINICAL PRESENTATION Most cases of cholera are mild and have minimal symptoms. Severe disease is characterized by profuse watery diarrhea ("rice water stools"), followed by vomiting, and leg cramps (stage I). Rapid loss of body fluids leads to dehydration and shock (stage II). Without aggressive treatment, death can occur within a few hours. Most patients improve spontaneously and recover (stage III).

DIAGNOSIS The diagnosis of cholera is typically based on clinical criteria; profuse, watery diarrhea and severe dehydration. If you suspect a case of cholera, send a rectal swab or stool specimen to the regional or district lab for culture confirmation.

TREATMENT Aggressive fluid resuscitation is the mainstay of therapy in cholera patients. Rehydration with oral rehydration solution (ORS) or intravenous fluid will effectively treat most cases. Consider the use of a "cholera bed," a cot covered with plastic sheeting with a hole in the center for drainage of watery stool. Tetracycline 500 mg QID or trimethoprim-sulfamethoxazole (two tabs BID for 3 days) can shorten the course.

PREVENTION Cholera is best controlled by vigilant attention to clean water and proper sanitation, especially in displaced and vulnerable populations. Chlorination or boiling water from an unsure source is important. Chemoprophylaxis with tetracycline in households where cholera has been identified may be useful, and adequate public health surveillance in vulnerable populations is essential. Two new cholera vaccines (Dukoral and Mutacol) provide better coverage than prior vaccines, but are not routinely recommended.

NEMATODE INFECTIONS

Nematodes, or round worms, cause many types of infections, from gastrointestinal to subcutaneous skin involvement. The worms are ubiquitous throughout the tropical world. The section will cover certain nematode infections in detail (onchocerciasis and dracunculiathis). The remainder are covered in Appendices 9.2 and 9.3.

ONCHOCERCIASIS (RIVER BLINDNESS)

River blindness is a chronic infection that can lead to skin changes and blindness. It is caused by a nematode that is transmitted by the bite of an infected female black fly, *Simulium* species. It is found predominantly in sub-Saharan Africa. Early treatment can prevent blindness and reduce the spread of the disease.

CLINICAL PRESENTATION Symptoms include:

- pruritus/dermatitis
- altered pigmentation/"leopard skin"
- nodules in the skin
- lymphadenopathy
- gradual visual impairment leading to blindness

The adult worms are found in the nodules, which occur several months after a black fly bite. Nodules are usually painless, and can grow up to 2 or 3 cm across.

DIAGNOSIS Diagnosis is made by demonstration of microfilariae on microscopic examination of fresh skin scrapings, nodule biopsies, or in the urine. A slit lamp examination may reveal microfilariae in the cornea, anterior chamber, or the vitreous.

TREATMENT

- Ivermectin (Mectizan), 150 *u*g/kg as a single dose, is the primary treatment, but does not kill the adult worm. The dose is then repeated in 6 months to suppress dermal and ocular microfilariae.
- Diethylcarbanazine citrate and suramin have been used in the past but have potentially serious side effects. Surgical removal of nodules can lower the incidence of worms, and surgical removal of nodules around the head can help prevent progression of visual impairment.

PREVENTION Avoid the bite of black flies by taking the same precautions as discussed in malaria above, including wearing protective clothing and using insect repellant which contains DEET. Insecticide spraying along breeding sites of the black fly may be effective, usually along fast-moving rivers and streams.

DRACUNCULIASIS (GUINEA WORM)

Guinea worm is a painful, debilitating worm infection found in parts of sub-Saharan Africa, India, and Yemen. The infection is acquired through drinking contaminated water. Prognosis is usually good unless the ulcer made by the worm becomes infected. International efforts are currently underway to eliminate this disease.

CLINICAL PRESENTATION Approximately a year after acquiring infection, a painful swelling starts usually on a lower extremity. After about a week a blister appears, and upon rupture the worm is ready to discharge larvae. Fever, itching, nausea, vomiting, and diarrhea may accompany sore formation. A 60-100 cm long female adult worm is found within the sore.

DIAGNOSIS Diagnosis is made by finding the adult worm in the sore or finding the larvae on a microscopic examination of fresh water.

TREATMENT There are no drugs available that kill the parasite.

- Tetanus toxoid should be given.
- Antibiotics can be given if secondary infection of the wound occurs.
- The worm can be removed slowly over a week or more by attaching a thread to the worm where it emerges from the skin, then pulling gently a little more each day. Roll the worm around a small stick. The worm may be over a meter in length so care must be taken not to break it as it is pulled out. Aseptic surgical excision can also be used to remove the adult worm.

PREVENTION

- Clean drinking water or filtering water through a fine mesh cloth is the most important preventive measure.
- When the worm has broken through the skin, it is ready to release larvae and will do so upon contact with water. People must be instructed not to enter water when they have blisters or open sores.
- Elimination of the intermediate host, a small crustacean, can also eliminate the worm.

INTESTINAL NEMATODES AND CESTODES

There are many different worms and other parasites that can infect the gastrointestinal systems of humans. Infection may range from minimal or no symptoms to life-threatening complications. Almost all of these organisms are contracted by eating undercooked food, or eating food or drinking water contaminated with feces. Good hygiene, clean water, and care when preparing foods can markedly decrease the likelihood of catching these diseases. See Appendix 9.3 for details on intestinal nematode infections, including Parastrongyloides, Strongyloides, and Trichinella.

ASCARIS (ROUNDWORM)

Ascaris is the most common helminthic infection of humans. Over 1 billion people in the world are infected. In total, all the roundworms in the world weigh as much as one million adult men and consume as much food as the country of France. Infection occurs at all ages but is most common in preschool and young school-aged children. Ascaris eggs can live for several years in moist, loose, sandy soil. Transmission in children is typically caused by ingesting infested soil (Fig. 9.2).

CLINICAL PRESENTATION Roundworm infection has minimal symptoms:

- The most common presentation is nonspecific abdominal pain or when live worms are passed in stools. Mothers will complain that their child has worms in the stools.
- A patient may have a dry cough or pneumonia as the young worm migrates from the lungs to the gut.
- A large concentration of worms can lead to malnutrition and weakness.
- A ball of worms can cause an obstruction in the intestines.

DIAGNOSIS The diagnosis is made by finding the egg or worms in the feces.

TREATMENT A number of medications are effective for roundworm, including:

- mebendazole 100 mg PO BID for 3 days or
- albendazole 400 PO as single dose, or
- pyrantel pamoate 11 mg/kg PO in a single dose
- Mebendazole and albendazole are not recommended during pregnancy.

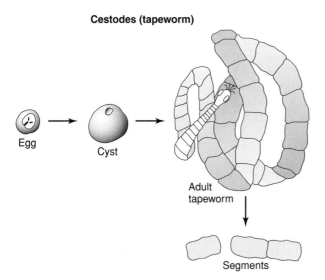

FIGURE 9-2 Drawing of a tapeworm

If intestinal obstruction occurs, piperazine citrate 75 mg/kg per day (no more than 3.5 g) may be used via NG tube. This paralyzes the worm and makes them pass per rectum. Surgical excision is rarely necessary.

PREVENTION Proper disposal of human feces, particularly if children are present, usually stops transmission. Handwashing after defecation helps in infection control. Wash food well with clean water.

ENTEROBIASIS (PINWORM, SEATWORM)

Pinworms are small intestinal parasites that are transmitted by the fecal-oral route, and can be acquired from contaminated objects such as toys, utensils, and bedding.

CLINICAL PRESENTATION Pinworms cause itching around the anus. The child will complain of intense perianal itching, especially at night.

DIAGNOSIS The diagnosis can be made by finding pinworms around the anus, or doing a Scotch tape test. Wait till the child is asleep, then roll the child on his or her stomach or side, and spread the buttocks apart to expose the anus. Place a 3–5 cm strip of cellophane tape directly on the anus, and press gently to adhere eggs. Pull the tape off and examine under a microscope.

TREATMENT

- mebendazole 100 mg PO single dose
- albendazole 400 mg PO once
- pyrantel pamoate 11 mg/kg daily for 3 days

Repeat the treatment in 2 weeks. The life of pinworms is short; good hygiene alone may eliminate the worm. Bathe the child frequently and cut his or her nails short to decrease the transmission of eggs from scratching.

PREVENTION Good sanitary habits can prevent this disease. Make sure that people wash their hands after defecating, and that there is proper disposal of feces.

TRICHURIASIS (WHIPWORM)

Whipworm is an infection of the large intestine. The infection is not transmitted from person to person, but by ingesting contaminated soil or vegetables.

CLINICAL PRESENTATION The infection is usually asymptomatic, but may cause bloody diarrhea or lead to rectal prolapse, anemia, and growth retardation in children with heavy infections. Children may present with symptoms similar to inflammatory bowel disease.

DIAGNOSIS The diagnosis is made by finding eggs in feces.

TREATMENT Antiworm medications, such as:

- mebendazole 100 mg BID for 3 days
- albendazole 400 mg PO for one dose

PREVENTION Good sanitary habits can prevent this disease. Make sure that there is proper disposal of feces. Wash food well with clean water.

HOOKWORM

Hookworm infection is a common disease of the tropics and subtropics and can cause significant problems for children. Chronic infection leads to severe anemia, loss of energy, and poor attention span in school-aged children. The infection is transmitted by direct contact (usually bare feet) with soil contaminated by human feces (Fig. 9.3).

CLINICAL PRESENTATION Presenting symptoms may be generalized malaise and anemia. There may be initial pruritus and localized rash at the site of worm entry ("ground itch"). Severe symptoms depend on the degree of blood loss, but can include stunted cognitive and physical development.

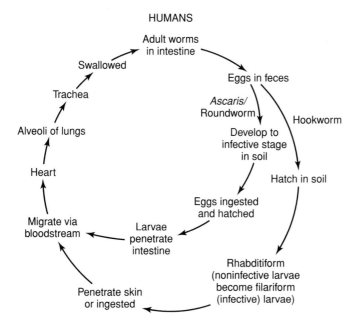

FIGURE 9-3 Hookworm and roundworm lifecycle

DIAGNOSIS Diagnosis is made by finding hookworm eggs on microscopic examination of feces using a potassium iodide stain. Eggs do not appear in the feces for 8 to 12 weeks after initial infection.

TREATMENT Antiworm medications, such as:

- mebendazole (100 mg PO BID for 3 days) or
- albendazole 400 mg PO once or
- pyrantel pamoate (11 mg/kg daily for 3 days)

Once the infection has been treated, treat iron deficiency anemia if needed with iron supplementation.

PREVENTION The worms penetrate through skin. Sanitary disposal of feces to prevent contamination of soil where people walk barefoot and children play can help prevent this disease. For other intestinal nematodes see Appendix 9.3.

CESTODES (TAPEWORMS)

There are a number of different organisms known as tapeworms (cestodes), but there are two basic types of infections: taeniasis and cystercercosis.

CLINICAL PRESENTATION Taeniasis is usually asymptomatic or associated with mild gastrointestinal symptoms such as diarrhea, weight loss, and abdominal pain. Ingestion of pork tapeworm (*Taenia solium*) eggs causes cysticercosis, where cysts (small sacs with baby worms) form throughout the body, including the brain. It can cause many problems, depending on the location of the cyst. In neurocystercercosis, patients may present with seizures, behavioral changes, or other neurological complications. Taeniasis is transmitted by eating undercooked beef or pork (Fig. 9.2 and Appendix 9.4)

DIAGNOSIS Diagnosis of *Taenia* is made by finding eggs or worm segments (proglottids) in the stool. Cysticercosis can be diagnosed by finding calcified cysts on radiographs.

TREATMENT Taeniasis:

- praziquantel 5–10 mg/kg PO in a single dose or
- niclosamide 2 g single dose

Cystercercosis: Treatment with albendazole or praziquantel has generally supplanted surgical excision. Secondary presentations such as seizures should be treated with standard anti-seizure therapy. Vasculitis and cerebral edema can be treated as above, with the addition of prednisone 60 mg daily for acute events.

PREVENTION These infections are normally acquired by eating raw or under-cooked meat. It is important to cook meat well, especially pork.

FLUKES

SCHISTOSOMIASIS (BILHARZIASIS OR SNAIL FEVER)

Schistosomiasis is caused by trematode (fluke) that migrates to kidney, bladder and intestines. People are infected through unbroken skin by contact with fresh water that contains the tiny, free-swimming larvae (cercariae) (9-4). Larvae are released from the intermediate host, an infected fresh-water snail which is infected by infected human feces. Symptoms are caused by scarring from the eggs that are deposited throughout the hosts. Schistosomiasis is found in Africa, the Middle East, South America, and parts of SE Asia. There are over 200 million people infected worldwide, with approximately 20 million suffering severe consequences (Appendices 9.5 and 9.6).

CLINICAL PRESENTATION Clinical symptoms generally depend on the infecting species and the site of infection. Infection causes variable manifestations, including central nervous system symptoms such as seizures.

- *Schistosoma hematobium* usually leads to painful urination, frequency, and hematuria.
- Other *Schistosoma* spp generally lead to abdominal complaints including diarrhea, abdominal cramps, and eventually portal hypertension.

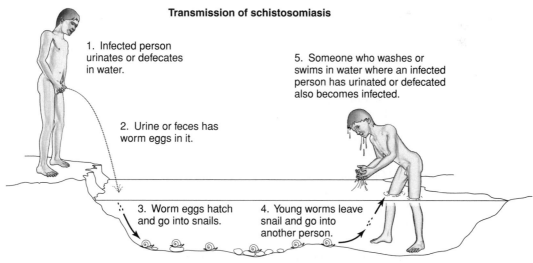

Transmission of schistosomiasis

1. Infected person urinates or defecates in water.

2. Urine or feces has worm eggs in it.

3. Worm eggs hatch and go into snails.

4. Young worms leave snail and go into another person.

5. Someone who washes or swims in water where an infected person has urinated or defecated also becomes infected.

FIGURE 9-4 Schistosomiasis (Trematode) lifecycle

- *Schistosoma japonicum* and *mekongi* can lead to severe abdominal disease including hepatosplenomegaly and jaundice.
- Chronic infection with *Schistosoma* spp can lead to bladder cancer.

DIAGNOSIS The diagnosis is made by finding fluke eggs in urine, stool, or a biopsy specimen. In endemic areas, consider testing anyone with blood in urine or stool for fluke eggs.

TREATMENT

- Praziquantel 40 mg/kg PO single dose works for all types of blood flukes.
- Oxamniquine 15 mg/kg in a single dose is effective against *S. mansoni*.

PREVENTION Most countries have found it difficult to nearly impossible to eliminate the watersnail that serves as the intermediate host. The most important preventive measures include proper sanitation, availability of fresh water, educating the population on prevention, and identification and treatment of infected individuals.

PROTOZOAL INFECTIONS

MALARIA—(see section above)

LEISHMANIASIS

Leishmaniasis is a granulomatous infection transmitted by sandflies and caused by invasion of the skin by several species of the protozoan *Leishmania*. The disease is widely distributed throughout Africa, Asian, and countries bordering the Mediterranean basin and Central and South America. The species of the infecting parasite affects the resultant pathology, which ranges from a localized self-healing lesion to a more widespread, persistent, and potentially destructive disease. The protozoan life cycle depends on one or more blood meals of the female sandfly for maturation of their eggs. The sandflies prefer dark, moist areas. They are small enough to pass through the mesh of mosquito netting, but their short mouthparts keep them from biting through clothing. Four major clinical syndromes are recognized:

- *Visceral leishmaniasis* (Kala-azar, Black fever)
- *Cutaneous leishmaniasis* (described under old world and new world classifications)
- *Mucocutaneous leishmaniasis* (espundia)
- *Diffuse cutaneous leishmaniasis*

CLINICAL PRESENTATION The clinical presentation varies and depends on the nature of the infecting parasite and the state of health of the patient. The incubation period is about 3 months for the visceral form and 2 to 24 months for others. The most common infection is the localized cutaneous form.

- A few weeks after the infected sandfly bite one or more painless itchy papules appear. There is surrounding inflammation and induration.
- After a few months the lesion(s) increase in size to form nodules 1 cm or more in diameter, then develop an adherent crust overlying a shallow ulcer.
- Most localized ulcers heal completely within 9 months even without treatment.

Signs and symptoms of infections in other areas of the body include:

- malaise
- failure to thrive in infants and children
- fever
- cough
- diarrhea
- GI bleeding
- organomegaly
- anemia
- nasal stuffiness
- nose bleeds

Spontaneous healing of skin lesions is less common in new world disease. Acute nodular necrosis is typical of the "wet," rural form (Baghdad boil), which is characterized by severe ulceration with serous oozing, much surrounding inflammation, and lymph node swelling. More chronic "dry" lesions (Oriental sore) are less dramatic and slower to heal. Mucocutaneous leishmaniasis is initially indistinguishable from localized disease, but months or years later metastatic lesions appear as fungating ulcers involving the mucocutaneous surfaces. Chronic progression leads to cartilage destruction, disfigurement, and death due to secondary infection. In *diffuse cutaneous leishmaniasis* there are extensive skin lesion, but no visceral lesions. The clinical picture is similar to leprosy.

DIAGNOSIS The physical exam will show chronic painless ulcerating or non-ulcerating lesions. The most important information to be obtained in diagnosing leishmaniasis is the location of the patient's home and travel history. Endemic areas known to harbor the disease will help to define the type of infection. Definitive diagnosis requires the demonstration of parasites in bone marrow aspirate, splenic aspirate, lymph node aspirate or biopsy, or on smears or sections taken from the border of the lesion.

TREATMENT Cutaneous leishmaniasis known not to be caused by *L. braziliensis*, may be left to heal. If infections with *L. braziliensis* are proven or suspected, they must be treated to prevent mucocutaneous disease. Visceral disease should also be treated. Medications include:

- sodium antimony gluconate (Pentostam) 100 mg Sb 5/ml IV/IM: single daily dose of 20 mg/kg/day for 20–30 days, or
- meglumine antimoniate (Glucantime) 85 mg Sb 5/ml, same dose and duration of treatment as above.

Relapses and incomplete responses should be treated with the same regimen for 40 to 60 days.

The addition of oral allopurinol 20–30 mg/kg/day in three divided doses has been effective. Relapses with drug-resistant organisms are usually treated with amphotericin B or pentamidine. Supportive care with blood transfusions, treatment of superinfections, bed rest, and good nutritional support are important. Some patients require splenectomy or reconstructive surgery.

PREVENTION Prevention is by wearing long shirts and pants to prevent sandfly bites, the use of pesticides against sandflies, insect repellants, permethrin-coated fine netting, early treatment of cases, and elimination of diseased dogs (Appendix 9.7).

AMEBIASIS

Amebiasis is found worldwide, and causes a wide range of clinical problems, from minimal to deadly. Transmission is fecal-oral. The disease is most severe in young children, the elderly, and pregnant women.

CLINICAL PRESENTATION An infected individual may have no symptoms, mild diarrhea, abdominal pain, dysentery (bloody diarrhea), fever, and chills. The most common presentation is that of gradually increasing diarrhea over 1 to 3 weeks. Eventually, patients develop abdominal pain, cramps, bloody diarrhea, and weight loss. Patients often develop fever, and have chronic, intermittent symptoms similar to inflammatory bowel disease.

Extraintestinal infection can include the liver, skin, lung, and the brain. Liver abscesses may present acutely with fever, right upper quadrant pain, or chronic vague abdominal pain with weight loss. Rupture of liver abscess can be fatal.

DIAGNOSIS The diagnosis is made by finding the organism, either as a motile form (trophozoites) or as cysts in the stool. Perform a normal saline wet mount of the stool within 30 minutes of collection to look for trophozoites, and also a fixative (polyvinyl alcohol) to look for the cysts. Intestinal amoebae have a diameter of about 10 *um*, and up to 8 nuclei. Ultrasound or CT scans may be useful to identify abscesses.

TREATMENT To treatment an amoeba infection, use the following:

- metronidazole (500 to 750 mg PO three times a day for 10 days) plus either iodoquinol (650 PO three times a day for 20 days) or
- paromomycin (25–35 mg/kg/day in three divided doses for 7 days or

- diloxanide furoate (500 mg PO three times a day for 10 days)
- alternately, tinidazole 600 mg PO three times a day for 3 to 5 days + iodoquinol or paromomycin or diloxanide furoate
- Chloroquine may be added for liver abscess; however aspiration may be needed for abscess.

PREVENTION As with any infection spread by the fecal-oral route it is important to protect drinking water from animal and human feces and to make sure that people wash their hands after defecating. Treat known carriers to prevent transmission of the organism.

GIARDIASIS

Giardia is a flagellated protozoan that infects the small intestine and biliary tract. It is found worldwide and transmitted by oral exposure to food or water contaminated by feces from humans and other mammals.

CLINICAL PRESENTATION Giardia may be asymptomatic, but more commonly causes very foul smelling, watery diarrhea without blood or mucus, abdominal cramps, bloating, and flatulence. Chronic infections cause weight loss and anemia (Appendix 9.8).

DIAGNOSIS The diagnosis of giardia is made by finding the organism, either as a motile form (trophozoites) or as cysts in the stool. As with amebiasis, do a wet mount and fixative stain on each sample. Three samples are recommended for study. Serologic tests exist, but are rarely available in locations with limited resources.

TREATMENT Patients can be treated with:

- metronidazole (250 mg PO three times a day for 5 days) or
- tinidazole (2 g PO as a single dose) or
- quinacrine (100 mg PO three times a day for 5 days)

PREVENTION It is important to protect drinking water from animal and human feces and to make sure that people wash their hands after defecating. For other protozoal infections, see Appendix 9.9.

SUMMARY

Parasitic diseases are found around the world, but the frequency and severity of disease caused by them are greatly increased in the tropics and subtropics. By following principles of disease recognition and knowledge of local endemic illnesses, many of these cases can be identified clinically. Simple preventive measures, especially in sanitation and handling of food and water, are the most important interventions.

APPENDIX 9-1 MALARIA (Protozoa)

ORGANISM (common names)	MODE OF TRANSMISSION/ VECTOR	GEOGRAPHIC LOCATION	CLINICAL FEATURES	DIAGNOSIS	TREATMENT	PREVENTION	COMMENTS
Plasmodium falciparum	Bite of an infected female *Anopheles* mosquito	Throughout the tropics	Primary infection: flulike illness including chills, headache, fever. Serious infection: coma, seizure, renal failure, pulmonary edema. Chronic infection: weakness, jaundice, splenomegaly	Demonstration of organism on blood smear	See above	Mosquito netting and repellants, avoidance behavior, mosquito control efforts, and chemoprophylaxis (usually for expatriates and pregnant women)	
P. malariae	Bite of an infected female *Anopheles* mosquito	Rare	See primary infection above	See above	See above	See above	Infection may persist up to 50 years
P. ovale	Bite of an infected female *Anopheles* mosquito	Mainly sub-Saharan Africa	See primary infection above	See above	See above	See above	Protracted incubation up to 8–10 months may occur; relapses may occur for up to 5 years
P. vivax	Bite of an infected female *Anopheles* mosquito	Tropics and subtropics	See primary infection above	See above	See above	See above	See *P. ovale* above

APPENDIX 9-2 NEMATODES

ORGANISM (common names)	MODE OF TRANSMISSION/ VECTOR	GEOGRAPHIC LOCATION	CLINICAL FEATURES	DIAGNOSIS	TREATMENT	PREVENTION	COMMENTS
Ancylostoma braziliensis, A. caninum (cutaneous larva migrans or creeping eruption)	Contact with damp, sandy soil contaminated with dog or cat feces	Tropics and subtropics	Snakelike tract in the skin; usually self-limited	By history and clinical examination	Cutaneous disease is self-limited; cure in weeks to months, or ivermectin 200 µg/kg orally for one dose or albendazole 200 mg orally b.i.d. for 3 days		Individual worms can be killed by freezing the area with ethyl chloride
Nematode larva of the subfamily *Anisakinae*	Eating raw or undercooked saltwater fish, squid or octopus	Ubiquitous in oceans	Nausea, vomiting, abdominal pain, stomach ulceration, and possibly perforated viscus	Recognition of the larvae in surgical specimen, on gastroscopy, or with migration of the larvae to the oropharynx	Endoscopic removal of larvae, or mebendazole 100 mg orally b.i.d. for 3 days or 500 mg once	Avoid eating raw or inadequately cooked salt water fish and mollusks	
Dracunculiasis medinensis (Guinea worm)	Drinking infected water	In certain areas of sub-Saharan Africa and parts of Asia (Yemen and India)	A painful blister appears, usually on a lower extremity, which ruptures and adult worm emerges; urticaria, fever, vomiting; diarrhea can also occur	Finding the 60–100 cm long adult worm in a blister; finding the microscopic larvae in water	Tetanus toxoid and antibiotics for the wound; aseptic surgical excision of adult worm just prior to worm emergence Metronidazole 250 gm TID × 10 days	Provide potable water, do not let people with blisters or ulcers enter drinking water; control numbers of intermediate host; small crustacean (copepod)	International efforts are underway to eradicate this disease; secondary bacterial infection can complicate ulcers

APPENDIX 9-2 NEMATODES *(continued)*

ORGANISM (common names)	MODE OF TRANSMISSION/ VECTOR	GEOGRAPHIC LOCATION	CLINICAL FEATURES	DIAGNOSIS	TREATMENT	PREVENTION	COMMENTS
"Filariasis" caused by a number of Filarioidea species, including Wuchereria bancrofti, Brugia malayi, B. timori	Bite of mosquito with infective larvae	Scattered around the world in most warm, humid areas	Asymptomatic to severe; includes recurrent fevers, lymphatic blockage (elephantiasis) and infection, chronic lung disease (tropical pulmonary eosinophilia syndrome)	Identification of microfilariae in peripheral blood	Diethylcarbamazine for 21 days: days 1 and 2, 50 mg t.i.d.; day 3, 100 mg t.i.d.; days 4–14, 2 mg/kg/day t.i.d. (possible severe reactions)	Identify and control vectors; wear long sleeves and long pants; mosquito repellents	Multiple mosquito species transmit the disease; medications clear microfilariae but not adult worms
Loa loa (eye disease of Africa, Calabar swelling)	Transmitted by deer fly— Chrysops species	African rain forest, especially Central Africa	Chronic disease; symptoms caused by migration of adult worm usually leading to localized pain, itching, and swelling	Demonstration of organism on blood smear; usually accompanied by eosinophilia	Diethylcarbamazine for 21 days: days 1 and 2, 50 mg t.i.d.; day 3, 100 mg t.i.d.; days 4–21, 3 mg/kg/day t.i.d. (possible severe reactions)	Wear protective clothing and use insect repellents; diethylcarbamazine 300 mg/wk orally	Symptoms may not occur for months to several years after exposure; adult worm may persist for years
Onchocerca volvulus (river blindness)	Transmitted by female blackflies, Simulium species	Scattered areas in Central and South America; sub-Saharan Africa, especially West Africa	Chronic, nonfatal disease; adult worm in subcutaneous nodules; microfilariae migrate and lead to blindness and chronic skin changes	Finding microfilariae on microscopic evaluation of skin biopsy incubated in water or saline or finding adult worms in nodules	Ivermectin 150 µg/kg orally for one dose; repeat every 6 months; if ocular involvement, start prednisone 1 mg/kg/day several days before ivermectin	Wear protective clothing and use insect repellents; control the vector (larvae elimination)	International efforts are underway to control this disease

APPENDIX 9-2 NEMATODES *(continued)*

ORGANISM (common names)	MODE OF TRANSMISSION/ VECTOR	GEOGRAPHIC LOCATION	CLINICAL FEATURES	DIAGNOSIS	TREATMENT	PREVENTION	COMMENTS
Toxocarias canis, T. cati (Gnathostoma spinigerum in Southeast Asia) (Visceral larva migrans, ocular larva migrans)	Fecal-oral, from soil contaminated with cat, dog, or human feces	Worldwide	Chronic, usually mild; can have significant eosinophilia, fever, chronic abdominal pain, hepatomegaly, pulmonary symptoms, loss of vision	Clinical suspicion	Mebendazole 100–200 mg orally b.i.d. for 5 days, albendazole 400 mg orally b.i.d. for 5 days, diethylcarbamazine 2 mg/kg orally t.i.d. for 10 days (possible severe reactions)	Hand washing after defecation; sanitary disposal of human and animal feces; deworm cats and dogs	May need steroids for severe disease; ocular disease, use prednisone 30–60 mg orally daily for 4 wk + subtenon triamcinolone 40 mg/wk for 2 wk
Trichinella spiralis	Eating raw or undercooked meat, especially pork	Worldwide, though variable depending on meat preparation practices	Asymptomatic to fatal; included myalgias, diarrhea, edema of face and eyelids, fever, abdominal pain, anorexia, severe brain or heart or kidney manifestations	Finding cyst in skeletal muscle biopsy	Albendazole 400 mg orally b.i.d. for 14 days, inebendazole 5 mg/kg orally b.i.d. for 10–13 days, use prednisone 40–60 mg orally daily with above medications	Adequately cook meat	Larvae migrate and become encapsulated in muscle; corticosteroids can be used to alleviate severe inflammatory reactions (e.g., encephalitis, myocarditis, or nephritis)

b.i.d., twice daily; t.i.d., three times daily.

APPENDIX 9-3 NEMATODES: INTESTINAL INFECTIONS

ORGANISM (common names)	MODE OF TRANSMISSION/ VECTOR	GEOGRAPHIC LOCATION	CLINICAL FEATURES	DIAGNOSIS	TREATMENT	PREVENTION	COMMENTS
Ascaris lumbricoides (roundworm infection)	Fecal-oral, from feces contaminated soil	Ubiquitous, though with highest prevalence in the moist tropics	Often asymptomatic; live worms may be seen in stool or mouth; migrating organisms may cause pulmonary symptoms; a large worm bolus may cause a hollow viscus obstruction	Finding the egg in feces or a migrating worm in stool, nose, or mouth	Albendazole 400 mg orally for 1 dose, or mebendazole 100 mg orally b.i.d. for 3 days, or pyrantel pamoate 11 mg/kg (max 1.0 g) for one dose	Hand washing after defecation; sanitary disposal of feces; protect food from dirt	
Capillaria philippinensis	May be from raw or inadequately cooked fish	Primarily in the northern Philippines and Thailand	Enteropathy with malabsorption and protein loss leading to cachexia	Organism (egg, larvae, or adult) found in the stool	Mebendazole 200 mg orally b.i.d. for 20 days or albendazole 200 mg orally b.i.d. for 10 days	Cook fish well; sanitary disposal of feces	Case fatality may be as high as 10%
Enterobius vermicularis (pinworm)	Predominantly fecal-oral	Ubiquitous	Perianal itching	Apply transparent adhesive tape to the perianal area and then microscopically examine for eggs	Albendazole 400 mg orally for one dose, or mebendazole 100 mg orally for one dose, or pyrantel pamoate 11 mg/kg (max 1.0 g) for one dose; see comments	Hand washing and good personal hygiene; reduce overcrowding	Repeat all treatments in 2 weeks. Pyrantel pamoate should also be repeated 2 weeks after repeat treatment

APPENDIX 9-3 NEMATODES: INTESTINAL INFECTIONS *(continued)*

ORGANISM (common names)	MODE OF TRANSMISSION/ VECTOR	GEOGRAPHIC LOCATION	CLINICAL FEATURES	DIAGNOSIS	TREATMENT	PREVENTION	COMMENTS
Necator americanus, Ancylostoma duodenale, A. ceylanicum, A. caninum (hookworm)	Organisms, from soil contaminated with feces, penetrate skin	Widely found in tropical and subtropical countries; prevailing organism varies by region	Chronic infection leading to hypochromic, microcytic anemia: symptoms variable depending on degree of anemia and coinfections	Finding hookworm eggs in feces	Albendazole 400 mg orally for 1 dose, or mebendazole 100 mg orally b.i.d. for 3 days, or pyrantel pamoate 11 mg/kg (max 1.0 g) orally daily for 3 days	Sanitary disposal of feces	
Parastrongylus (angiostrongylus) cantonensis	Eating of raw or undercooked slugs or land snails, fish, or crabs that have eaten the slugs/snails, or vegetables contaminated by slugs/snails	Endemic in Southeast Asia and Pacific Islands, but has also been found in Africa, Australia, Japan, and Puerto Rico	Meningeal involvement: headache, neck or back stiffness, low-grade fever, various paresthesia, possibly transient facial paralysis	CSF usually exhibits white blood cells with >20% eosinophils	Mebendazole 100 mg orally b.i.d. for 5 days, or thiabendazole 22 mg/kg orally b.i.d. for 3 days	Control rats (a reservoir for the larvae); thoroughly cook or freeze snails, fish, crabs, prawn	A related nematode found in the Americas Parastrongylus (Angiostrongylus) costaricensis causes an appendicitis-type syndrome

ORGANISM (common names)	MODE OF TRANSMISSION/ VECTOR	GEOGRAPHIC LOCATION	CLINICAL FEATURES	DIAGNOSIS	TREATMENT	PREVENTION	COMMENTS
Strongyloides stercoralis, S. fulleborni	Larvae, from moist soil containing feces, penetrate skin	Throughout tropical and temperate areas, especially if warm and moist	Often asymptomatic; may lead to diarrhea or constipation, nausea, vomiting, weight loss, perianal rash with itching	Identify larvae in concentrated stool specimens	Ivermectin 200 μg/kg/day orally for 2 days, or albendazole 400 mg orally daily for 3 days, or thiabendazole 25 mg/kg orally b.i.d. for 2 days (max 3 g/day) (use for 7–10 days for hyperinfection syndrome)	Sanitary disposal of feces; use of footwear in endemic areas	Treat all infections because of risk of autoinfection and dissemination
Trichuris trichiura (whipworm)	Fecal-oral, from soil contaminated with feces	Worldwide	Large intestine infection, usually asymptomatic but large infections can cause bloody diarrhea, possibly anemia and growth retardation	Finding eggs in feces	Albendazole 400 mg orally for one dose, or mebendazole 100 mg orally b.i.d. for 3 days.	Hand washing after defecation; sanitary disposal of feces	As a general rule, women should not be treated during first trimester; repeat treatment may be needed for heavy infestations

b.i.d., twice daily.

APPENDIX 9-4 CESTODE INFECTIONS

ORGANISM (common names)	MODE OF TRANSMISSION/ VECTOR	GEOGRAPHIC LOCATION	CLINICAL FEATURES	DIAGNOSIS	TREATMENT	PREVENTION	COMMENTS
Diphyllobothriasis latum, D. ursi, D. dalliae, D. pacificum, D. dendriticum, D. klebanovskii (broad or fish tapeworm)	Eating raw or undercooked freshwater fish	Fresh water areas worldwide, including subarctic, temperate, and tropical areas	Generally a long-term, asymptomatic infection; large infections may cause diarrhea	Finding eggs or segments (proglottids) of adult worm in feces	Praziquantel 10 mg/kg orally for one dose	Thoroughly cook or freeze freshwater fish	Can be found in other flesh-eating mammals such as cats and dogs
Echinococcus granulosus (hydatid cyst disease, unilocilar echinococcosis)	Food or substances contaminated with dog feces	Ubiquitous where humans and dogs are in close contact, especially if in proximity with intermediate host (e.g., sheep)	Long-duration illness with slowly growing mass (cyst); symptoms depend on location of cyst; if cyst leaks, an anaphylactoid reaction or daughter cysts may occur	Definitive diagnosis is by microscopic material obtained from surgery or aspiration	Surgery of isolated cysts Albendazole 400 mg b.i.d. × 1–6 months	Hand washing after exposure to dog feces; prevent dogs from eating uncooked herbivore viscera	Dogs can be asymptomatic with the infection; use hypertonic saline or ethanol to kill worm at time of surgery; if there is cyst spillage at surgery, praziquantel should also be used
Echinococcus multilocularis (alveolar hydatid disease, multilocular echinococcosis)	Food or substances contaminated with dog, cat, or fox feces	Limited areas of the Northern Hemisphere: former Soviet Union, Central Europe, Japan, Alaska, Canada	Highly invasive and destructive disease, usually found in the liver, but metastasis can occur	See above	Surgery less successful; albendazole may be used as for *E. granulosus* but efficacy not clear	Hand washing after exposure to dog or cat feces	Disease is often fatal

APPENDIX 9-4 CESTODE INFECTIONS *(continued)*

ORGANISM (common names)	MODE OF TRANSMISSION/ VECTOR	GEOGRAPHIC LOCATION	CLINICAL FEATURES	DIAGNOSIS	TREATMENT	PREVENTION	COMMENTS
Echinococcus vogeli (polycystic hydatid disease)	Food or substances contaminated with bush dog feces	Central and South America	Symptoms depend on cyst location; cyst may proliferate without rupture	Definitive diagnosis is by microscopic material obtained from surgery or aspiration			
Hymenolepis nana (dwarf tapeworm)	Fecal-oral, including water and food contaminated with feces	Ubiquitous	Often asymptomatic; large numbers of worms can cause diarrhea, abdominal pain, weight loss, fatigue	Finding eggs in feces	Praziquantel 25 mg/kg orally for one dose	Hand washing after defecation; sanitary disposal of feces	
Taenia saginata, T. solium (taeniasis, cysticercosis))	Usually from eating raw or undercooked beef (*T. saginata*) or pork (*T. solium*); occasionally fecal-oral	Worldwide	Intestinal: from asymptomatic to weight loss, anorexia, abdominal pain Tissue: cysticercosis, depends on location of cyst formation; may cause serious or fatal neuropsychiatric symptoms	Finding eggs or segments (proglottids) of adult worm in feces or anal swabs; finding cysts (cysticerci) on biopsy or x-ray if calcified	Intestinal: praziquantel 10 mg/kg orally for one dose; tissue-surgical excision of cyst Central nervous system: hospitalize and use praziquantel 50 mg/kg/day orally divided t.i.d. for 15 days or albendazole for 8–30 days: >60 kg 400 mg orally b.i.d. with meals, <60 kg, 15 mg/kg/day orally divided b.i.d.	Sanitary disposal of feces; adequately cooking or freezing meat	Taeniasis is an intestinal infection with the adult worm; cysticercosis is a tissue infection with the larvae of *T. solium*; may need to use dexamethasone or antiseizure medications to control CNS effects from cyst death related to inflammation

b.i.d., twice daily; t.i.d., three times daily.

APPENDIX 9-5 FLUKES: INTESTINAL, LIVER, & LUNG

ORGANISM (common names)	MODE OF TRANSMISSION/ VECTOR	GEOGRAPHIC LOCATION	CLINICAL FEATURES	DIAGNOSIS	TREATMENT	PREVENTION	COMMENTS
Clonorchis sinensis, Opisthorchis viverrini, O. felineus (Chinese or Oriental liver fluke disease)	Eating raw or undercooked freshwater fish	Southeast China and other parts of Southeast Asia (*O. felineus, O. felineus,* in Europe and Asia)	Anorexia, diarrhea, abdominal discomfort, jaundice from bile duct obstruction; may be asymptomatic	Finding eggs in feces	Praziquantel 25 mg/kg orally t.i.d. for 1 day Albendazole 10 mg/kg × 7 days	Thoroughly cook freshwater fish	Frequently a chronic disease, and is a risk factor for cholangiocarcinoma
Fasciola hepatica, F. gigantica	Eating uncooked aquatic plants in water contaminated with herbivore feces and containing the intermediate host (a snail)	Sheep- and cattle-raising areas throughout the world, and some areas of Africa and Western Pacific for *F. gigantica*	Predominantly affects the liver causing right upper quadrant pain, jaundice	Finding eggs in feces or bile	Treatment is generally unsatisfactory; bithionol 30–40 mg/kg (max dose 2 g/day) every other day for 10–15 doses	Avoid using sheep/cattle dung for fertilizer; educate public on hazards of eating raw aquatic plants	
Fasciolopsis buski	Eating uncooked aquatic plants in water containing the intermediate snail that has been contaminated with swine feces	Rural Southeast Asia	Predominantly affects the small intestine and may lead to diarrhea or constipation, nausea, vomiting, anorexia, intestinal obstruction, ascites, anasarca	Finding eggs or worms in feces	Praziquantel 25 mg/kg orally t.i.d. for 1 day	Avoid using swine dung for fertilizer; educate public on hazards of eating raw aquatic plants	

APPENDIX 9-5 FLUKES: INTESTINAL, LIVER, & LUNG *(continued)*

ORGANISM (common names)	MODE OF TRANSMISSION/ VECTOR	GEOGRAPHIC LOCATION	CLINICAL FEATURES	DIAGNOSIS	TREATMENT	PREVENTION	COMMENTS
Paragonimus westermani, P. skrjabini, P. africanus, P. uterobilateralis, P. mexicanus, other *Paragonimus* species (lung fluke disease, pulmonary distmiasis)	Eating raw or undercooked freshwater crabs or crayfish	Worldwide; China is now the major endemic country	Primarily affects the lungs causing cough, hemoptysis, pleuritic chest pain; extrapulmonary disease can occur throughout the body	Finding eggs in sputum or feces	Praziquantel 25 mg/kg orally t.i.d. for 1 day Bithionol 30–50 mg/kg on alternate days × 10–15 doses	Avoid eating raw or inadequately cooked freshwater crabs and crayfish; sanitary disposal of feces; control intermediate host (snails)	

t.i.d., three times daily.

APPENDIX 9-6 FLUKES: BLOOD

ORGANISM (common names)	MODE OF TRANSMISSION/ VECTOR	GEOGRAPHIC LOCATION	CLINICAL FEATURES	DIAGNOSIS	TREATMENT	PREVENTION	COMMENTS
Schistosoma hematobium (bilharziasis, snail fever)	Transcutaneously acquired from water contaminated with the free swimming larva forms (cercarie) that have developed in intermediate snail host, *Bulinus* species	Tropical and North Africa and the Middle East	Commonly blood in the urine especially at the end of urination, painful urination, and increased urination	Diagnosis is made by demonstrating eggs in stool, urine, or biopsy specimen	Praziquantel 40 mg/kg/day in 2 doses × 1 day	Interruption of life cycle or organism, sanitary disposal of feces and urine; protect water supplies from feces and urine; treat known carriers	Schistosomiasis (all organisms) affects more than 200 million worldwide, of which 20 million suffer severe consequences
S. mansoni (bilharziasis, snail fever)	As above, intermediate snail host, *Biiomphalaria species*	Tropical Africa and parts of South America and the Caribbean	Commonly leads to abdominal complaint: diarrhea, abdominal cramps and portal hypertension late in disease	See above	Praziquantel 20 mg/kg orally t.i.d. for 1 day (oxamniquine 15 mg/kg orally for one dose (in North and East Africa 20 mg/kg daily for 3 days)	See above	
S. intercalatum (bilharziasis, snail fever)	As above, intermediate snail host, *Physopsis species*	Parts of Central and West Africa (rare)	See above	See above	Praziquantel 20 mg/kg orally t.i.d. for 1 day	See above	
S. japonicum, S. mekongi (bilharziasis, snail fever)	As above, intermediate snail host, *Oncomelania* species	Southeast Asia	See above, also leads to severe abdominal disease (jaundice and hepato-splenomegaly	See above	Praziquantel 20 mg/kg orally t.i.d. for 1 day	See above	

t.i.d., three times daily.

APPENDIX 9-7 LEISHMANIASIS (Protozoa)

ORGANISM (common names)	MODE OF TRANSMISSION/ VECTOR	GEOGRAPHIC LOCATION	CLINICAL FEATURES	DIAGNOSIS	TREATMENT	PREVENTION	COMMENTS
Old World: *Leishmania tropica L. major, L. aethiopica* (Aleppo evil, Baghdad or Delhi boil, Oriental sore) New World: *L. braziliensis, L. mexicana* (Uta, Chiclero ulcer, Espundia, mucosal form)	By the bite of infected female sand flies (phlebotomines); rarely via blood transfusion or from sexual contact	Africa, India, Middle East, Central and South America	Cutaneous and mucosal. Starts as a papule that typically enlarges to an indolent ulcer. Can be single or multiple, and can cause destructive mucosal lesions (usually in the New World)	Microscopic demonstration of the intracellular (amastigote) form on stained specimens from lesions, or culture of the motile, extracellular (promastigote) form	Antimony (stibogluconate or meglumine antimonate) 20 mg/kg/day in two divided doses IM or IV for 28 days. Mucosal: amphotericin B, 1 mg/kg IV every other day for 20–30 doses. Cutaneous: pentamidine 2 mg/kg IV every other day for seven doses or 3 mg/ kg IV every other day for four doses	Elimination of known animal reservoirs; insecticide spraying to eliminate sand flies; wear long sleeves and pants and use insect repellents, especially dusk to dawn	If ulcers become infected, treat with antibiotics. Most cutaneous infections resolve without treatment
L. donovani, L. chagasi (Kala-azar)	See above	See above	Visceral. Hepato-splenomegaly, anemia, lymphadenopathy, leukopenia, thrombocytopenia, intermittent fever, usually fatal	See above	Antimony (stibogluconate or meglumine antimonate) 20 mg/kg/day in two divided doses IM or IV for 28 days. May also use amphotericin B, but dosage depends on the formulation	See above	These organisms can also cause cutaneous disease

IM, intramuscularly; IV, intravenously.

APPENDIX 9.8 PROTOZOA: INTESTINAL INFECTIONS

ORGANISM (common names)	MODE OF TRANSMISSION/ VECTOR	GEOGRAPHIC LOCATION	CLINICAL FEATURES	DIAGNOSIS	TREATMENT	PREVENTION	COMMENTS
Balantidium coli (balantidiosis, balantidial dysentery; ciliary dysentery)	Fecal-oral route, often from contaminated water	Ubiquitous, though human disease is unusual	Asymptomatic, or intermittent diarrhea and constipation, abdominal pain, nausea, and vomiting	Demonstration of cysts or mobile forms (trophozoites) in fecal specimen	Tetracycline 500 mg orally q.i.d. for 10 days, and possibly metronidazole 750 mg orally t.i.d. for 5 days	Hand washing after defecation; sanitary disposal of feces; protect water supplies from feces; treat known carriers	Swine are reservoirs
Cryptosporidium parvum	Predominantly fecal-oral	Ubiquitous	Symptoms can include nausea, vomiting, diarrhea, cramping abdominal pain, fever, anorexia malaise	Finding oocysts on fecal smears	No specific treatment	Hand washing after defecation; sanitary disposal of feces; protect water supplies from feces	Prolonged course in immuno-suppressed individuals; cattle are reservoirs
Cyclospora cayetanensis	Appears to be waterborne	Has been found in Asia and the Americas	Symptoms can include diarrhea, nausea, cramping abdominal pain, anorexia, weight loss	Finding oocysts, similar to large *Cryptosporidium* species on fecal smear	Possibly trimethoprim + sulfamethoxazole DS one tablet orally b.i.d. for 7 days	Protect water supply	Trimethoprim + sulfamethoxazole DS one tablet orally q.i.d. for 10 days then one tablet orally three times/week in immunosuppressed individuals

APPENDIX 9-8 PROTOZOA: INTESTINAL INFECTIONS *(continued)*

ORGANISM (common names)	MODE OF TRANSMISSION/ VECTOR	GEOGRAPHIC LOCATION	CLINICAL FEATURES	DIAGNOSIS	TREATMENT	PREVENTION	COMMENTS
Entamoeba hystolytica (amebiasis)	Predominantly fecal-oral	Ubiquitous	Usually seen in young adults; ranges from mild bloody diarrhea to fulminant dysentery; spread via bloodstream may cause abscess in liver, lung, or brain	Demonstration of cysts or mobile forms (trophozoites) in fecal specimen	Asymptomatic cyst passer: paromomycin 500 mg orally t.i.d. for 7 days or iodoquinal 650 mg orally t.i.d. for 20 days diloxanide furoate 500 mg orally t.i.d. for 10 days. Patient with diarrhea or dysentery: metronidazole 750 mg orally t.i.d. for 10 days or tinidazole 1 g orally every 12 h for 3 days or ornidazole 500 mg orally every 12 h for 5 days. Follow with metronidazole, tinidazone, or ornidazole with treatment for asymptomatic cyst passer. Patient with extraintestinal infection: metronidazole 750 mg IV t.i.d. for 10 days or tinidazole 600 mg orally b.i.d. for 5 days either medications should be followed by iodoquinol 650 mg orally t.i.d. for 20 days	Hand washing after defecation; sanitary disposal of feces; protect water supplies from feces; treat known carriers	*E. hartmanni*, *E. coli*, *E. dispar* are similar but nonpathogenic organisms; aspiration or surgical intervention may be needed for liver abscesses

APPENDIX 9-8 PROTOZOA: INTESTINAL INFECTIONS *(continued)*

ORGANISM (common names)	MODE OF TRANSMISSION/ VECTOR	GEOGRAPHIC LOCATION	CLINICAL FEATURES	DIAGNOSIS	TREATMENT	PREVENTION	COMMENTS
Giardia lamblia, G. intestinalis, G. duodenalis (giardiasis)	Fecal-oral, including water and food contaminated with feces	Ubiquitous	Predominantly affects the upper small intestine and may lead to chronic diarrhea, cramping, abdominal pain, bloating, pale and fatty stools, fatigue, weight loss	Demonstration of cysts or mobile forms (trophozoites) in fecal specimen or in duodenal fluid (string test)	Metronidazole 250 mg orally t.i.d. for 5 days or albendazole 400 mg orally daily for 5 days or tinidazole 2 g orally for 1 day or quinacrine 100 mg orally t.i.d. after meals for 5 days; treatment not always successful regardless of drug	Hand washing after defecation; sanitary disposal of feces; protect water supplies from feces	Children infected more commonly than adults

q.i.d., four times daily; t.i.d., three times daily; DS, double strength; IV, intravenously.

321

APPENDIX 9-9 PROTOZOA: OTHER INFECTIONS

ORGANISM (common names)	MODE OF TRANSMISSION/ VECTOR	GEOGRAPHIC LOCATION	CLINICAL FEATURES	DIAGNOSIS	TREATMENT	PREVENTION	COMMENTS
Babesia microti and other *Babesia* species	Transmitted from the bite of an *Ixodes* tick	North America and Europe	Severity ranges from asymptomatic to fatal; manifestations include fever, chills, myalgias, and hemolytic anemia	In red blood cells, identify parasites on thick or thin blood smears; appears similar to *Plasmodium falciparum*	Consider combination of clindamycin 600 mg orally t.i.d. + quinine 650 mg orally t.i.d. for 7 days	Control rodents (reservoir) and prevent tick bites	
Pneumocystis carinii (PCP)	Unclear, possible airborne	Worldwide	Symptoms include cough, shortness of breath, cyanosis	Finding organism on bronchial washings or lung biopsy	See Chapter on infectious diseases for specific treatment protocols	Prophylaxis with TMP-SMX or aerosolized pentamidine in immuno- compromised individuals	Causes pneumonia in immuno- compromised people (such as with HIV)
Toxoplasma gondii	Ingestion of infected food items (milk, undercooked meat); children may acquire by ingesting oocysts in dirt or sand where cats have defecated or transplacental (mother to fetus)	Worldwide	Acute infection: fever, lymphadenopathy Congenital: multiple symptoms in unborn child, including fetal death Immuno- compromised: cerebritis, rash, myocarditis	Based on clinical findings and demonstration of organism on biopsy	Pyrimethamine 25–100 mg/day × 3–4 weeks + Sulfadiazine 1.0–1.5 g qid × 3–4 weeks	Educate women about risk from cat feces; dispose of cat feces properly; wash hands after handling raw meats; cook food thoroughly	Definitive hosts are cats and felines; children may acquire by ingesting oocysts in dirt or sand where cats have defecated; can be deadly in immuno- compromised people

APPENDIX 9-9 PROTOZOA: OTHER INFECTIONS *(continued)*

ORGANISM (common names)	MODE OF TRANSMISSION/ VECTOR	GEOGRAPHIC LOCATION	CLINICAL FEATURES	DIAGNOSIS	TREATMENT	PREVENTION	COMMENTS
Trichomanas vaginalis	Sexual intercourse	Worldwide	Foul, greenish yellow vaginal discharge	Identification in vaginal secretions	See chapter on sexually transmitted diseases	Public education of safe sex behavior	
Trypanosoma brucei gambiense, T. b. rhodesiense (African trypanosomiasis or sleeping sickness)	Bite of an infected *Glossina* species tsetse fly	Tropical Africa; *T. b. gambiense,* West Africa; *T. b. rhodesiense,* East Africa	Initially a papule, then a chancre, then nodule at site of bite; fever, rash, headache, lymphadenopathy, anemia, local edema, leading to somnolence, wasting and death	Finding trypanosomes in blood, lymph, or cerebral spinal fluid	Early infection with normal CSF: suramin 100–200 mg (test dose) IV then 20 mg/kg IV days 1, 3, 7, 14, 21 (max dose 1.0 g) Late infection with CNS involvement: melarsoprol 2–3.6 mg/kg/day or IV for three days, repeat after 1 week and again after 10–21 days	Wear protective clothing and use insect repellents; control the vector; can use pentamidine isethionate 3 mg/kg IM every 6 months for *T. b. gambiense* only	Melarsoprol can induce encephalopathy; prednisolone 1 mg/kg/day orally may decrease this; pentamidine isethionate 4 mg/kg IM × 10 days or eflornithine 100 mg/kg every 6 h IV for 14 days and then 75 mg/kg orally for 21–30 days can be used but is effective only against *T. b. gambiense*

APPENDIX 9-9 PROTOZOA: OTHER INFECTIONS *(continued)*

ORGANISM (common names)	MODE OF TRANSMISSION/ VECTOR	GEOGRAPHIC LOCATION	CLINICAL FEATURES	DIAGNOSIS	TREATMENT	PREVENTION	COMMENTS
Trypanosoma cruzi (American trypanosomiasis or Chagas disease)	Bite of an infected *Reduviidae* species cone-nosed bug or kissing bug	Central and South America	Asymptomatic or with fever, malaise, lymphadenopathy, hepatosplenomagaly; long-term sequelae include cardiac dilatation with conduction disturbances, megacolon, or megaesophagus	Finding trypanosomes in blood	Nifurtimox 8–10 mg/kg/day orally divided four times/ day after meals for 120 days (ages 11–16 yr: 12.5–16 mg/kg/day orally divided four times/ day for 90 days <11 yr: 15–20 mg/kg/day orally divided four times/ day for 90 days) or benznidazole 5–7 mg/kg/day orally divided twice daily for 60 days	Wear protective clothing and use insect repellents; control the vector	Avoid tetracycline and steroids with benznidazole

t.i.d., three times daily; IV, intravenously; IM, intramuscularly.

APPENDIX 9-10 MALARIA TREATMENT REGIMENS

USAGE	DRUG	ADULT DOSAGE	CHILD DOSAGE	COMMENTS AND PRECAUTIONS
Chloroquine-sensitive *P. falciparum*, and most infections with *P. malariae, P. ovale,* and *P. vivax*	Chloroquine phosphate	25 mg of chloroquine base/kg administered over a three-day period Day 1: 10 mg/kg initially (~600 mg), base then 5 mg/kg (~300 mg) 6 hours later Day 2: 5 mg/kg (~300 mg) Day 3: 5 mg/kg (~300 mg)	See adult dosage	Organism drug sensitivity varies area to area. Every effort should be made to find out what is the best treatment for malaria in the area where the infection was acquired.
Chloroquine-resistant *P. falciparum,* or *P. vivax* acquired in Oceania	Mefloquine	750 mg followed by 500 mg/2 hrs later	15 mg/kg PO followed by 10 mg/kg PO 12 hrs later	Not recommended for individuals with seizure disorders, severe psychiatric disorders, cardiac conduction abnormalities, or known allergy to mefloquine
Chloroquine-resistant and mefloquine-resistant (or patient unable to take mefloquine) *P. falciparum*	Pyrimethamine-sulfadoxine in combination with Quinine	Three Tablets as a single oral dose (75 mg pyrimethamine + 1,500 mg sulfadoxine)	5–10 kg: ½ tablet 11–20 kg: 1 tablet 21–30 kg: 1½ tablet 31–45 kg: 2 tablets >45 kg: 3 tablets	Should not be used if allergic to sulfa drugs
	Quinine + doxycyline or tetracycline or pyrimethamine sulfadoxine	Quinine: 30 mg/kg/day divided in three doses for 3–7 days depending on where infection was acquired. Doxycycline: 100 mg twice a day for 7 days Tetracycline: 250 mg four times a day for 7 days	25 mg/kg/day divided in 3 doses × 3–7 days <8 yrs: 2 mg/kg/day × 7 days >8 yrs: 6–25 mg/kg qid × 7 days	Doxycycline and tetracycline should not be used in pregnant or nursing women and children under 8 years; can cause photosensitivity
	Atovaquone/ proquanil	2 adult tablets (250 mg/100 mg each) bid × 3 days	11–20 kg: 250 mg/100 mg × 3 days 21–30 kg: 500 mg/200 mg × 3 days 31–40 kg: 750 mg/300 mg × 3 days	For acute uncomplicated *P. falciparum*

APPENDIX 9-10 MALARIA TREATMENT REGIMENS *(continued)*

USAGE	DRUG	ADULT DOSAGE	CHILD DOSAGE	COMMENTS AND PRECAUTIONS
Severe malaria infections	Quinine dihydrochorlide	20 mg/kg base, diluted in 500 mL normal saline or glucose, administered over 2–4 hours; may repeat in 8 hours at 10 mg/kg	See adult dosage	If used >48 hours, and unable to monitor drug levels, reduce by 30%. Hypoglycemia is a common side effect. Quinine is not available in the United States; use quinidine. Convert to oral medications as soon as able to tolerate.
P. vivax or *P. ovale* infections	Primaquine	26.3 mg (15 mg base)/day × 14 days	0.3 mg base/kg/day (~15 mg base) for 14 days	The use of primaquine is decided on a case-by-case basis. Consider after prolonged exposure. Use after initial therapy due to risk of intrahepatic infection. Do not use in pregnancy (consider chloroquine until postpartum). Check for G-6-PD enzyme deficiency.

APPENDIX 9-11 MALARIA PREVENTION REGIMENS (CDC 1999–2000)

DRUG	USAGE	ADULT DOSAGE	CHILD DOSAGE	COMMENTS AND PRECAUTIONS
Mefloquine	In areas with chloroquine-resistent *Plasmodium falciparum*	228 mg base (250 mg salt) orally, once/week	<15 kg: 4.6 mg/kg (base), 5 mg/kg (salt) 15–19 kg: ¼ tablet/week 20–30 kg: ½ tablet/week 31–45 kg: ¾ tablet/week >45 kg: 1 tablet/week	Start one week before and continue until 4 weeks after visit to malaria-risk area; not recommended for individuals with seizure disorders, severe psychiatric disorders, cardiac conduction abnormalities or known allergy to mefloquine
Doxycycline	An alternative to mefloquine	100 mg orally, once/day	>8 years of age: 2 mg/kg orally/day up to maximum adult dose	Start 1 or 2 days before and continue until 4 weeks after visit to malaria-risk area; should not be used in pregnant or nursing women and children under 8 years; can cause photosensitivity
Chloroquine phosphate	In areas with chloroquine-sensitive *Plasmodium falciparum*	300 mg base (500 mg salt) orally, once/week	5 mg/kg base (8.3 mg/kg salt) orally, once/week up to maximum adult dose	Start 1 week before and continue until 4 weeks after visit to malaria-risk area
Hydroxy chloroquine sulfate	As an alternative to chloroquine	310 mg base (400 mg salt) orally, once/week	5 mg/kg base (6.5 mg/kg salt) orally, once/week up to maximum adult dose	Start one week before and continue until 4 weeks after visit to malaria-risk area
Chloroquine + proguanil	A less effective alternative for use in Africa, only if mefloquine or doxycycline cannot be used	Weekly chloroquine dose (as above) + proguanil dose of 200 mg orally, once/day	Weekly chloroquine dose (as above) + proguanil dose <2 years: 50 mg/day 2–6 years: 100 mg/day 7–10 years: 150 mg/day >10 years: 200 mg/day	Seek medical care immediately after treatment if individual develops fever of flulike symptoms.

APPENDIX 9-11 MALARIA PREVENTION REGIMENS *continued)*

DRUG	USAGE	ADULT DOSAGE	CHILD DOSAGE	COMMENTS AND PRECAUTIONS
Pyrimethamine-sulfadoxine	Self-treatment drug to be used if medical care is not available within 24 hours.	Three tablets orally as a single oral dose (75 mg pyrimethamine + 1,500 mg sulfadoxine)	5–10 kg: ½ tablet 11–20 kg: 1 tablet 21–30 kg: 1½ tablet 31–45 kg: 2 tablets >45 kg: 3 tablets	Seek medical care immediately after treatment; should not be used if allergic to sulfa drugs

Sources:

Benenson AS, ed. *Control of Communicable Diseases Manual*, 16th ed. Washington, DC: American Public Health Association, 1995.

Binford CH, Connor MD, eds. *Pathology of Tropical and Extraordinary Diseases, An Atlas*. Washington, DC: Armed Forces Institute of Pathology, 1976.

Centers for Disease Control and Prevention. *Health Information for International Travel 1999–2000*, Atlanta: DHHS.

Gilbert DN, Moellering Jr RC, Sande MA. *The Sanford Guide to Antimicrobial Therapy, 1999*, 29th ed. Hyde Park, VT: Antimicrobial Therapy, Inc, 1999.

Werner D, Thuman C, Maxwell J. *Where There Is No Doctor, A Village Health Care Handbook*, revised ed. Berkeley, CA: Hesperian Foundation, 1992.

Guerrant, RL, Walker D, Weller P. eds. *Essentials of Tropical Infectious Diseases* Philadelphia, PA: Churchill Livingstone, 2001.

CHAPTER 10
Pediatric Emergencies

Thomas D. Kirsch

Infant and childhood mortality is a major health problem in developing countries. Children with acute illnesses and injuries can present to any health-care setting. Therefore, health workers must be familiar with the assessment and treatment of pediatric emergencies.

The approach to children is much different from the approach to adults. Because children are not as able to express their problems as well as adults the clinician must rely on observation and a careful physical examination. The clinician also must be very aware of the development stages of children so that they can identify deviations from the norm.

PREVENTION

Children die of preventable causes at tremendous rates in developing countries and refugee situations. Once disease or injuries occur, the ability to cure them is limited. Prevention is the key.

PREVENTING INFECTIOUS DISEASES

The prevention of infectious diseases requires sanitation, cleanliness, and immunization. Equally important is the education of patients and health-care staff regarding the basics of prevention. Physicians are responsible for ensuring the implementation of these preventive measures (see Chapter 11 for details).

VITAMIN A SUPPLEMENTATION

Supplementation with vitamin A has been shown to have a significant impact on reducing childhood deaths from measles, diarrhea, and other infections. Consider vitamin A supplementation in refugee populations and during measles vaccination programs.

PREVENTING INJURIES

Injuries are now the leading cause of death in children 1 to 15 years of age in all but the least developed countries. Physicians must make sure that injury prevention is an integral part of their activities and patient education.

Primary prevention means ensuring that the environment is safe by eliminating hazards. This is the most effective form of injury prevention. Secondary prevention means lessening the severity of the force as the injury event occurs. The best example of this is seatbelts. Ensure that the environment where you work is a safe one, both in the health facility and in the surrounding community.

> Use each patient encounter to educate patients and their family regarding safety issues, including
>
> - Traffic safety
>   - Seatbelt use
>   - Driving with lights on at night
>   - Avoiding overloading vehicles
>   - Motorcycle and bicycle helmet use
>   - Pedestrian safety
> - Home safety
>   - Controlling access to open fires
>   - Storage of medicines, chemical, pesticides, etc.
>   - Controlling access to open wells
>   - Electricity safety

NUTRITION

Proper nutrition is essential to a child's health. Breast-feeding is the key for infants and children less than two years old. As children grow, a balanced diet is equally important and families must be educated about healthy eating habits (see Chapter 5 for details).

BREAST-FEEDING

Perhaps the single best health intervention for an infant is breast-feeding. It is the best and safest nutrition and provides protection against some infectious diseases, including diarrhea and otitis media. It also has some natural contraception properties for the mother that help to space births farther apart.

DID YOU KNOW?

The only nutritional deficit of breast milk is vitamin D. Therefore, women should be encouraged to expose their children to light to enhance the natural production of vitamin D. Alternately, 400 IU of vitamin D supplementation can be provided daily.

Contraindications to breast-feeding are few. The most important ones are certain infectious diseases of the mother, or the use of some medications. Maternal infectious disease contraindications include active chickenpox, pertussis, and tuberculosis (untreated). HIV infection is a relative contraindication, and infected mothers should avoid breast-feeding only if adequate, clean sources of formula are available.

There are relatively few medications that are absolutely contraindicated in a lactating woman. Major contraindicated drugs include

- Antibiotics
  - Chloramphenicol
  - Clindamycin
- Others
  - Cimetidine (H_2 blocker)
  - Clonidine (antihypertensive)
  - Cyclophosphamide
  - Thiouracil
  - Ergotamine

For other medications, such as ethambutol, isoniazid, and indomethacin, alternatives should be sought when available.

The introduction of food supplements is not recommended until at least 4 to 6 months of age. This supplementation is most useful to replace iron stores, so foods containing iron should be encouraged. Good sources of iron include meat, beans, peas, nuts, and eggs. Generally, small amounts of semisolid foods can be introduced during breast-feeding and the amounts gradually increased over the ensuing few months. Breast-feeding can be continued for 12 to 24 months. As foods are introduced, cleanliness in preparation and serving is critical to avoid the transmission of gastrointestinally transmitted diseases. Proteins, carbohydrates, and fats are all important parts of a child's diet.

GENERAL ASSESSMENT OF GROWTH AND HEALTH IN CHILDREN

Infants are defined as those children up to 1 year of age; *neonates* are those infants under 30 days of age (see Tables 10-1 to 10-3).

TABLE 10-1 A FEW CALCULATION TRICKS

To estimate children's weight: weight (kg) = 2 (age) + 8. This is true
   for whites, but less in other races.
A child's systolic BP = 2 (age) + 80.
A child's blood volume is estimated at 80 mL/kg.
"4/40/40": A 4-year-old weights 40 lbs (18 kg) and is 40 inches tall.

TABLE 10-2 NORMAL PEDIATRIC VITAL SIGNS

	RESPIRATIONS		**PULSE**		**BLOOD PRESSURE**	
	NORMAL	**RANGE**	**NORMAL**	**RANGE**	**NORMAL**	**RANGE**
Newborn	mid-40s	35–55	160	90–205	Sys 70	60–80 (by palpation)
Infant (1–11 mo)	30	25–45	130	110–150	90/50	80/40–110/70
Toddler (1–4 yr)	25	20–35	110	90–130	90/60	80/50–110/80
10 years	20	18–25	80	60–100	110/65	90/55–130/85
15 years	15	14–20	70	60–80	120/70	90/60–140/90

TABLE 10-3 A FEW IMPORTANT DIFFERENCES BETWEEN CHILDREN AND ADULTS

Respiratory differences between children and adults
   Infants are obligate nose breathers with very small airways. Small amounts of secretions or blood
   may cause respiratory distress.

Anatomic differences
   Children have relatively short necks and large heads and so do not need to be hyperextended to
   open the airway.
   They also have more flexible tracheas and overextension can occlude the airway.

Physiologic differences
   Children have large body surface areas, and heat is lost quickly (the younger the child, the more
   rapid the heat loss). Keep children warm.
   A child can lose up to 40% of blood volume and still maintain a normal BP. Check the pulse and
   capillary refill to assess shock.
   They have a high vagal tone, which predisposes to bradycardia.
   Higher basal metabolic rates and oxygen consumption leads to rapid hypoxia.

Therapeutic considerations
   Some drugs are metabolized differently (faster or slower); beware of dosing recommendations for
   children.
   Fluid boluses should begin with 20 mL/kg of NS or LR, and repeat boluses given as needed.

DRUG ADMINISTRATION

Calculating drug doses for a child during an emergency situation is difficult and fraught with errors. Because it is unlikely you will remember all the correct doses, keep preprinted tables readily available (preferably posted on the wall, so that everyone can see them). The Broselow system uses preprinted tapes that are laid next to the child's body and give accurate estimates of height and weight, and list the exact doses of all resuscitation medicines.

> **KEY POINT:**
>
> Use preprinted, weight-based tables for the doses of common pediatric drugs.

MAINTENANCE FLUIDS

To calculate daily maintenance for a child, see Table 10-4. For maintenance, a solution of 0.2 normal saline (NS) with 5% dextrose ($D_5 0.2$ NS) is used routinely, add K^+ when necessary.

KEY ADDITIONS TO THE PEDIATRIC HISTORY AND PHYSICAL EXAMINATION

In addition to the standard history and physical examination in adults, other key areas must be covered in children. An accurate history can lead to most diagnoses before even conducting a physical examination. See Table 10-5 for important additions to the pediatric history.

PEDIATRIC RESUSCITATION

> **KEY POINT:**
>
> Most pediatric cardiac arrests are from respiratory problems—treat with oxygen first.

TABLE 10-4 CALCULATING PEDIATRIC MAINTENANCE FLUID REQUIREMENTS

For the first 10 kg of the child's weight use	4 mL/kg/h
For the next 10–20 kg of weight add	2 mL/kg/h
For each kg above 20 kg add	1 mL/kg/h

TABLE 10-5 KEY AREAS TO COVER IN A PEDIATRIC HISTORY AND PHYSICAL

History
  Prenatal history
    Mother's obstetric history
      No. of pregnancies
      No. of births
      No. of miscarriages
      No. of living children
    Mother's health during pregnancy
      Infections
      Vaginal bleeding
      Tetanus immunization
      Medications taken
  Birth history
    Weeks of pregnancy to birth
    Problems during labor (including prolonged labor)
    Type of delivery (vaginal, cesarean section, forceps, etc.)
    Birthweight
  Neonnatal history
    Complications after birth
    Congenital anomalies
    Jaundice
  Feeding history
    Breast or bottle fed?
    Frequency
    Amount (or time on breast)
    Strength of the suck (to assess neonatal tetanus)
    Type of formula and how prepared (boiled water?)
    Frequency and amount of spitting up (try differential from active vomiting)
    Age that solid foods were introduced (what foods?)
    Current weight (and weights at 3 mo, 1 yr, 2 yr, and 5 yr)
  Activity routine
    Frequency and duration of sleep (remind mothers not to let babies sleep on their stomachs)
    Frequency and duration of crying (what consoles the baby?)
    Frequency of urination
    Frequency, amount, and color of stools
  Developmental history
    Age when slept through the night (normal = 2–3 mo)
    Age when first rolled over (4 mo)
    Age when first crawled (8–10 mo)
    Age when first walked (12–14 mo)
    Age when first used words (15–16 mo)
  Immunizations
    Assess if up to date (based on the country's schedule)
Physical exam
    Weight, length, and head circumference (compared with population-specific norms, use a
      growth chart to follow the trends)
    The size and fullness of the fontanelles
    Check for the eruption of the teeth
    Palpate the liver and spleen (the latter for malaria)
    Assess males for descended testicles
    Check the spine for straightness and a proper lordotic curve

Like all resuscitation situations, learning a simple, step-by-step plan for pediatric resuscitation ensures better adherence to protocols and improved outcomes. Study and practice resuscitations with the entire staff prior to an actual emergency. Always follow the steps of *Airway*, *Breathing*, and *Circulation* (ABCs) in any resuscitation situation.

AIRWAY

The most critical intervention, particularly in children, is to ensure the patency of the airway. Respiratory arrests usually precede cardiac arrests in children. If you prevent the respiratory arrest, the cardiac arrest may be avoided.

- The tongue is the most common cause of airway obstruction in unconscious children (it's big and their airway isn't).
- Don't manipulate the airway of an awake child in distress. Allow the child to sit comfortably.

CRITICAL ACTION:

The main cause of pediatric cardiac arrest is due to repiratory compromise. Always aggressively manage the pediatric airway first.

ASSESS THE AIRWAY

If a child is unconscious, first assume there is an airway problem. If a child is awake, assess the airway by looking and listening.

- Looking
    - Count the respiratory rate
    - Assess the level of distress (normal, anxious, agitated, lethargic, unconscious)
    - Look for retractions, nasal flaring and accessory muscle use.
    - Cyanosis is an ominous sign of impending respiratory failure.
- Listening
    - Upper airway problems present with stridor
    - Lower airway problems present with wheezing, rales, and grunting.

See Table 10-6.

OPEN THE AIRWAY

HEAD POSITIONING The first and most important step in an unconscious and uninjured child is to properly position the head.

TABLE 10-6 IMPORTANT CAUSES OF UPPER AIRWAY DISTRESS IN CHILDREN

	AGES AFFECTED	FINDINGS
Croup	3 mo to 3 yr	Barking cough especially at night; relief with humidity
Foreign body aspiration	8 mo to 4 yr	May have a history of choking followed by respiratory distress and wheezing; aspirations deep into the lung may present with pneumonia
Epiglottitis	1–7 yr	Very ill-appearing child with rapid onset of fever, dysphagia, drool
Other infections (tonsillitis, bacterial tracheitis, abscesses)	Various ages	Various presentations

- For an unconscious child, the head tilt/child lift is the best method to open the airway (but it is not used in the conscious child) (Fig. 10-1).
- The jaw thrust is also useful, especially in trauma when the possibility of a neck injury exists (Fig. 10-2).

Avoid hyperextension of the neck because the flexible pediatric airway can actually be obstructed by hyperextension.

ARTIFICIAL AIRWAYS A nasal or oral airway may be considered if the tongue is causing obstruction. A nasopharyngeal airway should not be used for children under age 3. To insert an oropharyngeal airway

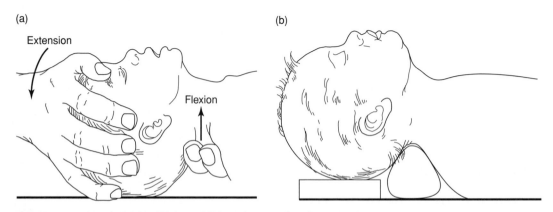

FIGURE 10-1 Head tilt/chin lift in a child, and proper head positioning.

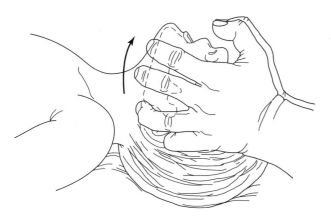

FIGURE 10-2 Jaw thrust to open a child's airway in trauma.

- The oropharyngeal airway should reach from the mandibular angle to the corner of the lip.
- Use a tongue depressor to hold down the tongue when placing an oropharyngeal airway and slide it gently over the tongue. Avoid the upside-down and twist technique.

SPECIFIC AIRWAY PROBLEMS

FOREIGN BODIES If these prior interventions do not work, assume that a foreign body is present. Foreign body aspiration can occur at any age, but it is most common in the very young and very old. Any object can be aspirated, but usually it is some type of food such as nuts or seeds, or a toy. In children the three most common areas for lodged esophageal foreign bodies are at the cricopharyngeus, the aortic arch, and the gastro-esophageal junction.

CLINICAL FEATURES Symptoms can range from asymptomatic to wheezing and acute respiratory distress. There is usually a history of a choking episode, but aspirated foreign bodies may present as new-onset wheezing, tachypnea, or pneumonia. Always keep foreign bodies in your differential diagnosis of new-onset asthma, particularly in children.

DIAGNOSIS A lateral and anteroposterior (AP) neck x-ray may identify the foreign body in the throat. If a neck x-ray, and a plain AP chest x-ray does not demonstrate the foreign body, then obtain inspiratory and expiratory views or lateral decubitus films. Look for collapsed lobes of the lung, paradoxical hyperinflation, or a midline shift.

TREATMENT For emergency treatment of an unconscious child

- Look in the mouth and pull out any visible foreign body (do not use the finger sweep). Use forceps (McGills are the best), pickups, tweezers, or whatever it takes.
- For infants: Administer five back blows while holding the infant draped upside down over your arm with the head hanging down (this can also be done on an awake, choking baby). Then lay the baby supine on a hard surface, or head tilted down on your arm and give five chest thrusts. The thrusts are sharper and at a slower rate than those given during cardiopulmonary resuscitation (CPR) (Fig. 10-3).
- For CHILDREN over 1 year of age: Administer repetitive abdominal thrusts to the upper abdomen. Direct the thrusts upward.
- Reexamine the airway to see if anything has been dislodged. Pull it out.
- If nothing is obvious, use a laryngoscope (particularly if the patient is unconscious). Remove the foreign body with a forceps.
- Intubate if the patient is unconscious.

If the patient is conscious but in respiratory distress

- Give oxygen by any means available. If the child deteriorates,
- Attempt bag-valve-mask (BVM) ventilation and then prepare for rapid sequence intubation (RSI).

For a stable child with a partial airway obstruction, the ideal method for dislodging the foreign body is with direct visualization under general anesthesia. If this is unavailable, visualization with a laryngoscope can be attempted with conscious sedation (preferably with ketamine; see Chapter 18). See Chapter 11 for discussions on epiglottitis and croup.

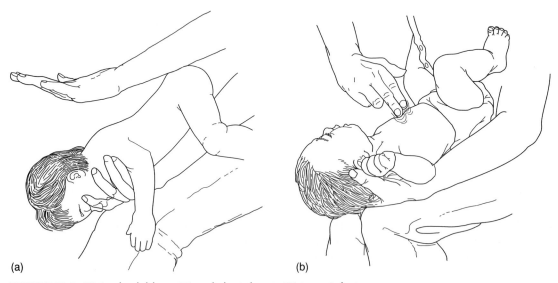

(a) (b)

FIGURE 10-3 Giving back blows (A) and chest thrusts (B) to an infant.

BREATHING

There are many respiratory problems specific to, or more significant in, children. Because the airway of the child is smaller and creates more resistance to airflow, diseases that affect the airway can lead to rapid respiratory compromise.

ASSESS BREATHING

This takes place simultaneously with airway assessment, as described earlier. Look for effort, rate, air entry, and color. Listen to the lungs for the presence of symmetric breath sounds, wheezes, rales, rhonchi, and other noises. In the early stages of respiratory distress, a child may appear anxious, but remain alert. As the respiratory problems worsen and hypoxia and hypercarbia develop, the child becomes more anxious, then combative, then lethargic, and finally unconscious. Other findings may include

- Tachypnea
- The use of accessory muscles to assist with breathing
- Intercostal, supra- and substernal, and supraclavicular retractions
- Nasal flaring
- Grunting (a serious sign of lower airway disease)
- Cyanosis (an ominous sign that is often followed by complete respiratory arrest)

Another clue to a child in respiratory distress is the position assumed. With upper airway disease (epiglottitis, foreign body), the child assumes the "sniffing position," which is sitting upright, leaning slightly forward with the neck and chin extended forward.

With lower airway disease, such as asthma, children (and adults) often sit in the "tripod position." They also sit upright and lean forward, but they fully extend their thorax by pushing their hands with extended arms against their thighs (or the edge of the bed).

BREATHING

For the unconscious and nonbreathing child, the first step is to administer mouth-to-mouth or BVM ventilation (Fig. 10-4).

- For either technique, ensure a good seal around the mouth, or proper lung inflation will not occur. Correct bagging technique is crucial. The most common problem when bagging is a poor seal so that the air is blown out in the cheeks and not down into the lungs. To prevent this, keep your fingers along the mandible or use one person to hold the mask with both hands and the other to squeeze the bag.
- First give two slow breaths while watching the chest rise.
- For infants and small children, breathe 20 times per minute.

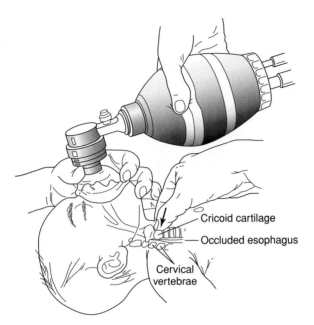

Cricoid cartilage

Occluded esophagus

Cervical
vertebrae

FIGURE 10-4 Bag-valve-mask technique.

INTUBATION

Intubation to control an airway is not available in many field settings. Even where there is the basic equipment [a laryngoscope, endotracheal tubes (ETTs), and a bag-valve mask], there is often not a mechanical respirator or monitor so the patient must be ventilated (bagged) by hand for the duration of the intubation. In ideal circumstances the optimum method for emergency intubation is rapid sequence intubation (RSI). However, it requires a great deal of training and experience with the techniques and drugs. It is therefore important that physicians who intubate be trained in and comfortable with performing the procedure, administering the drugs, and addressing the complications of the techniques. The major exceptions to using RSI are not being familiar with the procedure, the pressure of facial trauma or other difficult airway anatomy, and a patient who already has complete muscle relaxation and does not respond to painful stimulus.

For children in respiratory distress but still breathing, the key to treatment is to diagnose the cause of the respiratory distress. The provider must decide if the problem is occurring in the upper or lower tract.

SPECIFIC AIRWAY PROBLEMS

UPPER AIRWAY

Epiglottitis: see Chapter 11
Croup syndrome: see Chapter 11

Retropharyngeal abscess: see Chapter 8
Bacterial tracheitis: see Chapter 11

LOWER AIRWAY

ASTHMA Management of asthma in the child is similar to that in the adult, but calculate pediatric doses based on the child's weight. Aerosolized beta agonists (Albuterol) are the mainstay of treatment for an acute exacerbation, but are often not available. Inhaled and oral steroids are used for longer-term control. See Chapter 7 for details.

BRONCHIOLITIS Bronchiolitis is a clinical syndrome of tachypnea, wheezing, and retractions that generally occurs in children 2 to 8 months of age, but may occur in children up to 2 years of age. It is usually caused by the respiratory syncytial virus (RSV) and occurs more commonly in winter and spring. It may respond to aerosolized bronchodilator therapy, but generally requires no treatment. Younger children are often more severely affected and may require hospitalization and oxygen therapy.

CIRCULATION

ASSESS THE CIRCULATION

Check for the brachial pulse in infants and small children. Tachycardia is the first finding, bradycardia is an ominous sign. Blood pressure stays stable despite severe insults because children can vasoconstrict and compensate so well to maintain blood pressure.

> Use capillary refill to assess perfusion. Normal cap refill is 2 seconds or less. Other ways to assess the peripheral circulation:
>
> Assess the patient's level of consciousness
> Skin color: pink, pale, or mottled
> Cold hands and feet
> Skin turgor, mucous membranes, and urine output

TREAT THE CIRCULATION PROBLEMS

Stop all bleeding immediately and obtain vascular access. Begin fluid resuscitation for patients with a weak pulse, hypotension, and/or slow capillary refill (signs of shock). Use NS or lactated Ringer's solution (LR).

■ Give an initial bolus of 20 mL/kg of NS or LR and start looking for the cause of the hypotension.

■ If the patient continues to demonstrate signs of shock (tachycardia, slow capillary refill, etc.), the bolus may be repeated two more times.

If no response to the fluid boluses

■ If bleeding is a possible cause of hypotension (trauma, gastrointestinal bleed), then transfuse 10 mL/kg of packed red blood cells.
■ If there is a possible cardiac cause, treat the underlying cause (arrhythmia) and/or begin pressor support with epinephrine, dopamine, etc.

For patients with no pulse or blood pressure, start CPR:

■ The chest compression rate for children is at least 100 per minute.
■ For infants, compress with two fingers one finger breadth below the intermammary line and compress 1.5 to 2.5 cm (½ to 1 inch), or one third to one half the depth of the chest.
■ For children 1 to 8 years of age, place the heel of the hand one to two finger breadths above the infrasternal notch and compress 2.5 to 3.5 cm (1–1½ inches).
■ The ratio of compressions to breathing is 5:1.

CARDIAC ARREST

Securing the airway and providing oxygen is the first treatment for cardiac arrest in children.

TREATMENT

■ The dose of epinephrine for cardiac resuscitation is 0.01 mg/kg, or 0.1 mL/kg of the 1:10,000 solution. Therefore, a 10-kg 1-year-old needs 1 mL. The dose is repeated every 3 to 5 minutes. If the first dose is ineffective, consideration should be given to increasing the dose 10 times to 0.1 mg/kg (1.0 mL/kg of the 1:10,000 solution or 0.1 mL/kg of 1:1,000).
■ Atropine has questionable use for bradycardia and asystole in pediatrics because they are almost always caused by hypoxia and are treated with oxygen. When needed, the dose is 0.02 to 0.03 mg/kg, with a 0.15-mg minimum and a 1.0-mg maximum dose.
■ There is no evidence to show a benefit from bicarbonate, but some physicians still recommend it if the pH is below 7.0. If it is used, the starting dose is 1 to 2 mEq/kg. In general, do not use it unless the pH is confirmed to be less than 7.0.

For blood pressure support in a hypotensive child, use a continuous epinephrine effusion. Use the "rule of point six" to calculate the dose:

> ### THE RULE OF POINT SIX:
>
> 0.6 × body weight (kg) = the amount (mg) to add to 100 mL of fluid. Then, 1 mL/h of this solution delivers 0.1 µg/kg/min. The same formula can be used with nor-epinephrine, Neo-Synephrine, and isoproterenol.

For dopamine or dobutamine use the "rule of six":

> ### THE RULE OF SIX:
>
> 6 × the body weight (kg) = the amount (mg) to add to 100 mL of fluid. At this strength, 1 mL/h delivers 1 µg/kg/min. This same formula can be used for lidocaine.

DELIVERING MEDICINES VIA ENDOTRACHEAL TUBE Remember "NAVEL" for medications that can be delivered by endotracheal route: Narcan, atropine, Valium (diazepam), epinephrine, and lidocaine.

- When giving epinephrine via the ETT, use 0.1 mg/kg or 0.1 mL/kg of 1:1,000.
- Dilute the medication with 5 to 10 mL of NS and squirt it rapidly into the ETT, followed by five positive pressure bagged breaths to diffuse the medicine into the alveoli.

SHOCK

Shock results from inadequate tissue perfusion and oxygen due to a circulatory problem. The primary cause of shock in children is dehydration due to diarrhea (see Chapter 11). Other causes include hypovolemic (bleeding, other causes of dehydration), cardiogenic (congenital, dysrhythmias), distributive (sepsis, anaphylaxis), obstructive (tamponade, tension pneumothorax), and toxic (carbon monoxide).

After initiation of fluid resuscitation for circulatory compromise, the cause of the shock must be identified and specific treatment targeted to correct it. If there is no history of trauma, then it is wise to consider infection as the cause and to begin intravenous (IV) antibiotic therapy without delay.

FLUID AND ELECTROLYTE RESUSCITATION GUIDELINES

Diarrhea and vomiting are the most common cause of dehydration in children, particularly in developing countries. Other causes include trauma, diabetic ketoacidosis, and burns. For a child presenting in shock or severe dehydration

- The initial bolus of NS or LR is 20 mL/kg.
- If the patient remains "shocky" (tachycardic and poor capillary refill), repeat the bolus.
- If shock continues after the third bolus, then other methods are needed.
  - In trauma (or other potential causes of blood loss) a blood transfusion of 10 mL/kg is given.
  - If the cause is cardiogenic, medically treat the pathologic tachycardia or bradycardia or use a pressor agent such as epinephrine or dopamine.

DRUGS TO SUPPORT BLOOD PRESSURE

- Epinephrine: Start at 0.05 to 0.1 μg/kg/min. At low doses the beta-1 and beta-2 effects predominate. Titrate doses higher to achieve more alpha effects and blood pressure elevation.
- Dopamine: Start at 2.0 to 5.0 μg/kg/min for the renal effects and to increase urine output. From 6.0 to 10.0 μg/kg/min the beta effects increase cardiac output. Above 10.0 μg/kg/min the alpha effects (vasoconstriction) are most prominent.

CARDIAC EMERGENCIES

EXAMINING THE HEART IN A CHILD

THE CARDIAC EXAMINATION A murmur that is heard in the first few days of life is usually significant. Murmurs from left to right shunts such as a ventricular septal defect may not be heard until 4 to 6 weeks of age. The intensity of the murmur does not necessarily correlate with the severity of the defect. Patients with a murmur should be referred to a medical center for further evaluation.

Cyanosis in an infant is a frightening finding that is usually indicative of severe pathology. Causes include cardiac, respiratory, and toxicologic pathology. Cyanotic heart disease is usually due to a right-to-left shunt.

CHEST X-RAY A chest x-ray is used to assess the shape and size of the heart and to evaluate pulmonary blood flow by the distribution and size of the vessels. Infants have a large, straight, thymic border that appears as cardiomegaly to untrained readers. Any abnormalities of the heart or blood flow require that the child be referred for a more complete evaluation, including an echocardiogram.

ELECTROCARDIOGRAM Electrocardiograms (ECGs) are rarely indicated in newborns and young children. If an arrhythmia is suspected, an ECG can be performed. Remember in the interpretation that

- Right axis deviation is normal in newborns.
- T-waves may be inverted in the precordial leads until adolescence.

■ A "sinus arrhythmia" may be misdiagnosed because of the extreme respiratory variation in the rate seen in children.

Cardiac monitoring is usually sufficient to diagnose a dysrhythmia and to tailor the appropriate treatment. If necessary, the patient can be monitored by using the defibrillator paddles.

DYSRHYTHMIAS Cardiac arrhythmias are rare in children, even in those with congenital cardiac defects. The most likely causes of hypotension in a child are infection, trauma, or dehydration. These occur far more often than cardiogenic causes (see Chapter 9 for details on treating dysrhythmias). If cardiac monitoring capabilities exist, then the interventions can be targeted to the specific dysrhythmia. ACLS (advanced cardiac life support) and PALS (pediatric advanced life support) guidelines should be followed.

SUPRAVENTRICULAR TACHYCARDIA Supraventricular tachycardia (SVT) is the most common childhood dysrhythmia, with rates of 220 beats/min and higher (although the most common rhythm at this rate is sinus tachycardia). Infants present with periods of lethargy, tachycardia, and tachypnea. Older children may complain of palpitations and chest pain. Most SVTs resolve spontaneously. If not, treat by

■ Vagal maneuvers, including ice to the face, abdominal pressure (push against the child's abdomen and tell him or her to push back), and rubbing the patient's eyeballs
■ Adenosine at an initial dose of 0.1 mg/kg in a rapid IV bolus followed by a flush of 2 to 5 mL of NS. Double the dose to 0.2 mg/kg and repeat if necessary. The maximum dose is 12 mg.

For the stable patient, synchronized cardioversion is rarely needed, but for an unstable patient, use 0.5 J/kg. Then double the dose if ineffective.

VENTRICULAR FIBRILLATION AND PULSELESS VENTRICULAR TACHYCARDIA

■ Start oxygen.
■ Defibrillate starting at 2 J/kg. For infants use 4.5-cm paddles and 8.0-cm paddles for older children.

If unsuccessful

■ Double to 4 J/kg; if unsuccessful, repeat again if needed.

If unsuccessful

■ Intubate and give
    ■ Epinephrine 0.01 mg/kg of 1:10,000 IV or intraosseously, then
    ■ Defibrillate at 4 J/kg

If unsuccessful

■ Start lidocaine with a bolus of 1.0 mg/kg IV, then
■ Defibrillate at 4 J/kg
■ If the dysrhythmia persists, repeat the epinephrine dose every 3 to 5 minutes. May also alternate with lidocaine to a maximum of 3 to 5 mg/kg, while continuing defibrillations.

VENTRICULAR TACHYCARDIA WITH A PULSE

If an IV is available

■ Lidocaine 1.0 mg/kg, if a successful conversion to normal sinus rhythm, then start a continuous drip of 20 to 50 μg/min.

If unsuccessful

■ Synchronized cardioversion at 0.5 J/kg, repeat at 1.0 J/kg if necessary.

If unsuccessful

■ Repeat the lidocaine bolus of 1.0 mg/kg IV, then start an infusion or repeat the boluses to a maximum of 3 to 5 mg/kg, then
■ Repeat synchronized cardioversion at 1.0 J/kg as needed.

BRADYDYSRHYTHMIAS

> Bradycardia is almost exclusively due to hypoxia or airway problems: Treat with oxygen, not atropine.

If airway maneuvers and oxygen is not successful

■ Reduce vagal stimuli (vomiting, nausea, etc.).
■ Start epinephrine 0.01 mg/kg of the 1:10,000 solution IV or intraosseously (the dose is 0.01–0.03 mg/kg for neonates). If this is not successful,
■ Give atropine 0.02 mg/kg IV (minimum dose of 0.1 mg) every 5 minutes, to a maximum of 1 mg.

CONGENITAL HEART DISEASE

Congenital heart problems occur in approximately 1% of births, although most will remain asymptomatic and undiagnosed. The goal of the physician working in the field is to identify a potentially serious cardiac murmur and to refer the case to a hospital for a more definitive diagnosis. Therefore, the physician must be aware of the potential for the disorders and for the treatment and stabilization of their acute presentations.

Beware of hypercyanotic episodes of children with tetralogy of Fallot (tet spells). To treat

- Give oxygen.
- Place the patient in the knee-chest position.
- Give IV morphine if needed.

Also prevent any IV air bubbles for a suspected right-to-left shunt, which can cause a cerebrovascular accident or myocardial infarction.

CHEST PAIN The most common cause of chest pain in preadolescents and teenagers is costochondritis or other musculoskeletal pain. The pain is usually located over the anterior costochondral junction, which is tender to palpation. Treatment is pain relief with a nonsteroidal antiinflammatory drug, such as ibuprofen. Consideration should be given to an ischemic event in areas with endemic Kawasaki disease.

SYNCOPE The most common cause of syncope in children and adolescents is a benign vasovagal reflex. Other causes include hypertrophic cardiomyopathy, aortic stenosis, tetralogy of Fallot, and cardiac arrhythmias such as prolonged QT syndrome, ventricular tachycardia, and sick sinus syndrome.

Cardiac monitoring may be indicated if an arrhythmia is suspected, if the patient has an irregular pulse, or if the patient has cardiac symptoms such as palpitations, chest pain, or shortness of breath that preceded the syncope.

SEIZURES

Seizures are caused by abnormal electrical discharges in the brain that lead to an involuntary change in consciousness, usually associated with motor activity. Approximately 5% of children will have at least one seizure. Most are benign febrile seizures, but most nonfebrile seizures are idiopathic. Often the history may be the only clue to determine the cause of seizures. The major causes of childhood seizures include:

- Idiopathic
- Brain injury/head trauma
- Hyponatremia due to ingesting water without electrolytes, usually when treating gastroenteritis
- Hypoglycemia (always perform a fingerstick glucose test)

STATUS EPILEPTICUS

Status epilepticus is a seizure or multiple seizures, lasting more than 30 minutes or without a lucid (conscious and cognizant) period between seizures. These can lead to long-term damage to the brain. The most common cause of status epilepticus is idiopathic. Other etiologies include brain trauma (including birth injury), infections (meningitis), toxins (organophosphate insecticides, isoniazid, theophylline, anticonvulsants, sympathomimetics, others), hypoglycemia, hypo- and hypernatremia, hypocalcemia, and metabolic disorders.

DIAGNOSIS Status epilepticus must be considered whenever multiple seizures occur or in any unconscious patient, because the stereotypical tonic-clonic seizure movements do not always occur. Examine all unconscious patients for more subtle signs of seizures such as minor tremors or eye twitching.
Attempt to identify the underlying cause:

- Perform a fingerstick glucose test.
- Check the temperature.
- Look for signs of trauma.
- Get a detailed history from the parents.
- Check the electrolytes and calcium levels.
- A brain computed tomography (CT) scan and toxicology screen are very useful but often are not available outside of large hospitals.

TREATMENT As with any critical patient, always consider the ABCs first:

- Clear the airway and give oxygen.
- Don't stick anything in the mouth.
- If the glucose is low, or the child is a known diabetic, give glucose 250 to 500 mg/kg, 1 to 2 mL/kg of 25% dextrose solution ($D_{25}W$), or 2.5 to 5.0 mL/kg of $D_{10}W$.

The initial treatment of choice for the seizures is a benzodiazepine (Table 10-7). When IV access is not available, then diazepam can be given per rectum or midazolam can be given intramuscularly (IM).
After the benzodiazepine controls the seizures, long-term anticonvulsant control is needed. If patients do not stop seizing, then other drugs are indicated. For both cases use

- Phenytoin (Dilantin) 1 mg/kg/min IV (maximum 50 mg/min) to a total dose of 10 to 20 mg/kg. It is effective within 30 minutes after the end of the infusion.

TABLE 10-7 DRUGS FOR THE CONTROL OF STATUS EPILEPTICUS

DRUG	DOSE	DURATION
Diazepam	0.2 mg/kg IV or 0.5 mg/kg per rectum Repeat every 2 min, maximum dose 10 g IV or 20 mg PR	5–15 min
Lorazepam	0.05–0.10 mg/kg IV Repeat every 15 min, maximum dose 4 mg	12–24 h
Midazolam	0.20 mg/kg IM	1–5 h

(Fosphenytoin has recently come on the market and can be loaded faster, but it is expensive. The dose is the same, but it can be given at 3 mg/kg/min), or

- Phenobarbital 1 to 2 mg/min IV to a total dose of 15 to 20 mg/kg. Onset is 10 to 20 minutes, or
- Paraldehyde 0.3 mL/kg per rectum to a maximum of 5 mL. This drug may be available in developing countries.

If the seizures cannot be controlled with the above drugs, consideration must be given to more aggressive methods, depending on the availability of resources. These include ETT intubation with general anesthesia with muscle paralysis and a barbiturate coma. This can only be accomplished in a monitored setting.

TREATMENT OF CHRONIC SEIZURES

The need for treatment for a single nonfebrile seizure is controversial because as many as 70% of "epileptic" patients become seizure free. Given the cost of medications, the difficulty in follow-up, and the frequent unavailability of CT and electroencephalography equipment, a single seizure may not require treatment.

Long-term therapy for seizures relies primarily on six major drugs for children: phenytoin, phenobarbital, carbamazepine, valproic acid, ethosuximide, and primidone. Single-drug therapy is sufficient for the majority of children. See Chapter 11 for a discussion of benign febrile seizures.

NEONATAL RESUSCITATION

PHYSIOLOGIC CONSIDERATIONS IN THE FIRST 28 DAYS

From the moment the umbilical cord is cut, the cardiac and respiratory physiology of the neonate transforms to an independent system. The ductus arteriosus is normally completely closed by 15 hours, systemic vascular resistance increases, and pulmonary blood flow increases.

IMPORTANT PHYSIOLOGIC CONSIDERATIONS

- Infants lose heat quickly.
- Cardiac output is controlled almost exclusively by rate.
- Pulmonary vascular resistance is labile, leading to right-to-left shunting with acidosis, hypoxia, and hypercarbia.
- Hypoglycemia can occur quickly because of low stores and high use.

The level of resuscitation must be decided in advance, prior to resuscitation at birth. This should be based on the available resources and abilities. The availability of a pediatric ventilator is probably the greatest determinate of the ability to resuscitate premature infants. Markedly premature infants (less than 25–27 weeks' gestation, or 650–750 g) require advanced care, often not available anywhere in developing countries. An Apgar score (Table 10-8) that remains below 3 to 5 at 5 minutes (or even 10 minutes) is an ominous sign.

A score of 7 or less indicates the need for more aggressive resuscitation. By 1 minute, a baby with an Apgar score of 0 to 2 requires intubation. A score of 3 to 6 requires either bagging or intubation.

As with any emergency situation, prepare for the worst, but hope for the best. Have basic resuscitation equipment ready for every birth and practice, and prepare yourself prior to the birth.

Identify high-risk births by asking the mother about

- Her expected delivery date or last menstrual period (high-risk if early or late)
- If she has seen meconium (high-risk if present)
- How long the labor has lasted (high-risk if prolonged)
- The nature and timing of contractions
- The possibility of twins

BASIC RESUSCITATION

- As the head emerges at birth, immediately suction the nose and mouth with a bulb syringe, suction catheter, or 5 mL syringe. If meconium is present, always suction the nose and mouth before bagging a nonbreathing neonate.
- Warming is essential from the moment of birth.
- Don't forget stimulation and drying.
- Calculate the Apgar score at 1 and 5 minutes to direct the level of resuscitation.

RESUSCITATION OF AN UNRESPONSIVE NEONATE

- If drying, warming, suctioning, and stimulation do not increase the Apgar score, then give oxygen by blowing it at the baby's nose and mouth.
- If that is unsuccessful, then begin bagging the baby to support respirations.

TABLE 10-8 THE APGAR SCORE

	0	1	2
Appearance (color)	Pale/blue	Body pink, limbs blue	Pink body/limbs
Pulse (palpate the cord)	Absent	100	100
Grimace (reflex)	None	Weak	Strong
Activity (muscle tone)	None/limp	Slight flexion	Spontaneous
Respiratory effort	Absent	Hypoventilation	Strong cry

- If the cord and/or femoral artery are pulseless, or the heart rate is less than 60 beats/min, start CPR at 120 breaths/min.
- Finally, if the resources are available, intubate and start ACLS drugs.

Use the umbilical vein for drugs and fluids (Fig. 10-5).

- Epinephrine is dosed at 0.01 to 0.03 mg/kg of the 1:10,000 every 3 to 5 minutes. Do not increase the subsequent doses.
- Naloxone is given if the mother received a narcotic for pain during labor, or is suspected of narcotic use. Give 0.1 mg/kg IV, IM, or by the ETT.

Beware of hypoglycemia; premature babies may have low glucose stores that are used up quickly. Give $D_{50}W$ IV bolus if low blood sugar is suspected.

SUDDEN INFANT DEATH SYNDROME

Sudden infant death syndrome (SIDS) is a common cause of death between 1 month and 1 year of life, but rates in developing countries are not well described. The peak incidence is 1 to 4 months of age, with 90% occurring by 6 months. Infants who sleep in the prone position (face down) are at the greatest risk for SIDS. Maternal smoking, prematurity, low birth weight, and male gender are also risk factors.

PREVENTION

> All mothers should be educated to have their infants sleep on their backs or sides and to avoid positioning their babies in the prone position.

Parental smoking also increases the risk of SIDS: counsel patients to stop smoking.

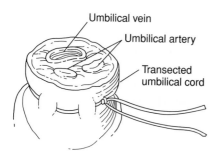

Umbilical vein
Umbilical artery
Transected umbilical cord

FIGURE 10-5 The umbilical vein for intravenous access.

CHILD ABUSE

Child abuse is a global problem and encompasses physical, psychological, and sexual abuse. Signs of physical abuse include the following:

- Bruises to lower back, buttocks, ears, or handprints to face are very suggestive.
- Beware of metaphyseal chips at the end of long bones from rotary forces.
- Unexplained spiral fractures
- Retinal hemorrhages, lethargy, and the "shaken baby" syndrome
- Glove-stocking patterns of burns

TREATMENT

There are no simple solutions to the problem of child abuse and there are many cultural complexities to the issue. The solution to child abuse is long term but there are some things that can be done immediately:

- Remove the child to a safe place if possible.
- Work with the local authorities if they are responsive to child abuse and there are enforceable laws protecting children.
- Work to educate families about appropriate discipline.
- Educate the population about child abuse.

APPENDIX 10.1: Advanced Pediatric Airway Management

Refer to Chapter 9 for further discussion of advanced airway management.

ANATOMIC CONSIDERATIONS WITH THE PEDIATRIC AIRWAY

The airway anatomy of young children is significantly different from that of an adult:

- The resistance of airflow increases markedly as the radius of the trachea is reduced. Therefore, even small changes in the already narrow pediatric airway drastically increases resistance and the work of breathing.
- The tongue is relatively larger, making visualization of the cords when intubating more difficult.
- The location and shape of the epiglottis leads to obstructions when infected. It may require the use of a straight blade to lift the epiglottis when intubating children.
- The cricoid cartilage just below the vocal cords is the narrowest area of the trachea. Therefore, uncuffed ETTs are used for children under 6 to 8 years of age.

- The trachea is very short; the distance from the cords to carina is 12 to 15 cm in adults but only 4 cm in newborns. This increases the risk of mainstem bronchus intubation and inadvertent extubation.
- Children have large adenoids, which is a relative contraindication to nasotracheal intubation.

STEPS FOR INTUBATION AND RAPID SEQUENCE INTUBATION

The reader is referred to Chapter 9 for further details regarding intubation. The following are modifications to the adult process that apply to children. The basic intubation steps are

1. Preparation
2. Pretreatment
3. Paralysis (RSI only)
4. Intubation
5. Protect/confirm

Table 10-9 provides information for intubating a child.

STEP 1: PREPARE TO INTUBATE

PREPARE THE PATIENT

- Position the child by placing the head in the sniffing position (neck extended/head tipped back/chin pointing up). A small pad under the occiput can be used to extend the neck in children over 2 years of age. Do not hyperextend the neck.
- If possible place a nasogastric tube prior to intubation to minimize gastric distention.
- Do not bag an awake patient—it fills the stomach with air and increases the risk of vomiting.

KEY POINT:

Preoxygenation for 3 to 5 minutes on 100% O_2 is particularly critical for children to allow for sufficient time to intubate.

TABLE 10-9 METHODS TO ESTIMATE THE SIZE OF THE ET TUBE FOR A CHILD

1. Use the tube that is the width of the fingernail of the 5th digit of the hand (the pinky)
2. Age (in years) + 16]/4 = ETT size
3. By the width of the child's nares

To estimate the depth to place an ETT: age (in years) + 12 cm

PREPARE THE EQUIPMENT A working suction is essential for children because they tend to have more secretions and an already small airway. Table 10-10 lists some of the equipment used in pediatric intubation.

STEP 2: PRETREATMENT See Table 10-11 for a complete listing of pediatric doses. Pretreat children under 6 years of age with atropine (0.02 mg/kg IV) to decrease secretions. Ketamine is a very useful pretreatment sedative for children and adults. It puts the patient in a dissociative state so that they are not aware of or responsive to their surroundings. Ketamine can be given IM prior to beginning the procedure (even starting the IV) to reduce the anxiety and pain of the child. See Chapter 18 for details on its use. The intubating dose of ketamine in children is 4 to 10 mg/kg IM or 2 to 4 mg/kg IV, followed by an infusion of 1 to 2 mg/kg/min.

STEP 3: PARALYSIS This step is taken for RSI only; see Chapter 9 for details.

STEP 4: INTUBATE Use a straight blade for children under 2 years of age.

STEP 5: CONFIRM AND PROTECT

■ Listen first over the stomach with the first bagged breath. If you hear a gurgle, stop bagging and attempt intubating again. If no stomach sounds,

TABLE 10-10 RECOMMENDED EQUIPMENT
FOR PEDIATRIC INTUBATION

- Laryngoscope handles (2)
- Laryngoscope blades
    Curved (MacIntosh)   2,3,4
    Straight (Miller)   0,1,2,3
- Uncuffed 2.5–8.0 ET tubes
- Cuffed 5.5–9.0 ET tubes
- Moldable stylets
- A suction device with a large-bore tip (Yankauer)
- Self-inflating ventilation bags (preferably with pop-off valve and an oxygen reservoir with pediatric and adult masks
- Nonrebreather face masks (neonate, infant, pediatric, and adult)
- Some type of monitor (cardiac or pulse oximeter)

Other useful equipment
- Pulse oximeter
- End-tidal CO_2 monitor
- A backup surgical airway tray (cricothyrotomy and/or tracheostomy)

TABLE 10-11 DRUG DOSES FOR PEDIATRIC INTUBATION

DRUG	DOSE	ONSET	DURATION
Pretreatment			
Atropine	0.02 mg/kg (0.1 mg minimum)	1 min	Not applicable
Pretreatment, Sedation			
Ketamine	1–2 mg/kg	1–2 min	20–30 min
Midazolam	0.05–0.2 mg/kg	1–2 min	30–60 min
Diazepam (Valium)	0.1–0.3 mg/kg slowly	3–5 min	45–90 min
Thiopental	4–6 mg/kg	30 s	10–30 min
Paralysis			
Succinylcholine	1.5–2.0 mg/kg	30–45 s	4–10 min
Pancuronium (Pavulon)	0.1 mg/kg	2–3 min	45–90 min

- Listen laterally to each side of the chest for equal breath sounds.
- Tape the ETT securely. You should also restrain the hands to prevent extubation.

SURGICAL AIRWAYS

The creation of an emergency surgical airway in the infant and child is also different from the adult techniques. A surgical cricothyrotomy is not recommended in children under 8 (some say 12) years of age because the cricoid cartilage does not provide sufficient support. Instead, needle cricothyrotomy can be attempted.

NEEDLE CRICOTHYROTOMY This technique uses a small-gauge port (a 14-gauge needle) to bag the child; therefore, this is a temporary solution, not a definitive airway.

- Attach a large-bore (12- or 14-gauge) angiocatheter (a needle with a plastic catheter over it) to a 10- to 20-mL syringe partially filled with liquid.
- The cricothyroid membrane is palpated and identified; the overlying skin is cleaned with iodine or other antiseptic.
- Insert the needle through the cricothyroid membrane while gently withdrawing on the syringe (look for bubbles).
- Draw back with a syringe to ensure that at least 10 to 20 mL of air returns.
- While holding the catheter steady, or advancing slightly, carefully pull the syringe and needle out.
- Attach the hub of the angiocatheter to a no. 3 or no. 3.5 pediatric ETT adapter (remove the tube). Attach the ambu bag to the adapter and begin bagging.
- A 3- or 5-mL syringe also may be used to make an adapter to attach to the bag.

The reader is referred to Chapter 9 for more information on cricothyrotomy.

APPENDIX 10.2: VASCULAR ACCESS FOR CHILDREN

Rapid vascular access is essential to resuscitate pediatric patients. In a resuscitation situation, take 10 to 15 seconds to look for the best vascular access. Then, if IV access is not available within 90 seconds try, alternative routes such as intraosseous, central, or open (cut down) access.

Besides the commonly used antecubital IV site, there are other areas (Fig. 10-6):

- Scalp veins in infants (Fig. 10-7)
- The interdigital area
- Hand vein between the fourth and fifth metacarpal dorsally
- Volar wrist veins
- Superficial veins on the dorsal-lateral aspect of the foot

CENTRAL VENOUS ACCESS

In an emergency situation, femoral vein access is easier than jugular or subclavian access because it doesn't interfere with CPR. However, resuscitation drugs are delivered more

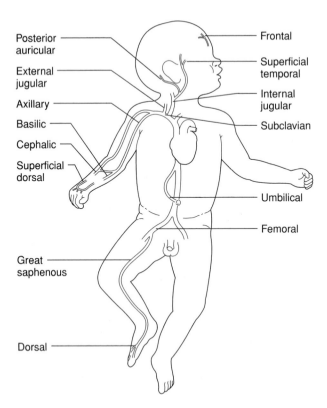

FIGURE 10-6 Common venous access sites in children.

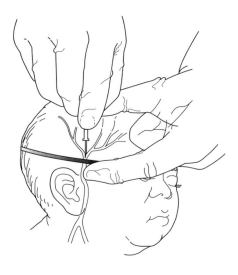

FIGURE 10-7 Scalp veins in children.

efficiently from lines above the diaphragm. Always prepare the site with betadine (or similar) solution.

For femoral access

■ Angle the needle 30 to 45 degrees superiorly and medially to the femoral pulse.
■ Insert slowly while gently aspirating the syringe.
■ When dark blood is found (bright red blood is probably arterial), advance the plastic catheter while holding the syringe and needle stable.
■ Withdraw the needle, then aspirate to see if the blood flows freely.
■ If so, attach the IV (NS or LR for resuscitation).
■ If not, start over from a slightly different position/angle.

For subclavian access, the reader is referred to Chapter 7.

INTRAOSSEOUS ACCESS

If two or three peripheral attempts are unsuccessful in the first 90 seconds, use an intraosseous or bone marrow needle for intraosseous access. The intraosseous route is rapid and effective for fluid resuscitation and all drugs. Study and practice this technique (chicken bones work well) prior to an emergency.

Critical steps for intraosseous access:

■ Locate the anterior tibial tuberosity just under the patellar ligament.
■ Prepare the skin with betadine.

- The needle entrance site is inferior and medial to the tibial tuberosity.
- Angle the needle downward (inferiorly) 45 to 60 degrees.
- Push the needle firmly while gently twisting back and forth.
- While pushing, stabilize your fingers against the bone to prevent deep penetration.
- You should feel a give or a slight pop as you enter the space. Then remove the trocar and flush with 5 mL of NS to assure flow.
- Connect the IV tubing to the needle.
- Stabilize the needle with tape or make a surrounding cardboard structure or tube to prevent it from being knocked out.

CHAPTER 11
Pediatric Infectious Diseases

Teresita Hogan and Thomas D. Kirsch

CRITICAL ACTIONS

When evaluating any patient, the ABCs (airway, breathing, and circulation) must be the first priority to ensure that you do not miss a critical problem (see Chapter 10 for details).

AIRWAY

In children the primary cause of cardiac arrest is hypoxia. Many infections can obstruct the airway, leading to hypoxia, including pseudomembrane of diphtheria, epiglottitis, or a peritonsillar abscess. It is critical to evaluate airway patency as your first step in any evaluation.

BREATHING

Ensure air exchange (breathing): Despite a patent airway, air exchange can be reduced or prevented by the infectious process. Bronchospasm can prevent adequate air exchange, as can pneumonia. Listen for clear, bilateral breath sounds and note the presence of wheezing, crackles, or diminished lung sounds. Pulse oximetry or arterial blood gases may be measured if the necessary equipment is available.

CIRCULATION

Adequate perfusion is assessed by the child's capillary perfusion, and the age-appropriate pulse and blood pressure. Remember that dehydration and sepsis are the most common causes of shock in children. Fluid boluses may be required to correct decreased circulating volume. The dose of fluid bolus is 20 mg/kg of normal saline (NS)-IV; this may be repeated every 5 minutes up to three times, depending on response.

If an infection is suspected as the cause of shock, then antibiotics should be administered immediately.

PREVENTION

Prevention is the most cost-effective disease management method. The prevention of infectious diseases requires sanitation, cleanliness, and immunization. Equally important is the education of patients and health-care staff regarding the basics of prevention. Physicians are responsible for ensuring the implementation of these preventive measures.

Sanitation means clean water and food, which means keeping these essentials away from feces. Physicians must familiarize themselves with the basic principles of sanitation, including water supplies and the use of latrines. It is their responsibility to make sure that these standards are observed at the facilities where they work. Personal cleanliness of the patient, health-care workers, and physician is also important. The single most important action is frequent hand washing while at work.

One of the greatest successes in the history of health care was the eradication of smallpox from the earth in 1979. The World Health Organization's (WHO's) Expanded Programme on Immunization evolved from that effort and now leads the fight against vaccine-preventable diseases. With the assistance of Unicef and national governments, approximately 80% of the world's children are now immunized against tuberculosis (TB), poliomyelitis, diphtheria, tetanus, pertussis, and measles. This translates to a saving of at least 2.7 million lives from measles, neonatal tetanus, and pertussis and the prevention of 200,000 cases of paralytic polio. Immunizations are also one of the most cost-effective of all health services, with an estimated savings of $5 to $30 per vaccine for each dollar spent. Unfortunately the coverage is not 100%, and vaccine-preventable diseases continue to kill millions of children, accounting for 20% to 35% of all deaths in children under 5 years of age. Measles alone still kills 1.5 million children annually. All health workers should promote childhood immunizations and be familiar with the recommendations and delivery of vaccines.

> Health-care workers should use every opportunity to immunize children. Upper respiratory infections (URIs; colds) and fevers of less than 38.5°C (101.3°F) are not contraindications to immunizations.

The primary vaccines of the Expanded Programme on Immunization protect against measles, diphtheria, tetanus, pertussis, and poliomyelitis. Some regions and countries use additional vaccines depending on their local disease epidemiology. These include Haemophilus b, Japanese B encephalitis, yellow fever, group A meningococcus, mumps, and rubella. Prior to embarking on any international work, health-care workers should familiarize themselves with local immunization schedules. When working in the country, cooperate with the local health centers to promote vaccine administration.

ACUTE FEBRILE ILLNESS IN CHILDREN

The standard definition of fever is a rectal temperature of greater than or equal to 100.4°F (38.0°C). Listen to parents: Their report that "my child feels hot" is a reliable indicator of actual fever. The level of fever is important. Children under the age of 24 months with a temperature of over 39.4°C (102.9°F) are at much greater risk for occult bacteremia. Most pediatric fevers result from infections, but noninfectious causes include environmental factors (high temperature in the summer, or overbundling in the winter), malignancy, recent immunizations, and prescription drugs. Even some non-prescribed drugs (aspirin), or drug overdoses may cause a febrile toxidrome.

FEVERS IN INFANTS UNDER 6 MONTHS OF AGE

When infants under 6 months of age present with fever, they should be considered sep-tic (bacteremic) until proven otherwise. Treat with antibiotics and then diagnose if they appear ill. The laboratory evaluation of these infants has been fairly well standardized, but not all of these modalities may be available in all conditions.

DIAGNOSIS

LABORATORY EVALUATION All infants under 3 months of age with fever, and those up to 6 months who look sick, generally need a full septic evaluation:

■ Complete blood count (CBC) with differential. A white blood cell (WBC) count of greater than 15,000/mm^2 is over 70% sensitive for predicting occult bacteremia. A differential cell count is not needed because increased bands are no more pre-dictive of bacteremia than the WBC count.
■ Blood culture (when available)
■ Blood chemistries are indicated for children with altered mental status, dehydra-tion, or seizure that may be due to hypoglycemia or hyponatremia.
■ Urinalysis and catheterized urine culture. Boys under 6 months of age and girls under 12 months of age have a high rate of urinary tract infections. More than 5 WBCs per high-power field (HPF) in spun urine are significant. Catheterized samples should be obtained when possible, especially if a culture will be done.

RADIOGRAPHIC STUDIES Chest radiography is used to rule out pneumonia, which may be present even without physical findings, particularly in infants. Chest radiography is specifically warranted if the child has tachypnea, grunting, flaring, retractions, or hypoxia.

LUMBAR PUNCTURE In children under 24 months of age, signs of meningitis are typically absent, making the physical examination unreliable (Fig. 11-1). Indications for lumbar puncture are as follows:

- All febrile neonates (essentially all febrile infants under 3 months of age)
- Persistent vomiting
- Irritability, lethargy, or other mental status change
- Full anterior fontanelle
- Seizure
- Petechial rash

Repeat lumbar puncture is indicated if the child continues to deteriorate after a normal lumbar puncture. The cerebrospinal fluid (CSF) result may change from normal to significant WBCs in as little as 30 minutes.

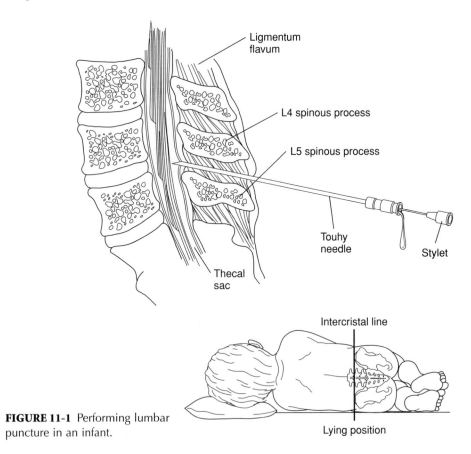

FIGURE 11-1 Performing lumbar puncture in an infant.

TREATMENT

FEVER REDUCTION Treating the fever makes the patient much more comfortable and may prevent febrile seizures. Alternating acetaminophen with ibuprofen may achieve greater reduction of fever than with either agent alone.

- The acetaminophen dose is 10 to 15 mg/kg every 4 hours.
- The ibuprofen dose is 10 mg/kg every 6 to 8 hours.

If a febrile seizure occurs, temperature reduction with a tepid bath and appropriate antipyretics must be initiated. Have the mother (or health worker) gently sponge the child with tepid (cool, but not cold) water across the forehead, chest, abdomen, and extremities.

ANTIBIOTICS Children suspected of having severe infections such as sepsis or meningitis require immediate administration of antibiotics. Antibiotic choices are discussed under each specific infection below.

OTHER ADJUNCTIVE CARE It is important to be familiar with and institute appropriate adjunctive measures to limit morbidity and mortality:

- Fluid administration is important to maintain hydration, circulation, and appropriate electrolyte balance.
- Immune globulin (when available) plays an important role in the prevention of hepatitis A and B, tetanus, rabies, and hemolytic disease of the newborn, as well as for conditions such as Kawasaki disease and idiopathic thrombocytopenic purpura (ITP).

FEBRILE SEIZURES

CLINICAL FEATURES Seizures are common with fever in infants and toddlers, and most of these febrile seizures are self-limited. However, febrile seizures also may be a manifestation of meningitis.

Benign febrile seizures usually last less than 5 minutes and are always generalized. They are commonly associated with a rapid increase in temperature at the onset of an illness (usually viral). Usually only one benign febrile seizure should occur per febrile illness. No neurologic deficits ensue. They occur in children 6 months to 5 years of age, with most in the age group of 9 to 24 months. Patients outside of this age range who experience seizures should undergo a more detailed examination for the cause. A family history of febrile seizures is common.

DIAGNOSIS Laboratory tests are unnecessary unless signs and symptoms of meningitis are present. No workup or therapy is needed if the child is febrile, is in the appropriate age group, and rapidly regains a normal mental status.

TREATMENT Reduction of the fever is the key to treatment (see above):

■ Do nothing for the first 5 minutes, other than ensuring the safety of the patient.
■ Do not stick anything into the patient's mouth to "protect the airway." The patient may aspirate the object.
■ No other treatment is needed if the child regains his or her normal mental status; if not, then evaluate and treat like a normal seizure.

Seizures lasting more than 5 minutes should be treated with intravenous (IV) or rectal benzodiazepines. Suggested medications are as follows:

■ Diazepam (Valium) 0.1 mg/kg IV or 0.3 mg/kg rectally
■ Lorazepam (Ativan) 0.1 mg/kg IV or rectally to a maximum dose of 4 mg

If seizures continue despite adequate dosing, then other anticonvulsants such as phenobarbital, dilantin (phenytoin), or fosphenytoin should be initiated. See Chapter 10 on seizure control for dosing.

INFECTIONS BY SYSTEM

SEPSIS

> **CRITICAL ACTION:**
>
> If you suspect sepsis, begin antibiotic treatment immediately. Do not wait for test results.

Sepsis, or septicemia, is the usually febrile state caused by microorganisms or their toxic products in the blood stream. Bacteria, viruses, fungi, and protozoa may all cause sepsis. Septic shock is a result of these infections causing vasodilatation and hypotension. Septic shock must be differentiated from other causes of shock. In neonates, cardiac diseases such as congestive heart failure or ductal-dependent lesions can mimic sepsis. Severe dehydration, botulism, and shaken baby syndrome all have similar presentations.

ETIOLOGY Age is extremely important in determining the etiology of sepsis. Different pathogens predominate as children mature (Table 11-1). In addition, the primary location of the infection, and the infections common to a given environment, will help identify the pathogen.

CLINICAL PRESENTATION Physical manifestations of sepsis vary with the age of the child and the stage of the disease. The younger the patient, the more atypical the presentation. Neonates and infants may simply present with poor feeding or hyperbilirubinemia. Older children are more likely to have a specific focus of infection.

TABLE 11-1 COMMON BACTERIAL CAUSES OF SEPSIS IN CHILDREN

■ **Neonates:** *Escherichia coli,* group B *Streptococcus pneumoniae,* and *Listeria monocytogenes* are the most common pathogens
■ **Infants >3 months:** *S. pneumoniae-* and *Haemophilus influenzae* (in un-immunized children), followed by *Neisseria meningitidis, Staphylococcus aureus,* group A beta hemolytic *Streptococcus* and gram-negative rods. The use of *H. influenzae* vaccine can have a dramatic impact on the causes of sepsis.
■ **Children 4 months to 4 years:** *S. pneumoniae, H. influenzae, S. aureus*
■ **Children 5–18 years:** *S. pneumoniae, N. meningitidis, S. aureus*

The following vital signs are characteristic of sepsis:

■ Fever or hypothermia (more common in younger children)
■ Tachycardia
■ Tachypnea (tachycardia and tachypnea out of proportion to the degree of fever may result from dehydration, sepsis, or cardiac abnormalities)
■ Wide pulse pressure
■ Hypotension is a late and ominous finding.

The following signs in the skin may be observed:

■ Initial flushing and warmth (cutaneous vasodilatation), to
■ Pallor and cyanosis as shock worsens
■ Petechiae [a late finding, particularly with meningitis or disseminated intravascular coagulopathy (DIC)]

The following mental status changes may be observed (vary with the progression of the shock):

■ Restlessness, then
■ Irritability, then
■ Confusion, then
■ Lethargy and unresponsiveness

There are various other symptoms, particularly in younger children:

■ Vomiting
■ Diarrhea
■ Diminished urine volume

Any primary focus of infection can spread to cause sepsis. This site should be sought because it can aid in the identification of the responsible organism.

DIAGNOSIS

LABORATORY EVALUATION The younger the child, the more likely the need for laboratory evaluation for diagnosis. In many field settings, these tests are not available. The most important thing in all cases is to treat empirically with antibiotics as soon as possible. The following studies should be considered:

- Rapid glucose (fingerstick) to assess for hypoglycemia
- CBC, urinalysis, electrolytes, blood urea nitrogen BUN, creatinine, and urine and serum cultures
- Chest radiography can be used to identify infiltrates, abscess, or tuberculin foci.
- Lumbar puncture should be performed if meningitis is a possibility.

TREATMENT Any young infant or child who is toxic appearing should be presumed to have sepsis and treated immediately before diagnosis. Antibiotic selection should be guided by age-appropriate pathogens (Table 11-2).

- Neonates generally respond to gentamicin and ampicillin.
- In older infants, a third-generation cephalosporin such as cefotaxime should be substituted for gentamicin.

MENINGITIS

CRITICAL ACTION:

As in sepsis, treat suspected meningitis with antibiotics immediately. Blood tests and lumbar puncture can be done later.

The manifestations of meningitis, from headache to frank shock, depend on the age of the patient, the pathogen, and the stage of disease presentation (early or late). The differential diagnosis ranges from simple headache to encephalitis or aneurysm. Toxic ingestion or traumatic brain injury also may be suspected when a child presents with an altered sensorium due to meningitis. Any patient presenting with sepsis or shock should be evaluated for meningitis.

Viral meningitis is more common than bacterial meningitis, but the bacterial variety has a more aggressive course and far worse prognosis. Bacterial etiologies vary with age (Table 11-3). In neonates, meningitis is associated with maternal infection or pyrexia at delivery.

CLINICAL PRESENTATION Like sepsis, meningitis in neonates and infants often presents with nonspecific findings, including fever or hypothermia, poor feeding,

TABLE 11-2 AGE-BASED TREATMENT OF SEPSIS

AGE	ANTIBIOTIC SELECTION
Neonate	Ampicillin 200 mg/kg/day divided every 8 h ***and*** Gentamicin 7.5 mg/kg ***or*** Cefotaxime 50 mg/kg/day
1–3 mo	Ampicillin 200 mg/kg/day divided every 8 h ***or*** Ceftriaxone 50 mg/kg/day divided every 12 h ***and*** Chloramphenicol 50 mg/kg/day

3–36 mo	Ampicillin 50 mg/kg/day divided every 8 h
	and
	Third-generation cephalosporin such as
	   Ceftriaxone 80 mg/kg/day divided every 12 h
	or
	   Cefotaxime 50 mg/kg/day divided every 4–6 h

Older than 36 mo	Cefotaxime 200 mg/kg/day divided every 4–6 h ***or*** Ceftriaxone 100 mg/kg/day divided every 12 h ***or*** Ampicillin 200 mg/kg/day divided every 8 h ***and*** Chloramphenicol 50–100 mg/kg/day divided every 6 h

dehydration, lethargy, irritability, or seizures. The diagnosis may not be established until lumbar puncture is performed.

Older children usually present with the more classic symptoms of headache, photophobia, nausea, and vomiting, as well as findings of nuchal rigidity with fever. They also may have altered mental status ranging from jitteriness and ataxia to lethargy. They

TABLE 11-3 COMMON CAUSES OF MENINGITIS BY AGE

- **Neonatal meningitis:** Group B *Streptococcus, Escherichia coli, Neisseria meningitidis, Listeria monocytogenes,* and *Haemophilus influenzae*
- **1–2 months:** Group B *Streptococcus, N. meningitidis,* and *H. influenzae*
- **Greater than 3 months:** *Streptococcus pneumoniae, N. meningitidis,* and *H. influenzae*

In some countries the use of *H. influenzae* vaccine is eliminating it as a predominant pathogen.

may manifest the classic Kernig sign (thigh pain on extension of the legs when hips are flexed to 90 degrees) and Brudzinski sign (flexion of the neck producing flexion at the knees and hips).

DIAGNOSIS See Chapter 8 for a discussion of the diagnosis of meningitis.

LABORATORY EVALUATION The only essential laboratory test for the evaluation of meningitis is lumbar puncture. See Table 11-4 for interpretation of the lumbar puncture results.

TREATMENT Definitive therapy for bacterial meningitis is immediate antibiotic administration. Antibiotics must penetrate the blood–brain barrier and act against the specific organism. Empiric therapy is always initiated prior to organism identification according to common etiologies in your patient population (Table 11-5).

In children the administration of corticosteroids in acute bacterial meningitis may lead to earlier symptom resolution and decreases the sequelae of hearing loss, but the

TABLE 11-4 LUMBAR PUNCTURE INTERPRETATION

TEST	NORMAL RANGE	MENINGITIS	OTHER FINDING/INDICATION
Color	Clear	Turbid	Bloody/trauma or hemorrhage >400 RBCs/mm^3 Cloudy/leukocytes >200 cells/mm^3
Opening pressure	50–150 mm/H$_2$O	>150 mm H$_2$O	Also increased with hemorrhage, mass effect, or CHF
Cell count	0–500 cell/mm^3	>500 cells/mm^3	
Differential	Leukocytes <5/mm^3	>5/mm^3 poor sensitivity if total cells <1,000	
	PMNs = 0	PMN > 1	
	Lymphocytes <50%	Lymphocytes >50%	
	Granulocytes = 1 > 2		
	Eosinophils = 0 > 1		
Gram stain	Negative	Bacteria seen	Identifies 80% of bacterial cases
Glucose	0.6:1 CSF:serum	Ration <0.5	Hyperglycemia = 0.4:1 CSF:serum
Protein	15–45 mg/dL	>150 mg/dL	Also increased in bleed, vasculitis, encephalitis, and neoplasm
India ink	Negative	Cryptococcus	See budding organisms in 33%
Cryptococcal antigen	Negative	Positive in 90% of cases	
CIE	Negative	Positive 95% specific with *Haemophilus influenzae*, *Neisseria meningitidis*, *Streptococcus pneumoniae*	

RBC, red blood cell; CHF, congestive heart failure; PMN, polymorphonuclear cell; CSF, cerebrospinal fluid; CIE, counter immuno electrophoresis

TABLE 11-5 MENINGITIS ANTIBIOTIC THERAPY
FOR INFANTS AND CHILDREN

AGE	ANTIBIOTIC	INITIAL DOSE
0-28 days	Ampicillin **and**	100 mg/kg
	Gentamicin	2.5 mg/kg
29-28 days	Ampicillin **and**	100 mg/kg
	Cefotaxime **or**	50 mg/kg
	Ampicillin **and**	100 mg/kg
	Ceftriaxone **or**	100 mg/kg
	Ampicillin **and**	100 mg/kg
	Chloramphenicol	25 mg/kg
>90 days	Cefotaxime **or**	50 mg/kg
	Ceftriaxone **or**	100 mg/kg
	Ampicillin **and**	100 mg/kg
	Chloramphenicol	25 mg/kg

dexamethasone must be given prior to antibiotics in a single dose of 0.6 mg/kg (but never delay antibiotics waiting for the steroids).

The following agents may be used for fungal meningitis:

■ Miconazole may be used in children under 1 year of age in a dose of 15 to 40 mg/kg/day divided every 8 hours to a maximum of 15 mg/dose.
■ Fluconazole may be used orally in children 3 to 13 years of age in a loading dose of 10 mg/kg. This is followed by a maintenance dose of 3 to 6 mg/kg every day.

PREVENTION

ISOLATION All patients should be placed in respiratory isolation to prevent transmission until they are no longer infectious (at least 48 hours of antibiotics).

CHEMOPROPHYLAXIS Five percent of household contacts develop bacterial meningitis. Therefore, treat the household contact (not just casual contacts) with the following:

■ Rifampin: adults 600 mg, children 10 mg/kg, and infants 5 mg/kg orally every 12 hours for four doses, or

- Ciprofloxacin 10 mg/kg one-time dose to a maximum of 250 mg; in adults a one-time 500-mg dose is given.
- Sulfadiazine: in children under 1 year of age, 500 mg every 24 hours for 2 days; 1 to 12 years, 500 mg every 12 hours for 2 days; adults, 1 g every 12 hours for 2 days

If household contacts become symptomatic, they should be immediately hospitalized and IV antibiotics administered. Rifampin prophylaxis only eradicates bacteria from the nasopharynx; it does not treat invasive disease. Health-care workers exposed to secretions from patients with meningitis also should begin a course of rifampin.

IMMUNOPROPHYLAXIS The use of *Haemophilus influenzae* type B vaccine drastically reduces the number of cases of pediatric meningitis, but it is not commonly used in developing countries. Vaccines effective against many pneumococcal serotypes and against group A and group C meningococci are available. The pneumococcal vaccine is targeted for prevention of pneumonia in populations such as the elderly, health-care workers, and the immunocompromised. Current use of the meningococcal vaccines is limited to established epidemic sites and to people who travel in countries with active epidemics. The costs of these vaccines limit their use in developing countries.

OTITIS MEDIA AND EXTERNA

Otitis media is an infection of the middle ear, whereas otitis externa is an infection of the external ear canal. It is a common infection that can lead to serious sequelae (meningitis, deafness) if untreated. It can be difficult to distinguish otitis media from otitis externa—both conditions can cause an erythematous tympanic membrane (TM) and discharge in the canal. In addition, both can cause edema of the canal that prevents adequate visualization of the TM. In equivocal cases it is prudent to treat for both.

Local trauma, foreign bodies, and mastoiditis can mimic symptoms of either form of otitis. In addition, infection of the teeth, sinuses, throat, or temporomandibular joint may all present a similar clinical picture.

OTITIS MEDIA Children are more susceptible to otitis media due to eustachian tube anatomy and dysfunction. The most common pediatric bacterial pathogens are *Streptococcus pneumoniae, H. influenzae,* and *Moraxella catarrhalis.*

CLINICAL PRESENTATION The classic presentation of otitis media is that of a febrile, irritable child pulling on his ear. However, many other nonspecific symptoms may occur, such as symptoms of URI, cough, poor appetite, and vomiting. Fever is not always present.

Physical examination reveals TM erythema dullness and lack of mobility. Pneumatic otoscopy (puffing air through the otoscope) is a sensitive modality for detecting a middle ear effusion indicative of otitis (use an insufflator, or blow through an IV tube extension attached to the otoscope to assess TM movement). Effusion fluid may obscure bony landmarks. Air fluid levels or bubbles may be seen.

DIAGNOSIS The diagnosis of otitis media is based on clinical findings, not on the results of tests or radiography.

TREATMENT Eighty percent of cases of acute otitis media resolve spontaneously without antibiotic therapy. However, serious complications may result from untreated otitis media such as hearing loss, tympanic perforation, cranial nerve paralysis, mastoiditis, brain abscess, and meningitis. Therefore, antibiotics are usually indicated. Recommendations for antibiotic selection and dosing are detailed in Table 11-6.

Intravenous antibiotics are generally given for 7 days, then treatment is continued orally for another 7 days. The duration of oral treatment is 10 to 14 days. Treatment failures occur most frequently in patients under 18 months of age and are usually due to antibiotic (β-lactamase)-resistant organisms or from viral etiology. In these patients, change to a β–lactamase-resistant antibiotic.

Patients should be instructed to return if no improvement occurs within 72 hours. The use of antihistamines, decongestants, or steroids does not improve clinical outcome.

OTITIS EXTERNA See Chapter 8 for a discussion on otitis externa.

EPIGLOTTITIS

Epiglottitis is an inflammation of the leaf-shaped mucosal structure covering the larynx, which can cause the complete and rapid obstruction of the airway. Airway protection is essential.

TABLE 11-6 ANTIBIOTIC THERAPY FOR PEDIATRIC OTITIS MEDIA

AGE	PATHOGEN	ANTIBIOTIC
0–2 mo	*Streptococcus pneumoniae* *Haemophilus influenzae* Group A streptococcus *Staphylococcus* Gram stain	Ampicillin 100–200 mg/kg/day divided every 4 h IV and Gentamicin 5.0–7.0 mg/kg/day divided every 8 h IV or Cefotaxime 50–100 mg/kg/day divided every 8 h IV
3 mo to 12 yr	*S. pneumoniae* *H. influenzae* *Moraxella catarrhalis* Group A streptococcus	Amoxicillin 30–50 mg/kg/day divided every 8 h orally or Erythromycin 30–50 mg/kg/day divided every 6 h orally and Sulfamethoxazole 100–150 mg/kg/day divided every 6 h orally and TMP 8 mg/kg/day divided every 6 h orally or Augmentin 20–40 mg/kg/day divided every 12 h orally

CLINICAL FEATURES The classic presentation of epiglottitis is that of a child 2 to 6 years of age with the rapid onset of a high fever and toxic appearance. In only a few hours, drooling, anxiety, and severe respiratory distress may develop. Children often sit in the "tripod" position (straight upright, neck extended and braced, with their arms pressed down against the bed or chair) and use accessory muscles to maintain respirations. Older children also may have a typical muffled voice.

DIAGNOSIS Children with suspected epiglottitis should not be agitated, which may promote obstruction. Therefore, blood tests and IV medications should be withheld until the airway is protected. Avoid any stimulation if the child appears in severe distress. Allow the child to assume the most comfortable position possible. Do not attempt to look into the throat of a child in distress without first being prepared for an emergency intubation or tracheostomy. A lateral soft tissue neck radiogram may be performed with the child seated upright.

TREATMENT In terms of airway maintenance, securing a stable airway is a priority in any child with epiglottitis. All children with epiglottitis require an artificial airway because more than 50% become obstructed. If epiglottitis is suspected, prepare for a tracheostomy immediately (call a surgeon to the location if possible; transportation is difficult and dangerous). Prepare for rapid sequence intubation (see Chapter 10). Fortunately, children with epiglottitis improve as quickly as they deteriorate. The average duration of intubation required is only 18 hours.

Blow-by oxygen can be provided in a manner least upsetting to the child. Some older children may tolerate a nonrebreather facemask.

The following measures should be taken if airway obstruction occurs:

- First try bagging the child using positive pressure bag-mask ventilation while preparing for intubation.
- Then attempt to rapid sequence intubate the patient. Paralysis is essential.
- If this method fails, attempt needle cricothyroidotomy or transtracheal jet ventilation (see Chapter 10).

Once the airway is secure, antibiotic treatment is required (Table 11-7). Steroid treatment and racemic epinephrine do not have any benefit in epiglottitis (and may be dangerous).

PREVENTION The infected child, as well as household and day-care contacts of children with *H. influenzae* epiglottitis, should be treated with rifampin. Doses are identical to those for meningitis prophylaxis. This will eradicate the carrier state and prevent invasive disease.

Haemophilus influenzae immunizations are effective in the prevention of *H. influenzae* epiglottitis.

- Dexamethasone 0.3 to 0.6 mg/kg may be given IV or intramuscularly (IM) or oral prednisone may be given in a dose of 2 mg/kg.
- If nebulized epinephrine is not available, subcutaneous epinephrine may be used in a dose of 0.01 mg/kg. Doses may be repeated every 20 minutes three times.

For severe symptoms and respiratory distress, the rare patient who does not respond to treatment may require intubation.

PREVENTION Respiratory isolation to limit respiratory droplet spread can reduce cases of infectious croup.

UPPER RESPIRATORY TRACT INFECTIONS

Upper respiratory tract infections (colds) are simple infections of the upper airway by viral organisms. They do not require treatment with antibiotics. The differential diagnosis should include infection by bacterial organisms, allergic rhinitis, and chemical irritation of the upper airway.

CLINICAL PRESENTATION Generally patients present with several days of rhinitis (runny nose), sore throat, and nasal congestion. Cough also may occur, but it is usually nonproductive or minimally productive. Fever, malaise, and myalgia may be present to varying degrees, but fevers are usually low grade. Typically there is exposure to other individuals with similar symptoms.

DIAGNOSIS Examination shows edema of the nasal and pharyngeal mucosa with a clear rhinorrhea. The pharynx may be erythematous, but exudates are rare. Lymphadenopathy is not common. The lungs should be clear, or occasionally have ronchi, but rales should not be present.

Laboratory evaluation is not indicated, except to rule out complications and bacterial suprainfections. Chest radiography should be performed if pneumonia is a possibility, particularly in the young and immunocompromised.

TREATMENT The most important thing to remember when treating a viral URI is that antibiotics are not indicated. In fact, antibiotic treatment may lead to the development of resistant bacterial strains that will compromise the patient in the future. It is a needless expense, associated with unnecessary complications that can be serious, and a threat to overall public health.

KEY POINT:

Do not treat a viral URI (cold, flu) with antibiotics. It is a waste of money and leads to antibiotic resistance.

Treatment is aimed at the alleviation of presenting symptoms:

- Antipyretics and anti-inflammatory drugs should be prescribed for fevers and myalgias. Throat pain also improves with these analgesics.
- Decongestants may alleviate nasal congestion and rhinorrhea.
- Saline nose drops can be used to clear nasal secretions in young children.
- Cough suppressants should be used if the cough is prolonged, interferes with sleep, or precipitates vomiting.
- Warm saltwater gargles or throat lozenges may relieve throat discomfort.
- Encourage oral fluids to keep patients well hydrated.

PREVENTION Patients should rest and avoid close contact with others. Hand washing prevents the contamination of surfaces with virus particles on hands. Patients should use disposable tissues for nasal secretions and not expectorate sputum. They should cover their mouth and nose during coughing and sneezing. Care should be taken not to share eating utensils with these patients unless they have been washed.

PNEUMONIA

Pneumonia is an infection of the lower respiratory tract that is differentiated from other pulmonary problems by the presence of a fever. It is most important to distinguish a URI (bronchitis) from a lower tract infection (pneumonia). Reactive airway diseases such as asthma also can present with chest pain, shortness of breath, and cough, but not fever. Aspiration of a foreign body should be considered if the history suggests it or if the patient is very young or very old. Costochondritis or pneumothorax also may be considered when patients present with chest pain and dyspnea.

Viruses cause 60% to 90% of pneumonia in children, with the exception of neonates, in whom bacterial pneumonia predominates. Pneumonia is most common in infants and toddlers, decreasing in incidence as children age. The etiology of pneumonia varies widely between countries. Table 11-8 lists the most common causative organisms by age group.

CLINICAL PRESENTATION The assessment of breathing and oxygenation is the first step for all patients. Use a pulse oximeter when available; otherwise, rely on the respiratory rate and the presence of retractions, accessory muscle use, rales, heart rate and presence of grunting or nasal flaring.

> **TIPS AND TRICKS:**
>
> Tachypnea of greater than 40 to 60 breaths/min in infants, or 30 to 50 breaths/min in older children, is the best single indicator of pneumonia.

As with other infections, younger children and infants present with less-specific symptoms. A cough is unusual with neonatal pneumonia, and the temperature can

TABLE 11-8 RANKED CAUSES
OF CHILDHOOD PNEUMONIA
BY AGE GROUP

Neonate
  Bacterial: Group B streptococcus, *Listeria monocytogenes,*
                Escherichia
  Viral: Respiratory syncytial virus (RSV), parainfluenza,
                herpes simplex, rubella, cytomegalovirus
1–4 mo
  Viral: RSV, parainfluenza
  Bacterial: *Streptococcus pneumoniae, Haemophilus,*
                Staphylococcus aureus
  Atypical: *Chlamydia trachomatis*
  Mycobacterium (tuberculosis)
4 mo to 5 yr
  Viral: Adenovirus, RSV, parainfluenza
  Bacterial: *H. influenzae, S. aureus, S. pneumoniae,*
                Bordetella pertussis
  Atypical: Mycoplasma
  Mycobacterium (tuberculosis)
5–8 yr
  Atypical: Mycoplasma
  Viral: Adenovirus, RSV, parainfluenza
  Bacterial: *S. pneumoniae*
  Mycobacterium (tuberculosis)

range from hypothermia to fever (fever is more typical in bacterial etiologies). Like any illness in infancy, poor feeding, irritability, vomiting, grunting, or lethargy may be the only symptoms of pneumonia. Abdominal breathing, retractions, and cyanosis are late and ominous findings.

As children age, symptoms become more specific. The classic symptoms of a fever with cough and pleuritic chest pain may occur. Vomiting after a coughing spell is common in preschool children. Wheezing may be present. Abdominal pain may occur due to irritation of the diaphragm.

DIAGNOSIS Infants with pneumonia may have a deceptively benign appearance at rest, for this reason infants with suspected pneumonia should be observed during feeding. Dyspnea during feeding is a significant finding. Auscultation is not reliable for detecting pneumonia in infants—don't rely on it.

LABORATORY EVALUATION When the diagnosis is clinically apparent, treatment may begin without radiologic or laboratory testing. Blood tests and cultures are rarely indicated. If a CBC is performed, leukocyte counts of greater than 15,000/mm^3 suggest a bacterial etiology.

RADIOGRAPHY Chest radiography is not routinely needed, particularly for older children in mild distress who will be treated with antibiotics anyway. Chest radiograph is recommended for all infants because of the unreliability of the physical examination. It is also indicated to look for active TB and if the diagnosis is not certain.

GRAM STAIN Sputum gram stain is the most specific, simple, and readily available test, but most children under 8 years of age are not able to produce an adequate sputum specimen. Suctioning can be used to obtain a good specimen. An adequate specimen must contain fewer than 10 epithelial cells and more than 25 WBCs per HPF. Look for the organism to determine the therapy. See Chapter 23 for a description of the gram stain technique.

TREATMENT The younger the child, the more likely the need for hospitalization. First determine the severity of the disease (remember the ABCs), then attempt to discover (or at least narrow) the etiology. Children with respiratory compromise as evidenced by decreased oxygenation, tachypnea, respiratory distress, dehydration, or any change in mental status require aggressive treatment. All severely ill children, infants under 3 months of age, or immunocompromised patients should receive IV antibiotics. All children with pneumonia should be followed closely, and hospitalized when in doubt. Failure of therapy may dictate a change of antibiotic.

For infants, antibiotic treatment should be instituted immediately, usually with ampicillin and an aminoglycoside. If infection with *Chlamydia trachomatis* or *Bordetella pertussis* is suspected, erythromycin should be added.

Fortunately, older children with mild to moderate bacterial pneumonia respond well to outpatient treatment. Because *Streptococcus pneumoniae* is the most common bacterial pathogen, treat as follows:

- Single IM dose of procaine penicillin, 25,000 to 50,000 U, followed by a 10- to 14-day course of penicillin V, 25 to 50 mg/kg day orally, divided into four doses, or
- Amoxicillin 25 to 50 mg/kg/day orally divided every 8 hours.

More severe illness should be treated as follows:

- Ampicillin can be given IV in doses of 150 mg/kg/day divided every 6 hours, or
- Erythromycin in oral doses of 40 to 50 mg/kg/day divided every 6 hours will treat bacterial pneumonia, mycoplasma, and chlamydia. Erythromycin also can be given to patients with penicillin allergy, as can sulfa [but it has many GI side effects (nausea, vomiting, and pain)].

Bronchodilators such as albuterol may be given if wheezing is significant. Proper hydration should be ensured.

PREVENTION Patients should be placed in respiratory isolation. Pneumococcal vaccine should be given to patients who are immunocompromised, have a chronic respiratory disease, or have an increased risk of exposure to the disease. Influenza vaccine also may be given to children with chronic disease. *H. influenzae* vaccine and pertussis vaccine should be administered to all children as part of routine immunization.

DIARRHEA/GASTRITIS AND ENTERITIS

Diarrhea is one of the leading causes of death in children globally, accounting for 5 to 10 million pediatric deaths annually. Infants are particularly susceptible to dehydration and sepsis from infectious diarrhea. Diarrhea is a symptom, not a disease, and has many causes, from infectious to metabolic to toxic. Gastritis is an inflammation of the gastric mucosa. Enteritis is an inflammation of the colonic mucosa. The key to treating diarrhea is to maintain adequate hydration and to understand when antibiotics are indicated.

Viral agents cause 30% to 40% of all pediatric gastroenteritis. Rotavirus results in up to 1 million deaths annually. Children in crowded living conditions are at increased risk for the oral-fecal spread of rotavirus. Neonates are more resistant to rotavirus because of maternal antibodies. Children up to 2 years of age are commonly affected.

CLINICAL PRESENTATION The purpose of the clinical evaluation is to determine if the patient requires antibiotics, IV fluids, hospitalization, or other therapy. Patients may present with symptoms ranging from intermittent loose stools to the cardiovascular collapse associated with cholera. It is most important to estimate the degree of dehydration and the patient's ability to tolerate oral fluids, and to rule out a significant intraabdominal process. Table 11-9 gives clues to assessing the degree of dehydration.

Viral gastroenteritis causes anorexia, low-grade fever, and vomiting. The vomiting lasts about 48 hours, with crampy abdominal pain and diarrhea lasting up to 6 days. The diarrhea is watery, nonbloody, and may be voluminous. Dehydration is a common presentation in these children.

Bacterial diarrheas tend to have a more rapid onset, with bloody stools, higher fever, and greater abdominal cramping.

Cholera is caused by infection with the gram-negative bacillus *Vibrio cholerae*, which leads to profound watery diarrhea with rapid depletion of fluid and electrolytes with minimal abdominal cramping. The majority of pandemics are caused by fecal-contaminated water. In endemic areas it is primarily a disease of children.

DIAGNOSIS

PHYSICAL EXAMINATION The general appearance of the patient helps to estimate the severity of the disease. Assess the mental status. Assess the degree of dehydration: Look for sunken eyes, sunken anterior fontanelle, and dry mucous membranes. Pinch the skin of the anterior chest for tenting (especially in children). The vital signs—with tachycardia, increased capillary refill, and orthostatic blood pressure changes—are important indicators of the degree of dehydration. The finding of decreased urine production is particularly worrisome, as is documented weight loss.

TABLE 11-9 DIAGNOSIS AND TREATMENT OF DEHYDRATION BY SEVERITY

SYMPTOMS	% DEFICIT	TREATMENT
Volume Deficit 5% Pulse: increased Urine: normal output/SG = 1.001–1.015 Mucosa: moist Skin: normal turgor Cap refill: 2 seconds Eyes: normal Fontanel: normal Sensorium: normal	5%	Oral fluids 50 mL/kg loss of weight plus maintenance fluid*
Volume Deficit 10% Pulse: resting tachycardia Urine: decreased output/SG = 1.020–1.025 Mucosa: dry Skin: doughy Cap refill: >3 seconds Eyes: sunken Fontanel: sunken Sensorium: depressed	10%	Oral fluids 100 mL/kg loss of weight plus maintenance fluid*
Volume Deficit 15% or greater Pulse: resting tachycardia Urine: decreased/no output/SG > 1.030 Mucosa: dry, no saliva Skin: doughy/tenting, cold, mottled Cap refill: >5 seconds Eyes: sunken, no tears Fontanel: sunken Sensorium: lethargic	15%	Intravenous fluids 110 mL/kg loss of weight plus maintenance fluid*

*See Chapter 10 for maintenance fluid requirements.

The abdomen may be tender, but there should be no rebound or guarding. The rectal examination provides important information for diagnosing and treating diarrheal disease, such as blood in the stools (more likely invasive or dysentery) and for staining for WBCs.

LABORATORY EVALUATION

- In general, blood tests are not warranted. Electrolytes may help to direct fluid replacement with severe dehydration.
- The most useful test is a smear of stool for fecal leukocytes, which indicates a bacterial cause of diarrhea. Fecal WBCs correlate with positive stool cultures in 85% to 90% of cases.

■ Heme-positive stools (by hemoccult examination) may indicate an invasive organism and are very suggestive of a bacterial infection.

A simple urine dipstick test may be used to look for ketonuria. This may suggest starvation ketosis or diabetes. A urine-specific gravity can indicate the degree of volume depletion.

■ Specific gravity of 1.001 to 1.015 = no to mild dehydration
■ 1.020 to 1.025 = moderate dehydration
■ >1.030 = severe dehydration

RADIOGRAPHY Radiography is rarely indicated unless the differential diagnosis includes a possible surgical abdomen (free air, obstruction, foreign body). In this case, upright and supine films should be obtained.

TREATMENT The WHO offers excellent treatment guidelines that are generally readily available in most countries. Rehydration and prevention of dehydration are the key to treatment. Usually oral rehydration is sufficient. Urine output is the key to assessing the hydration status. Admit patients if they are significantly dehydrated, if you are not sure of the diagnosis, or for multiple serial abdominal examinations.

HYDRATION For unstable patients, IV hydration is needed (Table 11-9). Give repeated boluses of 20 mL/kg of NS, lactated Ringer's solution, or Hartmann solution. Reassess for improvement of volume status after each bolus, up to 60 to 80 mL/kg, then consider another cause of shock.

Once improvement is seen, change the solution to D5 ½ NS at a rate to correct the volume deficit over 8 hours. Be careful in the hydration of hypernatremic patients. In these cases, the deficit should be slowly corrected over a minimum of 24 hours to prevent central nervous system complications.

For stable patients, oral fluids should be given in small amounts frequently. In young children this means 5 to 10 mL every few minutes. Use fluids that contain sugar and salts [oral rehydration fluids, oral rehydration salts, oral rehydration solution (ORS), etc.; see Table 11-10 for a common formula for ORS). Homemade soup (sugar, fluid, salt) or other sugar-containing fluids work well, but avoid fluids with a high osmolality, such as soda pop. Free water may result in hyponatremia. For children unable to take fluids, ORS may be passed through a feeding or nasogastric tube into the stomach.

ANTIBIOTICS Antibiotics are not indicated in most cases of diarrhea; only infectious diarrhea should be treated empirically with antibiotics. The most common antibiotics include the following:

■ Trimethoprim/sulfamethoxazole (TMP/SMX) double-strength, one tablet orally twice daily for 5 to 7 days is usually sufficient; alternatives include:
■ Ciprofloxacin 500 mg orally twice daily, or

TABLE 11-10 ORS

There are many formulas for ORS. Here are two:
Combine:
- 1 L water
- 2 level tablespoons of sugar (or honey)
- ¼ teaspoon of salt
- ¼ teaspoon of baking soda (bicarbonate of soda; if unavailable, use another ¼ teaspoon of salt)

To make the drink more palatable add a ½ cup of orange juice, coconut water, or a mashed ripe banana.

Or:
- 1 L water
- ½ teaspoon of salt
- 8 heaping teaspoons of one of the following:
  - Powdered rice cereal
  - Ground maize
  - Wheat flour
  - Cooked and mashed potatoes

Boil together for about 5 minutes and then cool. This mix will spoil in a few hours in hot weather, so only make what you can use rapidly.

- Noroxin 400 mg orally twice daily

See the section below on Specific Treatments by Etiology of diarrhea for more details on treatments.

ADJUVANT THERAPY

- Antiemetics may be needed for those unable to tolerate oral fluids.
- Antidiarrheal agents such as kaolin-pectin agents or bismuth subsalicylate (Pepto-Bismol) are not very effective, even at very high doses.
- Antimotility agents such as loperamide (Imodium) and diphenoxylate HCl-atropine (Lomotil) may be used in toxigenic diarrheas but should generally be avoided in most infectious diarrheas.

SPECIFIC TREATMENTS BY ETIOLOGY

The specific etiologies vary between region and country:

- *Campylobacter* is a common cause of infectious diarrhea, particularly in children over 2 years of age in developing countries. It can cause outbreaks from food contamination. Antibiotics are not usually needed; if necessary, treat with erythromycin, tetracycline, or quinolones.
- *Vibrio cholerae*: Once relatively uncommon, it is now endemic in much of the world following a pandemic in the early 1990s. The key to treatment is prompt

(often massive) fluid and electrolyte replacement. Tetracycline 12 mg/kg four times daily (500 mg four times daily in adults) is the primary antibiotic treatment. TMP/SMX or erythromycin may be given.

- *Salmonella* is associated with exposure to eggs, turkeys, unpasteurized milk, and animals, especially dogs and cats. The infection is usually self-limited, so antibiotics are not indicated, except in children under 2 years of age and in immunocompromised patients. In these cases, use ampicillin or amoxicillin (but resistance is common), TMP/SMX, or a quinolone.
- *Shigella* is a common cause of bloody diarrhea, as well as diarrheal deaths among children 6 months to 10 years of age. Outbreaks are common. *Shigella* infection should be treated with antibiotics even if the patient is asymptomatic when cultures return. Antibiotics include TMP/SMX, quinolones, and ampicillin.
- Enterohemorrhagic *Escherichia coli* 0157:H7 (EHEC): ETEC enterotoxigenic *Escherichia coli* and EHEC are common causes of childhood and traveler's diarrhea in developing countries. It causes bloody diarrhea. Hemolytic-uremic syndrome and TTP are serious complications. Fluid resuscitation must be aggressive. Antibiotics are generally not needed and there is much antibiotic resistance, but TMP/SMX, doxycycline, and quinolones can be used if started early.
- Rotavirus is a common cause of diarrhea in children, leading to a protracted watery diarrhea. There is now a vaccine for rotavirus indicated for children, although it is relatively expensive. Antibiotics are not indicated.
- *Yersinia enterocolitica* can produce an appendicitis-like picture. Antibiotics include TMP/SMX or a quinolone, or an aminoglycoside if septic.
- *Vibrio parahemolyticus* is a common cause of diarrhea in Asia and Japan, and results from inadequately cooked seafood; it is not spread between humans.
- *Giardia* is a parasite that commonly causes diarrhea worldwide. Symptoms vary widely from none to intermittent malodorous diarrhea to acute diarrhea with abdominal pain and fever. Treat with metronidazole or tinidazole or a similar agent.
- Amebiasis occurs commonly in travelers and is transmitted by contaminated water. Acute illness includes malodorous diarrhea associated with abdominal pain and fever. The course may be prolonged with intermittent symptoms. There is also a carrier state, especially in immunocompromised patients. Treat with metronidazole followed by iodoquinol, paromomycin, or diloxanide furoate.
- Antibiotic-associated colitis (pseudomembranous colitis) is caused by *Clostridium difficile* overgrowth in the gut after antibiotic use. It is most common after use of a broad-spectrum antibiotic, particularly those active against anaerobes, such as clindamycin, ampicillin, or cephalosporins. Treatment is with oral metronidazole or vancomycin (IV antibiotics do not work).

PREVENTION Purification of water supplies and improved human waste management are the most important mechanisms to prevent the spread of gastroenteritis. The use of latrines and a clean water source are essential in any community setting. Oral-fecal spread also accounts for many outbreaks, so frequent hand washing and careful food handling is important.

> **KEY POINT:**
>
> The best way to prevent diarrhea in infants is to encourage breast-feeding.

A rotavirus vaccine has been developed, and is becoming more available.

Prophylactic antibiotic use when entering certain endemic areas may decrease infection in travelers, but is not practical when staying for long periods of time.

VACCINE-PREVENTABLE DISEASES

POLIOMYELITIS

There is now an international effort to eradicate the poliovirus from the globe. Polio is spread by the fecal-oral and possibly the oral-oral route. The incubation period is 3 to 6 days for the infection and 7 to 21 days for paralysis to develop. In temperate climates, outbreaks of paralytic poliomyelitis were common in the summer and fall, but there is less seasonality in the tropics. Because of the goal of eradication, any suspected case of polio should be immediately reported and two stool cultures provided in the first 3 weeks of the disease.

CLINICAL FEATURES Approximately 90% to 95% of infections are completely asymptomatic. A nonspecific viral illness with fever, myalgias, and URI-like symptoms develop in 4% to 8% of patients. Some patients develop severe myalgias, particularly of the back. A transient asymmetric flaccid paralysis occurs in 2% of all infected patients, but only 0.1% develop permanent flaccid paralysis. The paralysis of polio is usually asymmetric (legs more often than arms) and develops with a fever present. The maximum extent of the paralysis occurs in only 3 to 4 days. The affected limb will be flaccid (no muscle tone and no reflexes). The disease must be differentiated from Guillain-Barré syndrome, which usually causes a symmetrical paralysis and has a more gradual onset (7–10 days).

TREATMENT There is no specific treatment for acute poliomyelitis, except for supportive measures, including respiratory support if the resources are available. Patients should be referred for rehabilitation early.

PREVENTION There are two basic types of poliomyelitis vaccines: a live, attenuated oral polio vaccine (OPV) and inactivated polio vaccine (IPV). Both provide 90% to 95% immunity. Until recently, the primary polio series in children has used OPV only. The benefit of OPV is that it prevents the excretion of the wild virus in the stool, whereas for IPV there is no risk of vaccine-associated paralytic poliomyelitis. As the incidence of wild poliomyelitis decreases, more countries are using IPV to prevent the rare cases of paralysis caused by OPV. Additional doses of vaccine are not harmful and are being recommended for children under 5 years of age as part of the eradication efforts.

In an outbreak, the surrounding population should be vaccinated for polio. Good sanitation also can reduce the transmission of the disease.

NEONATAL TETANUS

Neonatal tetanus is predominantly seen in underdeveloped countries, especially those with tropical climates. In the early 1990s, approximately 580,000 cases of neonatal tetanus deaths were reported annually. The differential diagnosis includes meningitis, dystonic reactions, encephalitis, hypocalcemia, strychnine toxicity, black widow spider envenomations, and subarachnoid hemorrhage.

Tetanus is caused by the exotoxin of *Clostridium tetani,* an anaerobic, encapsulated, gram-positive bacillus. Tetanus spores are ubiquitous and are found in soil, house dust, and animal and human feces. Spores are resistant to heat, desiccation, and disinfectants. The disease is transmitted when the spores are introduced into the body through a wound, usually a puncture. Neonatal tetanus is caused by unsterile handling of the umbilical cord at birth. The spores germinate under anaerobic conditions, so good wound care can prevent the disease.

CLINICAL PRESENTATION Newborns present with poor feeding and continuous crying, usually at 3 to 14 days of age. The umbilical cord may show signs of infection. Trismus (the inability to open the mouth) and irritability then develop. A low-grade fever is common. Babies experience excessive crying and facial grimaces. The tight, "sneering" mouth position known as risus sardonicus may be evident (Fig. 11-2).

Over 24 to 48 hours the contractions spread to the extensor muscles of the arms and legs, leading to postural rigidity and opisthotonus (head, neck, and back arched posteriorly in a bow shape). These contractions may produce intense pain. Touch, light, or sound may trigger reflex spasms. Severe contractions of abdominal musculature may

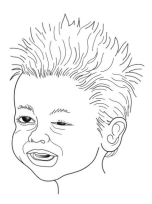

FIGURE 11-2 A neonate with risus sardonicus.

produce abdominal rigidity. Seizures without loss of consciousness are a poor prognostic sign.

DIAGNOSIS There is no test for tetanus, and the diagnosis is based on clinical findings.

TREATMENT Prevention of respiratory complications mandates prophylactic intubation in approximately 70% of patients. Because stimulation of the cords may result in severe laryngospasm, rapid sequence intubation with paralysis is indicated.

ANTITOXIN Antitoxin should be administered to neutralize any toxin that has not yet penetrated the central nervous system. Human tetanus immune globulin (HTIG) has replaced bovine or equine serum products in some countries. Only one dose of 3,000 to 10,000 U IM is needed for clinical tetanus. Intrathecal antitoxin use is controversial.

WOUND CARE Wound debridement should be delayed until after antitoxin is administered because of the potential toxin release from manipulation of the site. If a wound or umbilical cord is the suspected site of infection, it should be debrided to remove infected tissue and to create an aerobic environment by leaving only healthy tissue edges behind.

PHARMACOLOGIC MANAGEMENT Muscle spasm should be treated with benzodiazepines or barbiturates, or even general anesthetics, centrally acting muscle relaxants, and neuromuscular blocking agents if needed:

- For mild spasms, diazepam in a dose of 0.1 to 0.8 mg/kg/day orally divided every 6 to 8 hours can be used.
- For more intense spasms, increase the dose to 0.1 to 0.3 mg/kg IV every 4 to 8 hours.

Antibiotics have been used to prevent further *Clostridium* growth and release of toxin. Penicillin G and metronidazole have both been used, with tetracycline as an alternative for patients allergic to the preferred antibiotics.

PREVENTION Neonatal tetanus may be eliminated by immunization of all women of child-bearing years, especially those already pregnant. Maternal immunity is active in the infant for many months. Tetanus toxoid is not a vaccine, but rather an absorbed bacterial toxin, and there is no contraindication to its use in pregnancy.

Improved conditions during labor and delivery can limit contamination with *Clostridium*. The primary mechanism of prevention is hand washing and the use of clean instruments. Sterilization is the preferred method, but boiling of instruments can be used if more sophisticated techniques are not available. Soaking instruments in decontamination solution is the preferred method. The umbilical stump must be kept clean until it dries and sloughs. Good cord care includes the following:

- Cut within 2 cm (¾ inch) of the abdomen.
- Cut only with a sterile, boiled, or extremely clean instrument.
- Keep the cord dry and only loosely covered.

Any abrasions or lacerations to the child should be well cleaned. Bathe the baby to remove blood and other secretions. Begin the diphtheria-tetanus-pertussis (DTP) vaccine series as soon as possible, usually at 6 to 8 weeks of age.

MEASLES (RUBEOLA)

Measles is one of the leading causes of mortality in the world. It is a highly contagious virus, transmitted by respiratory droplets. The virus is found in nasopharyngeal secretions, blood, and urine. Virus particles can remain active on environmental surfaces at room temperature for at least 34 hours. Measles infects about 90% of susceptible family contacts. Rash and fever of measles is similar to rubeola and may be seen in rubella, coxsackievirus, adenovirus, infectious mononucleosis, toxoplasmosis, meningococcemia, scarlet fever, Kawasaki disease, drug rashes, and serum sickness. The rash of roseola can be distinguished because it appears as the child defervesces. Measles rash and fever increase together.

CLINICAL PRESENTATION Measles is characterized by three stages. During the 10- to 12-day incubation stage, the patient is infectious but has minimal to no symptoms. The prodromal second stage is marked by 3 to 5 days of moderate fever with the three C's: cough, coryza, and conjunctivitis. The third phase of measles includes the development of a rash and a sudden high fever, often as high as 40% to 42°C, placing children at risk for febrile seizures.

Conjunctival inflammation (red eyes) and photophobia are often the first clinical manifestations of measles. Periorbital edema may be seen. During the second or third day of the prodromal phase, Koplick spots may appear for 12 to 18 hours. These are grayish white dots the size of grains of sand on an erythematous base found in the mouth over the buccal mucosa, typically opposite the second molar.

The measles rash begins as faint macules on the face and upper neck, usually at the hairline and posterior cheeks. There is little or no itching. Over 24 hours the lesions become darker and increasingly papular and spread to involve the entire face, neck, and upper torso. Lesion density is greatest above the shoulders, where lesions may coalesce. The lymph nodes at the angle of the jaw and in the posterior neck are usually enlarged. During the second to third day, the rash spreads downward over the mid-torso and pelvis, eventually involving the legs, and may reach the feet. The measles rash involves both the palms and soles. The rash lasts 4 to 6 days, then begins to fade from the face downward in the same sequence as it appeared. Skin desquamation and brown discoloration then replace the rash, disappearing in 7 to 10 days. Complete recovery from measles generally occurs within 7 to 10 days after rash onset. A hemorrhagic type of "black measles" causes petechiae and bleeding into the skin, and may be associated with epistaxis or gastrointestinal bleeding.

COMPLICATIONS Complications occur most commonly in undernourished or immunocompromised children, although they can be seen in healthy children as well. Complications include encephalitis, otitis media, and pneumonia. Encephalitis symptoms begin 2 to 5 days after appearance of the rash. Measles encephalitis has a 10% mortality rate.

Measles pneumonia occurs more commonly from a secondary bacterial superinfection, but may result from the virus itself. In immunocompromised children, especially those with malnutrition and HIV, measles pneumonia is often fatal. DIC is a rare complication but is also very serious. A keratitis may occur, leading to blindness.

DIAGNOSIS The diagnosis is based on clinical findings. Chest radiography may be needed if there is a possibility of pneumonia. Blood tests are rarely indicated. If a CBC is obtained, the white blood cell count is low, with a relative lymphocytosis. In suspected measles encephalitis, the lumbar puncture shows increased protein, a small lymphocytosis, and normal glucose.

TREATMENT Supportive care is required during the prodromal and rash phases. Antipyretics are important for comfort, and to prevent febrile seizures. Adequate hydration must be maintained. Bed rest and a darkened room ease the fatigue and photophobia, respectively. Complicating bacterial superinfection should be treated with appropriate antibiotics.

Treatment with oral vitamin A in doses of 400,000 U daily reduces morbidity and mortality in developing countries.

PREVENTION Active immunization should be given to all infants from 9 to 15 months of age, depending on country recommendations. This may be lowered to 6 months in an outbreak, but a repeat dose should be given at the routinely scheduled time. A second immunization is indicated at 5 to 6 years of age. In HIV-infected children the vaccine is safe and may be life saving. In a refugee setting, measles vaccination is often given to all children under 5 years of age, and sometimes even to all children under 15 years of age, even those who report previous vaccination.

Respiratory isolation should be observed in all known cases during the infectious period, but transmission to susceptible contacts often occurs before diagnosis of the index case. Isolation precautions must be maintained from the seventh postexposure day until 5 days after the rash has appeared.

Following an exposure, immune serum globulin, 0.25 mL/kg IM, will prevent disease and is mostly indicated for immunocompromised patients. However, it must be given early to be effective, and will usually only attenuate symptoms if given more than 5 days after exposure. If not administered until day 9 or 10 postexposure, gamma globulin has little effect.

PERTUSSIS (WHOOPING COUGH)

Whooping cough is a common disease in developing countries and leads to considerable morbidity and mortality. The characteristic respiratory infection can be lethal in infants under 2 years of age. The differential diagnosis includes asthma, bronchitis, bronchiolitis, croup, and pneumonia.

ETIOLOGY Bordetella pertussis is an aerobic gram-negative coccobacillus transmitted by respiratory droplets. It forms a mucopurulosanguinous exudate in the lower respiratory tract. This compromises the small airways, especially in infants, and predisposes the patient to pneumonia. The disease is highly contagious; if exposed, 80% to 90% of susceptible people will contract the disease.

CLINICAL PRESENTATION The classic presentation is that of a child with a protracted cough that becomes so severe that children vomit after a coughing episode (post-tussive emesis). There are three stages to the infection: incubation, catarrhal, and paroxysmal. The child is asymptomatic during the incubation stage of 7 to 10 days. The catarrhal stage lasts 2 to 7 days and usually presents as a mild URI. There may be a low-grade fever (<38°C), or the child may be afebrile. Rhinorrhea, poor appetite, and mild cough are also noted. This is the stage where the disease is most often transmitted.

The paroxysmal stage is the most characteristic and lasts for 6 to 8 weeks. It is marked by chronic, severe paroxysms of coughing. A characteristic inspiratory gasp or whoop occurs between coughs, resulting in the term *whooping cough*. This is seen in children 6 months to 6 years of age. Feeding may provoke coughing in infants. Any exertion may precipitate a spasm of coughing. This may result in malnutrition and dehydration, especially in infants. Hypoxia usually develops but may be difficult to detect clinically. Still, a significant percentage of children will present with cyanosis and apneic spells. Cough may result in subconjunctival and soft palate hemorrhages/petechiae.

COMPLICATIONS A secondary bacterial pneumonia develops in 25% of children under 4 years of age. Seizures can be seen in infants and may warn of hypoxia or cerebral hemorrhage from the violent coughing spells. Encephalopathy may develop.

DIAGNOSIS Laboratory tests are rarely indicated. A CBC usually shows an elevated WBC count, from 20,000 to 40,000 cells/mm^2 with a profound lymphocytosis of greater than 70% lymphocytes. Blood cultures are usually negative and therefore not indicated. The former gold standard for diagnosis is a culture of nasopharyngeal swab from the deep nasopharyngeal space, plated on Bordet-Gengou agar. Unfortunately, positive results are found in only 15% to 40% of cases, and the results require too long to be clinically useful. Direct fluorescent antibody studies of deep nasopharyngeal swabs are positive in 40% to 80% of patients, and results are available in minutes. Specimens obtained in the first 3 weeks of disease are best. Enzyme-linked immunosorbent assay is becoming the new gold standard, but is rarely available outside of university settings.

TREATMENT Macrolide antibiotics are the drugs of choice with substitution of sulfa drugs in macrolide allergic patients. Erythromycin is given at a dosage of 30 to 50 mg/kg/day divided four times daily, with a maximum of 2 g/day. Treatment should continue for 14 days. It is preventive if begun within the first 10 to 14 days but not proven to prevent disease beyond this time frame. TMP-SMX at a dosage of 5 mg/kg/day can be given twice daily for 14 days.

PREVENTION Respiratory isolation is indicated for known cases for at least the first 5 days of antibiotic therapy. Suspected cases should just be isolated from other children, particularly those in children under 2 years of age and among the unimmunized. Contacts of known cases should receive prophylactic antibiotics and be kept from public places (such as schools) for the first 5 days of the therapy.

Vaccination is effective with either the older killed vaccine or the new acellular vaccine. It should be administered following the county recommendations. A booster should be given at 4 to 6 years of age. Multiple doses are essential for immunity.

Oral erythromycin for 14 days is recommended for prevention of disease in household or other close contacts.

DIPHTHERIA

Diphtheria is an acute infection affecting the respiratory tract and skin that is most noted for its pseudomembrane in the posterior pharynx. The manifestations of the disease are caused primarily from the effects of an exotoxin, which cause local tissue necrosis, neuritis, myocarditis, and focal damage to the kidneys, adrenal glands, and liver. It can lead to cardiovascular collapse and shock. The spread of the pseudomembrane to the lower airway can cause death from airway obstruction or from increased absorption and spread of the exotoxin.

Infections occur in both epidemics and sporadic cases. Recently, there have been epidemics of diphtheria in countries of the former Soviet Union, South America, and Southeast Asia. In each of the epidemics the majority of the cases were among adults. Inapparent infections are more common than clinical cases. In tropical climates cutaneous infections are more common than respiratory diphtheria. These infections are usually secondary to scabies, impetigo, or other forms of dermatitis.

ETIOLOGY Corynebacterium diphtheria is an aerobic gram-positive bacillus that causes respiratory and skin infections. It is spread by respiratory droplets or contact with infected skin or environmental surfaces. Transmission through contaminated milk and food also occurs. Asymptomatic carriers are important in transmission.

Complications of both forms of diphtheria include myocarditis, which is seen in 66% of patients but clinically significant in only 10% to 25%. Symptoms include cardiac dysrhythmias (atrial fibrillation, ventricular tachycardia), variable heart block, and right-sided cardiac failure with hepatic enlargement. Most diphtheria patients who develop dysrhythmias die, so continuous cardiac monitoring is required. Permanent cardiac damage results from cardiac fibrosis in survivors of diphtheria.

Congestive heart failure is also common. Treat the congestive heart failure with diuretics alone because digitalis and quinidine are associated with risk of dysrhythmias.

Neuritis may strike peripheral or cranial nerves in 15% to 20% of patients. Renal tubular necrosis and thrombocytopenia also may result.

CLINICAL PRESENTATION

RESPIRATORY DIPHTHERIA Respiratory tract diphtheria primarily affects the tonsils or pharynx and occasionally the nose and larynx. The distinguishing feature is the pseudomembrane, which occurs in 50% to 90% of patients, who present with a sore throat. During the incubation period of 2 to 4 days, local inflammation and discomfort develop, and nausea and vomiting may be common with children. Fevers of up to 39°C occur, but half of patients are afebrile. In infants, a serosanguinous, purulent, erosive rhinitis may be seen. These shallow ulcerations of the external nares and upper lip are an obvious external finding that should raise suspicion of diphtheria. Soft tissue swelling and lymphadenopathy in the neck can cause the classic "bull neck" appearance. Patients may appear toxic, pale, and profoundly weak.

Pseudomembrane formation is the classic physical finding of respiratory diphtheria and results from the exotoxin causing tissue necrosis. The pseudomembrane appears as a thick gray-brown or gray-blue sheet over the oropharyngeal mucosa. Unlike the exudate of a streptococcal infection, it spreads beyond the tonsillar pillars, and the removal of the pseudomembrane is difficult and may cause bleeding.

Remember the ABCs when evaluating these patients. Airway compromise is a constant life threat.

CUTANEOUS DIPHTHERIA Cutaneous diphtheria appears as a slow, superficial, nonhealing ulceration covered with a gray-brown membrane. These may be difficult to distinguish from streptococcal or staphylococcal impetigo. In most cases, an underlying lesion, such as an abrasion, burn, or impetigo, becomes secondarily infected with diphtheria.

DIAGNOSIS The primary diagnosis of diphtheria is clinical in nature:

- A methylene blue stain of throat scrapings can be used to identify the organism.
- A CBC shows a nonspecific leukocytosis, so is not useful.
- Plain radiographs of the neck show a normal epiglottis and normal diameter of the trachea on lateral views (absent steeple sign).
- Cultures of the scrapings use either Loffler medium or regular blood agar and may be positive within 12 hours.

TREATMENT The airway must be protected, usually by intubation and vigilant suctioning to prevent occlusion of the tube with the pseudomembrane. Cardiac monitoring is essential due to the frequent associated dysrhythmias.

ANTITOXIN THERAPY Antitoxin should be administered to all patients with diphtheria when it is available. Early administration of antitoxin is critical, because the exotoxin binds irreversibly to tissues and antitoxin binds only free exotoxin. First determine the patient's sensitivity to horse serum antitoxin. Give three intradermal injections:

- One with 0.02 mL of saline
- A second with 0.02 mL of histamine
- A third of 0.02 mL of 1:100 saline-diluted antitoxin

The test is read at 15 to 20 minutes. An immediate reaction is a wheal with circumferential erythema at least 3 mm larger than the saline control injection. Anergy is noted by no response to the histamine control, which should produce swelling. Desensitization must be performed in patients with immediate reactions. Use the schedule in Table 11-11 to desensitize, with doses given every 15 minutes.

Even patients with a negative sensitization test should be given the antitoxin cautiously. First give 0.5 mL of antitoxin diluted in 10 mL of NS over 5 to 10 minutes. Then observe for 30 minutes. If no reaction occurs, the remaining dose is diluted 1:20 with NS and given at a rate not to exceed 1 mL/minute. The empiric doses of antitoxin are given in Table 11-12.

Approximately 10% of patients have a hypersensitivity to the antitoxin and 8% develop serum sickness. Always be prepared to manage an anaphylactic reaction with epinephrine and steroids during desensitization and prior to complete dosing.

TABLE 11-11

DOSE	DILUTION OF ANTITOXIN	VOLUME OF INJECTION
1–3	1:1,000	0.1, 0.3, 0.6 mL
4–6	1:100	0.1, 0.3, 0.6 mL
7–9	1:10	0.1, 0.3, 0.6 mL
10–13	Nondilute	0.1, 0.2, 0.6, 1.0 mL
14	Nondilute	Remainder of total dose

TABLE 11-12

CLINICAL PRESENTATION	ANTITOXIN DOSE (U)
Cutaneous lesion only	20,000–40,000
Pharyngeal disease <48 hours' duration	20,000–40,000
Nasopharyngeal exudate	40,000–60,000
Extensive disease or >72 hours	80,000–100,000
Bull neck	80,000–100,000

ANTIBIOTIC THERAPY Antibiotics are indicated to eradicate the organism and prevent further exotoxin formation. There is no evidence that antibiotics have any impact on outcome.

Antibiotics should be given for 14 days. Recommendations include the following:

■ Erythromycin 40 to 50 mg/kg/day (maximum of 2 g/day).
■ Procaine penicillin 25,000 to 50,000 U/kg/day IM divided in two doses.
■ If resistance to erythromycin exists, clindamycin, rifampin, and tetracycline may all be given.

PREVENTION Any patient with pharyngeal diphtheria should be placed in strict isolation for 14 days. Those with cutaneous diphtheria require contact isolation. Isolation is maintained until the completion of 14 days of antibiotic therapy or the return of two negative cultures. All articles that have contacted the patient must be disinfected and sterilized. All contacts of the patients should receive a single dose of penicillin IM or a 7-day course of erythromycin and be closely observed for 7 days.

Even patients who have had an active infection must complete a diphtheria toxoid series to assure immunity. All children should be immunized as early and quickly as possible. A booster is required at 4 to 6 years of age. For unimmunized patients over 7 years of age, use three 0.5-mL doses—two doses 4 to 8 weeks apart and a third dose 6 to 12 months later. After completion of the initial series, a booster dose should be given once every 10 years.

MUMPS

Mumps is one of the most common causes of viral meningitis in unimmunized populations. It is caused by a paramyxovirus found in nasopharyngeal secretions, blood, and urine. The incubation period ranges from 14 to 24 days. Transmission may occur as early as 1 day before or 3 days after the appearance of parotid swelling.

CLINICAL PRESENTATION The characteristic clinical picture of mumps is fever and parotid gland enlargement. Children rarely have a mumps prodrome. The disease usually presents with fever (although 20% may be afebrile), headache, and an earache (which is the interpretation of a young child with pain and swelling in one or both parotid glands). The parotid swelling begins in the posterior gland and extends inferiorly and anteriorly. The surrounding skin also may become edematous, which makes the swelling even more visually striking. The swollen tissue can displace the earlobe superiorly and posteriorly. Edema of the soft palate and pharynx occurs and may displace the tonsil medially. Pain is increased by salivation. Both parotid glands swell in 20% to 25% of patients, and both submandibular glands become inflamed in 60% of cases. The swelling may progress rapidly over hours, peaks in 1 to 3 days, and then slowly subsides over 3 to 7 days.

COMPLICATIONS The most frequent complication of childhood mumps is meningoencephalitis, occurring in up to 10% of children with mumps. The CSF shows fewer than 500 cells/mm^3, with lymphocyte predominance. Permanent sequelae are rare, and the mortality rate is less than 1 in 10,000.

Orchitis and epididymitis are rare in children but may be seen in up to 35% of adolescents and adults. Sterility is very rare.

Mumps is the leading cause of unilateral nerve deafness. Incidence is 1 in 15,000. Hearing loss may be transient or permanent.

DIAGNOSIS Laboratory tests are not indicated; the diagnosis of mumps is clinical.

TREATMENT Mumps requires supportive care. Analgesics should be given for pain, and hydration must be maintained. Diet should be adjusted to the patient's ability to chew; foods and liquids (such as citrus) that stimulate salivation should be avoided to prevent discomfort.

PREVENTION The mumps vaccine is not often used in developing countries. When used, the vaccine should be given at 12 to 15 months of age and again at 4 to 6 years of age unless the patient is immunocompromised. Adolescents should also receive a booster. Immune globulin is not effective for mumps. Pregnant women should never receive live virus mumps vaccine.

Droplet precautions should be maintained until 9 days after the onset of parotid swelling in normal children. Immunocompromised children should be excluded from areas where mumps-infected children are found for at least 26 days after the onset of parotid swelling in the last infected child.

RUBELLA (GERMAN OR 3-DAY MEASLES)

Rubella epidemics occur every 6 to 9 years in unimmunized populations. Infection during the first trimester of pregnancy can result in congenital rubella syndrome, producing anomalies including cardiac defects, blindness, deafness, and mental retardation. The rash and fever of rubella should be differentiated from that of measles, scarlet fever, mononucleosis, erythema multiforme, Kawasaki disease, and rickettsial disease.

The rubella virus may be found in nasopharyngeal secretions, blood, urine, and feces, but is usually transmitted by respiratory droplets. Patients are infectious from 7 days prior to the development of the rash until 7 to 8 days after resolution of the rash.

CLINICAL PRESENTATION Rubella has a 2- to 3-week incubation period. Rubella causes mild constitutional symptoms such as a URI. Fever seldom exceeds 38.8°C. The most characteristic finding is extreme postoccipital, retroauricular, and posterior cervical lymphadenitis. In half the patients, an erythematous rash develops 5 days after the URI-like symptoms. Polyarthritis may occur, most often in the small joints of the hands, particularly in older girls and women. The rash starts as discrete rose-colored spots

(Forschheimer spots) on the soft palate. The rash begins on the face and forehead and spreads downward to the trunk and extremities. The rash may become confluent, particularly over the face. During the second day it may appear as fine and pinpoint, mimicking that of scarlet fever. The rash can be pruritic. The rash may evolve so quickly that it fades from the face as it appears on the trunk and usually disappears by the third day, without sequelae.

COMPLICATIONS Complications in children are fortunately rare. Encephalitis occurs in 1 of 6,000 cases. It is the complications of infections in pregnant women that are of the greatest concern. Congenital rubella syndrome can result in the birth of a child with devastating malformations and severe disability.

DIAGNOSIS Rubella is a clinical diagnosis. Laboratory testing is nonspecific. Diagnosis may be confirmed by seroconversion, but this is indicated only in exposure of pregnant nonvaccinated women.

TREATMENT The treatment of rubella is supportive. Acetaminophen should be given for fever and aches. Diphenhydramine may be given to control itching.

PREVENTION Patients with rubella should remain in contact isolation in a private room. Patients should remain out of the public for 7 days after the rash begins. Pregnant women should strictly avoid any contact with infected patients.

Most developing countries do not use the rubella vaccine because of its cost, the difficulties with the cold chain, and because almost all adults are immune through natural infections. This prevents infection during pregnancy and therefore prevents congenital rubella syndrome. When available and part of a national program, the live virus vaccine against rubella should be given at 12 to 15 months of age. Immunization also should be given to any susceptible women of child-bearing age. The live vaccine should not be given to pregnant women, but there have been no malformations found when it has been used in pregnancy. For pregnant, nonvaccinated women who have been exposed, passive immunization with immunoglobin 20 to 30 mL IM should be given.

CHAPTER 12

Gynecology and Women's Health

Jeff Hardesty and Kathleen Clem

INTRODUCTION

Women's health issues are some of the most prevalent and misunderstood health issues in the field setting. As health-care providers in remote settings, doctors, nurses, and health workers must be aware of essential issues in women's health, including gynecologic illnesses and complications of pregnancy. Gender-specific hormonal, nutritional, and emotional needs also require some special knowledge and different treatment than medical conditions that affect both sexes. The following sections address these female-specific health issues.

GYNECOLOGIC CAUSES OF ABDOMINAL/PELVIC PAIN

Diseases involving the organs of the reproductive tract should be high on the list of possible diagnoses when encountering a female patient with complaints of lower abdominal pain. Developmental abnormalities, infections, complications of pregnancy, and reproductive tract tumors may all involve pain as the presenting symptom. The diagnostic and clinical features of these diseases and their treatment are discussed in this section.

ECTOPIC PREGNANCY

A pregnancy that implants in any location other than within the uterine cavity is ectopic. The increased incidence of sexually transmitted diseases resulting in salpingitis and the efficacy of antibiotic therapy in preventing total tubal occlusion following salpingitis are related to the increasing rate of ectopic pregnancy. About 95% of ectopic

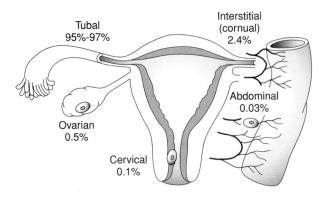

FIGURE 12-1 Sites ad incidence of ectopic pregnancy.

pregnancies occur in the oviduct. The remaining 5% may occur on the ovary, cervix, or peritoneal cavity. For a successful treatment prior to tubal rupture, the examiner must have a high index of suspicion so that the diagnosis can be made early (Fig. 12-1).

The clinical features of ectopic pregnancy depend on the site and duration since implantation, but the classic symptoms are unilateral lower abdominal pain that occurs following a delayed onset of menses. Pelvic examination usually reveals a mildly tender uterus that is less enlarged than appropriate for a normally implanted gestation, bleeding from the cervix, and the presence of a very tender adnexal mass or fullness. In situations where rapid, sensitive human chorionic gonadotropin (hCG) testing or ultrasonography is not available, culdocentesis is a useful technique for identifying the presence of intraperitoneal bleeding. An 18-gauge spinal needle attached to a 30-mL

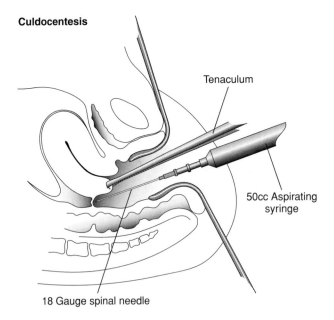

FIGURE 12-2 Culdocentesis. An 18-inch spinal needle is inserted through the posterior fornix and enters the cul-de-sac between the uterosacral ligaments.

syringe is inserted through the posterior fornix of the vagina under the cervix into the cul-de-sac between the uterosacral ligaments (Fig. 12-2). The finding of nonclotting blood upon aspiration confirms the presence of intraperitoneal bleeding. It does not distinguish whether this blood is from a hemorrhagic ovarian cyst, ruptured viscera, or ectopic pregnancy, but it does confirm the need for surgical intervention.

If tubal rupture has occurred, the onset of abdominal pain may be sudden and intense. The abdomen becomes rigid, and shoulder pain from diaphragmatic irritation due to hemoperitoneum may occur. The patient may have pallor with signs of shock and blood loss. This condition is a life-threatening emergency, and all the available means for resuscitation with intravenous (IV) fluids, blood replacement, and rapid surgical treatment should be instituted without delay. Surgical removal of a ruptured ectopic pregnancy should not be performed under spinal anesthesia because the vasodilatation that occurs with this type of anesthetic may put the patient into irreversible shock. General inhalational anesthesia with endotracheal tube placement is preferable, but the surgery may be performed under local anesthesia with light IV sedation if the situation is critical. Usually it is necessary to remove the ruptured portion of the tube to control the bleeding (Fig. 12-3).

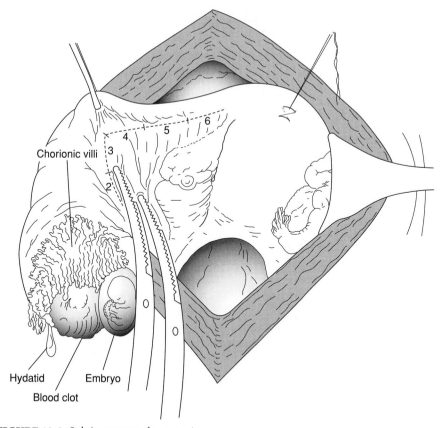

FIGURE 12-3 Salpingectomy for ectopic pregnancy.

Two major advances in technology have made possible the early diagnosis and thus the potential for nonsurgical treatment of ectopic pregnancy. The use of highly sensitive, rapid beta hCG serum assays with high-resolution ultrasonography has enabled physicians to determine an hCG zone where at a certain level of hCG a normal intrauterine pregnancy may be seen via ultrasonography. This level is 2,000 mIU/mL when using transvaginal ultrasonography and 6,500 mIU/mL when using transabdominal scanning. At hCG levels above the discriminatory zone, if ultrasonography fails to demonstrate an intrauterine pregnancy or determines signs of an ectopic pregnancy (gestational sac in the tube or free fluid in the cul-de-sac), then medical treatment for the ectopic pregnancy may be considered. Intramuscular (IM) injection of methotrexate can be initiated if the patient's condition is stable. If the hCG level is below the discriminatory zone and her condition is stable, then a repeat hCG and pelvic ultrasonography should be performed after 48 hours. In a normal intrauterine pregnancy, the hCG should increase by at least 66% during this interval. Methotrexate given in a single IM injection at a dosage of 50 mg/m^2 of body surface area has been shown to yield a success rate of better than 90% in the treatment of unruptured ectopic pregnancy. If the hCG level is over 10,000 mIU/mL, the chances for success decrease significantly, and surgical treatment should be undertaken (Table 12-1).

TABLE 12-1 METHOTREXATE TREATMENT PROTOCOL
FOR UNRUPTURED ECTOPIC PREGNANCY

The patient *must*:
  Be hemodynamically stable
  Have a tolerable level of pain
  Have hCG <15,000 mIU/mL
  Be able to return for follow-up care

The patient *must not*:
  Have a known allergy to
  methotrexate
  Have an underlying hepatic,
  renal, or hematologic dysfunction
  Continue breast-feeding

Treatment
  Day 1:
  Perform ultrasound, hCG, CBC, BUN, creatine, and liver function tests
  Administer 50 mg/m^2 BSA and methotrexate IM
  Days 4 and 7, then weekly:
  repeat hCG level until in nonpregnant range

  If hCG does not increase by at least 15% between days 4 and 7, or
  If hCG does not continue to decline to nonpregnant range, then:
  a second 50 mg/m^2, BSA dose of methotrexate should be given IM

  If patient develops intolerable pain, becomes hemodynamically unstable, or
  develops other signs of pending rupture, then medical treatment has failed and
  surgery should be performed.

hCG, human chorionic gonadotropin; CBC, complete blood count, BUN, blood urea nitrogen; BSA, body surface area; IM, intramuscularly.

ENDOMETRIOSIS

The presence of endometrial glands and stroma outside the uterus occurs in 7% to 10% of women in the general population, although it produces symptoms in only about half of these women. Ectopic endometrium is present in 40% of women with infertility and in 80% with chronic pelvic pain. Endometriosis is usually confined to the pelvis, but also may occur in distant sites throughout the body. The extent of the disease does not correlate with the amount of symptoms it causes in a given patient.

The typical clinical features are a worsening dysmenorrhea (painful menses) that radiates to the lower back. A deep, spasmodic pain that begins a day or two prior to the onset of menses and lessens toward the end of menstruation is often reported. Pelvic pain that occurs during sexual intercourse is also frequently present. Premenstrual spotting that occurs 3 to 7 days before the start of menses is also a relatively consistent sign of endometriosis. If the lesions extend into the colon or bladder, then cyclic, perimenstrual tenesmus, hematochezia, or hematuria can occur. Tender nodules in the posterior fornix of the vagina are classic findings in the presence of endometriosis. If the ovaries are involved, adhesions and tender cystlike structures filled with old blood (chocolate cysts) may occur. An endometrial cyst can leak, causing considerable pain, or it can rupture and produce acute, severe pain much like that seen with a ruptured ectopic pregnancy, tuboovarian abscess (TOA), or appendicitis.

The definitive diagnosis requires surgical intervention to obtain a biopsy sample of the lesions, but usually medical treatment is started once a clinical diagnosis is made based on the patient's symptoms and findings. Pelvic ultrasonography may be helpful in identifying endometrial cysts, but it cannot be used to identify adhesions or small implants of the disease. Diagnostic laparoscopy is helpful, if available.

Medical treatment (Table 12-2) involves the use of pain medications (usually nonsteroidal antiinflammatory drugs; NSAIDs) and hormonal manipulation to suppress estrogen levels. The use of gradually increasing higher doses of oral contraceptive pills (OCPs) used to be a popular treatment, but caused major side effects of weight gain, breast pain, nausea, headaches, and irregular bleeding. Continuous high-dose progesterone administration is often used as the first line of treatment. This therapy relieves the symptoms and produces amenorrhea, but may not cause the disease to regress. Danazol, a synthetic steroid compound that lowers estrogen levels, is effective for both relieving the symptoms as well as decreasing the extent of the disease, but has major potential androgenic side effects such as weight gain, acne, decrease in breast size, and deepening of voice. Inhibition of the hypothalamic–pituitary–ovarian axis by the use of gonadotropin-releasing hormone (GnRH) agonists results in extremely low estrogen levels, which causes the endometriosis implants and cysts to shrink. The problems associated with estrogen deprivation (mainly hot flushes and bone loss) can be ameliorated with the concomitant use of norethindrone (0.35–3.5 mg/day), but for these reasons GnRH agonist therapy is usually limited to 6 months of treatment.

Surgical treatment is indicated for correction of pain, infertility, or other symptoms in patients with extensive endometriosis, or when hormonal manipulation therapy fails to adequately treat the problem. In those patients who have completed their childbear-

TABLE 12-2 TREATMENT FOR ENDOMETRIOSIS

TREATMENT	DOSAGE	PRECAUTIONS
Monophasic OCPs	Start at two pills/day; increase at biweekly intervals until amenorrheic or maximum of 12 pills per day	Potent side effects have made this therapy unpopular
Progestins		
Medroxyprogesterone-acetate	30–50 mg orally daily or 100 mg IM every 2 wk for 3 mo then 200 mg IM monthly	Breakthrough bleeding, irritability, and edema can occur; use for 6 mo or longer
Megestrol 40 mg orally daily		Breakthrough bleeding, irritability, and edema can occur; use for up to 2 yr
Danazol	Start at 400 mg orally b.i.d. for 2 mo then decrease to 400 mg daily if remains amenorrheic	Androgenic side effects and hot flushes can occur; use for up to 8 mo; must also use barrier contraception
GnRH agonists		
Naferelin 0.2 mg intranasal b.i.d.		Estrogen deprivation side effects; add back norethindrone 0.35–3.5 mg daily; use for up to 6 mo
Leuprolide	3.75 mg IM monthly or 11.25 mg IM every 3 mo	
Goserelin	3.6 mg SC monthly	
Surgery	Conservative or definitive	Depends on future child-bearing wishes

OCP, oral contraceptive pill; IM, intramuscularly; GnRH, gonadotropin-releasing hormone; b.i.d., twice daily; SC, subcutaneously.

ing and have severe symptoms from endometriosis, a total abdominal hysterectomy with bilateral salpingo-oophorectomy (TAH/BSO) and resection of endometriosis lesions can be offered as definitive therapy for the disease.

REPRODUCTIVE TRACT NEOPLASMS

Both benign and malignant tumors occur in the female reproductive tract and often present with lower abdominal pain

Ovarian cysts are a common cause of unilateral lower abdominal pain. A careful, thorough pelvic examination is the main way to evaluate for the presence of an ovarian cyst. Getting the patient to cooperate with the examination by palpating the nontender areas first is helpful. A combined rectovaginal examination is often the easiest way to feel the cyst. Any adnexal mass encountered should be assessed in regard to location, size, mobility, consistency, surface irregularity, and degree of tenderness when palpated. If available, ultrasonography is a great aid in evaluating ovarian cysts and may be the only successful nonsurgical way to do so in an obese patient. Plain radiography can be helpful, especially if teeth or cartilage are present within the cyst, as in benign teratoma (dermoid cyst).

Evaluating whether the mass is most likely benign or malignant will determine the treatment plan. If the cyst is less than 6 cm in diameter, is smooth, mobile, and only moderately tender, then it is most likely a benign physiologic cyst. These cysts are caused by failure of a follicle to ovulate or to regress and are sometimes associated with irregular menstrual cycles. The patient with a suspected physiologic ovarian cyst should be reassured, but should have the cyst examined monthly over the next 2 months to see if it spontaneously regresses. The use of OCPs should prevent new follicular cysts from arising, but do not hasten the regression of a physiologic cyst. If the cyst remains persistently enlarged or grows even bigger over a 2-month period, then it should be surgically removed.

Ovarian cysts greater than 6 cm in diameter or those that are irregular, fixed, or solid should be considered potentially malignant and require surgical removal. Postmenopausal females do not produce physiologic cysts, and the development of a palpable adnexal mass in a woman in this age group requires surgical removal because the chance for malignancy is high.

A sudden onset of severe pain in the area of an ovarian cyst may be due to adnexal torsion, which requires emergency surgery to untwist it and reestablish its blood supply. A torsed adnexa that has become necrotic requires surgical removal.

Another cause for lower abdominal pain in women is uterine tumors. Leiomyomata (fibroids) are the most common tumors of the female reproductive tract and are especially prevalent in women of color. Because these benign smooth muscle tumors only rarely become malignant (<1 per 1,000), they do not require treatment unless they become very large (>14 weeks size), cause excessive bleeding, exert pressure on surrounding organs, interfere with pregnancy, or cause serious abdominal pain. Fibroids are usually easily palpated on combined abdominal and pelvic examination as solid masses arising from the uterine walls. Ultrasonography can be helpful in distinguishing fibroids from the potentially more serious ovarian masses.

The growth of uterine fibroids is dependent on estrogen production, and they tend to shrink during the menopausal years. In neglected cases, these tumors can attain a very large size, even exceeding that of a term pregnancy. GnRH agonists administered over 3 to 4 months can shrink these tumors by up to 50%, but they will regain their original size several months after the GnRH is discontinued. However, GnRH therapy is useful in allowing a patient's anemia to resolve prior to surgical removal of the fibroids. A patient with symptomatic fibroids who has completed her childbearing may desire to have a hysterectomy, or may choose to have the fibroids removed surgically (myomectomy).

Pain is not a common complaint in women with cervical tumors unless it is due to an advanced stage of cervical cancer. Cervical tumors usually present with problems of abnormal vaginal bleeding, or a profuse, malodorous vaginal discharge. A careful speculum examination and bimanual pelvic examination should be performed on any woman with these complaints. Cervical cancer often appears as an exophytic, cauliflower-like growth with an irregular, firm texture around its borders. Any suspicious lesion of the cervix should be examined via biopsy. If a cervical cancer has become invasive in the pelvis, radiation treatment usually yields better results than surgery. The benefits of having annual cervical cytology [Papanicolaou (Pap)] smears to screen for premalignant neoplasms of the cervix (often associated with the human papillomavirus) should be emphasized for all women once they have become sexually active.

Problems of infection, cysts, depigmented areas, and tumors involving the vulva are frequent causes for women to seek medical care. Careful inspection of the vulva with good lighting and, if available, using magnifying lenses or colposcopy aid in diagnosing the cause of the vulvar lesion. Lesions of uncertain diagnosis should be examined via biopsy. For small lesions, a Keyes biopsy punch is helpful; for larger lesions, a scalpel can be used for perineal biopsy.

INFECTIONS

Infections involving the vulvar area may be due to fungal (tinea or *Candida*), viral (herpes, condyloma, or molluscum), or bacterial causes (syphilis, chancroid, lymphogranuloma, granuloma inguinale, hidradenitis, or bartholinitis).

Fungal infections of the vulvar area usually cause an intense pruritus and irritation. The skin may appear beefy red and thickened acutely, or in chronic cases may be leathery with an overlying grayish sheen. Roundish satellite lesions (ringworm) also may be present. The diagnosis is suspected by the symptoms and typical appearance. Using a microscope to view hyphae in a KOH wet mount of surface scrapings from the affected skin is helpful to confirm the diagnosis. Treatment involves decreasing the humidity in the local area (cotton underwear during the day and none at night) and the use of antifungal medicines. A single application of 1% gentian violet solution will give rapid relief of symptoms. This should be followed by the application of nystatin, clotrimazole, or terconazole creams three times daily for 2 to 3 weeks. Patients with recurrent fungal vulvitis should be tested for diabetes mellitus and human immunodeficiency virus (HIV). For women who are prone to fungal vulvovaginitis following antibiotic usage, a single 150-mg oral dose of flucanazole is helpful.

Suppurative hydradenitis is an acnelike infectious process involving the apocrine sweat glands of the vulva, but also may occur in the axillae, breasts, and perirectal areas. Draining pustules with deep interconnecting sinuses may form, causing scarring and recurrent abscesses. Cultures usually grow *Staphylococcus* or *Streptococcus* species. Treatment involves the application of topical clindamycin cream twice daily and oral isotretinoin at 1 mg/kg/day for up to 4 months. Severe cases may require surgical excision.

A Bartholin abscess occurs when the duct leading from the gland to the vaginal opening develops an infectious obstruction. A tender, tense, bulging mass filled with the entrapped purulent mucus forms under the mid-labia. Trauma, gonococcus, or other bacteria may be the cause for the blockage of the duct. Treatment involves making a small skin incision under local anesthesia over the area of swelling just outside the hymenal ring and through the abscess wall to drain it. Placing a Word catheter or other drain through the incision keeps the duct open until the infection subsides (Fig 12-4). A cephalosporin antibiotic orally for 10 to 14 days is also usually prescribed.

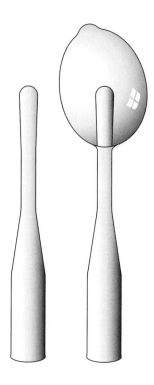

FIGURE 12-4 The Word catheter (left) is inserted into the Bartholim duct cyst through a vaginal incision. The bulb is inflated with saline solution (right), and the end of the catheter is placed in the vagina.

For recurrent cases of Bartholin abscess or cysts, a marsupialization procedure can be performed under local anesthesia (Fig. 12-5). A vertical skin incision is made over the cyst just external to the hymenal ring. After opening the cyst wall and draining its contents, the edges of the cyst's lining are turned out and sewn back against the skin incision with absorbable sutures.

A white lesion in the vulvar area may be caused by loss of melanocytes in the skin (vitiligo), by a benign inflammatory atrophic reaction of the skin (lichen sclerosus), or by either premalignant (vulvar intraepithelial neoplasia; VIN) or malignant disease (squamous cell cancer).

Vitiligo causes patchy depigmentation of the vulvar skin and hair, but does not cause itching or change the normal anatomic features of the vulva. This disorder tends to run in families. No treatment except for reassurance is necessary.

Lichen sclerosus is usually the cause when a postmenopausal woman develops a pruritic, thickened, pale white discoloration on the skin over the perineum, periclitoral, or perianal areas. If left untreated over time, the involved areas shrink from the atrophic process, causing retraction of the clitoris and diminution in the size of the vaginal introitus. Treatment with twice-daily application of 2% testosterone cream relieves the atrophic changes to a degree. Better symptomatic relief of the itching and irritation is achieved by applying highly potent topical steroid creams (0.05% clobestasol proprionate or 0.05% betamethasone diproprionate) twice daily to the affected area for 1 month, then nightly for 2 months, then twice weekly for 3 months, and then as needed.

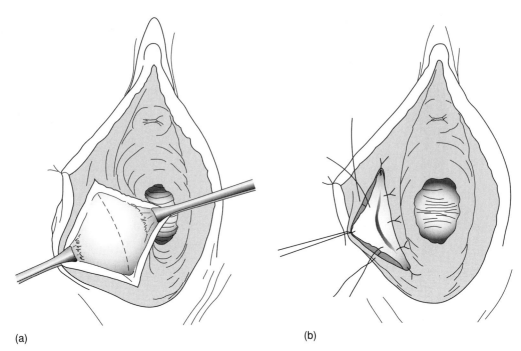

(a)   (b)

FIGURE 12-5 (A) Incision for marsupialization. (B) Marsupialization.

Vulvar intraepithelial neoplasia and squamous carcinoma of the vulva are associated with the human papillomavirus and cause both pruritus and pain. The appearance is that of raised, irregular, whitish, or colored skin lesions. Colposcopy is helpful in making the diagnosis. Biopsy from the worst-looking areas is necessary to confirm the diagnosis. VIN may be treated by wide local excision, laser vaporization, or twice-daily application of 5% 5-fluorouracil cream for up to 10 days followed by once-per-week application. Carcinoma of the vulva requires vulvectomy and groin lymph node excision.

VAGINITIS, CERVICITIS, AND PELVIC INFLAMMATORY DISEASE

Infections involving the vagina, cervix, and upper reproductive tract are described in this section. The most common complaint that prompts women to seek medical attention is vulvovaginitis. Symptoms include vaginal discharge, pruritus, and odor. Table 12-3 lists typical symptoms, signs, and clues to help make the correct diagnosis and prescribe the appropriate treatment for the various causes of vaginitis.

PELVIC INFLAMMATORY DISEASE

Pelvic inflammatory disease (PID) occurs when sexually transmitted pathogens penetrate the cervical mucus barrier and infect the uterus, fallopian tubes, or ovaries. PID

TABLE 12-3 VAGINITIS

INFECTION TYPE	SYMPTOMS	SIGNS	CLUES	DIAGNOSTIC METHODS	TREATMENT
Monilial (*Candida*)	Pruritus, nonodorous discharge	Thick, white, clumpy discharge	More common in tropical climate, pregnancy, diabetes, HIV, or HIV, or after antibiotic use	Hyphae or spores on KOH wet mount, pH <4.5	Intravaginal or oral imidazole or preparations work best (miconazole, clotrimazole, butacanazole, ketocanazole, or flucanazole); nystatin or boric acid can be used
Bacterial vaginosis	Malodorous discharge	Thin, homogeneous, whitish gray discharge	Associated with preterm delivery and pelvic inflammatory disease	Clue cells on saline wet mount; fishy odor on whiff test	Metronidazole 500 mg, orally for 7 days, or 5 g of 0.75% gel intravaginally b.i.d. for 5 days; clindamycin 300 mg orally b.i.d. for 7 days or 5 g of 0.75% cream intravaginally b.i.d. for 7 days; tinidazole 500 mg orally b.i.d. for 5 days
Trichomonas	Pruritus; malodorous discharge; dysuria	Copious, frothy, yellow-green discharge	Erythema of vaginal mucosa and strawberry cervicitis; postcoital bleeding	Motile trichomonads on saline wet mount; fishy odor on KOH whiff test, pH <4.5	Metronidazole 2 g single oral dose or 250 mg t.i.d. for 7 days; sexual partners also need treatment
Enterobius (pinworm)	Nocturnal pruritus	Yellowish discharge; perineal erythema	Caused by migrating pinworms from anus to vagina in young girls	Place adhesive tape on anus then onto glass slide to see ova on microscopy	Single oral dose of 100 mg mebendazole, or 11 mg/kg of pyrantel pamoate suspension; siblings also need treatment
Chemical	Nonodorous discharge	Clear discharge; vaginal erythema	Many possible causes for chemical irritation of the vaginal mucosa	WBCs but no pathogens seen on wet mount pH <4.5	Eliminate exposure to the chemical irritant; may apply steroid cream to areas of external erythema
Physiologic	Nonodorous discharge	Clear discharge; no erythema, odor, or pruritus at time of cycle	Increased vaginal secretions, especially periovulatory	Only lactobacilli and epithelial cells on wet mount, pH 3.8–4.2	Diagnosis of exclusion; treatment is reassurance; may douche

b.i.d., twice daily; t.i.d., three times daily.

may result in TOA, chronic pelvic pain, infertility, and increased chance of ectopic pregnancy. *Neisseria gonorrhoeae* and *Chlamydia trachomatis* are the most likely organisms to cause PID, but once the upper genital tract has been invaded, a polymicrobial superinfection with anaerobic and gram-negative bacteria often occurs.

The most common presenting history for acute PID is a sudden onset of lower abdominal/pelvic pain accompanied by a purulent vaginal discharge that begins soon after the completion of the first menses following a new sexual contact. Fever, nausea, and vomiting also may occur. Pelvic examination usually reveals cervical motion tenderness and bilateral adnexal tenderness. A palpable adnexal mass in this setting is most likely to be a TOA. If the proper equipment is available, laboratory testing for PID should include wet mount of the vaginal discharge, gram stain of the cervical discharge, with testing for *Chlamydia* and gonococci, complete blood count, erythrocyte sedimentation rate, urinalysis, pregnancy test, VDRL testing, and HIV screen. If available, ultrasonography can be helpful if TOA is suspected.

Outpatient treatment for PID may be given if the patient is afebrile, has no evidence of TOA, is adequately pain free, is not vomiting, and is willing and able to return for reexamination within 72 hours. Otherwise she should be hospitalized for inpatient therapy with parenteral antibiotics and IV fluids. The sex partners of patients with PID should be empirically treated with a single dose of azithromycin 1 g orally or doxycycline 100 mg orally twice daily for 10 days plus a single dose of ciprofloxin 500 mg orally or ofloxacin 400 mg orally. This will cover the patient's partner for both *Chlamydia* and gonococci (Tables 12-4 and 12-5). A barrier method of contraception also should be prescribed to decrease the chance of reinfection in the future.

Surgical treatment is usually reserved for patients who have failed medical management or for those with surgical emergencies such as peritonitis from a ruptured TOA. Laparoscopy is helpful if the diagnosis of PID is uncertain. TAH/BSO is the definitive surgical treatment for PID. Posterior colpotomy, a transvaginal technique for draining a fluctuant pelvic abscess that is bulging into the posterior cul-de-sac, is a useful procedure that can be performed even in primitive situations as long as adequate anesthesia is available.

The abscess should be carefully palpated on pelvic examination under anesthesia or sedation and its size and location noted. The posterior lip of the cervix is then grasped and elevated with a tenaculum. Culdocentesis (Fig. 12-2) is then performed to confirm that the palpated mass does indeed contain pus. A transverse incision is then made through the

TABLE 12-4 CDC REGIMENS FOR OUTPATIENT THERAPY OF PELVIC INFLAMMATORY DISEASE

Regimen A
  Cefoxitin 2 g IM with probenecid 1 g orally, or
  Ceftriaxone 250 mg IM, or
  Another third-generation cephalosporin (ceftizoxime or
    cefotaxime, plus
  Doxycycline 100 mg orally b.i.d. for 14 days

Regimen B
  Ofloxacin 400 mg orally b.i.d. for 14 days, plus
  Clindamycin 450 mg orally q.i.d. for 14 days, or
  Metronidazole 500 mg orally b.i.d. for 14 days

CDC, Centers for Disease Control and Prevention;
IM, intramuscularly; b.i.d., twice daily; q.i.d., four times daily.

TABLE 12-5 CDC REGIMENS FOR INPATIENT THERAPY
OF PELVIC INFLAMMATORY DISEASE

Regimen A
  Cefoxitin 2 g IV every 6 hours, or
  Cefotetan 2 g IV every 12 hours, plus
  Doxycycline 100 mg orally or IV every 12 hours for 14 days
  The cephalosporin may be discontinued 48 hours after the
    patient has made substantial improvement.

Regimen B
  Clindamycin 900 mg IV every 8 hours, plus
  Gentamicin 2 mg/kg IV loading dose followed by 1.5 mg/kg
    every 8 hours
  This regimen may be discontinued 48 hours after the patient
    made substantial improvement and then followed with
    either doxycycline 100 mg orally b.i.d. for 14 days or
    clindamycin 450 mg orally q.i.d. to complete 14 days of
    therapy.

CDC, Centers for Disease Control and Prevention; IV, intravenously; b.i.d., twice daily; q.i.d., four times daily.

vaginal mucosa just below the juncture of the posterior vaginal fornix with the cervix. The cul-de-sac peritoneum and abscess wall are then punctured with a tonsil clamp. Pus should be seen draining out through the incision. After suctioning out the abscess, an index finger should be inserted to bluntly break up any adhesions that may be loculating pus in separate chambers in the abscess (Fig. 12-6). A drain should then be inserted into the abscess cavity and anchored with absorbable sutures to permit easy removal a few days later.

Tuberculosis PID is a common cause of infertility and pelvic pain in developing countries. Miliary seeding of the mucosal and peritoneal surfaces of the pelvic organs occurs. The fallopian tube is the most common pelvic organ to be infected. The typical patient has a positive tuberculin skin test and may appear to be in poor general health. The development of a TOA in a virgin with a prior history of pulmonary tuberculosis is highly suspicious for tuberculosis PID. See Table 12-6 for medical treatment of female genital tuberculosis.

EVALUATION OF VAGINAL BLEEDING

When a patient presents with vaginal bleeding, the health worker must determine whether the bleeding is due to normal menses or is abnormal bleeding associated with a disease process.

Menstruation is the physiologic shedding of the endometrium with associated uterine bleeding that occurs at monthly intervals from menarche to menopause. Regular menstruation is dependent on the complex, interrelated, and intact functioning of the hypothalamic–pituitary–ovarian–uterine axis (HPOUA). Any disease state that affects these organs can result in abnormalities of menstruation.

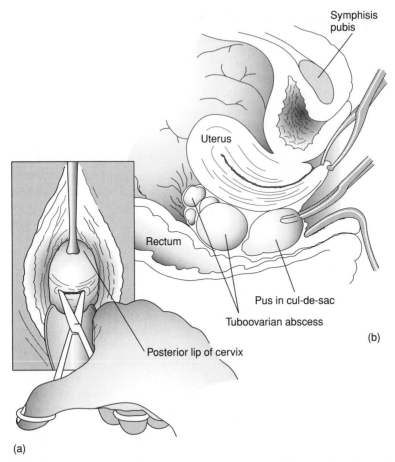

FIGURE 12-6 Posterior colpotomy. (A) A transverse incision is made through the vaginal mucosa at the junction of the posterior vaginal fornix with the cervix. (B) A tonsil clamp is thrust through the abscess wall.

Clotting disorders such as von Willebrand disease (factor deficiency) or idiopathic thrombocytopenic purpura (functioning platelet deficiency) account for about 20% of menorrhagia complaints in adolescent girls. Any form of hemophilia, acute leukemia, or liver dysfunction can cause excessive menstrual bleeding. The use of anticoagulants such as heparin or coumadin also may cause menorrhagia. Usually patients with clotting disorders have abnormal bleeding at other body sites, demonstrate easy bruising, or have a history of previously requiring blood transfusions. However, abnormal vaginal bleeding may be the first sign of the underlying disorder.

Pregnancy-related bleeding is one of the most common causes of abnormal vaginal bleeding. Threatened abortion, ectopic pregnancy, and hydatidiform moles all usually present with abnormal bleeding. A high level of suspicion for possible pregnancy should be maintained when evaluating any woman with vaginal bleeding.

TABLE 12-6 MEDICAL THERAPY FOR FEMALE GENITAL
TUBERCULOSIS

Regimen A (for mild, asymptomatic cases)
   Ethambutol 15 mg/kg orally daily for 2 months
   Isoniazid 300 mg orally daily for 9 months
   Rifampin 600 mg orally daily for 9 months

Regimen B (for advanced cases with tuboovarian masses)
   As above, plus if palpable adnexal masses persist after the
      9 months of therapy, TAH/BSO should be performed.
      Isoniazid and rifampin are then continued for an additional
      6 months postoperatively.

TAH/BSO, total abdominal hysterectomy/bilateral salpingo-
oophorectomy.

Reproductive tract tumors such as endometrial polyps or uterine fibroids are common causes of abnormal vaginal bleeding for women in the 40 to 50 age group. Malignant tumors of the vagina, cervix, uterus, or ovary also may present with bleeding problems.

Reproductive tract infections such as cervicitis, endometritis, or PID can cause abnormal vaginal bleeding. These may be the result of exposure to sexually transmitted diseases (STDs) or may be caused by a postpregnancy infection. Patients usually have associated pain, fever, or other signs of inflammation.

Pelvic trauma with potential lacerations of the vulva, vagina, or cervix causes abnormal vaginal bleeding. Sexual molestation, forcible rape, or straddle injuries are frequently encountered causes of pelvic trauma. A thorough history and high level of suspicion also may elicit the diagnosis of domestic violence, which has become the number one cause of injury to women in the United States. If this problem is not diagnosed or intervention is not implemented, the violent attacks usually escalate and many battered women die as a result.

Dysfunctional uterine bleeding is diagnosed when there is abnormal bleeding in the absence of anatomic lesions of the uterus. This is most commonly caused by a hormonal imbalance that results in lack of regular ovulation and therefore no cyclic production of progesterone. Anovulation leads to a state of chronic, unopposed stimulation of endometrial growth by estrogen, which causes unpredictable, often heavy bleeding due to uncoordinated endometrial sloughing. It is a condition that is seen most frequently at the extremes of menstrual life and is associated with either immaturity or aging of the HPOUA. This condition usually responds well to hormonal therapy.

Postmenopausal bleeding is a warning sign that either a precancerous growth or cancerous growth of the endometrium may be present. Histologic sampling of the endometrium by either endometrial biopsy or uterine curettage should be performed. Perimenopausal women beginning hormone replacement therapy (HRT) with combined estrogen/progestin regimens often have mild, intermittent vaginal bleeding during the first few months of use. This does not usually merit endometrial sampling unless the irregular bleeding persists longer than 6 months.

Diagnostic methods to evaluate abnormal vaginal bleeding range from the simple (speculum examination, pregnancy test, and hematocrit) to the sophisticated (hysteroscopy and hormone assays) (Table 12-7). A thorough history and a careful pelvic examination enable the health-care worker in even the most remote location to make a good working diagnosis and treatment plan.

The first step is to determine if the patient is ovulating regularly because the treatment differs based on this finding (Table 12-8). If she is ovulating and has menorrhagia, then anatomic abnormalities of the uterus are suspected and the need for surgical intervention is more likely. If she is anovulatory, then dysfunctional uterine bleeding amenable to hormone therapy is most likely present. If the patient reports that her menses occur at regular intervals and are preceded by breast tenderness and accompanied by uterine cramps, then she is almost certainly ovulating regularly. If she reports that her menses occur at irregular intervals, are not accompanied by cramps, and are unpredictable as to onset, duration, and amount of bleeding, then she has anovulatory bleeding.

On speculum examination, the bleeding should be confirmed to be coming through the cervix. Pap smears are preferably performed when the patient is not bleeding heavily. If the cervix has a bluish purple color and is softer than usual to the touch, then the patient is likely pregnant. Any uterine enlargement or adnexal mass should be carefully palpated. In virginal adolescents, a digital rectal examination may be substituted for the pelvic examination. If the equipment is available, this examination may be augmented by simultaneous transabdominal ultrasonography.

TABLE 12-7 DIAGNOSTIC METHODS TO EVALUATE
ABNORMAL VAGINAL BLEEDING

All patients with abnormal bleeding should have:
   Careful history and physical (including bimanual pelvic/rectal exam)
   CBC with platelet count and hCG

Patient with suspected anovulatory bleeding:
   TSH, prolactin, progesterone
   Endometrial biopsy

Patients with ovulatory bleeding
   Bleeding time (if adolescent or has symptoms of coagulopathy)
      Pelvic ultrasonography (saline infusion sonography is best to see small endometrial polyps or submucosal fibroids)

Treatment possibilities include hormonal therapy, blood clotting factor transfusions, tamponade techniques, and surgical procedures, depending on the cause of the bleeding and the severity of the patient's condition.

CBC, complete blood count; hCG, human chorionic gonadotropin; TSH, thyroid-stimulating hormone.

TABLE 12-8 TREATMENT OF ABNORMAL VAGINAL BLEEDING

Ovulatory profuse bleeding with unstable vital signs, acute anemia, or pregnancy related
Large-bore IV line for fluid resuscitation
Cross-match blood
Emergency suction curettage or operative D&C
If curettage not available, insert a 30-mL Foley catheter throughout the cervix into the uterine cavity then inflate the bulb to create tamponade; transport patient in MAST suit to hospital for curettage

Anovulatory profuse bleeding with stable vital signs and moderate anemia
Premarin 25 mg IV every 4 h or premarin 25 mg orally every 6 h until bleeding subsides; then place on monophasic 50 μg ethinyl estradiol OCPs daily for 2 weeks, or monophasic 50 μg ethinyl estradiol OCPs orally q.i.d. for 7 days, then one daily for 2 more weeks

Profuse bleeding with a prolonged bleeding time

Large bore IV for fluid resuscitation
Cross-match fresh whole blood or PRBC with FFP and platelet packs (if thrombocytopenic)
IV desmopressin (DDVAP) at 0.3 μg/kg over 20 min to increase Factor VIII in patients with von Willebrand disease
If patient is pregnant or has anatomic abnormalities within uterus perform D&C

IV, intravenous; D&C, dilatation and curettage; OCP, oral contraceptive pill; q.i.d., four times daily; PRBC, packed red blood cells; FFP, fresh-frozen plasma.

A bleeding time can be obtained almost anywhere. A blood pressure cuff is inflated to 400 mm Hg, and three forearm punctures are made with a lance. The three bleeding sites are then touched (not blotted) every 15 seconds to remove any visible blood. The time when the last site no longer bleeds is the patient's bleeding time. A bleeding time of 2 to 8 minutes virtually excludes serious clotting disorders.

PELVIC ORGAN PROLAPSE

The "falling out" of a woman's reproductive organs is being seen more commonly in developed countries as women's life spans continue to increase. The cause of pelvic organ prolapse is multifactional, but is related to damage during childbirth, hereditary factors, and age-related weakness of muscles and connective tissue, and is often exacerbated by estrogen deficiency following menopause. Activities that constantly exert pressure against the pelvic organ support systems, such as manual labor with heavy lifting, frequent coughing, obesity, or chronic constipation, also tend to worsen prolapse problems. Many women tend to ignore the prolapse until it causes functional problems of the bladder or rectum.

Treatment for mild prolapse involves exercises of the pelvic floor muscles (Kegels) and using intravaginal estrogen cream 2 g applied weekly if the patient is menopausal. For more advanced prolapse problems, vaginal pessaries are helpful to correct the acute problem, but in the long term, if the patient's health is otherwise good, corrective surgery should be undertaken.

FEMALE GENITAL MUTILATION

In various parts of the world, but especially in certain Muslim countries of Africa (e.g., Sudan), the practice of female circumcision is performed traditionally to every girl when she nears the age of puberty. It is often performed using crude instruments and without anesthesia. It involves excising the clitoris and sometimes part or all of the labia. Narrowing of the vaginal opening is often then performed by suturing the cut edges of the labia together (infibulation). As a result, these girls experience reproductive and urinary dysfunction, and are both physically and psychologically scarred for life. Some girls die as a result of bleeding or infection following the procedure.

Successful techniques for defibulation under local anesthesia have been developed. It is important to explain fully the procedure and obtain the woman's informed consent before performing a defibulation procedure (even at childbirth), because the cultural influences that promote this behavior are very strong.

EFFECT OF FEMALE REPRODUCTIVE STATUS ON HEALTH

Although it may vary between societies and different parts of the world, the average age for the onset of menses (menarche) is about 13 years. The average menstrual cycle length is 28+ days although it is often irregular during the first 2 years after menarche and the 3 years prior to menopause due to anovulatory cycles. The average age for menopause to occur is 51 years. Therefore, the average woman has menses and may possibly be subject to menstrual disorders for about 38 years of her lifetime (Fig. 12-7).

NUTRITIONAL NEEDS AND REPRODUCTIVE TRACT STATUS

Because of hormonal factors, women have specific nutritional needs that are distinct from men. The prevention of osteoporosis should begin with ensuring proper calcium consumption in children, and should continue through reproductive years into menopause. Vitamin D supplementation also may be necessary.

During the reproductive years, women require adequate amounts of iron-rich foods to prevent anemia from monthly blood loss. For women in the childbearing years,

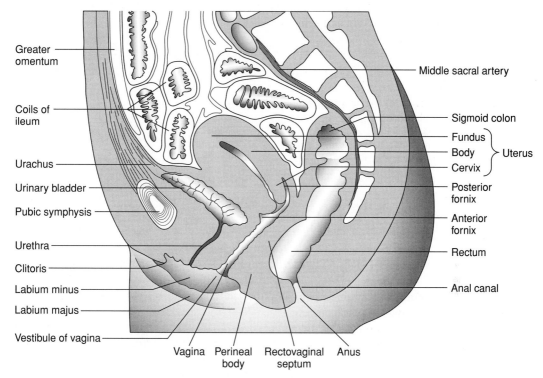

FIGURE 12-7 Sagittal section of the female pelvis.

supplemental folic acid before conception has been shown to decrease the incidence of neural tube defects. During pregnancy, adequate calorie and protein intake is important to ensure normal growth and development of the fetus. Finally, for postmenopausal females, dietary supplementation with calcium and vitamin D help to decrease osteoporotic fractures.

ROLE OF MATERNAL AND CHILD HEALTH WORKERS

In most developing countries and in rural or isolated areas of developed countries, the majority of routine health-care delivery for women and children is done by nonphysician maternal and child health (MCH) workers. The training and education of MCH workers may vary from simple health promotion training (village health workers) to fully trained advanced practice nurses (nurse practitioners, certified nurse midwives, or clinical nurse specialists). MCH workers form an essential component of the health care in many rural communities. For the most part, MCH workers recognize the limitations of their abilities and refer patients for treatment or consultation by a medical doctor as necessary (Table 12-9). As a health-care provider for women, it is important to recog-

TABLE 12-9 FUNCTIONS OF MATERNAL
AND CHILD HEALTH WORKERS

Providers of primary and preventive health care (e.g., Pap
smears and vaccinations)
Colaborers and extenders of medical doctors (particularly
in areas of physician shortage)
Counselors and teachers on issues specific to maternal and
child health (e.g., nutrition and family planning)
Advocates for improving health status of mothers and
children (e.g., formulate, administer, and potentiate
government health-care initiatives)

nize the contribution of community health workers and develop a working relationship
with them (see Chapter 13).

MENSTRUAL-RELATED DISORDERS

Certain health problems that are directly related to fluctuations of hormone levels
throughout the menstrual cycle include premenstrual syndrome, menstrual headaches,
catamenial seizures, and dysmenorrhea.

Premenstrual syndrome (PMS) refers to the cyclic appearance of dysphoric symptoms in the 7 to 10 days prior to menses. Over 100 symptoms have been related to PMS.
The most common are depression, irritability, anxiety, mood swings, headaches, breast
tenderness, bloating sensation, and backache. A sense of loss of control of both emotional and physical functions is commonly reported.

The occurrence of PMS may be just as strongly affected by a woman's cultural
beliefs and family history of problems related to menstruation as it is by a hormonal or
biochemical change. Two drugs have demonstrated effectiveness in relieving symptoms:
the antidepressant fluoxetine (Prozac) at doses of 20 to 60 mg daily, and the short-acting benzodiazepine alprazolam (Xanax) at a dose of 0.25 mg two to three times a day
during the luteal phase. A variety of herbal remedies, including evening primrose oil and
St. John's wort, are also popular treatments for PMS.

Menstrual headaches refers to all headaches that occur just before or during menstrual flow. Sixty percent of women who experience vascular (migraine) headaches
report an increased incidence during menstruation. Many women have headaches that
occur exclusively with menses. Other types of headaches, such as tension (muscle contraction) or psychologic stress-related headaches, also appear more commonly during
menses. Typically menstrual headaches can be effectively treated with acetaminophen,
aspirin, or other NSAIDs. For more severe forms of menstrual headaches, eliminating
menstruation by the daily intake of 10 mg of medroxyprogesterone acetate or by taking
OCPs on a continuous regimen (omitting the inactive pills) may be helpful.

Catamenial seizures refers to the worsening of seizure activity that occurs with
menses in about 50% of epileptic women. Progesterone is known to have a sedative

TABLE 12-10 NSAID DOSAGES FOR DYSMENORRHEA

Propionic acid derivatives	
Flurbiprofen (Ansaid)	200–300 mg/day divided b.i.d./t.i.d./q.i.d.
Ibuprofen (Motrin, Advil, Nuprin, Rufen)	200–600 mg q.i.d. or 800 mg t.i.d.
Ketoprofen (Orudis, Actron)	50–75 mg t.i.d.
Naproxen (Naprosyn, Aleve)	250–500 mg b.i.d.
Naproxen sodium (Anaprox)	275–550 mg b.i.d.
Oxaprozin (Daypro)	1,200 mg daily
Fenamate family	
Meclofenamate (Meclomen)	50–100 mg t.i.d./q.i.d.
*Mefenamic acid (Ponstan)	500 mg q.i.d.
*Flufenamic acid	
Cyclooxygenase-2 inhibitors	
Rofecoxib (Vioxx)	25–50 mg daily

*Not available in the United States.
NSAID, nonsteroidal antiinflammatory drug; b.i.d., twice daily; q.i.d., four times daily.

(antiepileptic) effect on the central nervous system. Depot injections of medroxyprogesterone acetate at 150 mg IM every 1 to 2 months has been shown to decrease seizure frequency by about 50%. Another treatment for catamenial seizures is to administer OCPs on a continuous regimen rather than cyclically.

Dysmenorrhea refers to the crampy lower abdominal pain that occurs with menses. Primary dysmenorrhea is due to myometrial contractions. Secondary dysmenorrhea is due to other pathologic conditions such as endometriosis, fibroid tumors, or PID. Due to their inhibition of prostaglandin synthesis, NSAIDs are the mainstay of treatment for dysmenorrhea (Table 12-10). Another good choice for therapy is OCPs, which also decrease the amount of menstrual flow and help to regulate menstrual cycles.

MENOPAUSE

Menopause is that point in time when menstruation permanently ceases, following the loss of ovarian activity. The perimenopausal period is when a woman passes through a transition from the reproductive stage of life to the postmenopausal years, a period marked by waning ovarian function. In developed countries the average woman spends about one third of her life in the postmenopausal state.

Perimenopausal symptoms directly related to declining estrogen production include the following:

1. Irregular menses with changes in amount of flow
2. Hot flushes
3. Anxiety, irritability, mood depression, and poor sleep patterns
4. Urogenital atrophy with resultant urinary control difficulties, vaginal dryness, and pain with intercourse

TABLE 12-11 PROS AND CONS OF HORMONE REPLACEMENT THERAPY (HRT)

ADVANTAGES OF HRT	RISKS OF HRT
Relief of hot flushes and urogenital atrophy Improved sense of psychological well-being Decrease bone fractures by 75% Decrease MI and strokes by 45% Significant decreases in macular degeneration of retina, colorectal cancer, memory disorders, and tooth loss	Two- to tenfold increase in endometrial cancer if not hysterectomized and on unopposed estrogen therapy Possible slight increase in breast cancer Contraindicated in patients with active thromboembolic disorders, known or suspected estrogen-dependent neoplasia, or undiagnosed abnormal vaginal bleeding Patients with impaired liver function or migraine headaches may require transdermal rather than oral route of administration

MI, myocardial infarction.

Health problems related to long-term estrogen deprivation include the following:

1. Osteoporosis with resultant increased rates of fractures and tooth loss
2. Atherosclerosis with increased rates of strokes and heart attacks
3. Acceleration of the aging-related reduction in muscular strength
4. Increased rates of bladder infections and urge incontinence due to urogenital atrophy

TABLE 12-12 RECOMMENDED HORMONE REPLACEMENT THERAPY REGIMENS

DAILY ESTROGEN	DAILY PROGESTIN
0.625 mg conjugated or esterified estrogens or estropipate or estrone sulfate, or	2.5 mg medroxyprogesterone acetate, or 0.35 mg norethindrone, or
1.0 mg micronized estradiol, or 0.05 mg transdermal estradiol	1.0 mg norethindrone acetate, or 100 mg micronized progesterone

SEQUENTIAL ESTROGEN	SEQUENTIAL PROGESTERONE
As above to take daily	5–10 mg of medroxyprogesterone, or 0.7 mg norethindrone, or 2.0 mg norethindrone, or 200 mg micronized progesterone for days 1–12 of each month

COMBINATION AGENTS

Both oral (Prempro, Premphase, or Ortho-prefest) and transdermal (Combipatch) combined estrogen and progesterone hormone preparations are currently available in the United States.
Unopposed estrogen: Only for hysterectomized patients without history of endometriosis
As above daily estrogen dosages, or may use injections of estradiol valerate 10–20 mg IM every 4 weeks

IM, intramuscularly.

The quality of life during these postmenopausal years may be greatly affected by health problems related to estrogen deprivation. Postmenopausal HRT should be viewed as specific treatment for postmenopausal estrogen deficiency symptoms in the short term and as preventive treatment for the health problems related to estrogen deprivation in the long term (Tables 12-11 and 12-12).

FAMILY PLANNING AND BIRTH CONTROL

Contraception is both a personal and social responsibility. Through effective contraceptive techniques, sex can be separated from procreation and thus provide couples greater control and enjoyment of their lives. It is also a critical element in limiting population growth, thereby preserving our planet's resources and improving quality of life for ourselves and for future generations.

Worldwide only 45% of married women in the reproductive age practice contraception, and 85% of these become pregnant within 1 year of ceasing contraception. Particularly in developing countries, the need for safe, affordable, effective, and easily accessible family planning methods is of paramount concern.

CONTRACEPTIVE TECHNIQUES

PERIODIC ABSTINENCE For certain religious or medical reasons, the only acceptable method of contraception for many people is to avoid sexual intercourse during the fertile (periovulatory) phase of the menstrual cycle. This "natural family planning" method must take into account that sperm remains viable within the female reproductive tract for 2 to 7 days and that the life span of the ovum postovulation is 1 to 3 days. This method requires commitment from both partners. It is not successful for women with irregular menstrual cycles, those with chronic vaginitis or cervicitis, people who cannot keep accurate records, or for couples who cannot part with sexual spontaneity. Up to 25% of women who use periodic abstinence techniques for contraception become pregnant within 1 year.

The rhythm or calendar method of periodic abstinence requires recording the length of the previous six menstrual cycles. By subtracting 18 days from the length of the shortest cycle, the beginning of the fertile period is estimated. By subtracting 11 days from the length of the longest cycle, the end of the fertile period is estimated. A woman with cycles of 27 to 31 days would then practice abstinence from the 9th day until the 20th day of the menstrual cycle.

The cervical mucus (Billings) method of periodic abstinence requires that the woman become aware of the estrogen-induced changes in cervical mucus that occur at the periovulatory time of the menstrual cycle. The woman should be instructed to use a clean finger to remove a small amount of mucus from the upper vagina daily (except when menstruating). By stretching the mucus out between her thumb and forefinger, she can check for the changes that occur during the fertile time. Practitioners of this method are not allowed to have intercourse on consecutive days during the preovulatory time of the cycle so that the seminal fluid will not obscure observation of cervical mucus changes. Abstinence begins when the mucus becomes wet, slippery, and stretchy (like a raw egg). Intercourse is permitted beginning on the 4th day after the last day of slippery, wet mucus.

The symptothermal method of periodic abstinence adds basal body temperature (BBT) monitoring of ovulation to the cervical mucus detection of the periovulatory fertile phase. To be accurate, the temperature must be taken immediately upon awakening each day. Specialized BBT thermometers that allow small changes in temperature to be easily discerned should be used for this purpose. The BBT rises by 0.2 to 0.4°C in response to the increasing levels of progesterone immediately after ovulation occurs. Abstinence begins when the mucus becomes slippery and moist. Intercourse is allowed to resume the night of either the third day of temperature elevation or the fourth day after the last day of slippery, wet mucus, whichever is later.

WITHDRAWAL (COITUS INTERRUPTUS) One of the earliest recorded methods of contraception (Onan in the Biblical book of Genesis) is also associated with a relatively high failure rate of about 20% per year. This is probably due to the release of some semen prior to the sensation of ejaculation in the male.

BARRIER CONTRACEPTIVES These methods are the oldest and most widely used contraceptive techniques of recorded history. In addition, they also provide some protection against sexually transmitted diseases.

The majority of condoms sold are made from latex, but "natural skin" (lamb intestine) condoms, and the newer polyurethane (Avanti) condoms also are available. The organisms that cause STDs and acquired immunodeficiency syndrome do not penetrate polyurethane or latex condoms, but can penetrate condoms made from intestine. When

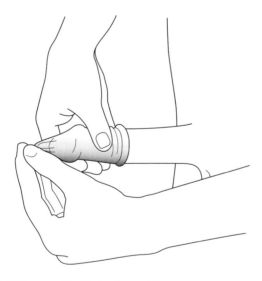

FIGURE 12-8 A male condom must be worn properly for it to work.

spermicides are used together with condoms, greater protection from STDs and pregnancy is achieved. Condoms must be properly used and worn for them to work effectively (Fig. 12-8). The foreskin must be pulled back if uncircumcised. Air should be squeezed out of the reservoir tip of the condom before unrolling it to the base of the penis. About a half inch of the pinched tip of the condom should extend beyond the penis to provide a reservoir to collect the ejaculate. The condom should be held at the base of the penis as it is withdrawn after intercourse so as not to allow any semen to leak or spill. Because oil-based lubricants degrade rubber, only water-based lubricants should be used with latex condoms.

> **DID YOU KNOW?** Worldwide approximately 20 billion *male condoms* will be manufactured and sold this year, making them one of the most popular methods of contraception. They have a typical failure rate of 14% during the first year of use.

The female condom was introduced in the United States in 1994. It consists of a thin polyurethane sheath with two flexible rings. The ring containing the closed end of the sheath is inserted into the vagina while the other ring containing the open end of the sheath remains outside the vagina (Fig. 12-9). The device is prelubricated with silicone, disposable after a single use, and is significantly more expensive than the male condom. Its failure rate of 21% during the first year of use is also significantly higher.

The vaginal diaphragm requires proper fitting and must be used with spermicidal jelly. It is a dome-shaped rubber cup that has a flexible spring-loaded rim. It should be removed within 24 hours but not less than 6 hours from the last intercourse. Most women use diaphragms 65 to 80 mm in diameter. A diaphragm fitting kit is available from the manufacturer. Three types of diaphragms are available. The flat spring has mild spring strength, the coil spring has moderate spring strength, and the arcing spring has the firmest spring strength. Those women with weaker vaginal muscle tone should use the stronger spring diaphragms. About one teaspoon of spermicidal jelly should be placed in the dome of the diaphragm prior to insertion. When the diaphragm is properly inserted, the leading edge is in the posterior fornix of the vagina and the front edge is behind the symphysis pubis with the dome completely covering the cervix (Fig. 12-10). As long as the patient has no allergies to latex, the only significant side effect of diaphragm use is an increased rate of urinary tract infections. The typical failure rate for diaphragms with spermicide is 20% during the first year of use.

The cervical cap is a soft, rubber cap with a deeper, smaller cup than the diaphragm. Its advantages over the diaphragm are that it may be left in place longer (up to 48 hours) and does not require repeated application of spermicide with each act of intercourse. Its disadvantages are that it is more difficult to fit and that it must be precisely and securely placed over the cervix by the wearer. Because it is only available in four sizes, about 50% of women cannot be properly fitted with the device. The cap must be evenly placed around the circumference of the cervix so that a slight suction fit is achieved (Fig. 12-11). The most common cause of failure of the cap is dislodgment from the cervix during intercourse. It has a typical failure rate of about 30% during the first year of use.

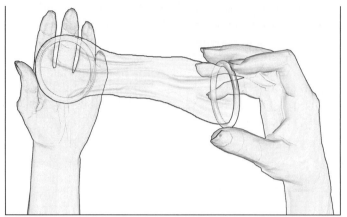

(a) **The Female Condom**

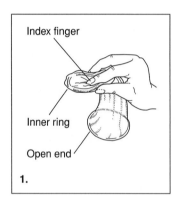

Index finger

Inner ring

Open end

1.

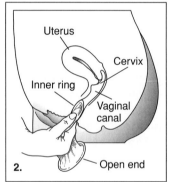

Uterus

Cervix

Inner ring

Vaginal canal

Open end

2.

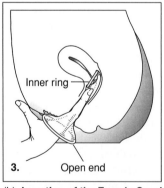

Inner ring

3. Open end

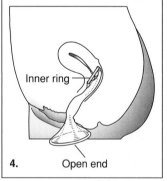

Inner ring

4. Open end

(b) **Insertion of the Female Condom**

FIGURE 12-9
(A) The female condom. (B) Insertion of the female condom.

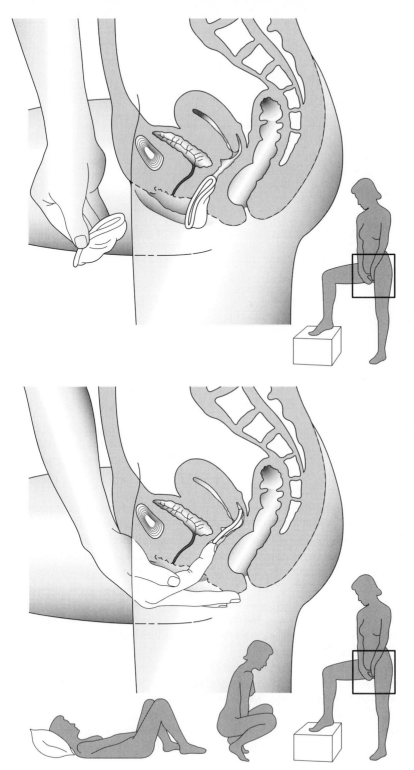

FIGURE 12-10 Diaphragm insertion technique.

423

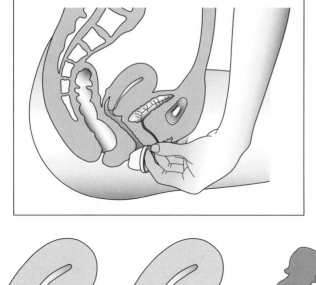

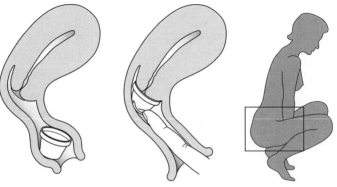

FIGURE 12-11
Insertion of a
cervical cap.

SPERMICIDES The vaginal contraceptive sponge (Today) serves as a sustained-released system for the spermicide nonoxynol-9. The sponge must be thoroughly moistened with water prior to insertion to activate the spermicide. It can be inserted immediately prior to intercourse or up to 24 hours beforehand, but must remain inside the vagina for at least 6 hours after intercourse (Fig. 12-12). In some parous women with weakened vaginal muscles or pelvic organ prolapse, retaining the sponge in the vaginal canal may be a problem, and a higher failure rate is observed in this group. There is no risk of toxic shock syndrome because the nonoxynol-9 actually retards staphylococcal replication and toxin production. The typical failure rate is about 30% during the first year of use of the spermicidal sponge.

Other vehicles for holding spermicide that can be placed intravaginally include vaginal contraceptive film, foams, jellies, creams, and suppositories. All spermicides require application at least 10 minutes prior to sexual intercourse. Tablets and suppositories remain effective for only 1 hour or less, whereas jellies, creams, and foam are good for as long as 8 hours. The principal minor problem is allergy or irritation related to either the vehicle or type of spermicide. Using a different type of product often solves the problem.

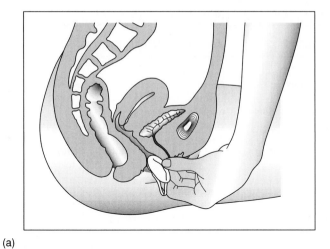

(a)

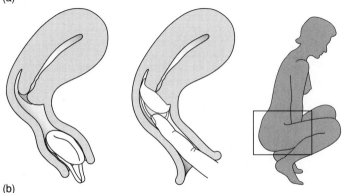

(b)

FIGURE 12-12
Insertion of a sponge. (A) The sponge is moistened with water (squeezing out the excess), folded upward, and inserted into the body and (B) placed firmly against the cervix.

ORAL CONTRACEPTIVE PILLS

Oral contraceptive pills are one of the most commonly used methods of contraception. All OCPs work by providing a progesterone-dominant hormonal state, which inhibits ovulation and implantation. Progesterone also thickens cervical mucus, making it relatively impervious to sperm. The estrogen component of OCPs also aids in inhibiting ovulation, but its main benefit is stabilization of the endometrium so that irregular bleeding can be controlled. The new low-dose preparations (<50 μg of estrogen) have proven to be just as effective as higher dose OCPs and have less unwanted side effects. For the occasional patient who requires an alternative to oral administration of contraceptive pills, the use of two pills placed daily high in the vagina has been shown to produce similar blood levels as a single pill taken orally. The typical failure rate for OCPs is 3% during the first year of use. Table 12-13 lists the contraindications for prescribing OCPs.

TABLE 12-13 TRUTHS ABOUT ORAL CONTRACEPTIVE PILLS (OCPs)

ABSOLUTE CONTRAINDICATIONS	RELATIVE CONTRAINDICATIONS
Thromboembolic disease, MI or CVA	Hypertension
Active liver disease such as hepatitis or hepatoma	Gallbladder disease
	Diabetes mellitus
Known or suspected breast or endometrium cancer	Migraine headaches
	History of obstructive jaundice of pregnancy
Smokers over age 35	Use of medications that reduce efficacy of OCPs: rifampin, phenobarbital, phenytoin, primidone, carbamazepine, felbamate, or topiramate
Undiagnosed abnormal vaginal bleeding	
Known or suspected pregnancy	Smokers under age 35

NONCONTRACEPTIVE BENEFITS	POTENTIAL SIDE EFFECTS
Decreased incidence of:	Breakthrough bleeding (manage by adding 1.25 mg conjugated estrogen or 2 mg estradiol daily for 7 days)
Ovarian cancer	
Endometrial cancer	
Benign breast disease	1% incidence of amenorrhea
PID	Nausea
Dysmenorrhea	Weight gain (not found with preparations containing <50 μg of estrogen)
Menorrhagia-related anemia	
Ovarian cysts	Hypertension (rare)
Symptomatic endometriosis	
Uterine fibroids	

Improvements in:
  Bone density
  Acne and hirsutism (especially the norgestimate-containing pills)

MANAGEMENT ISSUES

Pills should be taken at the same time each day.
If one pill is missed, then take missed pill as soon as possible and next pill at usual time.
    If two pills are missed during the first 2 weeks, then take two pills on each of the next 2 days and use barrier contraception for the next 7 days.
If two pills are missed in the third week or if more than two pills are missed at any time, then immediately start a new packet of pills and use barrier contraception for the next 7 days.

MI, myocardial infarction; CVA, cerebrovascular accident; PID, pelvic inflammatory disease.

PROGESTIN-ONLY PILLS

Progestin-only pills have twice the failure rate of other OCPs, and should only be used in women who are over age 40, or are breast-feeding, or others for whom the estrogen component of OCPs is contraindicated (history of an estrogen-dependent neoplasm or thromboembolic, cerebrovascular, or cardiovascular disease). Progestin-only pills should be started on the first day of menses and need to be faithfully taken at the same time each day. If the user is more than 3 hours late in taking a pill, then a barrier method of contraception should be used for the next 2 days. The main reason why women discontinue use of these pills is the increased incidence of unpredictable and irregular menstrual bleeding.

POSTCOITAL EMERGENCY CONTRACEPTION

Three new options in the field of emergency contraception have been developed. First, the insertion of a copper intrauterine device (IUD) up to 7 days after unprotected intercourse or up to 5 days after ovulation has been shown to lower the pregnancy rate to 1%. This method should not be used, however, in nulliparous women or in those at risk for sexually transmitted infections (multiple sexual partners or rape victims) (Fig. 12-13). Second, a dedicated emergency oral contraceptive product (Preven) may be used. It consists of four combined OCPs and a urine pregnancy test. Third, a progestin-only regimen has been shown to be more effective and yet significantly less likely to cause gastrointestinal upset than the combined oral emergency contraceptive regimens. The pregnancy rate of the progestin-only regimen is 1.1%, whereas the combined regimen pregnancy rate is 2% to 3%. Concomitant use of antiemetics is often needed in the combined regimen due to frequent occurrence of nausea (50%) and vomiting (20%). If vomiting occurs within 2 hours of taking the emergency contraceptive dose, then a repeat dosage is necessary. All patients should be advised to use these regimens for emergencies only and to adopt a reliable method of traditional contraception. Table 12-14 lists regimens for postcoital emergency contraception.

NORPLANT

The system consists of six flexible Silastic tubes (34 × 2.4 mm), each containing 36 mg of dry crystalline levonorgestrel designed to provide contraception for 5 years. After subdermal placement is performed in the upper, inner arm, the levonorgestrel diffuses through the wall of the tubing into the surrounding tissues, where it is absorbed (Fig. 12-14). During the first year of use, the implants release a total of 85 μg of levonorgestrel daily, which is about the same as the daily dose delivered by the progestin-only contraceptive pill. The rate of release gradually declines to 30 μg daily by year 5. The same medicines that induce liver enzymes and reduce the effectiveness of OCPs also reduce the effectiveness of Norplant. Because the progestin levels after the first year of use are already low, the use of these medicines (mostly antiepileptics) may lower the level below the contraceptive range. Therefore, Norplant is not generally recommended for women who have seizure disorders.

Both placement and removal of the implants is usually performed under local anesthesia as a minor surgical procedure. Scar tissue typically forms around the implants,

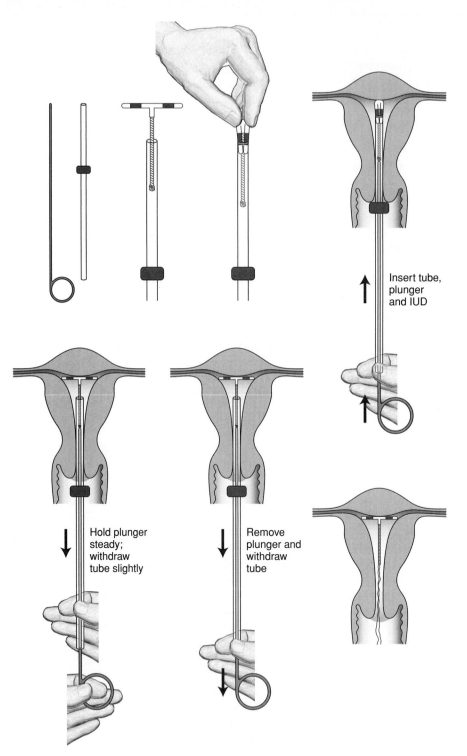

Insert tube,
plunger
and IUD

Hold plunger
steady;
withdraw
tube slightly

Remove
plunger and
withdraw
tube

FIGURE 12-13
Insertion of the
copper T 380
IUD for
postcoital
pregnancy
contraception
uses the same
insertion
technique
recommended
at any other
time.

TABLE 12-14 POSTCOITAL EMERGENCY ORAL CONTRACEPTIVE REGIMENS

TRADE NAME	FORMULATION	NO. OF PILLS WITH EACH DOSE
Ovral	50 μg ethinyl estradiol 500 μg norgestrel	2 (white pills)
Lo-Ovral	30 μg ethinyl estradiol 300 μg norgestrel	4 (white pills)
Nordette or Levlen	30 μg ethinyl estradiol 150 μg levonorgestrel	4 (light orange pills)
Triphasil or Tri-Levlen	30 μg ethinyl estradiol 125 μg levonorgestrel	4 (yellow pills)
Preven	50 μg ethinyl estradiol 250 μg levonorgestrel	2
Ovrette	75 μg norgestrel	20 (white pills)
*Microlut	30 μg levonorgestrel	25 (white pills)

First dose is given within 72 hours of coitus and second dose is given 12 hours later.
*Not available in the United States.

and removal causes more discomfort than does placement. Unlike oral contraceptives, the progestin levels maintained by Norplant are not high enough to suppress follicle-stimulating hormone, so some users develop benign functional ovarian cysts. Because these simple cysts usually regress within 1 month spontaneously, removal of the Norplant or the cyst is only necessary in those cases where the cysts are persistently large or painful. The typical failure rate within the first year of use is only 0.05%.

Depo-Provera (depot medroxyprogesterone acetate) is a 150-mg solution of progestin that is administered by a deep IM injection every 3 months. It is ideally initiated within 5 days of the onset of menses, thus preventing ovulation and eliminating the need for backup contraception. It also may be initiated immediately after abortion or childbirth because it does not increase the risk of thromboembolism, nor does it have a deleterious effect on lactation. If a woman shows up for her next injection more than 14 weeks after the initial shot, she should undergo a pregnancy test first and then be advised to use a backup method for 1 week following reinjection.

As with all progestin-only methods, abnormal menstrual bleeding commonly occurs and may persist for months after discontinuation. After 1 year (four injections) half of women develop amenorrhea and eventually three fourths of women cease to menstruate while using this method. A 10- to 18-month delay in return to fertility after discontinuing Depo-Provera may occur. Because Depo-Provera efficacy is not impaired

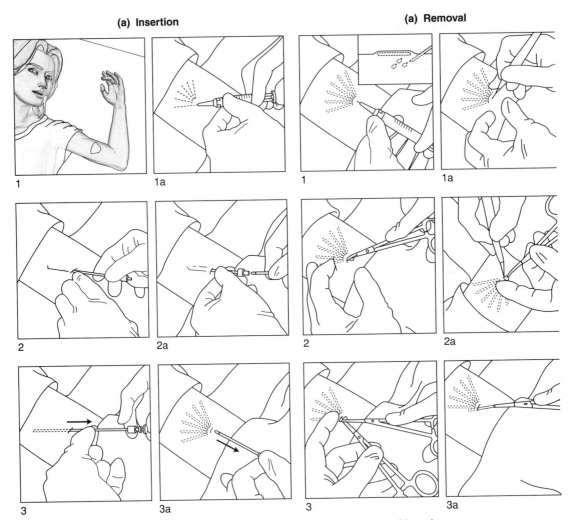

(a) Insertion

1

1a

2

2a

3

3a

(a) Removal

1

1a

2

2a

3

3a

FIGURE 12-14 The techniques for Norplant insertion (A) and removal (B), although not difficult, should be first learned under the guidance of a trained instructor.

by liver enzyme–inducing medications, it may be safely used in women with seizure disorders. Its typical failure rate is 0.3% during the first year of use.

INTRAUTERINE DEVICES

Intrauterine devices are the most cost-effective and most commonly used reversible form of birth control in the world. Because of their convenience and effectiveness, IUDs

TABLE 12-15 IUD INDICATIONS AND CONTRAINDICATIONS

IUDs ARE INDICATED FOR WOMEN WHO:	IUDs ARE CONTRAINDICATED FOR WOMEN WHO:
Are in a mutually monogamous relationship	Are pregnant or may be pregnant
Cannot tolerate estrogen	Have had postpartum endometritis or infected abortion in the past 3 months
Are breast cancer survivors	
Are smokers >35 years of age	Have a history of PID or STDs
Have active liver disease	Have a partner who has multiple sex partners
Have coronary or cerebrovascular disease	Have abnormal genital bleeding of unknown etiology
Have increased risk of thromboembolism	
Have lipid disorders	Have known or suspected uterine or cervical malignancy
Have diabetes mellitus or lupus	
Have anovulatory cycles	Have untreated acute vaginitis or cervicitis
Are breast-feeding	Have genital actinomycosis
Have dysmenorrhea or menorrhagia (progesterone IUD only)	Have conditions associated with increased susceptibility to infections, including leukemia, AIDS, and IV drug use
	Have abnormalities of the uterus resulting in distortion of the uterine cavity
	Have Wilson disease or known allergy (copper IUD only)
	Have a history of ectopic pregnancy or a condition that predisposes to ectopic pregnancy (Progestasert IUD only)

IUD, intrauterine device; PID, pelvic inflammatory disease; STD, sexually transmitted disease; IV, intravenous.

represent an excellent alternative to sterilization for many women. They are also useful in women for whom hormonal types of contraception are contraindicated. Many types of IUDs are in use throughout the world, but the most commonly used ones contain either copper or progesterone on a plastic frame that fits within the uterine cavity and has a monofilament string tail to aid in removal. The major mechanism of action for IUDs is to create a sterile, inflammatory environment in the endometrium that prevents sperm from reaching the fallopian tube. In addition, the progesterone IUDs also make the endometrium atrophic and less susceptible to implantation while at the same time thickening cervical mucus to prevent sperm penetration. See Table 12-15 for indications for using IUDs.

Intrauterine devices may be inserted at any time during the menstrual cycle as long as it is ascertained that the patient is not pregnant (Fig. 12-15). The advantages of inserting the IUD during menses include a dilated cervical canal, the masking of insertion-related bleeding, and the assurance that the patient is not pregnant.

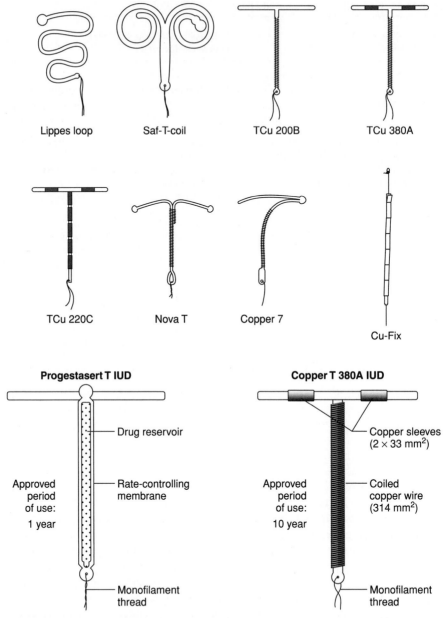

FIGURE 12-15 Although there are many IUDs used worldwide, only the Progestasert T and the copper T 380A are available in the United States.

MENSTRUAL REGULATION

This method of contraception has been extensively and successfully used in Eastern European countries for decades. It is also known as menstrual extraction, endometrial aspiration, or mini-abortion. It is of interest that in many Muslim countries where abortion is illegal this technique is permissible and widely practiced. A woman who is 7 to 10 days late for her regular menses is a candidate for this procedure. A flexible plastic cannula attached to a 20- or 50-mL syringe is inserted through the cervix into the endometrial cavity and negative pressure is applied by withdrawing the plunger of the syringe. Rotation of the syringe to ensure aspiration from all surfaces of the endometrium is required. Usually neither cervical dilation nor analgesia is necessary. If menstruation does not ensue within 1 week, then a pregnancy test should be performed. This is a rapid, low-cost procedure that is easy to perform. Patients may resume their normal activities the same day, and the complication/failure rates are low (2%–5%). However, this may be an unnecessary procedure for many patients (studies show that pregnancy was actually present in only about half of the patients), ectopic pregnancies are not addressed by this procedure, and the complications that do occur are of a more serious nature (perforation, infection, bleeding, retained products of conception, and continuing intrauterine pregnancy). Menstrual regulation has a 5% failure rate per year of use.

STERILIZATION TECHNIQUES

Female sterilization is the most popular method of contraception currently in use in the United States. Male sterilization (vasectomy) is cheaper, safer, easier, and more effective than female sterilization techniques. Despite these advantages, the volume of female sterilization procedures performed in the United States outnumbers vasectomy by nearly 3 to 1.

The development of laparoscopic and mini-laparotomy female sterilization techniques has resulted in a tremendous increase in convenience for women as well as a large savings in medical care costs as compared with older techniques.

Laparoscopic female sterilization can be performed with local anesthesia and IV sedation, but is usually performed under general anesthesia due to the greater pain from peritoneal irritation caused by the CO_2 gas insufflated before and during insertion of the laparoscope. Unipolar or bipolar electrocautery is commonly used for laparoscopic tubal sterilization, but Silastic rings and clips also may be applied (Figs. 12-16 and 12-17).

Even though failure rates are extremely low for sterilization procedures, patients should be counseled that pregnancy may still occur and that if pregnancy occurs, there is a high risk (1 out of 3) for it to be ectopic. A few women may experience menstrual abnormalities poststerilization, which is thought to be due to changes in ovarian steroid function brought on by decreased blood supply from the ligated tubes. Female sterilization has a 0.4% failure rate.

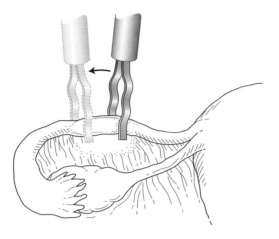

FIGURE 12-16 Laparoscopic bipolar electrocauterization of the fallopian tube. A full-thickness burn for at least 3 cm distance should be done.

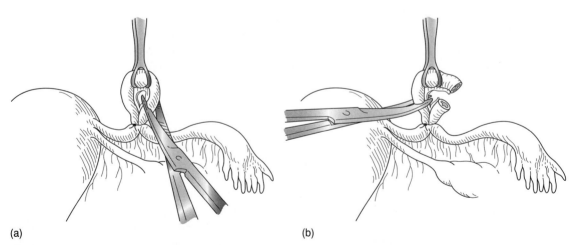

(a)

(b)

FIGURE 12-17 Pomeroy method of tubal ligation. (A) A loop of the isthmic portion of the tube is elevated and ligated at its base with one or two ties of #1 plain catgut suture. If performed through a minilaparotomy incision, these ties should be held long to prevent premature retraction of the tubal stumps into the abdomen when the loop of tube is transected. (B) A fenestration is bluntly created through the mesentery within the tubal loop, and each limb of the tube on either side of this fenestration is individually cut. The cut end of the tube is inspected for hemostasis and allowed to retract into the abdomen.

Tubal ligation via a small periumbilical incision for a recently postpartum woman or via a mini-laparotomy performed suprapubically can be accomplished with local anesthesia, but most commonly is done under regional or general anesthesia. Techniques that involve ligation, transection, and removal of a portion of the tubes include Pomeroy-Irving, and Uchida. Tubal occlusion with clips (Hulka or Filshie) and Silastic rings (Falope) have about the same efficacy rates as the transection techniques, but offer the advantage of potentially higher rates for successful tubal reanastomosis. Nevertheless, sterilization should only be offered to those patients who have made a permanent decision for no further childbearing. Most techniques for tubal ligation also can be performed through a vaginal incision, but the main disadvantages are significantly higher infection and failure rates.

Male sterilization via vasectomy is a much less invasive procedure than female sterilization. It is extremely effective once the supply of remaining sperm in the vas deferens is exhausted. Virtually all men are sterile after 15 ejaculations or 6 weeks postprocedure. Hematomas and infection rarely occur and are amenable to treatment with heat, scrotal support, and antibiotics. Contrary to popular opinion, there are no longterm adverse effects from vasectomy. There are no increased rates of prostate cancer or psychological disease, and sexual function is unchanged. Men do not even notice a change in the volume or velocity of their ejaculate because the other constituents of semen are made downstream from the vasectomy site. Vasectomy reversal is also easier to accomplish than tubal reanastomosis. Male sterilization has a 0.15% failure rate.

Lidocaine 1% is injected on each side of the scrotum where a small incision is then made to isolate, occlude, and resect a portion of the vasa. Incision closure usually requires only one or two sutures. A no-scalpel technique uses an instrument that punctures the scrotal skin and sheath of the vas. The vasa are then identified and vasectomy performed in the usual way, but no sutures are required for skin closure.

ABORTION

The termination of pregnancy prior to sufficient fetal development to sustain independent life is often considered to be an abortion. However, by strict definition, the gestation should be less than 20 weeks, and the conceptus should weigh less than 500 g and be less than 16.5 cm in crown-to-rump length to be an abortion. There remains substantial social and ethical debate over induced abortion. This section addresses the medical aspects of pregnancy termination.

Induced abortion, either medical or surgical, is the most common surgical procedure performed in the United States, with about 25% of all pregnancies being ended with this procedure. The death rate from legal induced abortion is about 0.6 per 100,000, whereas the death rate for childbirth is about 10 per 100,000. In general, the earlier in gestation that the abortion is performed, the lower the associated morbidity and mortality. Major complications of induced abortion include uterine perforation, anesthesia-related problems, hemorrhage, sepsis, and retained tissue. These may require further surgical procedures or hospitalization to treat. Minor complications include mild infection, cervical lacerations, and development of cervical stenosis, which can cause obstruction to subsequent menstrual flow. Rh-negative women should be given Rh immunoglobulin to prevent sensitization.

Vacuum curettage is the most common method of inducing abortion and may be performed up to 14 weeks of gestation. Osmotic dilators are placed in the cervix about 4 hours prior to the procedure, a paracervical block using local anesthetic is given, then the products of conception are removed by suction evacuation, and completeness of the procedure is confirmed with sharp curettage. Examination of the uterine aspirate for villi helps to prevent missing the diagnosis of an ectopic pregnancy. After 14 weeks' gestation, induced abortion can be accomplished by either surgical or medical means.

Dilatation and evacuation (D&E) is the surgical method used for second trimester abortions. It is considered to be safer, faster, and less expensive than medically induced abortions. D&E can be performed up to about 20 weeks' gestation depending on the training, experience, and skill of the surgeon. The availability of anesthesia services, emergency medical support, and hospitalization facilities are also important factors. The incidence of serious complications such as uterine perforation, infection, hemorrhage, amniotic fluid embolism, and anesthetic reactions are higher with advanced gestational age. D&E is performed by inserting laminaria into the cervix, which are left in overnight. This is followed by further dilation of the cervix with mechanical dilators to 2 cm, followed by extraction of the fetus in pieces using a combination of specially designed forceps, sharp curettage, and suction instruments. The development of cervical incompetence, which can affect the ability to carry a subsequent pregnancy to term, is a potential late complication of D&E.

Medically induced abortions can be performed in either the first or second trimester. With the availability of prostaglandin analogues and antiprogestogens, the use of intraamniotic instillation of urea or hypertonic saline to induce abortion has declined. Two successful regimens for first trimester medically induced abortion have been recently developed that have safety and efficacy rates comparable to those of vacuum curettage. The first regimen uses IM methotrexate 50 mg/m^2 of body surface area followed 3 to 7 days later by 800 mg of the prostaglandin misoprostol (Cytotec) given either orally or as a vaginal suppository. If abortion does not occur within 7 to 10 days, a second dose of misoprostol is given. Side effects of the medicines used include nausea, diarrhea, and vomiting. Vacuum curettage may be necessary for the 2% to 8% who only incompletely abort using this regimen.

A second method for medical induction of first trimester abortion uses the antiprogestogen mifepristone (RU-486) followed by administration of misoprostol. Three 200-mg tablets of mifepristone are taken orally, followed by two 200-µg oral tablets of misoprostol 36 to 48 hours later. Most women abort within 4 hours after the misoprostol dosage. If the abortion does not occur within 7 to 10 days, either a second course of misoprostol is given or vacuum curettage can be done. The regimen has been shown to be 95% successful in achieving a completed abortion for pregnancies at less than 10 weeks' gestation. Complications of abortion are listed in Table 12-16.

TABLE 12-16 COMPLICATIONS OF ABORTION: CAUSES, DIAGNOSES, AND TREATMENT PLANS

COMPLICATIONS	CAUSES	DIAGNOSES	TREATMENT PLANS
Unsuccessful termination pregnancy	Inadequate response to medical induction of abortion	No tissue passed	Uterine curettage
	Inability to open cervix	Cervical stenosis	Repeat laminaria or use misoprostol adequately with dilators
	Ectopic pregnancy	No villi in curettings	Surgical treatment or methotrexate; hCG remains elevated; ultrasonography
Infection	Endometritis	No fever; mild uterine tenderness; vaginal discharge	Augmentin 875 mg orally b.i.d. for 14 days or doxycycline 100 orally mg b.i.d. plus metronidazole 500 mg b.i.d. for 14 days
	Endomyometritis	Fever, severe uterine tenderness, malodorous vaginal discharge	Hospitalization, cefotetan IV 2 g every 12 hours and doxycycline 100 mg IV or orally every 12 hours
	Urinary tract infection	Dysuria with or without fever	Ciprofloxacin 500 mg orally b.i.d. or Septra DS orally b.i.d. or amoxicillin 1 g orally then 500 mg t.i.d.
Prolonged or excessive bleeding	Uterine atony	Nontender, soft, boggy uterus; excessive bleeding	Uterine massage, oxytocin 20–40 U/L of IV fluid over 30 minutes; methergine 0.2 mg IM; carboprost (Hemabate) 250 μg IM
	Cervical laceration	Speculum examination	Figure-of-8 sutures with 0 chromix and assistant to aid with visualization
	Retained products of conception	Tissue plus blood in cervix shows tissue in uterus	Ultrasonographic guidance, ultrasonographic vacuum, and sharp curettage
	Uterine perforation	Tender, firm uterus with or without hematuria Ultrasonography shows free fluid in abdomen/ pelvis	Laparoscopy or laparotomy under general anesthesia; check bowel and bladder

TABLE 12-16 COMPLICATIONS OF ABORTION: CAUSES, DIAGNOSES, AND TREATMENT PLANS
(continued)

COMPLICATIONS	CAUSES	DIAGNOSES	TREATMENT PLANS
	Coagulopathy	History of bleeding; nontender, firm uterus with nonstop bleeding; bruising or bleeding at IV sites; CBC, PT, PTT platelet count, fibrinogen or fibrin degradation products	Transfuse whole blood or PRBC to keep Hb >8; platelet transfusion if <50,000/mL; fresh frozen plasma 10–15 mL/kg if fibrinogen <100 mg/dL if PT/PTT are prolonged; check for sepsis or retained products of conception
Shock	Blood loss	Postural changes in vital signs; anemia; oliguria; heavy vaginal bleeding	As above
	Sepsis	Hypotension at rest; fever; granulocytosis, chest radiography; gram stain of cervix for *Streptococcus* or *Clostridium*	Triple antibiotics: ampicillin 2 g IV every 6 h, gentamicin 120 mg IV every 12 h, + clindamycin 900 mg IV every 8 h; IV fluids
	Cardiogenic	Dyspnea; auscultation; minimal vaginal bleeding; chest radiography; rare in gravidas without prior history of breast disease	Diuretics, inotropic agents, hemodynamic monitoring, and ventilatory support

hCG, human chorionic gonadotropin; b.i.d., twice daily; IV, intravenously; DS, double strength; t.i.d., three times daily; IM, intramuscularly; CBC, complete blood count; PT, prothrombin time; PTT, partial thromboplastin time; PRBC, packed red blood cells.

BREAST DISEASE

In Western cultures the female breast is associated with sexual attraction and stimulation, whereas in many other cultures the breast's purpose is utilitarian and its only function is for feeding infants. In almost all countries the leading cancer killer for women is breast malignancy. It is for these reasons that concerns about breast problems are a leading cause for women to seek medical care.

NONMALIGNANT CONDITIONS OF THE BREAST

Because the breast is a glandular organ, it is affected by hormonal fluctuations that occur with the onset of puberty, the menstrual cycle, pregnancy, lactation, and menopause. An exaggeration of the normal physiologic response to cyclic hormone levels may cause pain, engorgement, and cyst formation in the breast. Benign neoplasms of the glands, ducts, or stroma may occur. Infection and vascular disease also may affect the breast

Fibrocystic change is the most common benign breast disorder and is present in nearly half of premenopausal women in the 30 to 50 age group. This condition causes pain (mastalgia) and a sensation of fullness. The upper, outer quadrants of the breasts are the areas most often involved. The pain is usually cyclic in nature and worsens during the 7 to 14 days of the premenstrual phase. The pain is caused by breast stromal edema, ductal dilation (cysts), and an associated inflammatory response. On examination the involved areas of the breast have a rubbery, lumpy texture with increased tenderness, nodularity, and engorgement. Intermittent nipple discharge may occur. The woman should be instructed to decrease caffeine intake, wear a well-fitted support bra, and to return for examination soon after the next menses is finished. If on reexamination there is a persistent dominant mass, it should either be aspirated if cystic or excised if solid.

Long-term treatment for fibrocystic change of the breast involves methods of reducing mastalgia, dietary changes, and hormonal manipulation. Analgesics such as ibuprofen, acetaminophen, or salicylates are helpful. The use of high-dose vitamin A or E was originally thought to be helpful, but recent studies show that the level of improvement with either of these substances was about the same as placebo. Limiting exposure to methylxanthines (caffeine) often gives subjective improvement in symptoms. The use of a mild diuretic for 3 days prior to each menses also may reduce the symptoms of breast tenderness and swelling.

Oral contraceptive pills have been shown to suppress symptoms in 70% to 90% of women with fibrocystic breast changes. Oral progestins (5–10 mg of medroxyprogesterone acetate) daily for 10 days postovulation also have been shown to be highly effective. Unfortunately, symptoms reoccur in about 40% of women when OCPs or oral progestins are discontinued. For more severe cases, the use of the estrogen-lowering agent Danazol (100–200 mg twice daily for 6 months) is highly effective in reducing both the tenderness and the nodularity of the breasts. Usually its beneficial effect persists for months after stopping therapy. Unfortunately, the androgenic side effects and high cost of this drug limit its use. For recalcitrant cases, the prolactin inhibitor bromocriptine or the estrogen antagonist tamoxifen may be helpful. Surgical treatment (mastectomy) for mastalgia should only rarely be undertaken, and only after psychiatric consultation.

Fibroadenomas are the second most common benign breast disorder and the number one cause of a breast mass in a women under age 25. They are painless, slow-growing tumors consisting of both stromal and ductal cells. They are usually solitary and stop growing after attaining 2 to 4 cm in diameter. Rarely they will grow larger (massive fibroadenoma) or occur in multiple sequential development throughout the entire extent of the breast. On examination, fibroadenomas are solid, nontender, rounded, freely mobile, and rubbery in texture. Ultrasonography reveals a characteristic appearance of smooth external borders and a homogeneous echo pattern within the solid mass. For women under age 25 in whom the diagnosis is confirmed by ultrasonography, careful observation is appropriate because up to 30% of such masses resolve spontaneously. Excision should be performed if the mass increases in size significantly or becomes psychologically disturbing. In women over age 25, a palpable fibroadenoma should be excised. They are usually easily shelled out through a cosmetic incision.

Phyllodes tumor is an uncommon solid lesion of fibroepithelial origin that may grow to be quite large (10–15 cm) and become tender. Although these are considered to be benign tumors, almost 10% have malignant potential and may metastasize. All phyllodes tumors should be treated by wide, local excision.

Intraductal papilloma commonly occurs in a patient's fifth decade of life and often presents with a serous, bloody, or turbid-type nipple discharge. Intraductal papilloma is caused by solitary, papillary benign lesions growing in one of the main ducts close to the nipple. Occasionally a palpable mass may be felt at the areolar margin. These lesions can be identified by a ductigram radiograph. Treatment is excision of the offending duct along with a small amount of surrounding tissue. Cytology of the nipple discharge can be performed, but is not a reliable way to determine the absence of malignancy and should not delay operation.

Fat necrosis is a benign condition that is associated with trauma to the breast. It occurs most commonly in perimenopausal women with large breasts. A firm, irregular, somewhat tender, fixed, and solid mass that may cause skin retraction is usually palpable. Because its presentation on both clinical examination of the breast and on mammography mimics that of carcinoma, these lesions require excisional biopsy.

Mondor disease is caused by a superficial thrombosis of a vein in the breast accompanied by inflammation. It occurs most commonly in puerperal women or in association with breast reduction or augmentation. A tender, erythematous, firm, cordlike structure that may cause dimpling or creasing of the overlying skin is most often located on the lateral surface of the breast. Treatment consists of heat and analgesics. The condition should resolve spontaneously within 6 months. If the diagnosis is uncertain, excisional biopsy should be performed.

Duct ectasia occurs when the terminal collecting ducts become obstructed, dilated, and full of secretions. Infection may ensue, and a thick, greenish black nipple discharge may be present. A tender, distended, erythematous mass adjacent to the areola is found in association with a burning or pulling sensation. This disorder is usually found in postmenopausal or perimenopausal women. Treatment is by excisional biopsy.

Galactocele usually occurs as a cystic, centrally located swelling developing shortly after the abrupt termination of lactation, but it also may arise during pregnancy. The sterile, inspissated milk within the galactocele may appear clear or whitish upon needle aspiration. It may require aspiration on several occasions to allow the walls of the cyst to adhere to one another and obliterate the space. Local excision may be necessary.

Mastitis usually presents as tenderness, induration, and erythema of the breast in a lactating woman. Fever and a generalized achy sensation also may be present. The common skin organisms of *Staphylococcus* and *Streptococcus* are usually the causative bacteria, so the patient should be treated with a cephalosporin or penicillinase-resistant penicillin such as dicloxacillin or augmentin. Patients should be encouraged to breast-feed their infants from the noninfected breast and to express then discard the milk from the infected breast. If the infection does not resolve and an abscess forms, then incision and drainage are mandatory. A drain may need to be placed in the wound and removed 24 to 48 hours later.

EVALUATION OF A BREAST MASS

One of the most frightening experiences for a women is when she discovers a lump in her breast. The very real danger that this may be a life-threatening or disfiguring malignancy may become an overwhelming and all-consuming dread. The role of the physician in assessing the lump in a knowledgeable, rational, and sensitive manner is key in allaying the patient's fears. An appropriate history should be obtained regarding the duration and onset of signs and symptoms, reproductive and menstrual history, medication and hormone usage, and details of her family history of breast disease. Visual examination should be performed while the patient is upright with her hands on her hips. Asymmetry, skin or nipple changes, and appearance of a mass should be noted. A fingertip examination of the entire breast and axillary regions should then be performed with the patient in both the upright and supine positions. Imaging studies of the breast with mammography is helpful for both screening and diagnosis of a breast mass. Ultrasonography is helpful in characterizing cystic areas seen by mammography or in young women with dense breasts that may obscure the mammographic ability to detect lesions. Needle aspiration of palpable cysts can be performed if resources are available, and local anesthesia is usually not necessary. The mass should be immobilized between the fingers and a 22- to 24-gauge needle inserted and the cyst fluid withdrawn. If the mass is solid, several passes should be made through the mass until tissue or fluid is seen within the syringe. The specimen is then placed on a slide for cytologic evaluation. If the cyst fluid is bloody or the mass does not completely disappear, or if there is an associated nipple discharge, then excisional biopsy needs to be performed promptly. The patient's history, physical examination, imaging studies, and cytologic evaluation are all helpful, but only histologic evaluation of the mass is definitive to rule out malignancy.

BREAST CANCER SCREENING AND PREVENTION

The death rate from carcinoma of the breast exceeds in total the number of cancer deaths from all other organs of the female reproductive tract combined. Although great strides have been made in the treatment of breast cancer, the greatest gains in survival are found when techniques for early detection and prevention are emphasized.

Breast self-examination techniques should be taught to every women once breast development (thelarche) occurs. It should involve both visualization and palpation of each breast and needs to be performed monthly, usually just after completion of menstruation. An annual physical examination of the breasts by a qualified health-care provider should be performed annually starting at age 18.

If available, baseline mammography should be performed between the ages of 35 and 40 for every woman, then regular screening examinations should be performed

TABLE 12-17 RISK FACTORS FOR DEVELOPING BREAST CANCER

Family history of breast cancer
Early menarche (before age 12)
Delayed child-bearing (>30 years of age)
Nulliparity
Obesity or high-fat diet
Alcohol consumption
History of high-dose radiation exposure
History of a breast mass that required biopsy
Late menopause (after age 53)
Increased age (peak incidence is ages 50–70)

after age 40. Between the ages of 40 and 49, mammography should be performed every 1 to 2 years depending on the patient's risk factors. After age 50, mammography should be performed annually.

Prevention should be discussed with all women because only 25% of those who go on to develop breast cancer have identifiable risk factors. Changes in diet, idealizing body weight, eliminating alcohol, bearing children before age 30, and breast-feeding each baby for at least 3 months are all helpful activities to lower the risk. The use of post-menopausal HRT and the risk of breast cancer is unclear at this time. It does appear that a long duration of use (>10 years) increases the risk slightly. However, if a woman who is using HRT develops breast cancer, it is diagnosed at an earlier stage, tends to be of a lower grade, and has a better prognosis than breast cancers in women who are not using HRT (Tables 12-17 and 12-18).

TABLE 12-18 BREAST DISEASE

CONDITIONS	SYMPTOMS	PHYSICAL FINDINGS	IMAGING STUDIES	TREATMENT
Fibrocystic change	Cyclic pain and fullness	Bilateral rubbery, lumpy, tender nodules usually found in the upper, outer quadrant	Mammogram: negative US: cystic nodules Aspiration of macrocysts	Excisional biopsy of any solid, dominant mass Diuretics, OCPs, progestins, NSAIDs, vitamin A or E, and caffeine; danazol, bromocriptine, or tamoxifen for more serious cases
Fibroadenomas	Painless mass rubbery, nontender	Usually solitary, mobile, circumscribed mass solid mass	Mammogram: well US: solid homogeneous mass	<25 years old: careful observation >25 years old: excisional biopsy

TABLE 12-18 BREAST DISEASE *(continued)*

CONDITIONS	SYMPTOMS	PHYSICAL FINDINGS	IMAGING STUDIES	TREATMENT
Phyllodes tumor	Large potentially painful mass	Solitary, large, firm, bossellated, solid mass	Mammogram: large circumscribed mass US: large, solid homogeneous mass	Wide local excision
Intraductal papilloma	Painless nipple discharge	Unilateral, uniductal, nontender nipple discharge	Ductogram radiograph may show the papilloma	Probe the affected duct and excise a wedge of tissue
Fat necrosis	Mildly painful, unilateral mass that does not increase in size	Firm, tender, indurated, solid mass with irregular borders	Mammogram: fine, stippled calcifications and stellate contractions	Excisional biopsy
Mondor disease (thrombophlebitis)	Painful streak along one side during the puerperium	Tender, erythematous, firm, linear, and cordlike structure usually found on the lateral surface	US: may show the thrombosed vein	Analgesics, heat, and observation
Duct ectasia	Unilateral, painful mass with dark-colored nipple discharge	Tender, erythematous hard mass adjacent to the areola	US confirms cystic nature	Excisional biopsy
Galactocele	Mass occurring during pregnancy mass or after lactation has ended	Centrally located, cystic	US: cystic mass with smooth fibrous walls	Aspiration and possibly local exicision
Mastitis	Unilateral pain and swelling while lactating	Tender, erythematous, indurated, and possibly febrile	US may help to rule out abscess	Antibiotics and possibly I&D of abscess
Breast cancer	Painless lump and possible nipple discharge	Firm, irregular, fixed mass with possible associated skin retraction and axillary node enlargement	Mammography: calcifications and stellate contractions	Lumpectomy with node dissection, radiotherapy, and possible chemotherapy. Large tumors may require mastectomy

US, ultrasonography; OCP, oral contraceptive pill; NSAID, nonsteroidal antiinflammatory drug; I&D, incision and drainage.

CHAPTER 13
Obstetrics

Karen Frush and Mony Mehrotra

EMERGENCY DELIVERY

BACKGROUND

Health providers in remote settings are frequently needed to evaluate pregnant and actively laboring patients. It is important to be familiar with the basics of emergency obstetrics and the initial management of third-trimester emergencies such as pre-eclampsia, eclampsia, and hemorrhage, because these complications have major consequences for maternal and child survival. This chapter describes the major issues in preparing for patients who present in labor or with complications of late pregnancy.

PREPAREDNESS

Whether patients deliver at home, in a rural health post, or in the hospital, it is important for health workers to be prepared to provide prompt, appropriate care for both mother and infant. Every health facility should have access to necessary supplies and equipment (Table 13-1), or at least a basic delivery kit (Table 13-2). In addition to the delivery kit, resources for the initial care and potential resuscitation of the newborn are essential.

   Another important feature of preparedness that is frequently overlooked is the training of medical staff in the management of pregnancy-related emergencies. It is likewise important to work closely with maternal child health workers and traditional birth attendants (TBAs) to provide appropriate care for women in labor and for newborn infants.

TABLE 13-1 SUGGESTED LIST OF SUPPLIES AND EQUIPMENT

Antiseptic soap (or any soap)
Clean brush for cleaning the hands and fingernails
Alcohol for rubbing on hands after they are washed
Clean cotton
New razor blade (Do not unwrap until you are ready to cut the umbilical cord. If you do not have a razor blade, have clean, rust-free scissors ready. Boil them just before cutting the cord.)
Sterile gauze or patches of thoroughly cleaned cloth for covering the navel
Two ribbons or clean strips of clean cloth for tying the cord
Both patches and ribbons of cloth should be wrapped and sealed in paper packets and then baked in the oven or ironed.
Flashlight (torch)
Suction bulb for sucking the mucus out of the baby's nose and mouth
Sterile syringe and needles
Several injections of ergonovine or ergometrine
Two bowls—one for washing hands and one for catching and examining the afterbirth
Fetoscope, or fetal stethoscope, for listening for the baby's heartbeat through the mother's belly
Blunt-tipped scissors for cutting the cord before the baby is all the way born (extreme emergency only)
Two clamps (hemostats) for clamping the umbilical cord or clamping bleeding veins from tears of the birth opening
Rubber or plastic gloves (that can be sterilized by boiling) to wear while examining the woman, while the baby is coming out, when sewing tears in the birth opening, and for catching and examining the afterbirth
Sterile needle and gut thread for sewing tears in the birth opening
1% silver nitrate drops, tetracycline eye ointment, or erythromycin eye ointment for the baby's eyes to prevent dangerous infection

CLINICAL PRESENTATION

Any pregnant woman beyond 20 weeks' gestation who arrives in the emergency department with signs of active labor should be carefully evaluated to determine the condition of the mother and the fetus. An important component is the medical and obstetric history of the patient, including parity and estimated date of confinement (EDC). If the last menstrual period (LMP) is known and a pregnancy wheel is not available, the EDC

TABLE 13-2 BASIC EQUIPMENT AND SUPPLIES FOR EMERGENCY DELIVERY

Surgical scissors	Cord clamps
Placenta basin	Sterile gloves
Rubber bulb syringe	Gauze sponge (4 × 4)
Neonatal airways	Syringes (10-mL)
Towels	Needles (23-gauge)
Hemostats	

List excludes standard adult and neonatal resuscitation equipment.

can be calculated by adding 9 months and 7 days to the LMP. Although useful for providing a rough estimate, ultrasonographic examination late in the third trimester is not an accurate predictor of gestational age, because estimates of EDC can vary by plus or minus 3 weeks. Fundal height also provides a rapid estimate of gestational age in the patient who does not recall LMP or EDC. Fundal height is measured in centimeters (cm = weeks gestation ± 2 weeks) from the pubic symphysis to the top of the fundus as palpated by the examiner, although this measurement can be greatly overestimated in obese patients. In addition to the obstetric history of the patient, it is important to obtain pertinent medical information, such as allergies, medications, drug and alcohol use, and prenatal care, and to elicit any past history of complications with prior deliveries or precipitous labor.

Every patient presenting with signs of active labor should receive immediate monitoring of maternal vital signs and fetal heart rate. Maternal blood pressure should be monitored closely while in the emergency department. Doppler heart tones are helpful to confirm normal fetal heart rate (120–160 beats/min). A persistent slow fetal heart rate (less than 100/min) is an indicator of fetal distress, and emergent obstetric consultation is necessary.

DISTINGUISHING TRUE VERSUS FALSE LABOR

The confirmation of true labor as opposed to false labor is an important initial step in the management of the term or near-term pregnant patient. False labor is defined as uterine contractions that do not lead to cervical changes. False labor is characterized by irregular, brief contractions usually confined to the lower abdomen. These contractions, commonly called Braxton-Hicks contractions, are irregular in both intensity and duration. False labor may be persistent for several days. It is most commonly treated by hydration and rest, but may uncommonly require admission with supportive care.

True labor is characterized by painful, regular contractions with steadily increasing intensity and duration leading to progressive cervical dilatation. True labor typically begins in the fundal region and upper abdomen and radiates into the pelvis and to the lower back. True labor also leads to progressive descent of the fetus into the pelvis in preparation for delivery, as well as cervical dilatation and effacement.

PHYSICAL EXAMINATION

Patients without vaginal bleeding should undergo a sterile speculum examination and a bimanual examination. Patients presenting with vaginal bleeding should be evaluated with ultrasonography prior to any speculum or bimanual examination to rule out placenta previa. If spontaneous rupture of membranes (SROM) is suspected, sterile speculum examination should be performed and digital examination avoided, because studies have shown an increased risk of infection after a single digital examination. It is particularly important to avoid digital examinations in the preterm patient in whom prolongation of gestation is desired. Sterile speculum examination allows confirmation of SROM, visualization of the cervix with estimation of dilatation, and collection of cervical cultures, particularly group B streptococci, *Neisseria gonorrhoeae*, and *Chlamydia* cultures. The typical method for pelvic examination is in the lithotomy position. Stirrups are not necessary, although they are helpful. Alternatively, a bedpan may be used to elevate the patient's buttocks enough to allow speculum examination. Lubricant should be avoided unless rupture of membranes has been confirmed, because lubricant may contribute to a false-positive nitrazine test result.

The abdomen should be inspected and palpated to determine fundal height. The cervix is then examined to determine effacement, dilatation, and station. Effacement of the cervix refers to the process of thinning that occurs during labor. Effacement has conventionally been described in terms of a percentage of normal cervical length. This method often has been confusing and poorly reproduced between examiners. More recently, the preferred method is to describe the degree of effacement in terms of actual length of remaining cervix in centimeters. Cervical dilatation describes the diameter of the cervical os and is an indicator of the progression of labor. The index and middle finger of the examining hand are used to determine the diameter, expressed in centimeters (fingertip to 10 cm). Ten centimeters indicates full dilatation. The station indicates the level that the fetus occupies in the pelvis, with the reference point being the maternal ischial spines, palpable on either side of the vaginal canal at about the 4 and 8 o'clock positions. If the fetus remains above the ischial spines, the station is described as negative. Once the fetal head has reached the level of the ischial spines, the station is 0, with further descent into the pelvis described as +1 or +2. A +3 station corresponds to visible scalp at the introitus, indicating a fetal position consistent with impending delivery.

Both digital examination and Leopold maneuvers provide information about the presentation of the child and can indicate a potential breech presentation or cord prolapse. Care should be taken to ensure that the pregnant woman does not remain flat on her back for a prolonged period of time, because compression of venous return by the gravid uterus can lead to hypotension in the mother and decreased blood supply to the fetus. After examination, the patient should be placed in the left lateral position.

RUPTURE OF MEMBRANES

Determining if membranes have ruptured is an important predictor of the likelihood of imminent labor, as well the potential for complications such as infection or cord prolapse. SROM occurs during the course of active labor in most patients, although it may occur prior to the onset of labor in 10% of third-trimester patients. SROM typically occurs with a gush of clear or blood-tinged fluid. Rupture of membranes can be confirmed by using nitrazine paper to test residual fluid in the fornix or vaginal vault while performing a sterile speculum examination. Amniotic fluid has a pH of 7.0 to 7.4 and will turn nitrazine paper a dark blue. Vaginal fluid typically has a pH of 4.5 to 5.5, and the nitrazine strip will remain yellow. False-positive test results may occur with blood, lubricant, or other contaminants. Another test used to confirm rupture of the membranes (ROM) is ferning, or observing sodium chloride crystals on a slide as amniotic fluid dries.

If membranes are intact, an amniotomy should not be performed in the emergency department setting, because this may lead to precipitous labor and the potential for cord prolapse. It is also important to note the presence of meconium after the ROM, indicated by the presence of thick greenish brown fluid. ROM that occurs prior to the onset of labor is called premature ROM. Prolonged ROM occurs if delivery does not occur within 18 hours of the beginning of ROM.

EMERGENCY DELIVERY

The initial step in the management of a woman in active labor is to obtain vital signs and initiate supportive therapy, including obtaining venous access and monitoring the mother and fetus if fetal monitoring is available. If the pelvic examination reveals no remaining cervix and fetal presentation at the introitus, then delivery is imminent. It is important to recognize that patients, particularly multiparous patients, can progress very rapidly. The stage of labor and the parity of the patient should be taken into account when considering transport of a laboring patient to another facility.

As the cervix becomes fully dilated and effacement becomes complete, the fetus continues to descend and the patient experiences the urge to push. Patients delivering in the emergency setting may have difficulty controlling these expulsive efforts, and they are in even greater need of assistance, reassurance, and instruction. Preoccupation with the delivery should not exclude the needs of the mother, nor minimize the importance of maternal cooperation to accomplish a controlled delivery.

Determination of fetal position is best accomplished in the emergency setting by evaluation of the presenting portion of the infant. Pelvic examination should provide evidence of the infant's position, including palpable skull sutures and fontanelles or, in the case of breech delivery, the infant's buttock or extremity. Confirmation may be accomplished by personnel familiar with Leopold maneuvers. Leopold maneuvers are the palpation of the fetus through the maternal abdomen to determine fetus position and presentation. Such maneuvers are relatively unreliable in inexperienced hands.

The typical delivery position is the dorsal lithotomy position, which allows maximum visualization and control of the delivery. As time allows, the perineum may then be prepared by washing with mild soap and water, and swabbing with povidone iodine. Drapes should be placed over the patient, and gowns, masks, and gloves should be donned by medical personnel attending the patient. Obstetric support should be notified as indicated.

The process of fetal descent during labor and delivery is described by six cardinal movements: (1) engagement, (2) flexion, (3) descent, (4) internal rotation, (5) extension, and (6) external rotation (Fig. 13-1). As the fetus descends through the birth canal and reaches the introitus, the perineum bulges to accommodate the fetal head. Once the head extends to open the vaginal introitus to a diameter of approximately 5 cm, drape a towel over one gloved hand to protect it from the anus. Delivery can be aided by

1.

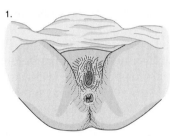

Mother should be encouraged to push.

2.

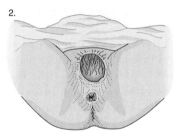

Gentle controlled pushing to prevent tearing. She should take short, fast breaths.

3.

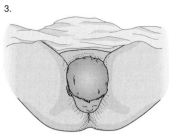

Suction infant nose and mouth.

4.

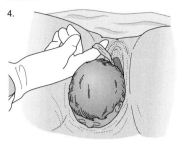

Check for cord around infant's neck.

5.

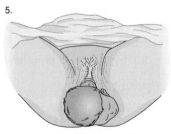

The infant's head turns to one side.

6.

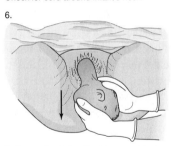

Delivery of anterior shoulder - encourage mother to push.

7.

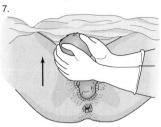

Delivery of posterior shoulder. The infant should now slide out easily. Keep a firm grip on the infant!

FIGURE 13-1 Vaginal delivery. (1) Encourage mother to push. (2) Gentle controlled pushing to prevent tearing. Mother should take short, fast breaths. (3) Suction infant nose and mouth. (4) Check for cord around infant's neck. (5) Infant's head turns toward side. (6) Delivery of anterior shoulder. Encourage mother to push. (7) Delivery of posterior shoulder. Infant should now slide out easily. Keep a firm grip on the infant.

gentle digital stretching of the inferior portion of the perineum. The perineum undergoes gradual thinning and stretching to enable the passage of the newborn.

Exert forward pressure on the chin of the fetus through the perineum just in front of the coccyx with one hand, while the other hand exerts pressure superiorly against the occiput. This allows for a more controlled delivery, with the base of the occiput rotating around the lower margin of the symphysis pubis as a fulcrum, while the face passes over the perineum. Wipe the face and aspirate the nares and mouth to minimize aspiration of amniotic fluid debris. Check for a nuchal cord by passing your fingers over the neck of the fetus. If a cord is present and loosely coiled around the neck, slip it over the head. If coiled too tightly, the cord should be cut between 2 clamps and the infant should be delivered promptly.

DELIVERING THE SHOULDERS

As the infant's head is delivered, it begins to rotate, so that the occiput turns toward one of the maternal thighs and the head assumes a transverse position. Most times, the shoulders then appear and are born spontaneously. If a delay occurs, grasp the head with two hands and apply gentle downward traction until the anterior shoulder appears under the pubic arch. Then deliver the posterior shoulder with a slight upward movement; the anterior shoulder usually drops down from beneath the symphysis. The rest of the body almost always follows easily. In the case of prolonged delay, apply gentle traction on the head and moderate pressure on the uterine fundus. Never pull on the head or twist or bend the infant's neck. Position the infant slightly head down while clearing the airway.

> **CRITICAL ACTION:**
>
> A point of practical concern is the need to maintain control of the newly born infant—do not drop the baby. The combination of amniotic fluid, blood, and white, cheesy desquamation called vernix makes for a very slippery infant.

It is useful to prepare for the delivery by placing the posterior (left) hand underneath the axilla of the infant prior to delivering the rest of the body. The anterior hand may then be used to grasp the ankles of the infant and ensure a firm grip. In obstetric training, students are often instructed to hold the infant close to their chest like a football.

The infant is then loosely wrapped in a towel and stimulated as it is dried. In the setting of an uncomplicated delivery, the mother may immediately hold the child while the cord is being cut, providing the child has responded well to initial stimulation and has a clear airway and good respiratory effort. The umbilical cord is double clamped and cut with sterile scissors, and the infant is further dried and warmed under an incubator, where postnatal care may be provided and Apgar scores calculated at 1 and 5 minutes after delivery. Scoring includes general color, tone, heart rate, respiratory effort, and reflexes.

In the case of suspected meconium aspiration, the infant is delivered, the cord is double clamped and cut immediately, and the infant is placed in an incubator for airway assessment and possible intubation prior to stimulating the child to breath spontaneously. Intubation allows for the trachea to be suctioned adequately prior to spontaneous breathing, thus reducing the risk of meconium aspiration. If a cyanotic or apneic child is delivered and does not respond immediately to stimulation, neonatal resuscitation is instituted.

CLAMPING THE CORD

Clamp the cord after thoroughly clearing the infant's airway, keeping the infant at or below the level of the introitus. Clamp the cord in two places, approximately 2 and 5 cm from the infant's abdomen. Cut the cord between the two clamps, and place the infant at the mother's breast. Sucking will stimulate contractions, aid in the delivery of the placenta, and help to control heavy bleeding.

DELIVERING THE PLACENTA

After delivery of the baby, the height of the uterine fundus and its consistency should be assessed. If the uterus is firm and there is no heavy bleeding, wait for the following signs of placental separation.

SIGNS OF PLACENTAL SEPARATION

- The uterus becomes globular and there is often a sudden gush of blood.
- The uterus rises in the abdomen.
- The umbilical cord protrudes farther out of the vagina.

Ask the mother to bear down to expel the placenta. Never pull on the cord to extract the placenta, which may result in inversion of the uterus. Examine the placenta, membranes, and cord carefully for completeness and anomalies.

The hour immediately following the delivery of the placenta is critical, for this is when hemorrhage, as a result of uterine relaxation, is most likely to occur. Frequently assess the uterus, and massage the fundus if it does not feel firm. Check the vagina and perineum every 5 to 10 minutes for evidence of excessive bleeding.

If heavy bleeding continues despite fundal massage, oxytocin agents may be helpful in achieving hemostasis. Oxytocin (Pitocin), ergonovine maleate (Ergotrate), and methylergonovine maleate (Methergine) are used to stimulate uterine contractions and reduce blood loss. These agents should be used cautiously, in most cases only after the placenta has been delivered. If given prior to placental delivery, they may cause entrapment and death of an undiagnosed (undelivered) twin. Table 13-3 describes the dosing regimen for these medications.

EPISIOTOMY

The use of routine episiotomy for a normal spontaneous vaginal delivery has been discouraged in recent years, and has been demonstrated to increase the incidence of third-

TABLE 13-3 MEDICATIONS FOR EMERGENCY DELIVERY AND INDICATIONS FOR USE

MEDICATION	DOSE	INDICATION
Oxytocin 10 U/mL	Infuse 2 L of 20 U/L 0.9 NS solution	Give routinely for uterine contraction and hemostasis immediately postpartum
Methyl ergonovine (Methergine)	0.2 mg IM	Control of postpartum hemorrhage
Hydralazine 20 mg/mL	5–10 mg IVP every 3–5 min to treat diastolic BP>110 mm Hg)	Control of hypertensive crisis (to diastolic BP 80–90 mm Hg)
Magnesium sulfate (50% solution: 5 g/10 mL)	Bolus 4–6 gr. IV over several minutes	First-line control of eclamptic seizures
Calcium gluconate 10%	1 ampule (10 mL) IVP	Magnesium toxicity
Phenytoin	10 mg/kg loading dose, followed by second loading dose of 5 mg/kg 2 h later	Second-line drug for eclamptic seizures
Terbutaline sulfate 1 mg/mL	0.25 SC every 3 h	Tocolysis
Fentanyl 50 µg/mL	50 µg/mL (1mL) every h	Short-acting narcotic analgesic
Lidocaine (Xylocaine) 1%	1–10 mL locally	Local anesthetic
Prochlorperazine (Compazine) 10 mg/2 mL	5–10 mg IV	Nausea and vomiting
Naloxone (Narcan) 0.4 mg/mL	0.8–2 mg IV	Narcotic overdose

and fourth-degree lacerations occurring at the time of delivery. If an episiotomy is necessary, it may be performed as follows (Fig. 13-2). Inject 5 to 10 mL of 1% lidocaine solution with a small-gauge needle into the posterior fourchette and perineum. As the head crowns, place the index and second fingers inside the introitus to expose the mucosa, posterior fourchette, and perineal body. Place scissors in the midline at the fourchette, and make a 3-cm incision either directly posteriorly (midline) or posterolaterally, at a 45 degree angle to the midline (mediolateral). Extend the incision up to 6 cm into the vaginal mucosa to ease delivery of the head. The incision must be supported with manual pressure from below, taking care not to allow the incision to extend into the rectum.

EPISIOTOMY REPAIR The episiotomy is most often repaired after the placenta has been delivered to allow undivided attention to the signs of placental separation. (Fig. 13-3). The surgical wound is repaired in layers, starting with the vaginal mucosa. Using 2-0 or 3-0 chromic catgut, place continuous sutures until the level of the hymenal ring is reached. Close the bulbocavernosus muscles at the midline, then pass the needle through the vaginal tissues to exit the perineal side of the episiotomy incision. Hold the

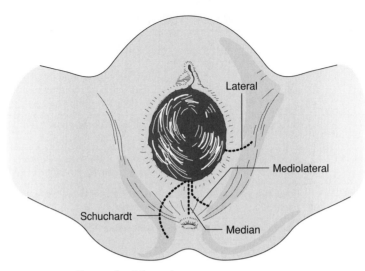

FIGURE 13-2 Types of episiotomies.

continuous suture at this point, and use interrupted sutures of 2-0 chromic catgut to approximate the muscles and fascia of the perineal body. Then return to the continuous suture and continue to close the subcutaneous layer of muscle and fascia. When the inferior margin of the incision has been reached, the suture is carried upward as a subcuticular suture to close the skin.

COMPLICATIONS OF DELIVERY

CORD PROLAPSE In the event that the bimanual examination reveals a palpable, pulsating cord, the examiner's hand should not be removed, but rather should be used to elevate the presenting fetal part to reduce compression on the cord. Immediate obstetric assistance is necessary, because a cesarean section is indicated. The examiner's hand should remain in the vagina while the patient is transported and prepared for surgery in order to prevent further compression of the cord by the fetal head. No attempt should ever be made to replace a prolapsed cord.

SHOULDER DYSTOCIA Shoulder dystocia is the impaction of fetal shoulders at the pelvic outlet after delivery of the head. Typically, the anterior shoulder is trapped behind the pubic symphysis, leading to delay of delivery of the rest of the infant. It usually occurs in the delivery of larger infants with disproportionately large shoulders compared with the fetal head. Although rare, shoulder dystocia should be a serious concern because of the risk of fetal morbidity and mortality if not managed promptly and appropriately. Complications of shoulder dystocia include brachial plexus injury from

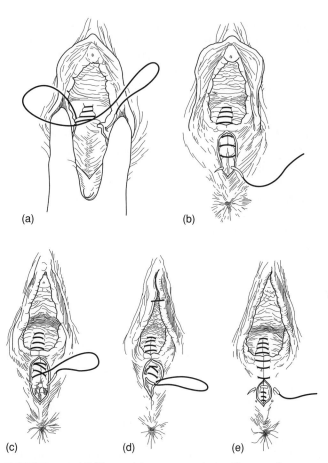

(a)   (b)

(c)   (d)   (e)

FIGURE 13-3 Midline episiotomy repair. A: Closure of mucosa and hymenal ring with continuous suture. B: Approximation of perineal musculature with interrupted sutures. C: Continuous suture to unite superficial fascia. D: Completion of repair by carrying continuous suture upward as a subcuticular stitch. E: Alternatively, closure of the superficial fascia and skin may be accomplished by a series of loosely tied interrupted sutures.

overly aggressive traction, fetal hypoxia from impaired respirations, compression of the umbilical cord, and compromised fetal circulation.

Shoulder dystocia is first recognized after the delivery of the fetal head, when routine downward traction is insufficient to deliver the anterior shoulder. After delivering the infant's head, it retracts tightly against the perineum (the turtle sign). After recognition of shoulder dystocia, the physician should suction the infant's nose and mouth and call for assistance to position the mother in the extreme lithotomy position, with legs sharply flexed up to the abdomen (the McRobert's maneuver), with the legs held by the mother or an assistant. The bladder should be drained if this has not already been done. A generous episiotomy may also facilitate delivery. Next, an assistant should apply suprapubic pressure to disimpact the anterior shoulder from the pubic symphysis. It is important to remember never to apply fundal pressure, which will further impact the shoulder on the pelvic rim.

To deliver the impacted anterior shoulder, a corkscrew maneuver (Woods maneuver) is the first manipulation attempted. The physician grasps the posterior scapula of the infant with two fingers and rotates the shoulder girdle 180 degrees in the pelvic outlet in an attempt to rotate the posterior shoulder into the anterior position and in the process deliver the shoulder. Gentle traction may then be applied as the patient pushes, and the infant is delivered through an oblique pelvic diameter. If the corkscrew maneuver fails to reduce the dystocia, the physician may then attempt to deliver the posterior shoulder. The examiner's hand is passed posteriorly in the vagina, and the infant's posterior arm is felt. The elbow is grasped and flexed, and the arm is delivered with the posterior shoulder, and the anterior shoulder usually follows.

BREECH PRESENTATION

Breech presentations occur in 3% to 4% of term pregnancies and are associated with a morbidity rate three to four times greater than that of cephalad presentations. Breech presentations most frequently occur in premature infants, because final rotation in the pelvis may not have occurred. The major concern in breech deliveries is head entrapment. In a normal cephalic delivery, the larger head dilates the cervical canal, thus ensuring that the rest of the infant follows. With breech deliveries, however, the head emerges last and may become trapped by an incompletely dilated cervix.

Emergency cesarean section is the procedure of choice for a breech presentation. If delivery is well underway and the buttocks are born, proceed with a vaginal delivery (Fig. 13-4). Place the mother in a bed in the lithotomy position, if possible. Breech presentations may be classified as frank, complete, incomplete, or footling. Frank and complete breech presentations serve as a dilating wedge nearly as well as the fetal head, and delivery may proceed in an uncomplicated fashion. The main point for the health worker to remember in a breech presentation is to keep hands away and let the delivery happen spontaneously. This allows the presenting portion of the fetus to maximally dilate the introitus prior to the presentation of the fetal head. It is recommended that the examiner literally refrain from touching the fetus until the scapula are visualized.

At this point the infant may be gently supported by wrapping a towel around the child's lower half. Gently rotate until one arm emerges, then rotate the opposite way to allow delivery of the other arm. Then, keeping the infant's head flexed, the physician should place the index and middle fingers over the infant's maxillary bones (not in the infant's mouth). This should allow the mother to expel the fetus. It is important not to pull on the fetus, which may impact the head in the pelvis or entrap the extended fetal arm. Footling and incomplete breech positions are not considered safe for vaginal delivery because of the possibility of cord prolapse or incomplete dilatation of the cervix.

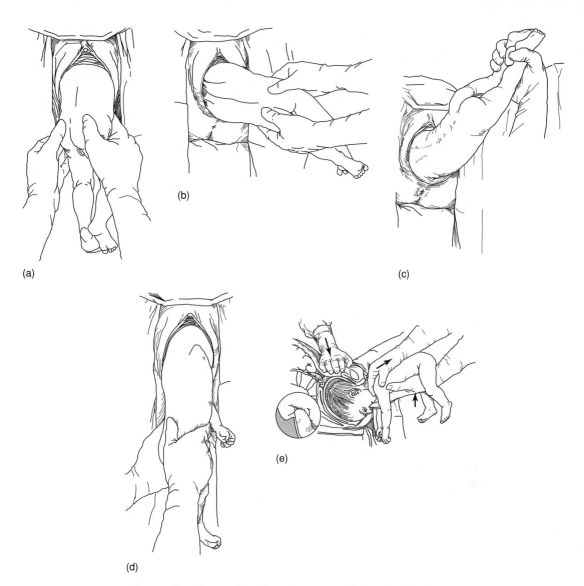

FIGURE 13-4 A: Hands are placed over the infant's sacrum to deliver the body. B: Rotation occurs as the scapulae emerge. C: Delivery of the posterior shoulder. D: Delivery of the anterior shoulder beneath the symphysis by traction. E: Delivery of the aftercoming head. While suprapubic pressure is applied by an assistant, the head is gently flexed by pressure on the mandible.

In any breech delivery, obstetric consultation should be obtained immediately. Support the infant's body until the head is delivered by flexion.

Always try to proceed to cesarean section for breech presentation, if possible. If a leg is showing at presentation, do not pull on it. Unless the infant has been delivered to the level of the umbilicus, there is time to prepare for cesarean section.

PRETERM DELIVERY

Preterm delivery is a major cause of precipitous childbirth and is often the cause of emergency delivery. Preterm infants also more often present in the breech position and are associated with greater incidence of infant morbidity and mortality. It is essential to carefully control the delivery to reduce the likelihood of trauma to the fragile preterm infant. Care must be taken to deliver the infant slowly and immediately dry and warm the infant while performing the initial assessment, because the premature infant is much more likely to require resuscitation. The decision whether to initiate resuscitative efforts in the emergency department is often difficult, because patients may deliver an extremely premature fetus of unknown gestational age. In general, even very premature infants (18–22 weeks) should receive initial resuscitative efforts until determination of viability is made.

MATERNAL COMPLICATIONS

Immediately after delivery of the infant, the umbilical cord is clamped and the placenta is delivered. The placenta should be allowed to separate spontaneously, assisted with gentle traction. Aggressive traction on the cord risks uterine inversion, tearing of the cord, or disruption of the placenta, which can result in severe vaginal bleeding.

After removal of the placenta, the uterus should be gently massaged to promote contraction. Oxytocin (20 U in 1 L of 0.9% normal saline at a moderate rate) is infused to maintain uterine contraction.

Uterine atony may follow a precipitous delivery and may lead to excessive vaginal bleeding. Additional oxytocin may be administered, as well as methyl ergonovine (Methergine) 0.2 mg (intramuscularly [IM] only) or prostaglandin $F_{2\alpha}$ (Hemabate) 0.25 mg IM. With significant postpartum hemorrhage, vigorous bimanual massage should be continued while administering contractile agents. Episiotomy or laceration repair may be delayed until an experienced obstetrician is able to close the laceration and inspect the patient for fourth-degree (rectovaginal) tears.

NORMAL POSTPARTUM CARE

Patients should be encouraged to breast-feed. A local health-care worker or midwife should be consulted to ensure support. Patients should report excessive bleeding and fevers over 38°C. Sexual activity may be resumed after puerperal bleeding has ceased. Provide patients with contraception for at least 1 year for child spacing. Ambulation should be encouraged, but return to full activity should be delayed for 6 weeks.

CESAREAN SECTION

Where surgical services and sterile conditions are available, cesarean section is a safe procedure, which is indicated in clinical situations posing a potential threat to mother or infant. These include abruptio placentae, placenta previa, fetal distress, footling or breech presentation, shoulder dystocia, and failure to progress. In underdeveloped countries or in the setting of limited resources, however, the risks for maternal and fetal morbidity and mortality are much higher. Proper equipment and instruments must be available to proceed with a surgical intervention, and the high risk of postoperative infectious complications due to unsanitary surroundings must be considered. In these settings, cesarean section is indicated only as a last effort to save a mother's life.

If possible, assemble a team of providers to be in attendance, including someone who is able to resuscitate the newborn infant. Rapidly prepare a sterile abdomen with available agents, and insert a catheter to decompress the bladder. These procedures are desired, but should not delay delivery when personnel and resources are limited.

There is some debate about the optimal procedure for cesarean section in suboptimal conditions. Most sources suggest a vertical skin incision, followed by a low transverse incision of the uterus.

Women in remote areas or developing countries may not be able to access medical care at the time of a future delivery, and a low transverse uterine incision will allow for a decreased risk of uterine rupture in subsequent pregnancies compared with a vertical uterine incision.

PROCEDURE FOR ABDOMINAL INCISION

A vertical incision of the abdomen is suggested because it can be performed rapidly and with minimal assistance. The risk of incisional hematoma is less than that with other procedures, and the vertical incision can be easily extended to allow access to the upper abdomen if necessary.

Perform a vertical incision from the level of the uterine fundus to the symphysis pubis, through the abdominal wall to the peritoneal cavity. Assess the uterus to determine the optimal location and direction of the incision. If the lower uterine segment appears wide enough to allow delivery of the fetus, a low transverse incision should be performed. This incision heals more strongly than a vertical uterine incision, decreasing the risk of uterine rupture in subsequent pregnancies.

Perform a lower uterine transverse incision with a scalpel, until amniotic fluid is obtained or until the uterine cavity is clearly entered (Fig. 13-5). Being very careful to avoid injury to the fetus, enlarge the incision with scissors to allow adequate room for delivery of the head (Fig. 13-6). Elevate the fetal head from the pelvis and maintain it in a flexed position, and ask an assistant to apply gentle fundal pressure to assist in delivery of the head. Grasp the head and deliver the shoulders one at a time. The rest of the infant's body usually follows easily. Aspirate the infant's nares and mouth with a bulb syringe, clamp the cord, and hand the infant to an assistant.

Remove the placenta manually, running a hand between the uterus and placenta along the cleavage plane. Alternatively, massage the fundus and apply gentle traction on the umbilical cord until the uterus is extracted. Fundal massage and oxytocin are usually adequate to control bleeding.

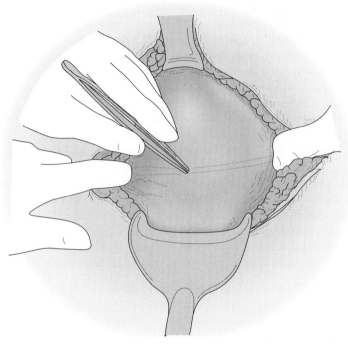

FIGURE 13-5 Uterine incision for cesarean section. The peritoneal flexion is identified on the lower uterine segment before creation of the bladder flap.

Close the uterine incision first (Fig. 13-7). It is easiest to exteriorize the uterus for repair. Use ring clamps along the edges of the uterine incision to contain bleeding. Carefully examine the internal uterine walls for retained placenta. Examine the entire uterine incision to identify any extensions of the incision, as well as possible involvement of adjacent structures. Use absorbable suture (e.g., no. 1 chromic gut, O Vicryl). First repair any extensions of the incision, sewing toward the initial incision in a running lock stitch. Make each stitch approximately 1 cm from the incision edge, and make 1 cm of progress with each stitch. Try to avoid incorporating the endometrial layer into the suture. Carry the suture line slightly beyond the lateral edge of the incision, taking care to avoid the broad ligament. If complete hemostasis is achieved with the initial layer of suture, no further uterine suturing needs to be performed. If hemostasis is not achieved, place a second layer between the first by placing vertical stitches 1 cm above and 1 cm below the incision, rolling the original suture line. Return the uterus to the abdominal cavity by elevating the abdominal wall, and turning the uterus to the right slightly, and put gentle pressure on the fundus. Remove clots from the abdominal cavity before the abdominal wall is closed. Next look at the drainage from the catheter. If the urine is grossly bloody, check the bladder for damage. If an obvious injury is not seen, sterile formula from the nursery can be irrigated into the bladder via the catheter and a careful search conducted for disruptions in the bladder wall. Repair is performed with double-layer closure with absorbable suture.

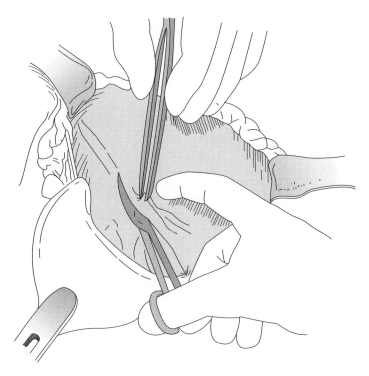

FIGURE 13-6 Enlargement of the uterine incision. The uterine incision is enlarged with scissors.

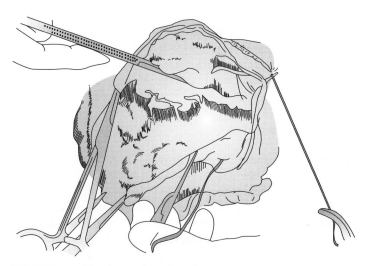

FIGURE 13-7 First layer of uterine closure.

461

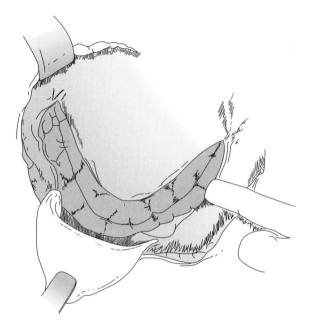

FIGURE 13-8 First layer of uterine closure completed.

Next close the abdominal wall (Fig. 13-8). Check the rectus muscle for bleeding and cauterize or suture ligate to prevent hematoma formation. Approximate the facial borders with a running absorbable suture. Begin the suture at the lateral margins and continue toward the midline. Use care to incorporate the edge and both layers of fascia in the initial sutures. This helps prevent hernia formation. Use 1-cm nonlocking stitches. Overly tight stitches can cause tissue necrosis. Check the subcutaneous tissue for bleeders and cauterize or suture ligate these. Close the skin with a subcuticular stitch of 4-0 nonabsorbable suture and skin adhesive strips (Steri-Strips) (Fig. 13-9). Wash the preparation solution from the patient and apply a sterile bandage. Express clots from the uterine cavity with a bimanual examination.

POSTOPERATIVE CARE

Make certain to provide relief for postoperative pain. Provide intravenous (IV) fluid at 125 to 175 mL/h until the patient can tolerate oral fluids, usually after about 24 hours. Replace blood loss with 3 mL of crystalloid for every 1 mL of blood loss. Transfuse blood if the mother is tachycardic or has orthostatic symptoms or difficulty with ambulation. Encourage ambulation within 12 to 24 hours of the procedure. Remove the catheter as soon as the patient can walk. Prophylactic antibiotics decrease but do not eliminate infection. Postoperative temperature elevation to 38.5°C or more, a tender fundus, and the absence of other localizing symptoms (such as engorgement) suggest endometritis.

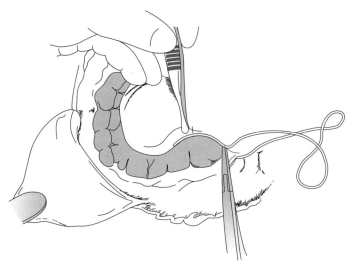

FIGURE 13-9 Second layer of uterine closure.

An elevated white blood cell count is not helpful—a count as high 35,000 may be normal postpartum. If the diagnosis of endometritis is made, use broad-spectrum antibiotics to treat a mixed aerobic-anaerobic infection. Ampicillin plus sulbactam, second-generation cephalosporins, or gentamicin plus clindamycin are some options. Good wound care is important.

Breast-feeding is encouraged. Before the patient leaves the hospital review the events leading to the cesarean delivery and set guidelines for future deliveries. Most patients will be able to perform routine baby care despite undergoing major abdominal surgery. The mother should avoid heavy lifting for 6 weeks.

THIRD TRIMESTER BLEEDING

> **KEY POINT:**
>
> Bleeding late in pregnancy (after 24–28 weeks' gestation) may be a sign of grave risk to the fetus and mother and should always be treated as an emergency. Profound shock can occur in minutes secondary to massive loss of blood.

The most common causes of late-pregnancy bleeding are placenta previa (20%) and abruptio placentae (30%), both of which are associated with significant increase in maternal morbidity and mortality, even in developed countries. Other causes include uterine rupture, cervical or vaginal infection or inflammation, bloody show (associated with release of mucous plug by the cervix just prior to the onset of labor), and polyps or other lesions of the reproductive tract. Many times the cause is not clear but may be

TABLE 13-4 DIFFERENTIATING ETIOLOGY OF THIRD TRIMESTER VAGINAL BLEEDING

EXAMINATION	PLACENTA PREVIA	PLACENTAL ABRUPTION	BLOODY SHOW
Vaginal discharge	Moderate to large amount of bright red blood	Varying amounts of dark clotted blood	Small amounts of blood or pink blood-tinged fluid
Abdominal examination	Nontender	Marked tenderness constant, nonremitting uterine pain	Nontender intermittent pain
Bimanual examination	Contraindicated	Contraindicated	Sterile examination
Laboratory tests	Possible decreased hematocrit	Coagulopathy, DIC picture	Normal
Confirmatory test	Ultrasonography	No accurate confirmatory test (ultrasonography <10% sensitive)	None
Fetal status	Generally normal	Fetal distress (HR<100)	Normal

related to small marginal separations of the placenta. See Table 13-4 to differentiate the etiology of third-trimester bleeding.

PLACENTA PREVIA

Placenta previa is defined as placement of the placenta over, or in close proximity to, the cervical os. The characteristic clinical presentation is that of painless, bright red vaginal bleeding. The bleeding is most often minor and intermittent initially, but it persists throughout the third trimester and becomes progressively severe. If a digital vaginal examination is performed, the placenta may become dislodged and cause massive, life-threatening hemorrhage. For this reason, do not insert a finger or object into the vagina if there is bleeding after 20 weeks' gestation.

Ultrasonography is the imaging modality of choice, but this may not be available in remote areas or developing countries. If placenta previa is suspected based on clinical presentation and risk factors (Table 13-5), the mother should be taken to an operating room

TABLE 13-5 RISK FACTORS FOR PLACENTA PREVIA

Prior cesarean section
Multiparity
Previous placenta previa
Multiple gestations
Multiple induced abortions

for vaginal evaluation, where it is possible to proceed emergently to cesarean section if necessary. Establish large-bore IV access, and draw blood for type and cross-matching and clotting studies, if these can be performed. Begin cardiac and fetal monitoring if possible. If the mother begins to bleed rapidly or blood pressure falls below 100 mm Hg systolic, emergency cesarean section must be considered. In a woman who is hemodynamically stable with scant vaginal bleeding, a careful perineal examination is indicated, followed by cautious examination of the vagina to identify other sources of bleeding.

ABRUPTIO PLACENTAE

Abruptio placentae is defined as premature separation of a normally implanted placenta from the uterine wall, causing obvious or "hidden" bleeding. Most often only a portion (<25%) of the placenta separates from the uterine wall, but in approximately 10% of cases the separation is severe (>50%), and fetal distress or death can result. The clinical presentation is that of painful uterine bleeding, characterized by dark or clotted blood and uterine tenderness. Hypertonic uterine contractions may be present, and signs of maternal shock may exceed the degree of visible vaginal bleeding. Fetal heart tones may be decreased or absent, depending on the degree of fetal distress. Table 13-6 lists the risk factors for abruptio placentae.

Diagnosis is made by clinical presentation; ultrasonography (if available) is used to exclude other causes of bleeding. Emergency management includes IV access to allow for rapid fluid resuscitation and blood replacement. Blood should be obtained for type and cross-match and a clotting profile if laboratory services are available. Fetal heart rate and maternal blood volume should be continually assessed. Immediate delivery by cesarean section is indicated for maternal hypotension, and RhoGAM should be considered.

UTERINE RUPTURE

Uterine rupture is an unpredictable event that occurs in late pregnancy. Vaginal bleeding may or may not be present, and in some cases there may be no maternal pain to suggest the diagnosis. The severity of the rupture ranges from minor dehiscence of a previous surgical scar to complete extrusion of the fetus. Significant fetal mortality is associated with moderate to severe uterine rupture, but maternal death is much less common. The primary problem is that of hemorrhage, which should be managed with fluid resuscitation and emergency surgical intervention.

TABLE 13-6 RISK FACTORS FOR
ABRUPTIO PLACENTAE

Maternal hypertension
Smoking
Increased maternal age
Greater than five previous deliveries
Trauma or blunt forces to the abdomen

PREECLAMPSIA AND ECLAMPSIA

PREECLAMPSIA

Preeclampsia is defined as the development of hypertension with proteinuria, edema, or both induced by pregnancy. This entity typically occurs in the second half of gestation (Table 13-7). It is more common in primagravidas (women with their first pregnancy) beyond 20 weeks' gestation and at the extremes of reproductive age. Preeclampsia is described as severe if the systolic blood pressure is greater than 160 mm Hg and the diastolic blood pressure is greater than 110 mm Hg. Other criteria include marked proteinuria (typically >1 g found in urine collected over 24 hours or 2+ on dipstick evaluation), decreased urine output, or evidence of cerebral compromise. The neurologic symptoms associated with severe preeclampsia include, but are not limited to, severe headache, occurrence of scotomata (spots in front of the eyes), and other visual disturbances. Other entities associated with severe preeclampsia include pulmonary edema, epigastric or right upper quadrant pain (due to subcapsular hepatic hemorrhage), liver dysfunction, and thrombocytopenia. See Table 13-8 for pharmacologic agents for antihypertensive therapy in preeclampsia.

> A good rule is to assume that the hypertensive pregnant patient is preeclamptic and to manage her accordingly.

ECLAMPSIA

Eclampsia is a condition in which a pregnant or recently pregnant patient develops convulsions (seizures or fits) that are not caused by a preexisting neurologic problem, and also meets the criteria for preeclampsia. This occurs in 0.5% to 4% of all deliveries. Approximately 25% of the time, eclampsia occurs during the first 72 hours postpartum. Women with preexisting hypertension are at greatest risk for these conditions. In 25% of these women, superimposed preeclampsia or eclampsia is found. The diagnosis of these entities in these women can be difficult, especially if the patient presents late in the course of her pregnancy and baseline blood pressures are not available for comparison.

TABLE 13-7 PREECLAMPSIA

Systolic blood pressure >160 mm Hg
Diastolic blood pressure >110 mm Hg
Edema
Proteinuria
Decreased urine output
Mental status changes
Epigastric pain
Right upper quadrant abdominal pain
Headache
Liver dysfunction
Thrombocytopenia

TABLE 13-8 PHARMACOLOGIC AGENTS FOR ANTIHYPERTENSIVE THERAPY
IN PREECLAMPSIA AND ECLAMPSIA

Magnesium sulfate	4 g IV over 20–30 min or may give IM; followed by a 1 to 3-g/h IV infusion or 1–4 g IM every 4 h	Follow reflexes, respiratory rate, and urine output. Give 1 g 10% calcium gluconate if hypo-reflexive or respiratory depression. Magnesium sulfate is contraindicated if renal disease is present.
Hydralazine hydrocholoride	2.5 mg IV, then 5–10 mg IV for 20 min up to 40 mg total dose; IV infusion 5–10 mg/h titrated; IM 10–25 mg every 4 h	Must wait 20 min for response between IV doses
Labetalol	20 mg IV, then 40–80 mg IV for 10 min to 300 mg total dose; IV infusion 1–2 mg/min titrated	Less reflex tachycardia and hypotension than with hydralazine
Sodium nitroprusside	0.25 μg/kg/min infusion, increase 0.25 μg/kg/min every 5 min	Potential cyanide toxicity; must protect from light.

Eclamptic seizures can be life threatening to both the mother and the fetus. The mother may succumb to musculoskeletal injury, hypoxia, and aspiration (the entry of stomach contents into the airways and lungs). She should be placed in a padded bed, restrained gently, started on oxygen, and given an IV. Fortunately, these seizures are usually self-limited. Treatment consists of magnesium sulfate therapy as previously described to prevent further seizures (Table 13-8). Fetal heart rate changes are common following and during maternal seizures. Bradycardia, tachycardia, and late decelerations may all occur. These can all be tolerated unless they occur for greater than 20 minutes, in which case fetal distress should be assumed and treated accordingly.

PREGNANCY-INDUCED HYPERTENSION

Hypertension in pregnancy is typically defined as a diastolic blood pressure greater than 90 mm Hg or a systolic blood pressure greater than 140 mm Hg. It also can be diagnosed by an increase in diastolic blood pressure of greater than 15 mm Hg from baseline or a similar increase of greater than 30 mm Hg in systolic blood pressure. These measurements should be confirmed by two separate readings at least 6 hours apart. The patient's blood pressure is lowest when she is lying down in the lateral decubitus position (lying on the left side), and at its highest when she is standing. Care also must be taken when choosing the size of the blood pressure cuff to be used because cuffs that are too small for the patient can give rise to falsely elevated readings.

Pregnancy-induced hypertension occurs in 5% to 10% of all pregnancies that proceed beyond the first trimester (Table 13-9). There is a 30% occurrence rate in women

TABLE 13-9 RISK FACTOR FOR DEVELOPMENT OF HYPERTENSION DURING PREGNANCY

Nulliparity
Age > 40 years
Prepregnancy hypertension
Chronic renal disease
African heritage
Diabetes mellitus
Multiple gestation

carrying multiple gestations regardless of how many pregnancies they have had in the past. Although the morbidity related to hypertension can be substantial and is directly correlated with the severity of blood pressure elevation, mortality is rare. Perinatal mortality, however, increases with each 5-mm increase in the mother's mean arterial blood pressure. This is due to a phenomenon known as uteroplacental insufficiency, which basically means that the fetus is deprived of the vital substances it needs to survive due to the physiologic changes seen in pregnancy-induced hypertension. Another severe complication, which can also severely compromise the fetus, is placental abruption, or abruptio placentae. This is the actual premature separation of the placenta from the wall of the uterus, which can lead to severe maternal hemorrhage and fetal compromise.

The evaluation of hypertension in pregnancy is multifactorial. The clinical history is of great value and should illicit any complaints of visual changes, severe or persistent headache, right upper quadrant abdominal pain, and any change in the level of consciousness or occurrence of seizures (Table 13-10). The physical examination should include checking vital signs and recording the patient's weight. Excessive or rapid weight gain also can be a signal to consider preeclampsia. Peripheral edema is common in pregnancy, but if it is persistent or does not resolve with lying down or propping the feet up, then it may be pathologic. Also, edema of the upper extremities and of the face is not common in normal pregnancies. Tenderness over the liver can imply a subcapsular hematoma. The funduscopic examination, when the examiner looks at the back of the patient's eyes by using an ophthalmoscope, may show vasoconstriction of the retinal blood vessels. The examiner should also check patellar (knee) and Achilles (back of the ankle) reflexes because hyperreflexia (brisker than normal reflexes) can be found in preeclampsia.

Laboratory tests can be very helpful in making the diagnosis of preeclampsia. One valuable maternal test is a complete blood count. An increasing hematocrit can imply a decreased amount of intravascular volume, which means that fluid is being shunted from blood vessels out into the tissue spaces. The platelet count also should be noted, because a low count signifies the occurrence of a coagulopathy, or dysfunction of the liver or the basic clotting mechanism. If available, the prothrombin time (PT) and the partial thromboplastin time (PTT) can be used to identify failure of the clotting mechanism as well. Liver function tests can be used to identify hepatic dysfunction, and

TABLE 13-10 DIAGNOSIS OF HYPERTENSION
IN PREGNANCY

History
    Visual changes—blurred vision
    Severe or persistent headache
    Right upper quadrant abdominal or epigastric pain
    Mental status changes
    Seizures
Physical examination
    Excessive or rapid weight gain
    Peripheral edema—persistent and not positional
    Edema of the upper extremities and face
    Tenderness over the liver
    Vasoconstriction of the retinal blood vessels
    Hyperreflexia
Diagnostic tests
    Increasing hematocrit
    Low platelet count
    Abnormal blood clotting tests
    Elevated liver function tests
    Elevated creatine
    Elevated urine protein (2+)
    Fetal bradycardia or tachycardia
    Intrauterine growth retardation
    Oligohydramnios
    Decreased fetal movement

creatinine can be obtained to evaluate kidney function. Analysis of maternal urine is a valuable test because significant urine protein (2+) can diagnose preeclampsia. Fetal testing can be performed through use of a Doppler machine to detect fetal heart tones. Heart rates that are too rapid or too slow can signify fetal distress. An ultrasonography machine can be used to look for intrauterine growth retardation, lower than normal amniotic fluid (oligohydramnios), and decreased fetal movement.

The management of preeclampsia must be a balanced one, considering the needs of both the mother and the fetus (Table 13-11). Maternal blood pressure must be closely monitored, and she should be observed for the physical sequelae of hypertension. The caretaker should intervene when the risks to the mother caused by her condition outweigh the risk to the fetus caused by the intervention. Intervention should also be undertaken when the risk to the fetus is greater in utero than it would be once delivery

TABLE 13-11 TREATMENT OF PREECLAMPSIA

Bedrest in left lateral decubitus position
Monitoring of maternal and fetal vital signs
Monitor maternal reflexes and mental status
Pharmacologic agents

is completed. The basic considerations to be evaluated are the severity of the preeclampsia and the maturity of the fetus. If preeclampsia is mild and the fetus is still immature, then strict bedrest in the lateral decubitus position, which maximizes fetal blood flow, should be prescribed for the mother. In most cases, this action will normalize maternal blood pressure. Bedrest can be observed at home rather than in the hospital if daily weighing, blood pressure checks, and fetal movement counts can be performed. The mother should also have ready access to medical care and be given a detailed set of criteria of when to come to the hospital or health center (i.e., significant increase in blood pressure, unusual weight gain, decreased fetal kick counts, severe headache, etc.). Hospitalization should be considered if the patient lacks transportation, is not motivated toward self-care, or if her blood pressure does not normalize with the above measures.

Worsening or severe preeclampsia or eclampsia must undergo medical treatment. This includes stabilizing the patient with magnesium sulfate, administering antihypertensive therapy, monitoring maternal and fetal vital signs, and delivering the child when indicated. Magnesium sulfate is used to prevent the convulsions, which define eclampsia. This medication has virtually no affect on maternal blood pressure. It can be administered either by IV or IM routes. The dose consists of a 4-g IV load over 20 to 30 minutes or the same amount IM. This is followed by a 1- to 3-g per hour IV infusion or 1 to 4 g IM every 4 hours. This will prevent convulsions in 90% of cases. Therapeutic blood levels of magnesium sulfate range from 4 to 7 μg/L, and there are predictable toxic consequences associated with higher levels. Because magnesium sulfate is a potent relaxant of smooth muscle, it can affect the patient's reflexes and respiration. The mother's patellar reflex should be checked at least every 2 hours while on the medication in order to determine whether she is becoming "magnesium toxic." If her reflexes are absent, her respirations become shallow, or her urine output decreases to less than 25 mL/h, then the magnesium should be reversed by a slow infusion of 1 g of 10% calcium gluconate. The patient should also be started on oxygen and her vital signs should be closely monitored and assisted if necessary. Antihypertensive therapy should be initiated if the diastolic blood pressure is greater than 110 mm Hg. The initial drug of choice is hydralazine. It should be administered in 5-mg doses, either IM or IV, and can be repeated every 20 to 30 minutes as needed. The goal is to reduce the diastolic blood pressure to 90 to 100 mm Hg. At levels lower than that, there exists the potential for decreased fetal blood flow. Several other antihypertensives also can be used (Table 13-8).

If the above listed measures are not successful and the mother is at significant risk for morbidity and mortality, then delivery of the fetus, either by induction or cesarean section, should be undertaken. There should be careful monitoring of blood loss because the preeclamptic mother already has a reduced blood volume. Close observation for 24 hours after delivery is also warranted because the risk for seizures persists for some time postpartum. In general, 25% of seizures occur before labor, 50% during labor, and 25% postpartum.

Finally, there exists an entity known as HELLP syndrome: *h*emolysis (destruction of red blood cells), *l*iver disease, and *l*ow *p*latelets. This occurs in 4% to 12% of severely preeclamptic patients. It is most often seen in multiparous, older, and less hypertensive patients. One should consider HELLP if the patient has right upper quadrant pain, signifying potential liver damage. The patient often has vague complaints of nausea, vomiting, and muscle aches. The patient with HELLP can be diagnosed by blood tests for liver dysfunction, decreased red blood cells, and a decreased platelet count. She should be transferred to a medical center equipped to handle high-risk patients. There she should undergo cardiovascular stabilization, correction of her clotting disorder, and expedient delivery. Of note, the patient should not receive pudendal or epidural anesthesia due to her existing bleeding disorder. She should also be transfused with platelets if her count is less than 20,000 or if it is less than 50,000 and she is to undergo cesarean delivery.

POSTPARTUM COMPLICATIONS

The postpartum period, or puerperium, is generally considered to be the 6 weeks after birth. This is the time frame during which the female reproductive tract returns to its normal state. This section will begin by briefly discussing the changes that take place and then will focus on potential complications of the puerperium and their management.

NORMAL POSTPARTUM CHANGES

The first process that occurs is the involution of the uterus. This begins immediately after delivery. Once the child and placenta have been delivered, the uterus is palpable halfway between the umbilicus, or navel, and the pubic bone. The smooth muscle cells of uterine arteries and arterioles also contract. This step is vital to controlling blood loss. Further involution occurs as cells, which compose the uterus, undergo a process known as autolysis, and shrink back to their prepregnant size. The uterus returns into the pelvis by 2 weeks and to its nonpregnant size in 6 weeks. Lochia is the discharge secreted after delivery has occurred. It consists of blood, debris, and the necrotic remains of membranes. The first 2 to 3 days postpartum it is known as lochia rubra, because blood makes up a significant component. As the amount of blood decreases, the discharge becomes browner and is called lochia serosa. The amount secreted is fairly heavy at first and then rapidly decreases over 2 to 3 days. It may continue for up to several weeks. By the end of the third week postpartum, the endometrium is reestablished in most women.

The cervix reforms several hours after delivery. By the end of the first week, it is closed to the extent that only one finger may be inserted. Its once round shape is permanently replaced by a transverse external os. The vulvar and vaginal tissues return to their normal state over the first several days.

Ovulation can occur as early as 4 to 5 weeks postpartum in non–breast-feeding women. The mean time to ovulation is approximately 10 weeks. Among breast-feeding women, the time varies according to how long they continue to lactate. This is because high levels of prolactin, the hormone that induces milk production, suppress ovulation. Estrogen levels decrease immediately after delivery and begin to increase 2 weeks afterward in nonlactating women.

HEMORRHAGE

The most common and potentially serious complication postpartum is hemorrhage, or blood loss. It can be sudden and profuse or slow and steady. Most women lose up to 500 mL of blood at the time of delivery. An amount greater then 500 mL is considered to be a significant hemorrhage.

UTERINE ATONY

The major cause of hemorrhage is uterine atony. This is when the uterus does not contract properly postpartum. Normally, the body of the uterus contracts promptly after delivery of the placenta. This process constricts arteries and prevents excessive bleeding. One predisposing factor to uterine atony is extraordinary enlargement of the uterus. This can occur with twin gestations or excessive production of amniotic fluid. Also, abnormal labor, such as a prolonged course or augmentation with oxytocin, can lead to hemorrhage. The existence of leiomyomas or other such intrauterine masses can interfere with mechanical contraction, thereby causing excessive bleeding. The diagnosis of uterine atony is a clinical one. When palpated, the uterus will have a "boggy" feel instead of a firm one. The cervix will be open as well. Bleeding will be massive or unrelenting and there may be a paucity of blood clots.

MANAGEMENT OF UTERINE ATONY

The management of uterine atony follows three courses of therapy: manipulative, medical, and surgical (Table 13-12). Once the diagnosis is made, the first step is to initiate

TABLE 13-12 MANAGEMENT OF UTERINE ATONY WITH RESULTANT HEMORRHAGE

Manipulative
  Massage
Medical
  2 large bore IVs
  Crystalloid IV fluids
  Oxytocin 20 U in 1 L of normal saline or lactated Ringer's,
    150 mL/h after delivery of placenta
  Type and cross for blood
  Transfuse (can use O-negative blood if cross-matched blood is
    unavailable)
  Methergine or methylergovine maleate IM 0.2–0.4 mg
    or 0.2 mg IV
  Prostaglandin $F_{2\alpha}$ IM or directly into the myometrium
Surgical
  Ligation of the uterine and/or hypogastric arteries or hysterectomy
    if bleeding continues (last resort)

uterine massage. This is done by making a fist and firmly pressing on the uterus in a circular fashion. It will likely be uncomfortable to the mother but should be continued nonetheless.

For external uterine massage

- Massage the abdomen until the uterus feels firm.
- Lift the uterus with one hand and massage its distal portion.
- Stop the massage when the uterus feels firm and the bleeding ceases.
- This procedure may have to be repeated several times.

Massage alone is often successful in causing uterine contraction and should be performed immediately while other measures are being undertaken.

When external massage is unsuccessful, use internal massage:

- Use sterile technique.
- Place a hand into the vagina inferior to the uterus.
- Make a fist and lift the uterus upward.
- With the other hand, grab the uterus through the abdominal wall.
- Massage the uterus and maintain pressure until bleeding stops.

Two large-bore, functioning IVs and typed and cross-matched blood, where available rapidly, should be attained. One can also use O-negative blood as well. If manipulation is unsuccessful, then medical management should be undertaken. It is normal practice to infuse oxytocin (20 U in 1 L of normal saline or lactated Ringer's solution run at 125–165 mL/h) once the placenta has been delivered. This promotes uterine contraction. This infusion can be continued once hemorrhage is diagnosed, but oxytocin should not be given as a bolus because it can significantly decrease blood pressure. Methergine, or methylergonovine maleate, is a potent constrictor and can cause uterine contractions within minutes. It can be given either IV or IM. Caution should be taken because it can cause high blood pressure. Prostaglandin also can be used to attempt uterine contraction. Prostaglandin $F2_\alpha$ can be given IM or directly into the myometrium, and prostaglandin E_2 can be delivered through vaginal suppositories. If these measures are all unsuccessful and life-threatening hemorrhage ensues, then surgical measures must be considered. This includes ligation, or tying off, of the uterine or hypogastric arteries and, ultimately, hysterectomy if bleeding continues.

LACERATIONS OF THE LOWER GENITAL TRACT

Another cause of postpartum hemorrhage is laceration of the lower genital tract. Predisposing factors include forceps delivery, manipulative delivery (i.e., a breech extraction), rapid delivery of the infant, or a large infant. Minor lacerations of the cervix and vagina are common, but if they are greater than 2 cm long or are actively bleeding, then repair is required. The genital tract should always be inspected after delivery and assistance is commonly required for good visualization. Repair is accomplished by placing interlocking, hemostatic sutures with resorbable material. Great care should be taken if the laceration is near the urethra. In this situation, it is often helpful to place a Foley catheter in the urethra to prevent accidental urethral injury. Always visualize the genital tract to look for lacerations and hematomas. Surgical consultation may be required.

RETENTION OF THE PLACENTA OR PARTS OF THE PLACENTA

Retention of the placenta or of parts of the placenta can also cause excessive maternal blood loss. See Table 13-13 for risk factors. Normally, the placenta cleaves off of the wall of the uterus in a single plane. It is then expelled by a series of strong contractions. A placenta is considered to be retained when this process is incomplete. Factors leading to this include previous cesarean section, uterine leiomyomas (fibroids), prior curettage, or accessory placental lobes. After delivery, it is important not to apply too much traction on the umbilical cord to prevent placental retention. A retained placenta can prevent adequate uterine contractions, thereby causing excessive bleeding (Fig. 13-10).

- Maternal analgesia and education is necessary.
- Use sterile technique.
- Follow the cord up into the vagina, maintaining the hand in a cone shape.
- Give oxytocin after the hand is in the uterus.
- Feel for the edge of the placenta.
- Pry the edge of the placenta away from the uterine wall by working fingers between these structures.
- Bring the placenta out into the palm of the hand.
- Perform external uterine massage.
- Give 1 g of cefazolin IM or IV.

After expulsion, care should be taken to inspect the placenta for missing cotyledons (sections). If retained tissue is suspected, two fingers can be inserted into the uterus through the cervical os and tissue can be manipulated out.

- Maternal analgesia and education is necessary.
- Use sterile technique.
- Fold a piece of strong sterile gauze with a tail over the fingers.
- Manually remove identified retained parts.
- Give 1 g of cefazolin IM or IV.

TABLE 13-13 RISK FACTORS FOR RETAINED PLACENTA

Previous cesarean section
Uterine leiomyomas (fibroids)
Prior curettage
Accessory placental lobes

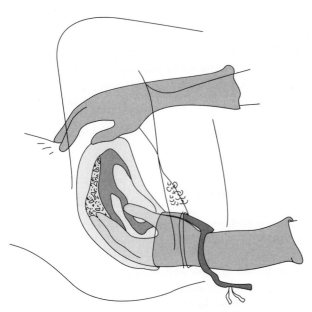

FIGURE 13-10 Manual removal of retained placenta. Use sterile technique. A: Follow the cord up into the vagina, maintaining the hand in a cone shape. Give oxytocin after the hand is in the uterus. B: Feel for the edge of the placenta and pry it away from the uterine wall by working the fingers between the placenta and the uterine wall. C: Bring the placenta out into the palm of the hand. Perform external uterine massage. Give 1 g cefazolin IM or IV.

An ultrasonography machine, if available, can be used to aid in diagnosis. A contracted uterus displays a stripe on ultrasonography. If this is absent, it could imply placental tissue or blood clots in the uterine cavity. If manual efforts to remove tissue are unsuccessful, curettage can be performed, with care taken not to perforate the uterus. In rare circumstances, a phenomenon known as placenta accreta can occur. This occurs when the placental villi penetrate the uterine lining, muscle, or through its entirety, and adhere. Because the placenta is "stuck," the uterus cannot contract, and life-threatening hemorrhage can occur. Hysterectomy is often required for placenta accreta.

HEMATOMAS

Hematomas can cause postpartum hemorrhage. These occur when a collection of blood develops between tissue planes. Hematomas can occur anywhere along the genital tract. They are commonly caused by birth trauma and are found on the lower aspect of the genital tract. The less accessible the hematomas are (i.e., the higher along in the tract), the greater the morbidity associated with them is. Hematomas are diagnosed by palpation, demonstrating exquisite pain and perhaps a mass at a particular site. There also may be changes in the mother's vital signs, which indicate significant blood loss. If hematomas are greater then 5 cm in size or if they are expanding, they should be managed surgically. This is accomplished by draining the hematoma at its most dependent aspect (i.e., at the point where it will drain the most effectively). The patient should be supported by closely following her vital signs and giving pain medication as needed. Ice packs also can be applied for pain control and to decrease bleeding into the site. If the bleeding occurs at the site of an episiotomy, then the sutures should be released and the bleeding vessel should be ligated.

COAGULATION OR BLOOD-CLOTTING DEFECTS

The mother may have a preexisting coagulation, or blood clotting defect. This can be diagnosed by laboratory testing (i.e., PT and PTT). Blood also should be sent for typing and screening. A baseline hematocrit is also helpful because it can help to quantify the degree of maternal blood loss. Finally, the patient's vital signs should be checked often during both delivery and the several hours following childbirth because an increasing pulse rate or decreasing blood pressure can be clues to occult bleeding.

LESS COMMON POSTPARTUM COMPLICATIONS

AMNIOTIC FLUID EMBOLISM This is a rare, sudden, and often fatal event caused by the entrance of amniotic fluid into maternal circulation. It leads to rapid cardiopulmonary failure and an extreme form of a coagulation defect known as disseminated intravascular coagulopathy. Treatment is supportive. Use IV fluids, mechanical ventilation, if available, and medications designed to assist with cardiovascular support, such as epinephrine IV drips when available.

UTERINE INVERSION Uterine inversion occurs when the uterus literally turns inside out and protrudes from the os or through the introitus. This can lead to severe and rapid hemorrhage. Treatment includes providing analgesia that induces uterine relaxation, or giving another relaxing agent such as IM terbutaline. Create a fist and push the uterus inward into its natural position to replace the body of the uterus. If this maneuver is unsuccessful, immediate surgical consultation should be obtained, because hysterectomy may be unavoidable.

MANAGEMENT OF POSTPARTUM HEMORRHAGE

In general, the management of postpartum hemorrhage, regardless of the precipitating cause, should provide rapid assessment and treatment. Essential steps are listed as follows:

1. Prompt evaluation. This includes identification of a probable cause (e.g., forceps delivery, retained placenta, identification of a coagulation defect, etc.).

2. Stabilize the patient. This entails frequent monitoring of vital signs, starting two large-bore IVs, applying oxygen, and obtaining laboratory work, such as the PT, PTT, and a complete blood count. Blood should also be typed and cross-matched, or O-negative blood should be obtained. Definitive on-site treatment should be rendered if possible. Use the steps outlined above for each specific complication.

3. Get help. In remote settings it may take time and arrangements for transport, so begin this process early if you anticipate the complications will be greater than can be managed with local resources. An obstetrician or surgeon will be needed if a hysterectomy must be performed. Remember that most bleeding is caused by uterine atony. A thorough physical examination checking for a boggy uterus, lacerations, and hematomas must be undertaken.

POSTPARTUM DEPRESSION

Many of the physical complications following delivery have been discussed above. One psychological problem also deserves mention: postpartum depression. Women at the highest risk for this are those who have an underlying psychological illness and those who have suffered from previous bouts of postpartum depression. The illness can range from a mild depression, which occurs in 50% of cases and resolves in 1 to 2 weeks, to frank depression, which occurs in 10% of cases and has a varied time course. In extreme cases, women can even have suicidal thoughts and may need hospitalization. The symptoms of depression include sleep disturbances, low self-esteem, irritability, mood swings, and even estrangement from the newborn. Both internal and external factors can contribute to depression. Women who do not cope well with stress, have a poor support system, are poor or abused, or have other young children at home are at an increased risk for depression. Care should be taken not to force the infant on the depressed mother because this may exacerbate symptoms. Psychiatric therapy and the use of antidepressant medication should be considered. Inpatient treatment should be considered if the patient does not demonstrate signs of improvement.

MIDWIFERY AND TRADITIONAL BIRTH ATTENDANTS

Midwives and traditional birth attendants are used in many places in the world to provide health care to women who are pregnant and giving birth. Traditional medicine is based on beliefs and practices that have been passed down from midwife to midwife, and across the generations for hundreds of years. Often, older, more experienced lay health-care workers teach the care of pregnant women and the birthing process to the younger midwives. Tradition and folklore can become entwined. It is important to separate traditions that are either helpful or do no harm, from those that may actually cause harm. Education addressing harmful traditions is necessary. Support or tolerance should be observed for other benign traditions.

    In many communities midwives staff the health centers providing prenatal care. The village traditional teaching can be enriched by the addition of modern medical

TABLE 13-14 THE USUAL SCOPE OF PRACTICE IS
FOR TRADITIONAL BIRTH ATTENDANTS
AND MIDWIVES

Prenatal care—once a month for 6 m, then twice a month during
  months 7 and 8, then every week until delivery
Nutritional assessment and education
Family and patient education
Psychological counseling
Checkups
Assessment of fetal lie
Care of the mother during normal labor, birth, and postpartum
Vaginal delivery
Episiotomies
Managing routine care and minor complications postpartum
Newborn care
Breast-feeding education
Infant care education
Family planning
Treatment of sexually transmitted diseases
Administration of specific medications related to pregnancy and birth

principles. By working closely with the midwife, the best of both traditional and modern medicine can be made available to the population served.

Although a midwife will probably spend most of her time with individual women, her work can affect the health of the entire family—either directly by prenatal care and delivery or indirectly by family planning and teaching. The scope of midwifery in the developing world is frequently greater than that practiced by midwives in more developed countries (Table 13-14). For example, it is considered within the range of practice of traditional birth attendants to deliver breech infants if a hospital or physician is not immediately available. By contrast, women identified as carrying a breech infant in more developed countries are referred to an obstetrician. Additional roles for traditional birth attendants include prenatal teaching on nutrition, hygiene, and immunizations, and prenatal care and delivery.

Health-care workers from developed countries should listen carefully and take seriously a midwife's request for consult or care of the pregnant patient. Experienced midwives are often experts in Leopold maneuvers (abdominal palpation for fetal lie), and the recognition of deviation from normal labor. Local health-care workers also can educate expatriate health-care workers regarding local customs regarding maternal and infant care. Failure to take these cultural aspects of care into consideration can lead to maternal and infant complications.

SELECTED READINGS

Burns AA, et al. *Where Women Have No Doctor.* Berkeley, CA: Hesperian Foundation, 1997.
Klein SA. *A Book for Midwives.* Berkeley, CA: Hesperian Foundation, Berkeley, 1998.

CHAPTER 14
Trauma Management

C. James Holliman

INTRODUCTION AND THE ABCDEs OF TRAUMA CARE

Injuries are the leading cause of death in the first four decades of life in all but the least developed countries. The incidence of traumatic injuries has increased rapidly as populations grow and people concentrate in large cities. The "golden hour" is essential to the survival of multiply injured patients. It means providing optimum care during the first hour after injury. A systematic approach to the trauma patient begins with five critical steps necessary to identify life threats:

1. Rapid primary assessment of the patient
2. Starting resuscitative measures
3. Secondary survey
4. Identifying surgical emergencies or the need to transfer for higher level of care
5. Definitive care and rehabilitation

Life threats from trauma are primarily due to either compromise of respiratory status or loss of circulation (shock) (Table 14-1).

TABLE 14-1 LIFE THREATS IN TRAUMA PATIENTS (FROM MOST SEVERE TO LEAST)

Loss of the airway (blood, vomitus, foreign body, or external compression)
Loss of breathing (due to pneumothorax, hemothorax, or lung injury)
Bleeding (internal or external), heart injury, arrhythmias, or an expanding intracranial mass.

> **KEY POINT:**
>
> If a patient has multiple injuries, first treat the one that is the greatest threat to life.

If a large number of injured patients arrive simultaneously, treat those with serious but survivable injuries first. Those with minor injuries can wait until the more serious are treated. Some may require quick interventions such as pressure dressing to stop bleeding. If multiple casualties do not exceed the capabilities of the facility, treat the patients with life-threatening or multiple injuries first.

Prior to any trauma resuscitation, all members of the trauma team should have "universal precautions" in place: gown, face mask or shield, eye protection, latex gloves, and shoe covers . Team members should remember to safely dispose of all sharp items.

RAPID ASSESSMENT AND TREATMENT: THE "ABCDE" SYSTEM

The basic principle of resuscitation is that the initial assessment and corrective interventions be done simultaneously as part of the primary survey. Treatment takes precedence over diagnosis (see Chapter 6 for more detail about the ABCs and primary resuscitation). Always follow this sequence, called the primary survey:

A = Airway (with cervical spine control)
B = Breathing
C = Circulation
D = Disability (neurologic status)
E = Expose and environment (completely undress the patient for examination, but keep the patient warm)

When there are multiple members of the trauma team, many initial resuscitation events should occur simultaneously, including

- Airway assessment and management
- Control of external hemorrhage
- Vital signs and monitoring
- Spine immobilization for blunt trauma (Fig. 14-1)
- Placement of intravenous (IV) line and sending initial blood studies
- Cervical spine films, chest radiograph, and pelvis film (for blunt trauma), when available

PRELIMINARY HISTORY

Obtaining the history is an important part of the trauma evaluation but should not interfere with the primary survey and stabilization. Therefore, initially:

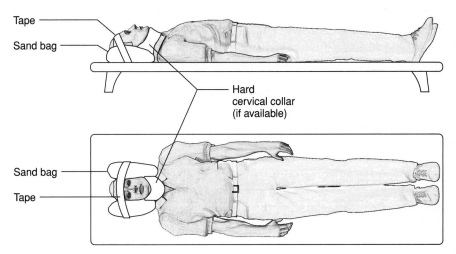

Tape

Sand bag

Hard
cervical collar
(if available)

Sand bag

Tape

FIGURE 14-1 Cervical spine immobilization.

- Ask few focused questions.
- Use other team members to obtain a more detailed history (nurses, residents).
- Get the more detailed history as part of the secondary survey.
- There are multiple sources of historical information: the patient, family, friends, bystanders, and prehospital personnel.

AIRWAY

Rapidly assess the airway by observing the patient's level of consciousness and checking for foreign bodies, as well as facial, mandibular, tracheal, or laryngeal injuries. These measures should always be performed while maintaining immobilization of the cervical spine; preferably using the chin lift or jaw thrust maneuvers (see Chapter 6 for further details).

AIRWAY RESUSCITATION TECHNIQUES

- Jaw thrust in an unconscious and nonbreathing patient
- Oral or nasopharyngeal airway in an unconscious, but breathing patient
- Supplemental oxygen for breathing patients
- Endotracheal intubation if no response to the other interventions

CRITICAL ACTION:

If there is any question of the stability of the airway, err in favor of intubating the patient.

BREATHING

Assess by auscultation, palpation, and inspection of the chest wall and lungs. Count the patient respirations yourself. Obtain pulse oximetry and cardiac monitoring if available. Use bag-valve-mask (BVM)–assisted ventilation if needed. Start oxygen by high-flow face mask on all patients. The emergent diagnoses that require immediate intervention are:

- Tension or open pneumothorax
- Massive hemothorax
- Flail chest

BREATHING RESUSCITATION TECHNIQUES

- BVM ventilation if needed
- Needle decompression of a tension pneumothorax (see later section on Chest Trauma)
- Tube thoracostomy (chest tube placement) is the definitive for pneumothorax and hemothorax (see section on Chest Trauma), but it is done after the primary survey is complete.

CIRCULATION

First control any external bleeding with direct pressure. Assess the circulatory status by palpation of pulses, noting skin color and level of consciousness. Be on guard for intraabdominal or intrathoracic injury, as well as fractures of the pelvis or femur.

CIRCULATION RESUSCITATION TECHNIQUES

- Establish two IV lines (16 gauge or larger), or
- Central venous access (Fig. 14-2),
- IV fluid therapy for tachycardia and hypotension,
- Blood transfusion if continued hypotension

DISABILITY

Always assume that all patients with trauma have a neck (cervical spine) injury until proven otherwise. Immobilize the head and neck. Conduct a rapid neurologic examination to assess the level of consciousness:

- Alert
- Responds to verbal stimulation

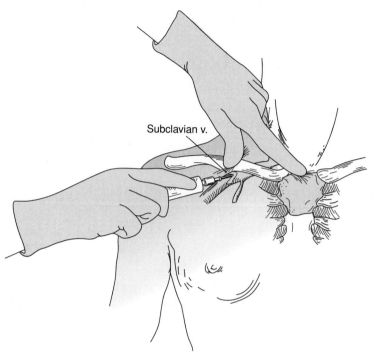

Subclavian v.

FIGURE 14-2 Subclavian vein access.

- Responds to painful stimulation
- Unresponsive (term preferred to comatose)

You also can use the Glasgow Coma Scale (GCS; Table 14-2) to follow changing neurologic status. The GCS assesses for head injury, shock, and decreased oxygenation.

TABLE 14-2 GLASGOW COMA SCALE (GCS)

EYE OPENING	(E SCORE)	BEST VERBAL RESPONSE	(V SCORE)	BEST MOTOR RESPONSE	(M SCORE)
Spontaneous	4	Oriented	5	Obeys commands	6
To speech	3	Confused	4	Moves toward stimulus	5
To pain	2	Inappropriate (garbled)	3	Withdraws to pain	4
None (closed)	1	Incomprehensible (grunts)	2	Flexion response to pain (decorticate posturing)	3
		None	1	Extensor response to pain (decerebrate posturing)	2
				None	1

Sum of the E, M, and V scores then is the GCS score number

DISABILITY RESUSCITATION TECHNIQUES Complete neck and head immobilization should be undertaken.

EXPOSURE/ENVIRONMENT

Patients must be completely undressed to facilitate complete examination. They should be protected from hypothermia with warm blankets and warm IV fluids if available.

> **CRITICAL ACTION:**
>
> Reassess primary survey before moving on to secondary survey.

SECONDARY SURVEY

The secondary survey includes a complete history and examination with initiation of diagnostic studies. The purpose of the secondary survey is to identify all injuries and to begin treatment. Begin with a complete head-to-toe examination and a thorough neurologic examination, including the GCS (Table 14-2).

HISTORY

Attempt to get more history about the injuring event to better understand the mechanism and the forces applied. (How far did the patient fall? Was the patient wearing a seatbelt?). Also ask about an "AMPLE" history:

    A = Allergies
    M = Medications
    P = Past illnesses
    L = Last meal (time)
    E = Events (preceding injury). Clarify the mechanism of injury.

PHYSICAL EXAMINATION

A brief examination from head to toe should be performed, or the organ system approach may be used:

HEENT examination
    Head: Examine and palpate the head for lacerations and fractures. Check the
        mastoids for bruising (battle sign: basilar skull fracture). Visualize and
        palpate the entire face for signs of fractures.
    Ears: Look in the ears for ruptured tympanic membranes (TMs), or hemo-
        tympanum (blood behind the TM, sign of a basilar skull fracture).

Eyes: Check extraocular movements for signs of entrapment from a 'blow-out' orbital fracture. Check visual acuity and examine the eye.

Nose: Look and palpate for signs of a fracture. Look in the nostril for a septal hematoma.

Throat: Ask the patient to bite and elicit whether it feels normal (if not, consider a mandible fracture). Palpate the entire jaw, check its range of motion. Check the stability of the teeth. Visualize the entire inside of the mouth.

Neck examination

At this point the patient's head and neck may still be immobilized, making the examination difficult.

Visualize the anterior neck to look for signs of injuries and for a midline trachea.

If the patient is neurologically intact and alert and conscious, palpate the back of the neck for tenderness or signs of fractures.

Neurologic examination

Assess patient's level of consciousness, pupils, cranial nerves, TMs, spinal cord, and peripheral nerves.

Absences of rectal tone may be the only indication of cord injury.

Palpate entire spine, with radiographs for any suspicion of injury.

Abdominal examination

Look for evidence of external trauma, absence of bowel sounds, distention, peritoneal findings, or evisceration.

Multiple, serial examinations increase the diagnostic accuracy.

Perform a diagnostic peritoneal lavage (DPL) for patients with blunt trauma and abdominal tenderness.

If available, consider abdominal computed tomography (CT) scan for stable patients and to evaluate the retroperitoneum and kidneys.

Surgery is needed for all gunshot wounds that penetrate the peritoneal cavity.

Start antibiotics if necessary.

Genitourinary (GU) examination

Look and feel for signs of injury.

Check the urine for gross and microscopic bleeding.

Chest examination

Observe the rate and quality of respirations (paradoxic or asymmetric expansion).

Palpate for rib fractures, subcutaneous air, and flail chest.

Auscultate for symmetric breath sounds.

Percuss for signs of hyperresonance (tension pneumothorax).

Cardiac examination

An ECG may be useful for victims of serious trauma. But remember: no specific ECG findings in patients with myocardial contusion or pericardial tamponade.

Musculoskeletal examination

Identify fractures by palpating for deformity, crepitus, swelling, pain, or tenderness.

Check the peripheral neurovascular function.

Reduce major joint dislocations (knee and hip) as soon as possible.

Don't forget to examine the back.

Skin and soft tissue examination

Lowest priority (except to control bleeding)

Inspect, irrigate, and dress all wounds.

Additional actions

Urinary catheter and nasogastric (NG) tube placement (unless contraindicated; see earlier sections on examination of the head and genitourinary area)

Definitive stabilizing procedures such as a tube thoracostomy (see later sections on specific injuries)

LABORATORY

The most important laboratory test is to type and cross-match the patient for blood transfusions if transfusion is available.

■ A complete blood count or hematocrit analysis also may be useful to assess and monitor blood loss.

■ A urinalysis that demonstrates gross blood can indicate a severe kidney injury that will require further advanced diagnostic studies.

RADIOGRAPHY

If available, consider obtaining the following radiographs: lateral cervical spine, chest radiograph, and anteroposterior (AP) pelvis. Further radiographs can include a complete cervical spine series (AP and odontoid) and films of possible fracture sites. Plain abdominal films are rarely useful in blunt trauma. Decide if special studies are needed (e.g., CT, angiography, or ultrasonography, if available). Figure 14-3 shows the normal structural relationships of the lateral cervical spine.

TREATMENT

■ Clean and close all lacerations.

■ Splint all fractures.

■ Provide tetanus toxoid if no immunizations have been given within 5 years. Tetanus immunoglobulin is needed if the patient has never been immunized.

■ Consider pain medications once the examination is complete.

■ Continue to reevaluate the patient and obtain vital signs frequently (at least every 15 minutes).

CRITICAL ACTION:

Frequent repetition of the primary and secondary surveys is critical to detect any deterioration in the patient's status.

(a)

(b)

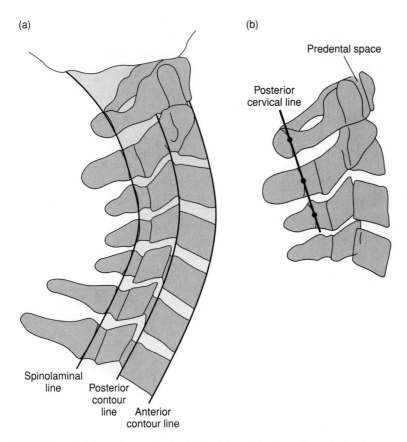

Predental space

Posterior
cervical line

Spinolaminal
line

Posterior
contour
line

Anterior
contour line

FIGURE 14-3 Normal structural relationships of the lateral cervical spine.

TRANSFER OF TRAUMA PATIENTS

After completion of the secondary survey, decide if the patient will need to be transferred to another medical facility for more advanced care. In transferring a trauma patient to another hospital, you should always follow the principle of "do no harm." Sometimes you cannot transfer a patient—there are no vehicles, you are too remote, etc. Then the goal is to provide the best possible care given the limited available resources.

Many aspects of the decision to transfer patients should be made in advance, preferably in the form of a written policy. This decision is based on the capabilities of your hospital and physicians: if you don't have a surgeon, you cannot operate; if you don't have equipment, you cannot intubate, etc. Therefore, some injured patients will need to be transferred to other facilities for more definitive care. Understanding the mechanism and resources for transferring in advance is crucial.

Choosing the transfer destination depends on the availability of multiple facilities, the types of service they provide, the type of care required, and how quickly the patient can be transferred.

If possible, the sending physician should speak with the receiving physician to discuss the case directly. Both doctors should decide on the mode of transportation (ground ambulance vs. aeromedical ambulance) and the personnel who should travel with the patient. Time is critical and the transfer should be arranged as quickly as possible.

Some essential steps must be completed prior to transfer:

- Manage all life-threatening problems.
- Complete the secondary survey.
- Stabilize any secondary injuries identified.
- Arrange the transfer.
- Provide a written summary of your findings and treatments.

AIRWAY MANAGEMENT FOR THE TRAUMA PATIENT

This section focuses on a few points specific to airways in injured persons (for further details on airway management, see the Airway section of Chapter 6).

Protection of the airway, prevention of hypoxemia, and provision of adequate ventilation take priority in all resuscitations. The airways of injured patients are especially difficult to manage because it is necessary to keep the neck and head immobile with the possibility of a cervical spine injury.

INITIAL AIRWAY MANAGEMENT TECHNIQUES

Do not move the head when protecting the airway (no head tilt). Instead, use the following maneuvers:

- Chin lift
- Jaw thrust
- Oropharyngeal or nasopharyngeal airway

> **KEY POINT:**
>
> Maintain cervical spine immobilization during all airway maneuvers.

DEFINITIVE AIRWAY TECHNIQUES (INTUBATION AND SURGICAL)

If you have the capabilities and the patient needs definitive airway protection, endotracheal intubation should be performed as early as possible. The most experienced person present should intubate.

OROTRACHEAL INTUBATION Orotracheal intubation is preferred for almost all patients, and paralysis makes intubation easier and more accurate and involves fewer complications. The head must remain immobilized during the entire procedure.

NASOTRACHEAL INTUBATION Nasotracheal intubation should never be attempted in a nonbreathing patient, in patients with mid-face or possible basilar skull fractures, or in those with a known coagulopathy. Although orotracheal intubation is almost always preferred, the decision on which technique to use depends on the training, experience, and comfort level of the physician.

SURGICAL AIRWAY Surgical cricothyrotomy is an excellent technique for rapid airway access in a patient with facial injuries, and does not require the head to be moved (should be used only in patients >12 years of age). Needle cricothyrotomy can only be used for short-term ventilation, but may help as you set up for the surgical cricothyrotomy.

Indications for a surgical airway include the following:

- Inability to intubate orotracheally or nasotracheally (usually from facial trauma)
- Uncorrectable upper airway obstruction above level of vocal cords

TRAUMA TEAM MANAGEMENT

The roles and responsibilities of the each person involved in trauma care should be decided ahead of time. Duties vary depending on the number and types of personnel available, the number of simultaneous trauma patients, and hospital resources. Personnel should practice their roles as part of a team in simulations and exercises. A team leader should always be designated in advance.

PREHOSPITAL TRAUMA MANAGEMENT

If it is possible, the hospital should be notified in advance of the arrival of an injured (or any emergent) patient. However, in many situations rapid access to communication (radio or telephone) is not possible. Prehospital personnel should provide information on the number and age of victims, mechanism of injury, major injuries, vital signs, treatments, and estimated time of arrival. If there has been warning of an injured patient coming, the response team should be assembled, and equipment (including universal precautions) should be prepared.

TRAUMA PERSONNEL ROLES AND RESPONSIBILITIES

Ideally, the trauma team is composed of 8 to 10 people. (Fig. 14-4). It is imperative that there is a single designated leader who controls all aspects of the evaluation and resuscitation. Important roles include:

- Team leader (physician leader/examiner/resuscitator)
- Airway control (anesthesiologist, emergency physician)

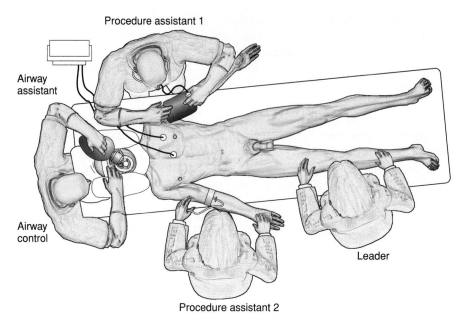

FIGURE 14-4 Positions of the trauma team members.

- Procedure person (IV access assistant/airway assistant/medications)

When additional personnel are available, other possible jobs include

- A separate examining physician
- A second procedure assistant to divide the first assistant's duties (left and right sides)
- A person to deliver medicine and record the resuscitation steps
- An x-ray technician

If possible, additional personnel can be mobilized for nursing floors, intensive care units, the operating room, and laboratory. Even the prehospital personnel can assist.

> **KEY POINT:**
>
> Know the capabilities of your facility, and pick a team and practice in advance.

Depending on the number of trauma team members, the trauma team leader either supervises all team members and does not examine the patient, or directly performs the examination/resuscitation while directing other team members to perform certain functions (placing IV lines, chest tubes, etc.). They also decide which imaging studies and procedures are needed.

In some situations the team leader also may be the airway manager, which entails assessing the patient's airway and intervening as indicated. They also are responsible for maintaining neck immobilization.

The procedures person starts an IV line in the right upper limb (or a central line if the patient presents in shock) and performs the initial blood draw and other procedures as directed by the leader (placement of NG tube, bladder catheter, etc). This assistant also can assist with log rolling the patient for examination of the back.

HEAD INJURIES

Head injuries are the leading cause of injury deaths. Delayed or prolonged effects (even from minor trauma) are headache, memory loss, and behavioral, learning, or psychological dysfunction. Types of head injuries include the following:

- Scalp lacerations, abrasions, and contusions
- Skull fractures (linear, depressed)
- Brain injuries
  Diffuse (concussion, diffuse axonal injury, cerebral edema)
  Focal (subdural, epidural, subarachnoid, parenchymal hemorrhages, brain lacerations)

ASSESSMENT

HISTORY The history should include the time and type of injury, whether the head was protected, if there was loss of consciousness, nausea, neurologic symptoms, seizure, alcohol or drug intake, prior head injuries or neurologic problems, and current medications and allergies.

PHYSICAL EXAMINATION Assessing the level of consciousness is the most important examination. A decrease in the level of consciousness implies a possible brain injury. Other causes include hypoxia, alcohol, drugs, hypoglycemia, cerebrovascular accident, hypothermia, and carbon monoxide.

- Vital signs: Signs of shock [low blood pressure (BP) and high pulse rate] in a head-injured patient are usually due to another injury. Uncommonly shock can be due to blood loss from a scalp laceration alone.
- A low pulse rate and increased BP may represent Cushing reflex, indicating increased intracranial pressure (ICP). This is an ominous finding.

NEUROLOGIC EXAMINATION The neurologic examination is essential to evaluating patients with head injuries. A detailed examination should include the cranial nerves, motor and sensory function, and fine motor function and gait. Components of the mini-neurologic examination include the following:

- Level of consciousness (e.g., awake, responds to verbal stimulation, responds to pain, unresponsive)
- GCS (Table 14-2)
- Pupil reactivity
- Deep tendon reflexes
- Unilateral extremity findings (loss of motor function in one limb or side of the body)

The GCS score can be interpreted as follows:

- Severe = GCS score of 3 to 8: high mortality, almost all require neurosurgery.
- Moderate = 9 to 12: variable mortality, up to 50% require neurosurgery.
- Mild = 13 to 15: low mortality, but significant morbidity; less than 3% require neurosurgery.

For a GCS score less than or equal to 8, most patients require intubation.

There are many factors that give falsely low GCS scores. For example, the eye may not be able to open due to an orbital injury. With a limb injury, the patient may not move the limb due to a fracture or other injury of the limb. Children may be nonverbal.

Other indicators of severe head injury are listed as follows:

- Unequal pupils
- Lateralizing motor response or posturing
- Open skull injury with cerebrospinal fluid (CSF) leak/exposed brain tissue
- Depressed skull fracture
- Deterioration in neurologic status (but always make sure that it is not due to hypoxia or shock first)

DIAGNOSIS

A CT scan is needed to definitively diagnose an intracranial injury, although the examination can provide valuable clues. Always make sure that it is not hypoxia or shock causing the changes in mental status.

Skull radiographs are generally useless to diagnose intracranial injuries. They are indicated under the following circumstances:

- A head CT is not available and the patient has a suspected depressed or open skull fracture by physical examination.
- A fracture may cross the middle meningeal artery area (occipitotemporal). If the fracture does cross this area, a head CT is indicated to look for an epidural hematoma.
- There is a large scalp hematoma through which the skull cannot be felt well enough to rule out a depressed fracture.

TREATMENT

The most important goal of treating brain-injured patients is to prevent secondary injury from hypoxia, hypotension, and increased ICP. Initial treatment of the head-injured patient includes the following:

- High-flow oxygen
- Maintain a systolic BP of at least 120 mm Hg (some authorities say 140)
- Check a fingerstick glucose and treat with IV 50% dextrose if low
- Check for hyper- or hypothermia
- If signs of increased ICP, treat by:
  Elevating the head of the bed
  Mannitol 0.25 to 1.0 g/kg IV and/or furosemide 1 mg/kg IV
  Hyperventilation at 14 to 18 breaths/min (controversial)
  Consider use of barbiturates (phenobarbitol 10–20 mg/kg loading dose or pentobarbital 3–6 mg/kg IV)
  Steroids are not indicated
- Antistaphylococcal antibiotics for penetrating skull injury
- Diazepam (0.2–0.3 mg/kg IV) or lorazepam (0.1–0.2 mg/kg IV) if seizures occur, followed by phenytoin 18 mg/kg at a rate of less than 50 mg/kg/min
- Repair of scalp lacerations

Frequent reassessment of the head trauma patient is extremely important to detect deteriorations or changes. Signs of dangerous neurologic deterioration are a decrease in the GCS score of 2 or more points, increased severity of headache, increased size of one pupil, and unilateral weakness.

DISPOSITION

The primary decision that needs to be made is whether the patient needs emergency neurosurgical consultation. High-risk patients include those with GCS scores of 8 or less, unequal pupils or lateralizing defects, or posturing. If possible, these patients should be intubated early with control of the cervical spine, hyperventilated, and resuscitated aggressively to prevent hypotension, and should have their ICP lowered.

If the patient's GCS score does not return to 15 after observation, if he or she remains confused, or if the GCS score was ever less than 13, then he or she needs to be transferred to a facility with a CT scan and a neurosurgeon. Patients whose GCS score improves to 15 in less than 6 hours should be observed overnight to ensure they don't deteriorate.

SPECIFIC HEAD INJURIES

SCALP LACERATIONS See Chapter 16 for a more detailed discussion. Scalp lacerations bleed profusely, so rapid control of bleeding is essential. Options include the following:

- Direct pressure
- Ligation of the bleeding vessels
- Injection of lidocaine with epinephrine into the bleeding areas
- Multilayer closure of the wound (always close torn galea)

SKULL FRACTURES Most skull fractures do not require specific treatment, except those that are depressed below the inner table of the bone. Indications for surgery include some open fractures and fractures that are depressed more than 3 to 5 mm.

BASILAR SKULL FRACTURES Basilar skull fractures are not seen well on skull radiographs. A CT scan, if available, is indicated. Physical examination signs of basilar skull fracture include the following:

- Periorbital ecchymoses (raccoon eyes; may not develop for 6–12 hours)
- Ecchymosis over the mastoid (Battle sign; may not develop for 6–12 hours)
- CSF leak from nose or ear
- Hemotympanum (blood behind the eardrum)
- Occasionally deafness from auditory nerve injury

Most basilar skull fractures require no treatment, but patients should be admitted for observation. The use of prophylactic antibiotics for an open skull fracture is controversial. Given the difficult situation in developing countries, it is probably best to treat with penicillin or an antistaphylococcal antibiotic until the CSF leak resolves.

CONCUSSION Symptoms include the following:

- GCS score of 14 or 15
- Brief loss of consciousness (<5 minutes)
- Headache
- Dizziness
- Nausea/vomiting
- Normal neurologic examination

Patients may need to be admitted if they have severe dizziness or persistent vomiting or confusion. Patients usually just need observation for 12 to 24 hours.

INTRACRANIAL HEMATOMA If suspected on physical examination or identified on CT, intracranial hematomas always require a neurosurgical consult, although most do not require surgery.

TRAUMATIC SUBARACHNOID HEMORRHAGE Patients with traumatic subarachnoid hemorrhage may present as normal to unresponsive. This condition is diagnosed by the detection of blood in the subarachnoid space on a head CT scan. There is no specific treatment other than to monitor and treat the ICP.

SUBDURAL HEMATOMA Subdural hematomas are associated with a high mortality rate (40%–60%) even with surgery, because there is usually underlying brain injury. They are treated by craniotomy and drainage (unless very small and bilateral). Symptoms of a subdural hematoma may not develop for weeks following an injury, so it should be considered in a patient with a history of a head injury who presents as confused or unresponsive.

EPIDURAL HEMATOMA Epidural hematomas are uncommon (occurring in <10% of unconscious head-injured patients). It is caused by a fracture in the temporo-occipital region that tears the middle meningeal artery. The mortality rate is 10% to 50% (better prognosis than subdural hematomas because there is usually less underlying brain injury).

The classic patient presentation (seen in only one fourth of cases) is loss of consciousness at impact followed by a normal, awake interval, then a progressive decline to unconsciousness as the hematoma expands. Physical findings include a dilated pupil on the side of the hematoma and paralysis of the limbs on the opposite side.

Emergency craniotomy is indicated to treat epidural hematomas. The causative artery usually needs ligation (and the hematoma drained). Emergently, bilateral burr holes can be made if normal efforts to reduce ICP do not resolve the dilated pupils or unresponsiveness. Holes should be made two fingerbreadths anterior and three fingerbreadths superior to the anterior tragus of the ear, starting on the side of the first dilated pupil.

CERVICAL SPINE TRAUMA

Manipulation of an unstable cervical spine can paralyze a patient; keep the head and neck immobilized until you have proven that he or she does not have a cervical spine injury. Sixty percent of cervical fractures occur at the C5/C6 level and 30% at the C6 or C7 level.

> **CRITICAL ACTION:**
>
> If cervical spine injury is suspected and radiography is not available, the patient must remain immobile on a backboard and fitted with a cervical collar and transferred to a facility with radiographic capabilities.

ASSESSMENT

PHYSICAL EXAMINATION Neurologic assessment should include the following:

- Motor strength in all four limbs (paralysis with a cord injury)
- Sensation in the trunk and limbs (may have paresthesia as the only symptom)

- Deep tendon reflexes (flaccid areflexia)
- Rectal sphincter tone (no tone with a cord injury)

The "quick and dirty" method of determining the level of the injury entails ascertaining the last working motor function:

- C4: Spontaneous breathing
- C6: Flexion at the elbow
- C8: Extension at the wrist
- L1: Flexion at the hips
- S2-4: Rectal sphincter tone

Other indicators of a possible spinal cord injury include the following:

- Diaphragmatic breathing
- Pain response above the clavicle only
- Motor response limited to forearm flexion
- Priapism (involuntary penile erection)
- Neurogenic shock (hypotension with a normal or slow pulse)

NECK EXAMINATION If the patient presents with paralysis or neurologic symptoms, do not remove the cervical collar to examine the neck: perform radiography first. If they are neurologically intact, examine the immobilized neck for tenderness, deformity, step-off, edema, ecchymosis, muscle spasm, abnormal head position, and tracheal deviation.

DIAGNOSIS

Cervical spine films should be obtained in all patients with blunt trauma to the head or neck (or general severe blunt trauma) along with the following:

- Neck pain or tenderness
- Decreased pain perception (head trauma, intoxication with alcohol or drugs, children <2 years of age, or mentally retarded)
- Penetrating trauma to the neck
- Neurologic root or cord symptoms or signs
- A concurrent, very painful "distracting" injury (making the patient a poor historian)

Generally, a standard three-view (lateral, open-mouth odontoid, and AP) set of radiographs is needed. The lateral cervical spine view is the most important one in assessment of cervical injuries and shows about 90% of fractures and dislocations. A neck CT, if available, should be performed for all radiographs suspicious for a fracture, or for those that do not adequately visualize the cervical spine. Other findings to seek on the lateral cervical spine radiograph include the following:

- Make sure you can see all seven cervical vertebrae and the top of the T1 vertebral body.
- Look at the three vertebral column lines for any step-off or line disruption. The line running up the anterior edge of the vertebral bodies, the line running up the posterior edge of the vertebral bodies, and the line running at the anterior edge of the spinous processes should be assessed.
- Measure the prevertebral space. It should be less than 5 mm between C2 and C4.
- Measure the predental space. This should be less than 3 mm in adults and less than 5 mm in children.
- Look at all the bony structures, including the facet joints for fractures.
- Look at the adjacent soft tissues.
- Look at the skull and mandible for associated bony injuries.

After the cervical spine has been cleared radiographically, it also must be cleared by examination. If the patient is completely awake and alert, gently remove the head immobilization and palpate the back of the neck for tenderness. If there is no midline tenderness, ask the patient to slowly flex, extend, rotate, and laterally flex the head. If no pain or neurologic symptoms are elicited with movement, then the patient is cleared.

If the injury remains mildly tender or induces pain with movement but no neurologic symptoms, then a flexion-extension lateral cervical spine radiograph and/or a neck CT should be performed to look for ligament instability.

- Have the patient slowly flex the head forward as far as possible (stopping if neurologic symptoms are elicited), then take a lateral radiograph. Repeat the process in full extension. There should be no subluxation on the films.
- If the patient has neurologic symptoms or severe point tenderness, a neck CT should be performed, not flexion-extension radiography.

TREATMENT

CERVICAL FRACTURE The treatment of cervical fracture entails the following:

- Maintain neck immobilization in a hard cervical collar.
- IV methylprednisolone 30 mg/kg bolus followed by an IV drip at 5.4 mg/kg/h for 23 hours, starting within 8 hours of the time of injury
- Avoid traction or distraction.
- Film the remainder of the spine (thoracic spine and lumbar spine) if any cervical level sensory or motor deficit is present.
- Support the circulation with IV fluid boluses and possibly vasopressors if there is neurogenic shock.
- IV antibiotics if there is an open fracture (as from a gunshot wound).
- Definitive care is provided by neurosurgery or orthopedic surgery.

TREATMENT OF NEUROGENIC SHOCK The loss of sympathetic stimulation leads to peripheral vasodilatation and venous blood pooling, resulting in hypotension and bradycardia. Treatment should include the following:

- IV fluid
- Alpha agonists such as dopamine or ephedrine
- Atropine may be needed for refractory bradycardia.
- IV methylprednisolone

Some specific types of cervical spine fractures are listed as follows:

- A Jefferson fracture is a burst fracture of the atlas (C1) that is mechanically unstable.
- A Hangman fracture is a bilateral pedicle fracture of C2. It often occurs from a blow to, or fall onto, the top of the head.
- Wedge fractures of the vertebral bodies are usually mechanically stable. There is loss of vertebral body height anteriorly, but no vertical fracture line. These often do not require specific therapy, except for pain medications.
- Vertebral body burst fractures are mechanically stable but cause spinal cord injury from bone fragments.
- A flexion teardrop fracture is a chip fracture of the lower anterior corner of the vertebral body. This is often associated with an anterior cord syndrome and is mechanically unstable.
- An extension teardrop fracture is a chip fracture of the upper anterior corner of the vertebral body and is unstable in extension.
- A unilateral facet dislocation is a displacement of the superior facet of one vertebra, which then rests in the intervertebral foramen. Such a dislocation is mechanically stable but requires reduction. The vertebral body is displaced less than one half the vertebral body width over the adjoining body.
- A bilateral facet dislocation is mechanically unstable and has a high incidence of cord injury. There is a significant degree of displacement of one vertebral body on the adjacent one.
- A clay shoveler's fracture is an avulsion fracture of the spinous process, most commonly at C6, C7, or T1. This fracture is mechanically stable and does not require treatment except for pain medication.

CHEST TRAUMA

Chest injuries cause 25% of injury deaths. Eighty-five percent of chest injuries are treatable by simple procedures such as tube thoracostomy, and only 15% of major chest injuries require surgery (thoracotomy). However, the majority of severe chest injuries require the advanced care of a thoracic surgeon and intensive care monitoring. There are many injuries to the chest and its contents. Table 14-3 categorizes them by their lethality.

Common mistakes in evaluating thoracic trauma include the following:

- Failure to completely undress the patient

TABLE 14-3 CHEST INJURIES BY SEVERITY

The 5 rapidly lethal injuries that must be found and treated
    during the primary survey:
1. Tension pneumothorax
2. Open pneumothorax
3. Massive hemothorax
4. Flail chest
5. Cardiac tamponade

The 6 potentially lethal chest injuries that should be identified
    on the secondary survey:
1. Aortic disruption or dissection
2. Myocardial contusion
3. Tracheobronchial disruption
4. Esophageal disruption or perforation
5. Pulmonary contusion
6. Diaphragmatic disruption

Other, usually nonlethal chest injuries:
1. Chest wall contusions
2. Simple rib fracture
3. Simple pneumothorax or small hemothorax
4. Sternoclavicular dislocation
5. Sternal fracture
6. Clavicle fracture
7. Scapular fracture

- Failure to observe and count the respirations yourself
- Failure to palpate the chest wall

ASSESSMENT AND MANAGEMENT OF SEVERE INJURIES DURING THE PRIMARY SURVEY

TENSION PNEUMOTHORAX Tension pneumothorax can develop from a traumatic disruption of lung tissue and accumulation of air in the pleural cavity and displacement of mediastinal structures.

DIAGNOSIS The diagnosis of tension pneumothorax is based on the following clinical findings:

- Respiratory distress
- Breath sounds are decreased or absent on the injured side.
- Hyperinflation of the injured side
- Tympanitic to percussion on the injured side
- Tracheal deviation toward the opposite side
- Neck veins may be distended.
- Hypotension (late finding)

TREATMENT Immediate needle decompression may be achieved using a 14- to 18-gauge needle inserted in the anterior second intercostal space in the mid-clavicular line along the upper edge of the rib (Fig. 14-5). Do not wait for confirmation of a tension pneumothorax by chest radiography. The definitive treatment is tube thoracostomy (placement of a chest tube), which is performed after the primary survey.

OPEN PNEUMOTHORAX Open pneumothorax is an open hole in the chest wall whose diameter is greater than two thirds the diameter of the trachea.

DIAGNOSIS

■ An obvious hole in the chest wall that inspires and expires air with each respiration
■ Decreased breath sounds on the affected side

TREATMENT Place an occlusive dressing of vaseline gauze over the hole that is taped down to the skin on three sides (Fig. 14-6). After the primary survey is completed, a chest tube is placed on the injured side, and the wound on the chest wall is repaired.

MASSIVE HEMOTHORAX With a massive hemothorax, greater than 1,500 mL of blood has leaked into the pleural cavity.

DIAGNOSIS

■ Shock
■ Respiratory distress

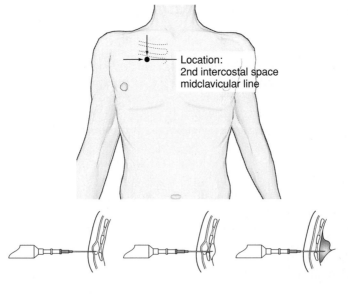

Location:
2nd intercostal space
midclavicular line

FIGURE 14-5
Needle
thoracostomy.

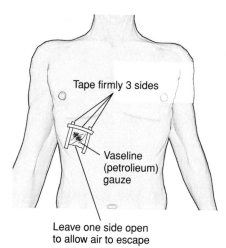

Tape firmly 3 sides

Vaseline
(petrolieum)
gauze

Leave one side open
to allow air to escape

FIGURE 14-6 A flap dressing for an open pneumothorax.

- Flat neck veins
- Decreased breath sounds on the injured side
- Dullness to percussion on the injured side

TREATMENT

- Rapid replacement of intravascular volume
- Obtain at least 4 units of blood for transfusion.
- The patient will eventually require a thoracostomy tube, but placing it too early may wash away the clot and the patient may then exsanguinate via the chest tube. If the patient is in severe respiratory distress, however, a chest tube should be placed immediately.
- After placement of the thoracostomy tube, the patient may require an emergent thoracotomy if the bleeding continues.

> **CRITICAL ACTION:**
>
> Respiratory distress with unilateral decreased breath sounds probably indicates a tension pneumothorax or massive hemothorax: perform needle decompression immediately.

FLAIL CHEST Flail chest as defined as three or more fractured ribs in two or more places. This causes a free-floating section of the chest wall that interferes with ventilation. There is usually an underlying pulmonary contusion.

DIAGNOSIS This diagnosis is often missed initially.

- Palpation of the chest may reveal multiple rib fractures.

■ Careful observation may demonstrate a section of the chest wall that moves opposite that of the rest of the chest with each respiration.

■ A chest radiograph will show multiple fractures of the same rib.

TREATMENT Most patients with flail chest can be treated as follows:

■ Initially, simply lay the patient on the affected side or lay a small sandbag on the area.

■ Broad adhesive taping of the flail segment

■ Give oxygen by face-mask.

■ Fluid restriction to reduce the pulmonary contusion

■ Good airway suction

■ Intracostal nerve blocks are helpful for pain control.

The patient may require intubation and ventilation with positive end-expiratory pressure under the following conditions:

■ They are over 65 years of age.

■ Other major injuries are present.

■ Significant respiratory distress

■ The PO_2 is less than 60 mm Hg on 40% oxygen by face mask or the PCO_2 is greater than 50 mm Hg.

■ There is preexisting lung disease.

CARDIAC TAMPONADE Cardiac tamponade results from blood (or other fluid) accumulating in the pericardial space. This may lead to rapid decrease in cardiac output and shock.

DIAGNOSIS Cardiac tamponade can be diagnosed by Beck's triad:

■ Hypotension

■ Distended neck veins (jugular venous distention)

■ Muffled heart tones

Blood pressure measurement may show the patient to have a pulsus paradoxis.

TREATMENT

■ Initially attempt to support the BP with IV fluid boluses.

■ If unsuccessful, use pressors (dopamine 2–10 μg/kg/min or epinephrine or norepinephrine).

■ Perform pericardiocentesis if no response.

> **KEY POINT:**
>
> Tension pneumothorax and cardiac tamponade are the only traumatic causes of shock associated with distended neck veins.

AORTIC DISRUPTION OR RUPTURE Aortic rupture after blunt trauma is usually rapidly fatal (90% die immediately) and difficult to treat.

PHYSICAL EXAMINATION Patients complain of retrosternal or interscapular pain. There may be a harsh murmur noted on the heart examination. Suspect the diagnosis if there is a pulse deficit in the left arm or there is a BP difference between the arms.

DIAGNOSIS First screen with a chest radiograph. However, the definitive test is emergency aortography, CT, or magnetic resonance imaging when available. Chest radiography shows the following findings:

- Widening of the upper mediastinum (>8 cm on an AP view at the level of the aortic knob)
- Blurring or haziness of the aortic knob shadow
- Left pleural effusion or left pleural cap
- Deviation of the trachea or a nasogastric tube to the right
- Depression of the left main stem bronchus
- Separation of a calcified aortic plaque from the edge of the aortic shadow of more than 5 mm
- Clouding of the aortopulmonary window

TREATMENT In general, these patients need advanced care and transfer to a thoracic surgeon. To stablilize the patient

- Keep the BP below 140/90 mm Hg (do not overresuscitate with fluid).
- Have at least 8 to 10 units of blood available.

DIAGNOSIS AND MANAGEMENT OF OTHER SERIOUS CHEST INJURIES

The following injuries can be diagnosed during the secondary examination, but should be treated immediately. Do not wait until the secondary examination is completed.

PULMONARY CONTUSION Pulmonary contusion is a common serious chest injury. Often patients have minimum symptoms and findings, and the contusion seen on a chest radiograph.

HISTORY AND PHYSICAL EXAMINATION Patients may present after a traumatic event with

- Mild to moderate respiratory distress
- Hemoptysis
- Slightly decreased breath sounds
- Dullness on percussion
- Hypoxemia

DIAGNOSIS A patchy, fluffy infiltrate appearance is noted on the chest radiograph, often associated with rib fractures.

TREATMENT Most pulmonary contusions resolve well with conservative treatment. Treat with oxygen, pulmonary toilet, restriction of fluids (if the patient is not in shock), and bronchodilators if the patient is wheezing. Be warned that up to 50% of patients develop pneumonia.

TRACHEOBRONCHIAL DISRUPTION Tracheobronchial disruption is associated with an extremely high mortality rate and requires emergent surgery and specialized equipment. It can be diagnosed by a persistent, large air leak in a chest tube that is placed for the pneumothorax. Most of these patients also have a large amount of subcutaneous air.

TREATMENT

- Place a second chest tube to stabilize for surgery.
- Essentially all patients need to be intubated.
- The definitive treatment is bronchoscopy or thoracotomy and surgical repair of the lacerated bronchus.

ESOPHAGEAL RUPTURE Esophageal rupture is most common with penetrating trauma but can occur from blunt trauma. Signs of this are dysphagia, a deep aching chest pain, subcutaneous or mediastinal air, and occasionally pneumothorax with a pleural effusion. It can cause a severe infection. A gastrograffin swallow or esophagoscopy should be performed to confirm the diagnosis.

TREATMENT

- A chest tube should be placed on the affected side to drain the infection.
- Broad-spectrum IV antibiotics
- Emergent surgical repair is indicated

DIAPHRAGMATIC DISRUPTION OR RUPTURE An uncommon, difficult to diagnose, and serious injury, diaphragmatic disruption or rupture should be suspected if the chest radiograph shows elevation or indistinctness of one hemidiaphragm or a basilar infiltrate on the affected side or if there are loops of bowel, stomach, or an NG tube in the chest.

TREATMENT Surgical repair is indicated.

MYOCARDIAL CONTUSION Myocardial contusion is an uncommon chest injury with a usually good prognosis. It is difficult to diagnose without monitoring and special equipment. Suspect myocardial contusion if a patient with chest injuries develops premature ventricular contractions, premature atrial contractions, has inverted T-waves, or elevated ST segments on their ECG.

TREATMENT Cardiac monitoring may be needed to identify arrhythmias. Administer lidocaine if the patient has ventricular arrhythmias. Careful fluid and dobutamine administration should be undertaken for hypotension.

DIAGNOSIS AND MANAGEMENT OF LESS SERIOUS CHEST INJURIES

These injuries can be treated either during the secondary survey, or after it. Some may be associated with other significant or underlying injuries.

SIMPLE RIB FRACTURES Rib fracture is the most common result of significant chest trauma (>50% cases). There is an increased risk for penetrating injury to the pleura, lung, liver, and spleen, especially with 9th to 11th rib fractures. Pneumonia from lack of deep breathing is a common preventable complication.

PHYSICAL EXAMINATION Tenderness, crepitus, ecchymosis, and local muscle spasm will be observed at the fracture site.

DIAGNOSIS Multiple rib x-rays are not indicated with suspected single mid-chest rib fractures, but may be indicated under the following circumstances:

- Suspected fractures of ribs 1, 2, or 9 to 12
- Suspected multiple rib fractures
- Elderly patient

TREATMENT

- Pain control for as long as 1–2 weeks
- Encourage deep respirations. After the patient takes the prescribed pain medications, have them hold a blanket against the affected side and then cough at least three to four times a day.

- Rib belts, tape, and binders are contraindicated. They restrict breathing.
- For multiple rib fractures you can attempt an intercostal nerve block with long-acting anesthetic.

OTHER INJURIES Simple pneumothorax or small hemothorax is a common chest injury. Patients may be asymptotic except for chest pain and mild dyspnea. Treat with simple aspiration or by chest tube.

A sternoclavicular dislocation can represent a serious injury if there is posterior displacement of the clavicular head, but there are usually no complications. With posterior displacement only, grasp the clavicular head with a towel clip and pull upward. An anterior sternoclavicular dislocation can be treated just with pain medications and a sling on the arm on the affected side.

A sternal fracture is not usually associated with myocardial contusion. It can be diagnosed by palpation or on the lateral chest radiograph. Treat only with pain medications. If there is marked inward displacement of the sternum, then surgical treatment may be required.

Clavicle fractures can usually be treated simply with a figure-of-eight soft bandage or a sling. Operative treatment is required only if there is an open fracture.

Scapular fractures may accompany other traumatic injuries. They usually heal well because they are completely surrounded by muscle. They usually do not require surgery unless involving the glenoid surface. They can usually be treated with pain medications and a sling only.

Traumatic asphyxia is caused by diffuse compression of the chest (such as being run over by a car). Signs of this are subcutaneous hemorrhages, petechiae, retinal hemorrhages, and facial edema. Unless other serious chest injuries are present, it usually does not require treatment but pain control.

Chest wall contusions (where the chest film does not show any rib fractures) are treated the same as rib fractures (pain medications only). The patient should be advised that this type of injury might be painful for an extended period (2 weeks to 3 months).

PROCEDURES FOR CHEST TRAUMA

TUBE THORACOSTOMY (CHEST TUBE PLACEMENT) Placement of a chest tube is indicated if there is tension pneumothorax, massive hemothorax, suspected tracheobronchial disruption, or suspected esophageal rupture. A small pneumothorax may be managed by aspiration and observation, unless the patient will undergo surgery under general anesthesia. Tubes are placed in the fifth or sixth interspace in the mid-axillary line. For trauma, adults require a 36 to 40 French tube and children a 16 to 32 French tube, depending on their size.

The insertion procedure for tube thoracostomy involves the following steps (Fig. 14-7). The preferred site is usually the fifth or sixth intercostal space in the mid-axillary line.

1. Prepare the side of the chest with iodine and apply sterile drapes.
2. Inject local anesthetic in the skin and intercostal muscle.

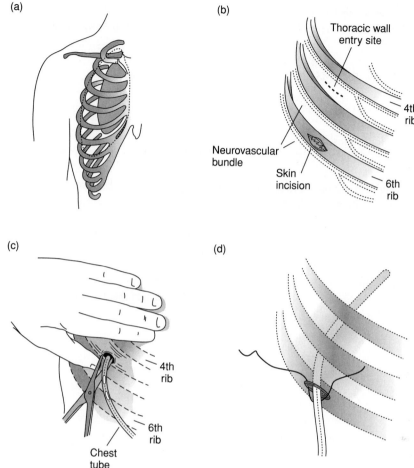

FIGURE 14-7 Chest tube insertion.

3. Make an approximately 2-cm long skin incision parallel to the rib.
4. With a large clamp tunnel up over the superior rib with a blunt clamp.
5. Incise the intracostal muscles above the rib.
6. Push the clamp forcefully (but carefully) to enter the pleural space.
7. Do a finger sweep in the pleural space to make sure the lung is not adherent to the opening in the pleura.
8. Place the thoracostomy tube into the pleural space using your finger as a guide.
9. Slide the tube posterior and superior to deep enough so that all ports are intrathoracic.
10. Suture the tube in place with heavy suture (000 silk or nylon).

11. Attach to water seal suction (Fig. 14-8).
12. Always check the tube position afterward by chest radiography to confirm proper placement.

PERICARDIOCENTESIS Ideally this is done with continuous cardiac monitoring.

1. Prepare the anterior and left chest around the xiphoid with iodine and drape with sterile drapes.
2. Consider local anesthesia.
3. Attach an ECG V-lead to the procedure needle. Watch the monitor for ST segment elevation.
4. Use a long catheter over a needle or a Seldinger placement technique.
5. Insert the needle just to the left of and below the xiphoid while aiming toward the tip of the left scapula.
6. Gently pull back on the syringe as the needle advances.
7. Stop advancing once you get blood return in the syringe or see an ST segment elevation on the ECG monitor (this signifies ventricular wall contact).
8. Slide the catheter off the needle and gently aspirate the fluid from the pericardial space. Attach a closed stopcock to the catheter so that recurrent aspiration can be performed if necessary.

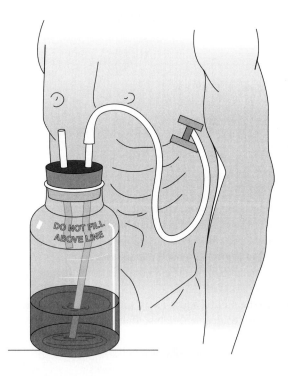

FIGURE 14-8 A basic water seal device.

9. The patient's BP should improve almost immediately.
10. Obtain a chest radiograph to look for a pneumothorax or other complication.

ABDOMINAL TRAUMA

Abdominal injuries account for 10% of all trauma deaths. Up to 30% of patients with major blunt abdominal trauma and 15% of those with gunshot wounds die. There is a progressive decline in mortality with more rapid transport for definitive treatment of abdominal injuries.

The etiology of abdominal trauma is categorized as either blunt or penetrating. The approach to each is different. In blunt trauma the most commonly injured organs (in order of frequency) are the spleen, liver, small bowel, and kidney. In penetrating trauma it is the liver, small bowel, stomach, and large bowel.

> **KEY POINT:**
>
> Multiple, repeated examinations are essential for the evaluation of abdominal trauma, especially for patients with altered mentation (drugs, alcohol, head, or other injuries).

The diagnostic and treatment priorities for abdominal trauma are as follows:

1. Address the ABCs.
2. Rule out external bleeding and chest trauma as the cause of shock.
3. Determine if the abdomen is the source for shock.
4. Determine if emergency laparotomy (surgical exploration and repair) is needed.
5. Complete the secondary survey and laboratory and radiographic studies to determine if an occult abdominal injury is present.
6. Conduct frequent reexaminations.

If an intraabdominal injury is suspected (or known), the patient almost always requires surgery, or at least intensive monitoring. Transfer or consult a surgeon as soon as possible.

HISTORY

The following historical points should be addressed:

■ Type or mechanism of injury
■ Time of injury
■ Associated injuries

- Prior abdominal problems or surgeries
- Drug or alcohol use
- Current medications and allergies

Important symptoms include the following:

- Lightheadedness implies hypotension.
- Shoulder pain (the Kerr sign) suggests hemoperitoneum, probably from a liver or splenic injury.

PHYSICAL EXAMINATION

The physical examination for the patient with abdominal trauma is part of the secondary survey and includes detailed abdominal, genital, pelvic, and rectal examinations, and careful assessment of the patient's back after log-rolling. The initial physical examination is only about 65% accurate. The physical examination is made even more unreliable in the presence of an altered level of consciousness or neurologic examination. Serial examinations increase the accuracy.

When performing a physical examination, check the following:

- Abdominal examination
  Look for abrasions, lacerations, ecchymosis, distention.
  Palpate for tenderness, guarding, masses, and crepitus. If there is tenderness, particularly if it is persistent over multiple examinations, then advanced diagnostic studies are needed.
  Auscultation: Absent bowel sounds may signify an ileus from an injury or bleeding. High-pitched sounds may signify bowel obstruction. Some vascular injuries might cause an audible bruit. Bowel sounds noted in the chest also might imply a ruptured diaphragm.
  Percussion: Tympany implies an ileus or bowel obstruction, dullness an intraabdominal bleed or fluid.
- The bony pelvis should be assessed for stability by placing hands on both iliac crests and compressing.
- GU examination: Inspect for blood at the urethral meatus, or for perineal/scrotal hematomas.
- Rectal: Check for prostate position (always prior to urethral catheterization), anal sphincter tone, tenderness/masses/lacerations, or blood in the stool.
- Vaginal examination for gross blood or tears with pelvic trauma.

Important additional physical findings include the following:

- Periumbilical ecchymosis (the Cullen sign) implies retroperitoneal bleeding.
- Flank ecchymosis (the Gray-Turner sign) implies retroperitoneal bleeding.

■ Lower rib fractures affect the spleen in 20% of left-sided injuries and the liver in 10% of right-sided injuries.

DIAGNOSIS

Laboratory studies may be useful to give some clues about the presence of an intraabdominal injury, but they are not very accurate, and a normal laboratory test does not exclude an abdominal injury.

■ Type and cross-match is the only essential laboratory study.
■ Complete blood count: The hematocrit usually changes late with acute blood loss, so is not a reliable indicator. The white blood cell count usually increases to 12,000 to 20,000 following severe trauma.
■ Amylase and liver function studies are not good indicators.

RADIOGRAPHIC EVALUATION

Initial radiographs to consider for the abdominal trauma patient when available include the following:

■ AP view of the pelvis for pelvic fractures
■ AP and lateral films of the lumbar spine if spinal tenderness or neurologic findings are present
■ Flat and upright films of the abdomen can be obtained if free air or bowel obstruction are suspected, but such films are of limited utility, leading to actual operative decisions in fewer than 5% of cases. Upright and chest radiographs are essential because the finding of free air is significant. The patient must sit up for 10 to 15 minutes prior to radiography.

ADVANCED DIAGNOSTIC STUDIES TO RULE OUT INTRAABDOMINAL INJURIES

Because of the unreliability of the physical examination, laboratory studies, and plain radiographs, advanced tests are often needed to identify the presence of intraabdominal injuries. These tests include ultrasonography, DPL, and CT scans. If these tests yield positive results, the patient almost always requires surgical repair. Therefore, before these tests are undertaken, a surgeon should be present, or at least immediately available. The indications for advanced diagnostic studies in blunt trauma patients include the following:

■ Abdominal tenderness
■ Unreliable examination (altered mental status, distracting injury)

- Unexplained hypotension
- Concomitant spinal cord injury
- Patients undergoing general anesthesia for other injuries (orthopedic, neurosurgical, etc.)

ULTRASONOGRAPHY Ultrasonography is a quick, accurate, and noninvasive procedure that detects free intraabdominal fluid and organ disruption. It is easily repeated multiple times to follow the patient's course. It is not very accurate for obese patients or for those with stab wounds to the abdomen. Four views are generally used:

- Morrison pouch (hepatorenal)
- Douglas pouch (rectopelvic)
- Left upper quadrant (spleen)
- Epigastric (pericardium)

DIAGNOSTIC PERITONEAL LAVAGE Diagnostic peritoneal lavage should not be performed without the immediate availability of surgery. It would generally be better to transfer a patient for their advanced studies than to perform DPL without surgery available (Fig. 14-9). DPL is particularly useful for penetrating trauma from a stab wound with no peritoneal signs, suspected diaphragm rupture, and penetrating trauma to the chest below the nipple or to the flank or back. It is relatively contraindicated for patients who have had a previous laparotomy (the chance of hitting bowel with the DPL needle or catheter is much higher) and for late-term pregnancy (use the supraumbilical approach if possible). There are three basic DPL techniques:

- Closed using the Seldinger needle technique (a catheter is threaded over a wire) with no surgical dissection
- Open using an incision and surgical dissection through the posterior fascia and then directly placing a plastic catheter into the abdomen
- Semiopen using an incision and dissection to the posterior rectus fascia, then using a needle to punch through.

Prior to performing DPL:

- Place a NG tube and suction to decompress the stomach and bowel.
- Place a urethral catheter to decompress the bladder.
- Check the upright abdominal films for free air (if present, the patient needs surgery, not DPL).

The procedure for closed (percutaneous) DPL should proceed as follows:

- Prepare the abdominal skin with iodine, and drape sterilely.
- Inject local anesthesia at the puncture site in the midline 1 to 2 cm below the umbilicus.
- Make a small skin incision with a no. 11 knife blade.

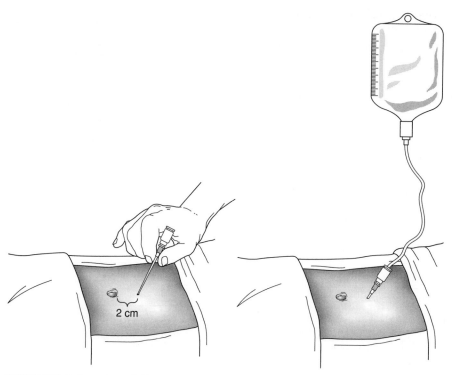

FIGURE 14-9 Location of diagnostic peritoneal lavage.

- Gently insert an 18-gauge needle at a slight angle downward toward the pelvis.
- Advance the needle till a second "pop" is felt as the needle penetrates the posterior rectus fascia and peritoneum.
- Insert the guidewire through the needle and withdraw the needle.
- Advance the catheter over the guidewire.
- Remove the guidewire.
- Pull back on the catheter with a syringe. If more than 10 mL of blood returns, the DPL is positive; call the surgeon and dress the wound (Table 14-4).
- If no blood is drawn back, attach the IV tubing and run in 1 L of normal saline or lactated Ringer's solution for an adult or 20 mL/kg for a child.
- After the fluid is in, lower the IV bag and tubing below the level of the patient and allow the fluid to run back out. The fluid should be sent for red cell and white cell counts, microscopic examination, and if possible for amylase and Gram staining. After the fluid stops returning, the catheter should be withdrawn and the small skin wound closed with a suture.

LOCAL EXPLORATION OF STAB WOUNDS Stab wounds can be locally explored by extending the wound under sterile conditions. The goal is to make sure that the wound

TABLE 14-4 POSITIVE DIAGNOSTIC PERITONEAL LAVAGE

	BLUNT TRAUMA	PENETRATING TRAUMA
Gross blood	≥10 mL	≥10 mL
Red blood cells (per mm³)	≥100,000	≥5,000 (90% sensitive for diaphragmatic penetration in low chest wounds)
		≥10,000 in evaluating flank, tangential, or low thoracic gunshot wound
White blood cells³	≥500	≥500
Feces	Any	Any
Bacteria (Gram's stain)	Any	Any
Bile	Any	Any
Vegetable fibers	Any	Any
Alkaline phosphatase	≥3 IU/L	≥3 IU/L
Amylase (IU/L)	Unknown	≥20 for small bowel perforation

Another positive indicator is lavage fluid originating in the chest tube, nasogastric tube, or urethral catheter.

does not penetrate the posterior fascia. This procedure can prevent up to 50% to 75% of unnecessary surgery.

The procedure should proceed as follows:

- Prepare and drape the wound.
- Inject local anesthetic (epinephrine) widely around the wound.
- Explore the stab wound tract gently and bluntly (finger, clamp, or cotton swab) to define its direction and depth.
- Slowly dissect down along the tract to the fascia, then dissect the tissue away from the fascia widely to ensure it is intact. If it is intact, you are done and the patient is cleared. If not
- Incise through the anterior fascia and bluntly dissect through the muscle to the posterior fascia to repeat the process.

This approach is useful for field management. It is still safest to admit the patient for serial examinations under the care of a surgeon to ensure that peritonitis does not develop.

TREATMENT

Any patient who has sustained significant trauma should be admitted for serial observations to ensure they remain stable and do not have any hidden chest or abdominal injuries.

Emergent (immediate) laparotomy is indicated for hypotension associated with penetrating injury or for uncorrectable and unexplainable (by other sources) hypotension with blunt trauma. Other indications for laparotomy include the following:

- Positive ultrasonographic, DPL, or CT results
- Essentially all abdominal gunshot wounds
- A deeply impaled foreign object
- Evisceration (exposed bowel)
- Signs of peritoneal irritation (peritonitis)
- Radiographic findings of pneumoperitoneum, retroperitoneal air, or interruption of diaphragmatic integrity, or cystography revealing interruption of bladder integrity
- Blood in the rectum after penetrating or blunt injury
- Blood from the stomach via the NG tube
- Positive local wound exploration (posterior fascia violated)

Antibiotics should be administered to patients with penetrating abdominal trauma:

- Ampicillin plus an antianaerobic antibiotic such as metronidazole or clindamycin, or
- A second-generation cephalosporin such as cefoxitin

Tetanus toxoid also should be administered for the usual criteria, and the patient should be treated with pain medications once the diagnostic tests are completed.

GENITOURINARY TRAUMA

The GU system is scattered all over the abdomen, mostly in the retroperitoneal area. It is therefore commonly injured, particularly with penetrating trauma.

The sequence of evaluation for GU trauma should include the following:

1. Perform a physical examination to include the flank, pelvis, external genitalia, peritoneum, and rectum and vagina.
2. Decide if there are any initial contraindications to passing a urethral catheter (as listed below).
3. If there are no contraindications, pass the urethral catheter.
4. If there are contraindications, then perform retrograde urethrography if available, and pass the catheter if there is no urethral lesion.
5. Consider performing cystography or IV contrast CT if available for delineation of other GU tract injuries.
6. Consider placement of a suprapubic catheter if urethral disruption exists.

A penetrating wound to the flank, pelvis, abdomen, or genitalia is also high risk for GU trauma.

PHYSICAL FINDINGS THAT RAISE SUSPICION OF A GENITOURINARY INJURY

- Lower abdominal or suprapubic tenderness
- Signs of a pelvic fracture (pain with compression of the pelvis or pubic symphysis)
- Ecchymosis in the perineum, scrotum, or penis (late finding)
- Abnormal prostate examination
- Vaginal laceration (if blunt trauma, look for a pelvic fracture)
- Blood at the urethral meatus
- Gross hematuria after urethral catheter placement
- Decreased urine output

The severity and site of GU trauma are not correlated with the amount of blood noted in the urine. Gross hematuria can sometimes occur from mild injuries, and there may be no hematuria with other types of severe injuries.

DIAGNOSIS

A urethral catheter can be diagnostic and therapeutic for GU trauma, but it is also contraindicated in some situations. In such situations, retrograde urethrography should be performed:

- Blood at the urethral meatus
- A penetrating injury in the vicinity of the urethra
- A high-riding or nonpalpable prostate on rectal examination
- A butterfly-shaped perineal hematoma
- A major scrotal hematoma

RETROGRADE URETHROGRAPHY

- Draw up 30 to 35 mL of 10% to 20% Conray or Renografin dye in a syringe.
- Place a small 12 to 14 French urethral catheter or tubing adapter on the end of the syringe.
- Place the end of the urethral catheter or adapter just into the urethral meatus. Slightly inflate the balloon if you are using the catheter.
- Stretch the penis superiorly and obliquely to eliminate urethral folding.
- Inject 20 to 30 mL while squeezing the tip of the penis to prevent extravasation of the dye. Have an assistant expose the radiographic film as most of the dye goes in.

If retrograde urethrography shows a urethral disruption, you should consult a urologist. Do not place a urethral catheter; instead, place a suprapubic catheter or tap the bladder (after skin preparation) with a small needle and syringe.

CYSTOGRAPHY (BLADDER RADIOGRAPHY)

- Verify that the urethra is intact by retrograde urethrography first.
- Place the urethral catheter into the bladder and inflate the balloon.
- Inject 100 to 200 mL of Conray or Renografin and clamp the catheter.
- Shoot one film.
- If no extravasation is noted, inject additional dye to a total of 300 mL and clamp the catheter.
- Shoot a second film.
- Unclamp the catheter. Drain the bladder, and shoot a third film, which is the postvoid film.

SPECIFIC GENITOURINARY INJURIES

EXTERNAL GENITALIA INJURIES For scrotal trauma it is important to rule out testicular torsion. This diagnosis should be suspected if the patient had any major discomfort with attempted rotation of either testicle. A ruptured capsule requires surgical repair. If there is any penetrating trauma to the scrotum, antibiotics will be needed.

For labial and vaginal introitus trauma, very shallow lacerations do not need suture repair. Deeper mucosal lacerations should be repaired with absorbable sutures and treated with antibiotics.

If the trauma originates from a sexual assault, then it is important to arrange counseling and crisis intervention for the patient and to notify the police and collect evidence. If possible, run gonococcal and chlamydial cultures, HIV antibody assay, and a Venereal Disease Research Laboratory (VDRL) test. Venereal disease prophylaxis and pregnancy prophylaxis also should be considered.

URETHRAL INJURY Urethral injuries are generally diagnosed by retrograde urethrography. If the injury is posterior to the urogenital diaphragm, the patient should be treated with a suprapubic catheter and delayed surgical repair. Injuries that are anterior to the urogenital diaphragm and only partial or noncircumferential can be treated with prolonged placement of a urethral catheter. Large anterior tears need to be treated with surgery with drains and a stented repair.

BLADDER INJURY Bladder injuries are generally diagnosed either by cystography or abdominal CT.

- Extraperitoneal rupture: requires placement of a suprapubic catheter, supravesicle, and antibiotics
- Intraperitoneal rupture: surgical repair at laparotomy and placement of a suprapubic catheter

URETERAL INJURIES Ureteral injuries are most common with retroperitoneal penetrating injuries and rare with blunt trauma. Most require surgery with suture repair over a stent.

RENAL INJURY Renal injuries can be classed into five groups based on the findings of CT or IVP:

1. Class I cortical contusion
2. Class II cortical laceration
3. Class III calyceal laceration
4. Class IV complete renal fracture
5. Class V vascular pedicle injury

TREATMENT

Types I through III often can be treated conservatively and do not require surgery. Some class IV injuries can be treated nonoperatively, but some of these require nephrectomy. For class V injuries, often the kidney is unsalvageable and nephrectomy is required.

PEDIATRIC TRAUMA

The primary resuscitation of an injured child follows the same ABCs as with general resuscitation. See Chapter 10 for a detailed description of the pediatric ABCs. Some of the unique considerations in assessing pediatric trauma patients are listed as follows:

- The heads of children are disproportionately larger than the heads of adults, and more prone to injury (resulting in airway and breathing compromise).
- Children have a less calcified skeleton, so often there may be internal damage without overlying bone fractures.
- The liver, spleen, bladder, and kidneys of children are less protected and therefore more prone to injury than those of adults.

ABC TRAUMA SPECIFICS

AIRWAY The high proportion of head injuries leads to frequent loss of airway function. Always focus the primary resuscitation on the airway first. Do not hesitate to intubate an injured child with altered mental status, which usually results from a head injury, not from hypotension.

- Do not tilt the head; use the jaw thrust maneuver and bag the child as needed.
- Intubate as recommended in Chapter 10 (keep the head and neck immobilized).

BREATHING The differential diagnosis and treatment for breathing emergencies is the same as for adults (see earlier section on Chest Trauma). Remember to correct breathing problems during the primary surveys.

CIRCULATION Assess and treat circulatory problems as recommended in Chapter 10. Children are able to compensate extremely well for blood loss with tachycardia and can maintain their BP until they "crash" and become severely hypotensive. The normal blood volume of the child is about 80 mL/kg or 8% of body weight. Rapid IV access is essential for trauma resuscitation—either peripheral, central, or intraosseous is acceptable. Emergent transfusion with 10 mL/kg of packed red cells should be performed if the patient does not respond quickly to multiple boluses of 20 mL/kg of lactated Ringer's solution or normal saline, or if blood loss is ongoing.

> **KEY POINT:**
>
> The initial fluid bolus in children is 20 mL/kg of lactated Ringer's solution or normal saline.

Signs of correction of shock in the pediatric trauma patient are listed as follows:

- The heart rate slows to less than 120 beats/min.
- The pulse pressure increases to more than 20 mm Hg.
- The limbs become warmer or less mottled.
- Mental status and behavior improve.
- Urinary output increases to more than 1 mL/kg/h.
- BP increases to more than 80 mm Hg systolic.

DISABILITY

Cervical spine injuries are relatively less frequent than in adults, but brain injuries are more common. Both require aggressive management. Do not move the child's head until you have radiographic confirmation that there is no neck injury.

It is usually easier to assess a child's mental status by using the AVPU system to measure their alertness: A = alert, V = responds to verbal, P = responds to pain, U = unresponsive. As with adults, frequent measurements are needed to identify changes.

EXPOSURE

Children get cold quickly—they have a higher body surface area. Prevention of hypothermia in the injured child is extremely important. Hypothermia can cause decreased mental status, hypotension, arrhythmias, coagulopathy, and ineffectiveness of administered medications.

- Keep the resuscitation room warm. Use heating lamps, blankets, and warm IV fluids.
- Cover the child after the secondary survey (but uncover the chest intermittently to reassess breathing).

THE SECONDARY SURVEY

The secondary survey is conducted in a head-to-toe format, as for adults.

SPECIFIC INJURY CONSIDERATIONS IN PEDIATRIC PATIENTS

HEAD INJURY Head injury occurs in 60% to 80% of major blunt trauma in children and causes 80% of all pediatric trauma deaths. However, 6% of cases require surgical intervention, compared with 30% for adults. Diffuse cerebral edema is more common, and focal intracranial hemorrhages are less common than in adults. As with adults, the goal is to prevent secondary brain cell death from hypoxia and hypotension.

> **KEY POINT:**
>
> The key treatment for major head injury in children is to maintain the BP and prevent hypoxia.

Hypotension is rarely due to intracranial bleeding, with the exception that some infants become hypotensive from blood loss into the epidural or subgaleal space. A bulging fontanelle in a baby may signify severe head injury and almost always is an indication to perform a CT scan of the head. Vomiting after head injury in children is common and does not always indicate a significant intracranial injury.

NECK INJURY Children occasionally can have cervical spinal cord injuries that are not detected on radiography. If a child has neurologic symptoms or physical findings, do not move the head, even if the radiographs look normal.

Children cannot communicate the presence of neck pain well, so you should maintain a low threshold to obtain cervical spine films in young pediatric trauma victims. Some unique cervical spine radiographic findings in young children are listed as follows:

- Pseudosubluxation of C2 on C3 or C3 on C4, where the anterior longitudinal line is offset but the line at the base of the spinous processes is not. This represents a normal finding and does not represent any type of neck injury.
- The predental space can be wider than in an adult; up to 5 mm is normal.
- The spinous process epiphysis can appear to be a fracture.

CHEST INJURY Children's chests are much more flexible than adults; therefore, rib fractures result from a greater force to the chest and are commonly associated with severe pulmonary contusions. Blunt aortic injuries in children are less common than in adults, but can still occur in severe trauma.

ABDOMINAL INJURY To assess abdominal injuries in children, the diagnostic and treatment priorities are basically the same as for adults.

There are some additional psychological considerations for the pediatric trauma victim. You should routinely explain procedures to children and be honest about the potential for pain or discomfort from these. You should treat their pain early once your examination is complete, and you should try to address any fears that the child expresses. If the parents are calm and cooperative, you should allow them to comfort the child after resuscitation.

CHILD ABUSE

Child abuse or child battering is a deliberate injury inflicted by a child's caretaker. It is a global problem that encompasses physical, psychological, and sexual abuse. It is extremely important to recognize child abuse because you may be able to save the child from what would be a fatal future injury. Signs of physical abuse include the following:

- The history is not consistent with the severity or type of injury.
- There is a delay between the time of injury and time of care seeking.
- A history of multiple prior injuries
- The history of injury differs between the caretaker and the child.
- The caretaker reaction is inappropriate for the situation.
- The child appears afraid of the caretaker.

The following physical findings indicated possible child abuse:

- Bruises to lower back, buttocks, ears, or handprints to face are suggestive.
- Bruises in different stages of development and in areas not over the bony prominences
- Unexplained spiral fractures
- Look for retinal hemorrhages and the "shaken baby" syndrome
- Glove-stocking patterns of burns are probably inflicted by dipping a child into hot water.
- Sharply demarcated burns
- Perioral, perineal, anal, or genital injuries
- Bizarre injuries such as cigarette burns, bites, or belt or rope marks

The following radiographic findings indicate possible child abuse:

- Multiple fractures in different stages of healing
- Multiple rib fractures
- "Bucket-handle" injuries, metaphyseal chip fractures at the end of long bones from rotary forces, and spiral fractures of long bones

If child abuse is suspected from either the history, examination, or radiographic features, the child should have multiple radiographs to rule out bony injuries to other unsuspected areas (a skeletal survey).

TREATMENT There are no simple solutions to the problem of child abuse, and there are many cultural complexities to the issue. The solution to child abuse involves long-term measures, but some actions can be taken immediately:

■ Remove the child to a safe place if possible (admit to the hospital for protection even if the injuries would not normally require admission).
■ Work with the local authorities if they are responsive to child abuse and there are enforceable laws protecting children.
■ Work to educate families about appropriate discipline.
■ Educate the population about child abuse.

PEDIATRIC TRAUMA SUMMARY

■ Care for the pediatric victim of trauma should follow the same priorities as for adults.
■ Vital signs should be interpreted carefully.
■ Fluid boluses and medications should be adjusted to the patient's weight.
■ Prevent hypothermia.
■ Pay attention early to psychological considerations for the child.
■ Be alert for child abuse as a cause for children's injuries.

TRAUMA IN PREGNANCY

The diagnostic and treatment priorities for injured pregnant patients are the same as for all other patients. However, there is another life and some significant physiologic changes with pregnancy to consider. The treatment of the mother takes precedence over treatment directed to the fetus, because the fetus's best chance of survival is with the successful resuscitation of the mother. Even minor trauma during pregnancy involves a 4% to 10% fetal complication rate, such as placental abruption, premature labor, and premature rupture of the membranes.

> **CRITICAL ACTION:**
>
> Treatment of the mother takes precedence over treatment for the fetus.

Standard trauma priorities include

- The ABCDEs: evaluate and treat emergency conditions.
- Secondary survey
- Deciding if radiographic or laboratory studies is needed
- Providing definitive trauma management

In late pregnancy, numerous physiologic, anatomic, and laboratory value changes occur that have relevance to trauma care.

PHYSIOLOGIC CHANGES

- Increased cardiac output
- Increased heart rate (normal is 100–105 beats/min).
- BP is slightly decreased in the second trimester, but normal in the third trimester.
- Blood volume is increased up to 50%.
- Increased respiratory rate and tidal volume
- Prolonged gastric emptying
- A tendency toward gastroesophageal reflux
- Relative venous hypertension in the legs

ANATOMIC CHANGES

- The uterus enlarges to displace and somewhat compress the large and small bowel.
- When the patient lies supine, the uterus also can compress the inferior vena cava.
- The synthesis pubis widens.
- The sacroiliac joints widen.

LABORATORY VALUE CHANGES

- The white blood cell count typically increases to 13,000 to 18,000.
- The hemoglobin and hematocrit levels decrease by about 10% due to hemodilution.
- The PCO_2 decreases to 30 to 36 mm Hg.

The duration of the pregnancy can be roughly estimated from the size of the uterus (Table 14-5).

The injured pregnant patient should undergo the same primary and secondary surveys as for other trauma patients. There are additional examinations that must be performed on the pregnant patient.

TABLE 14-5 ESTIMATING GESTATIONAL AGE
BY THE ABDOMINAL EXAMINATION

UTERINE SIZE	GESTATIONAL AGE
Enlarged on pelvic examination	8 w
Pelvic brim	12 w
Umbilicus	20 w
Above umbilicus	1 cm per week over 20 wk

ADDITIONS TO THE PRIMARY SURVEY

- The most important alteration of the primary survey is that as part of the circulation evaluation, compression of the vena cava by the uterus must be avoided (it can cause serious hypotension). If there is no potential for spinal injury, then the patient could be placed in the left lateral decubitus position. If necessary, the entire backboard can be tilted to the left with the patient still immobilized on it.
- Uterine blood flow decreases earlier than maternal hypotension, so the fetus can be in shock before the mother is. Therefore, early, aggressive fluid treatment is important for pregnant trauma patients. Vasopressors should generally be avoided because they reduce uterine blood flow.

KEY POINT:

Hypotension in the pregnant patient can be a sign of vena caval compression by the uterus—safely move the patient to her left side.

ADDITIONS TO THE SECONDARY SURVEY

- The abdominal examination should include measuring the fundal height, listening for fetal heart tones (with a stethoscope or via Doppler sonography), palpating for fetal movement, assessing for uterine contractions and irritability, and assessing the fetal position.
- Consider performing a pelvic examination, including a speculum examination. However, if the patient is known to have or suspected of having a placenta previa (this might be manifest by painless, bright red bleeding in the third trimester), then a speculum or digital vaginal examination is contraindicated.
- When performing DPL, use the supraumbilical approach to avoid the uterus.
- The risk of fetal radiation exposure from plain radiographs is extremely small, and radiographs should be performed if indicated. Remember the health of the fetus is dependent on the treatment of the mother.

ADDITIONAL STUDIES

- Abdominal ultrasonography is an extremely valuable examination for injured pregnant women to assess the uterus and fetus for trauma.
- Continuous fetal heart monitoring helps to identify fetal distress. The heart rate and its relationship to uterine contractions should be followed for at least 4 hours and up to 24 hours. Signs of fetal distress that should be monitored include
  Bradycardia with a heart rate of less than 110 beats/min
  Tachycardia with a heart rate more than 160 beats/min
  Late decelerations
  Loss of beat-to-beat variability
- Count the number of uterine contractions per hour. More than eight uterine contractions per hour means that there is a 10% rate of adverse pregnancy outcome. If there are less than eight uterine contractions per hour during the first 4 hours, there is no increased risk of adverse outcome.

Additional criteria for admitting pregnant trauma patients include the following:

- Any vaginal bleeding
- Any uterine contractions or uterine irritability
- Any abdominal pain, tenderness, or cramps
- Hypovolemia
- Changes in fetal heart rate or other evidence for potential fetal distress
- Any leakage of amniotic fluid

Unique complications of trauma in pregnancy include the following:

- Rh isoimmunization can occur in Rh-negative mothers if their blood is exposed to fetal blood cells. If this is suspected, patients should receive Rh immunoglobulin (Rhogam) 300 μg intramuscularly within 72 hours of the trauma event.
- Amniotic fluid embolism can occur from blunt trauma and may manifest as disseminated intravascular coagulation, severe bleeding, or shock. Treatment involves emergent cesarean section.
- Abruptio placenta is the separation of the wall of the placenta from the uterus, resulting in bleeding. It is a leading cause of fetal death after blunt trauma to the abdomen. This may manifest by dark red vaginal bleeding associated with uterine tenderness, uterine rigidity, or maternal shock. Ultrasonography is the best test to determine if an abruptio placenta is present.

GUNSHOT AND LAND MINE EXPLOSION INJURIES

Gunshots and land mine injuries are a frequent cause of mortality and morbidity in a number of countries. Explosions from buried land mines are a major problem in much of southeast Asia, Afghanistan, the Balkans, and central and southern Africa. The smaller types of land mines typically cause severe injuries limited to the feet, but the medium to larger land mines can cause injuries to multiple extremities, as well as death.

BALLISTICS

The damage caused by a bullet is more dependent on the velocity of the bullet than its size. Handguns are generally low velocity, whereas rifles (particularly military weapons such as the AK-47 and the M-16) are high velocity. The kinetic energy of a bullet when it strikes the victim is turned into heat, vibration, mechanical, and vacuum forces, and these cause tissue damage. High-velocity bullets cause damage from cavitation and shock waves, as well as the direct damage for its mass. This effect can rupture blood vessels, nerves, and even bone. This cavitation effect is why high-velocity bullets are so damaging and cause such high fatality rates.

HISTORY

The most important history is to determine the type of weapon, at least if it was a pistol or rifle. This gives an indication of the size and velocity of the bullet. Other important information includes the following:

- Range and direction of the shooter
- Number of shots fired
- Patient's tetanus immunization status
- Presence of allergies to antibiotics
- Other concurrent trauma (such as spine trauma from a fall that occurred as a result of the gunshot injury)

TREATMENT

The treatment priorities in the emergent management of the gunshot wound victims are as follows:

- The ABCs of resuscitation
- Hemorrhage control
- High-flow oxygen
- Obtaining IV access and starting IV fluid resuscitation
- Type and cross-match for blood if available
- Neurovascular examination

■ Using radiographs to locate the bullet (generally both AP and lateral films should be obtained to locate the bullet)

Definitive treatment for gunshot wounds involves careful wound exploration of the gunshot wound and removal of any embedded foreign bodies such as clothing. Bullets are not sterile, so all bullet wounds should be considered grossly contaminated. Some low-velocity wounds may be safely closed primarily with suture. High-velocity wounds should not be surgically closed but should be debrided and have a delayed closure. Antibiotics should be used for almost all cases, and generally a first-generation cephalosporin is appropriate.

SPECIFIC INJURIES

For extremity wounds, assess pulses frequently and maintain high level of suspicion for compartment syndrome. Signs of compartment syndrome are listed as follows:

■ Pain
■ Pallor
■ Paresthesia
■ Paralysis
■ Pulselessness (late)

HEAD WOUNDS If possible, intracranial debris and bullet fragments should be surgically removed. Usually bullets that enter one side of the head, and cross to the opposite side cause nonsurvivable injuries. Gunshot wounds to the eye are usually not salvageable, and enucleation should be performed to prevent sympathetic ophthalmia from developing in the other eye.

For maxillofacial gunshot wounds, primary closure for hemorrhage control may be necessary. The patient may require early tracheostomy, as well as ligation of the external carotid artery to control bleeding. Some of these patients have concurrent cervical spine trauma and should be assessed for this.

NECK All gunshot wounds of the neck should be surgically explored. If the carotid artery is injured and there is no neurologic deficit, then carotid artery repair should be undertaken. However, if there is a complete preexistent neurologic deficit from a carotid injury, then generally the carotid artery should be ligated. If the jugular vein is injured, it is important to prevent air embolism. It is also important to verify that the esophagus is uninjured either through direct surgical exploration or use of esophagoscopy or gastrograffin swallow where available.

CHEST Most gunshot wounds to the thorax require treatment with a thoracostomy tube alone. Thoracotomy should be performed, however, for major degrees of blood loss, major air leak, suspected cardiac tamponade, or esophageal injury as detailed earlier in the section on Chest Injury.

ABDOMEN Generally all gunshot wounds of the abdomen, even if they are tangential, should be treated with exploratory laparotomy. Often the only preoperative test needed is a so-called "one shot" IV pyelogram to assess the ureters for injury.

PREVENTION

- Teach children to stay away from guns.
- Keep guns locked safely up, and keep the ammunition stored separately.
- Mine safety programs are essential for areas with land mines.

CHAPTER 15

Orthopedic Trauma

C. James Holliman

Orthopedic injuries or bony injuries are among the most common presenting problems to the rural or urban health center, dispensary, or hospital. Correct initial management of these injuries is even more important in cases where the patient will be unable to obtain specialist follow-up care. After initial treatment (reduction and stabilization) by the emergency care provider, many of the injuries described in this chapter should have follow-up care with an orthopedic specialist if available.

The objectives of this chapter are for the reader to identify life- or limb-threatening extremity injuries, prioritize management of extremity injuries in relation to other injuries, determine whether extremity injuries require surgical management, and manage simple fractures, dislocations, and soft tissue injuries.

CRITICAL ACTIONS

The following critical actions should be undertaken for extremity injuries:

- Stop external hemorrhage.
- Assess for vascular and nerve damage.
- Recognize life- and limb-threatening injuries.
- Treat injuries, close wounds as necessary.
- Reduce fractures and immobilize the extremity.

ASSESSMENT

Extremity injuries should be quickly assessed to determine if they are life or limb threatening. Life-threatening extremity injuries are those with active bleeding from major vessels, severe crush injuries, severe open fractures, amputation, and multiple limb fractures. Limb-threatening extremity injuries are arterial injury or occlusion, compartment syndrome, open fracture, limited crush injury, and joint dislocation.

The general management of extremity injuries as part of the primary survey is to control hemorrhage with direct pressure dressings. As part of the secondary survey, assess the neurovascular status of each limb. Identify all potential sites of fractures/dislocations. Apply splints, especially to potentially unstable injuries. Identify all soft tissue wounds. Decide on the radiographic films needed. As part of final definitive management, perform relocation or fracture reduction via closed or surgical techniques, and repair the wounds.

Ask the patient about the time of the injury, the mechanism of injury, if any dislocation was already reduced, prior limb injuries or problems, estimated blood loss at the scene, allergies and current medications, and tetanus immunization status.

Physical examination of each limb should include inspection for deformity, swelling, ecchymosis, and skin wounds. Palpate the entire length of the limb for tenderness and crepitus. Assess the distal pulses, capillary refill, sensation, motor strength, and active range of motion (ROM) of joints (don't perform passive ROM if there is a possible fracture or dislocation). Assess tendon function and integrity.

EVALUATE FOR ASSOCIATED INJURIES

Common associated injury patterns include a fracture of one of a pair of long bones with dislocation of the other paired bone. A femur fracture may have an associated hip dislocation. A calcaneus fracture from a jump or fall injury may have an associated lumbar spine compression fracture. An ankle fracture may be associated with high fibular fracture. It is important to evaluate the joint above and below the injury by examination and radiography.

OPEN (COMPOUND) FRACTURES

Open (compound) fractures represent communication of skin wound and bone fracture site. The patient is at risk for development of osteomyelitis and soft tissue infection. Be suspicious if there is any skin wound in the vicinity of a fracture. Most need to be treated (irrigated, debrided, and fracture fixed) in the operating room. All patients should receive intravenous (IV) antistaphylococcal antibiotics and should be referred for surgical treatment.

Potential signs of arterial injury include a nonpalpable pulse (but presence of a pulse does not exclude major vascular injury). Suspect arterial injury with unexplained pain (perhaps out of proportion to the apparent injury), decreased pulse, capillary refill of greater than 3 seconds, loss of nerve function, duskiness of the limb, and decreased motor function.

Dislocations commonly associated with vascular injuries are those of the knee with injury to the popliteal artery, of the elbow with injury to the brachial artery, of the hip with ischemia of the femoral head, and of the ankle with injury to the dorsalis pedis or posterior tibial arteries. Displaced long bone fractures also may injure the adjacent artery. Emergent reduction of these dislocations may be needed to restore perfusion to the distal extremity.

TO X-RAY OR NOT TO X-RAY

Physical examination alone cannot accurately predict the presence or absence of an extremity fracture. However, in the field setting, there is often not ready access to radiographic equipment. Many extremity injuries can be treated as fractures by splinting and will heal well without reduction or surgery. You should obtain radiographs for patients with the following injuries:

- Deformity of the injury site
- Large swelling and bruising over the site
- Altered vascular status (decreased pulses or capillary refill)
- Decreased motor function
- Possible embedded foreign body

COMPARTMENT SYNDROME

Compartment syndrome is increased tissue pressure within muscle compartments, usually as a result of a severe crush injury, fracture, gunshot wound, circumferential burn, or arterial injury. Untreated, compartment syndrome can lead to decreased perfusion and tissue death. The signs are swelling and pain (especially with passive stretch of the muscle of the involved compartment), and the patient may have weakness, paralysis, tenderness, and decreased distal capillary refill (same signs as for possible arterial injury).

The best method to confirm the diagnosis of compartment syndrome is to measure the muscle compartment pressure directly with a needle or wick catheter apparatus. A pressure of greater than 30 mm Hg implies the need for emergent fasciotomy (surgical release of fascia to decrease compartment pressure). A pressure measuring device may not be available, and the diagnosis of compartment syndrome is made on the basis of clinical examination.

FASCIOTOMY

In the event of a crush injury, you may be the only health-care provider, and time is of the essence. Delay will lead to tissue ischemia, loss of limb, and possibly death. If the patient has the physical findings for compartment syndrome, emergency fasciotomy is required. Perform emergent fasciotomy for treatment of compartment syndrome as follows:

- Provide general or regional anesthesia; ketamine is a good alternative.
- Surgically prepare the site.
- Make the surgical incision longitudinally through the skin and muscle fascia.
- Pack gently with saline dressings.
- Keep the wound clean, properly hydrate the patient, and maintain good urine output (below) and transfer, if necessary, for definitive surgical management and eventual wound closure.

An additional danger with major crush injuries (and from compartment syndromes) is rhabdomyolysis and resultant renal failure from the hemoglobin and myoglobin released into the circulation and filtered out by the kidneys. Acute rhabdomyolysis can be diagnosed by elevated serum creatinine phosphokinase (CPK) or the presence of urine myoglobin. A simple test is a urinalysis to detect blood in the urine with few accompanying red cells. This may indicate the presence of myoglobin. Urine is typically a red-brown color.

If muscle destruction and myoglobinuria is suspected, use aggressive rehydration to prevent renal damage. Use IV fluid resuscitation to generate urine output of more than 50 mL/h (2 mL/kg/h in children). Give IV bicarbonate ($NaHCO_3$) (50 mEq boluses, or one ampule in each bag of IV fluid) or mannitol (1 g/kg IV), which may assist in establishing urine flow.

TRAUMATIC AMPUTATIONS

The first priority in caring for an amputated limb is to stop the hemorrhage with a pressure dressing to the stump. Save the amputated part and place it in a sealed plastic bag on iced saline (do not freeze). Decide if reimplantation is possible. You will need to consult with a surgeon. Do not promise reimplantation to the patient (the surgeon may decide that it is not possible). Give antibiotics, tetanus immunization, and pain medication.

Contraindications to reimplantation of amputated limbs are preexistent medical conditions causing inability to tolerate prolonged general anesthesia, finger amputation distal to the distal interphalangeal (DIP) joint crease, warm ischemia time of greater than 4 hours, or a mangled or crushed wound (usually should be a sharply incised wound for reimplantation to succeed).

FRACTURE CLASSIFICATION

It is important to be able to describe a fracture, because the characteristics of the fracture impacts the treatment plan. The parameters for fracture description and classification are listed as follows (Figs. 15-1 and 15-2):

- Closed: a fracture with no disruption of overlying skin
- Open: disruption of overlying skin and wound contamination
- Single: one localized fracture
- Comminuted: more than one bone fragment at the fracture site
- Location: location along length of bone may be proximal, distal, mid-shaft, or intraarticular.
- Orientation: transverse, oblique, spiral, greenstick (break of cortex on just one side), torus (cortex buckling without discontinuity), or segmental (two parallel fractures in same bone)

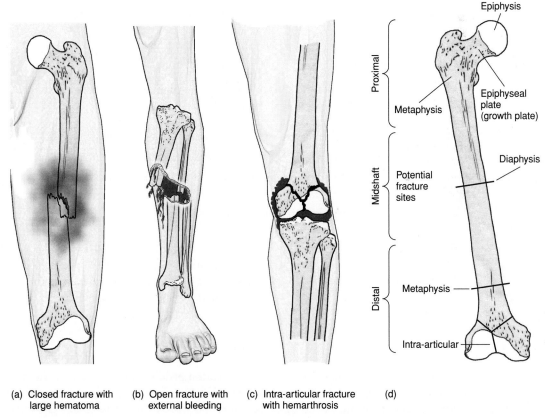

(a) Closed fracture with large hematoma

(b) Open fracture with external bleeding

(c) Intra-articular fracture with hemarthrosis

(d)

FIGURE 15-1 Open and closed fracture sites. A: Closed fracture with large hematoma. B: Open fracture with external bleeding. C: Intra-articular fracture with hemarthrosis. D: Potential fracture sites.

Fracture patterns

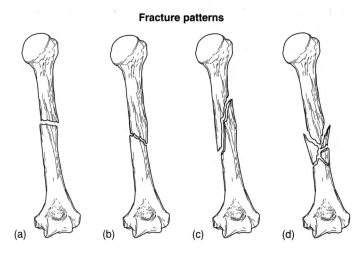

(a)   (b)   (c)   (d)

FIGURE 15-2
Fracture patterns.
A: Transverse.
B: Oblique.
C: Spiral.
D: Comminuted.

- Displacement: extent to which the ends are offset (express as millimeters of displacement or percentage of width of shaft)
- Shortening: overlap of the ends of the bones (in millimeters or centimeters)
- Impaction: jamming together of bone ends
- Angulation: degree and direction of deformity
- Growth plate disturbance: In children, a fracture through the growth plate (epiphyseal plate) may lead to growth impairment; this is described by the Salter-Harris classification.

PRINCIPLES OF SPLINTING AND CASTING

The purpose of casting is to create a comfortable form of immobilization to allow the fracture to heal (Fig. 15-3). Without immobilization, a fracture will not heal, leading to disability and loss of function. The most versatile casting material is plaster. You can mold plaster to fit, creating a durable, cheap, light form of immobilization.

CASTING

Prepare the fracture site by wrapping it with cotton padding (Webril) next to the skin, so that the plaster is not in direct contact with skin. You should usually overlap each "roll loop" by 50%. Use extra padding on bony prominences. Using strips of soft cloth may be an alternative.

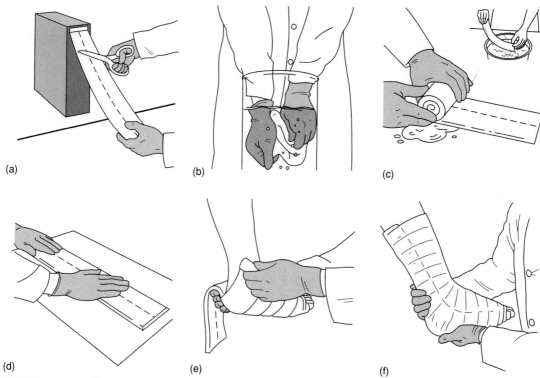

FIGURE 15-3 Application of plaster. A: Measure appropriate length. (Note that plain plaster slabs shrink a few inches when wet. Measure the length slightly longer because the excess may be folded back on itself if necessary.) B: Submerge until bubbles stop (do not oversoak). C: Roll and squeeze excess water from the premade splint. Inset: If using plain plaster slabs, allow the water to drip off. D: Smooth the sheets to remove wrinkles, and mix the plaster throughout the layers. E: Apply the splint and secure it with an elastic bandage. F: Mold the splint to fit the contour of the extremity—a very important step. (Specialist J-splint. Drawings courtesy of Johnson & Johnson Products, New Brunswick, NJ.)

Choose the size of plaster roll (available in 1-inch- to 6-inch-wide rolls). Usually 2-inch- to 3-inch-wide rolls are good for the hand, and 4-inch- to 6-inch-wide rolls are better overlying the long bones. Dunk the plaster roll in the water bucket, and hold under water until bubbling stops. Knead the roll somewhat while in the water, squeeze out excess water, and start roller application. Hot water causes plaster splints to set faster and is not recommended. Warm water is better for plaster casts because they require more molding and surface preparation. Wear gloves, and put down splash barriers.

For the second and subsequent layers, be sure to knead each layer so it bonds into the layers below. You can roll back the end of Webril after the first plaster layer applied in order to create a nice padded edge. Don't leave any unpadded plaster against the skin.

You usually need at least six (often eight) plaster roll layers for adequate strength. After allowing the initial plaster to set, try to indent the splint with finger pressure. If it indents, then it needs more plaster layers. Be sure to leave nailbeds and distal digits exposed to allow capillary refill assessment. The patient should not put any pressure on the splint for at least 1 to 2 hours.

An option for extremity splints is to use prepadded plaster rolls (just cut to proper length and soak the whole splint to set). Another option is to unroll a plaster roll into several flat layers and place on top of Webril. Either type should be finally molded and held in place with elastic (Ace) wrap.

SPLINTING

Splinting of suspected fractures should be done as part of the secondary survey and should precede moving the patient (for radiography, etc.). Splinting is important for reducing pain. It also may lessen blood loss, especially for femur fractures splinted with a traction splint. You should always reassess distal circulation after a splint is applied. Remove and adjust the splint if the patient complains of increased pain, numbness, or if there is possible circulatory compromise. Keep fingers and toes exposed to check for proper circulation. Examples of plaster splints are shown in Figures 15-4 to 15-9.

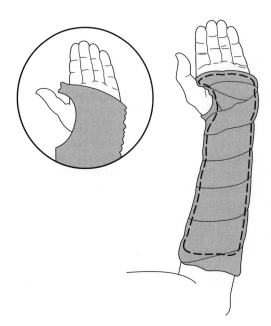

FIGURE 15-4 The volar forearm splint extends from the distal metacarpals to the proximal forearm and allows the thumb and fingers to remain free. For fractures an additional dorsal slab may be used to create a bivalve splint. The wrist is placed in slight (10–20 degree) extension. A thumb spica is added to immobilize a navicular fracture. (Reprinted from Howes DS, Kaufman JJ. Plaster splints: techniques and indications. *Am Fam Physician* 1984;30:215; with permission.)

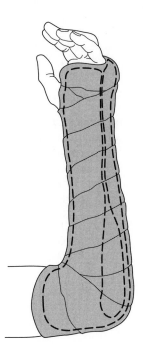

FIGURE 15-5 The sugar-tong forearm splint immobilizes the forearm and wrist and eliminates pronation or supination. The elbow is positioned in a 90 degree angle, and the forearm is in a neutral (thumb up) position. The splint extends to the distal metacarpals (volar and palmar), and the thumb and fingers have normal movement. (Reprinted from Howes DS, Kaufman JJ. Plaster splints: techniques and indications. *Am Fam Physician* 1984;30:215; with permission.)

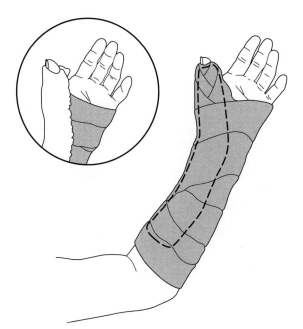

FIGURE 15-6 The thumb spica (gutter) splint extends from the thumbnail to the mid-forearm. The thumb is held in abduction with 4-inch plaster. (From Howes DS, Kaufman JJ. Plaster splints: techniques and indications. *Am Fam Physician* 1984;30:215; with permission.)

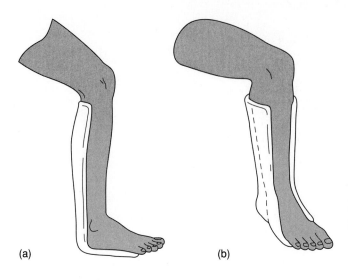

(a)   (b)

FIGURE 15-7 The short leg posterior splint is used alone or in conjunction with a stirrup splint. (Specialist J-splint. Drawing courtesy of Johnson & Johnson Products, New Brunswick, NJ.)

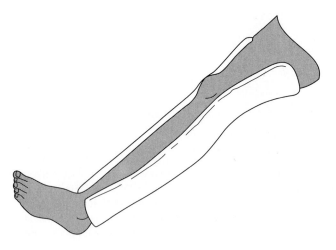

FIGURE 15-8 Posterior gutter. The knee is immobilized with either a long leg posterior gutter splint or parallel lateral slabs from the proximal thigh to the distal leg. Many prefer to use the easily removable Velcro knee immobilizer as an alternative. (Specialist J-splint. Drawing courtesy of Johnson & Johnson, New Brunswick, NJ.)

(a)

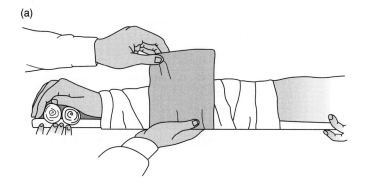

(b)

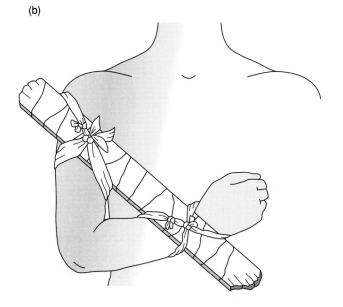

FIGURE 15-9
Methods for temporary splinting in the field.

If a cast is placed too tightly, or a patient complains of increased pain and numbness or diminished circulation, the cast may need to be split. You can use a rotary cast cutter to remove or split casts. The blade vibrates back and forth (not circular spin motion) so it will not cut the skin unless held down too hard. Incise the cast longitudinally along its entire length down to Webril, then spread with a cast spreader. You may need to incise on the opposite side longitudinally to fully release the cast.

HAND INJURIES

EXAMINING AN INJURED HAND

Hand injuries can result in significant loss of function if they are not treated properly, so it is important to perform a thorough examination of the injured hand. Check the position of the fingers at rest and their alignment when flexed to diagnose tendon injuries or angulated fractures. Look for overlapping fingers. Common hand injuries include a fifth metacarpal fracture (Boxer fracture). Be sure to reduce broken digits or metacarpal bones prior to immobilization.

TENDON INJURIES

Tendon injuries can lead to permanent loss of function unless properly repaired. Suspect tendon injuries in penetrating hand injuries, lacerations, or severe hand trauma. Examine the hand for tendon function before repairing a hand laceration. In general, extensor tendon lacerations can be repaired and splinted. Flexor tendon injuries are more likely to heal poorly and may need specialized surgical repair.

FINGER (PHALANGEAL) INJURIES

Fingertip skin avulsions can usually be treated with nonadherent dressing (if bone is not exposed) and allowed to heal by granulating in. For lacerations of the nailbed, do a digital block, remove the nail, repair the nailbed with fine absorbable sutures, and replace the nail to maintain nail fold edges.

Blood under the nail from trauma (subungual hematoma) can be very painful. Relieve the pressure by draining the blood with a needle. Drill through the nail (just twist back and forth an 18 gauge needle against the nail till a hole is drilled through the nail and the blood is released).

Skier's thumb or gamekeeper's thumb (injury to the thumb ulnar collateral ligament) should be suspected if there is decreased thumb abduction strength. Treat the patient with either a thumb spica cast or surgical repair of the ligament.

Finger dislocations (proximal interphalangeal or DIP joints) are usually easily reducible with traction after digital block (Fig. 15-10). Check ROM, then apply a padded dorsal splint. Mallet finger injury (disruption of the insertion of the extensor tendon on the distal phalanx) should be treated with a DIP extension splint for 6 weeks.

Injury to the more proximal extensor tendon can result in a boutonniere deformity. If this central slip extensor tendon disruption is suspected, the patient should be treated with a finger splint for 4 weeks. Paint or grease gun injection injury to the hand is a surgical emergency. It requires surgical debridement in the operating room.

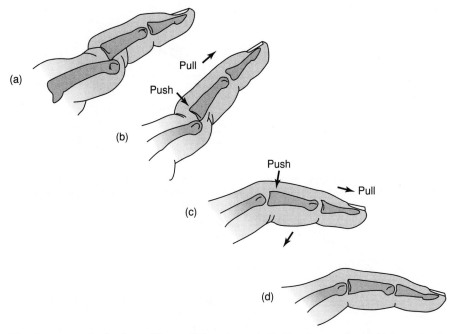

FIGURE 15-10 Reduction of finger dislocations. A–D: Traction method of joint reduction. Complete anesthesia using a regional block should precede reduction attempts. Exaggeration of existing deformity method. First exaggerate the deformity that is present, then to steady traction, push the joint back into position. (Reprinted from Carter P, ed. *Common hand injuries and infections.* Philadelphia: WB Saunders, 1983:109, 110; with permission.)

PERFORMING A DIGITAL BLOCK

Prepare both sides of the finger (or toe) with iodine or alcohol (Fig. 15-11). Inject a small bleb of 1% or 2% lidocaine (without epinephrine) just beneath the skin surface toward the volar side of the finger. Insert the needle until the phalanx is contacted. Back the needle out 1 to 2 mm and then inject 1 mL lidocaine (this should be in the vicinity of the digital nerve). Back the needle out further and then angle the needle upward and inject a subcutaneous lidocaine bleb across half of the dorsum of the digit. Repeat the procedure for the other side of the digit. If properly placed, you should not have to wait for anesthetic effect. Place a loop tourniquet (rubber tubing or unrolled 4 × 4 gauze) around the base of the digit to help hold the lidocaine in place and prolong the duration of the anesthesia. Remove the tourniquet after completion of suturing or fracture reduction.

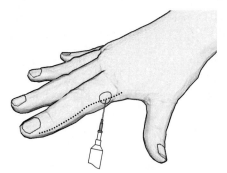

1. Inject small skin bleb just above web space crease (dots show path of digital nerve).

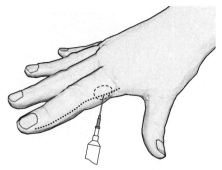

2. Inject 1cc of local anesthetic next to phalanx (in the vicinity of the digital nerve).

3. Back needle out to just beneath the skin surface and then inject a subcutaneous bleb across the dorsum of the finger (this anesthetizes the small dorsal sensory nerve).

4. Repeat same 3-step procedure on the other side of the finger to anesthetize the other digital nerve.

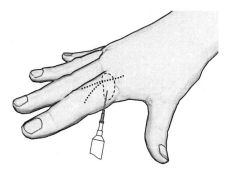

5. Apply tourniquet around base of finger at the metacarpal head to hold the anesthetic in place.

FIGURE 15-11 Digital anesthetic block.

WRIST INJURIES

If there is any tenderness over the anatomic snuffbox, treat as a possible scaphoid fracture, even if the first radiograph is negative, and place a thumb spica splint or cast. Repeat radiography in 7 to 10 days to try to detect demineralization at the fracture site. If the second radiograph is also negative, treat as a wrist sprain. On the anteroposterior (AP) radiograph of the wrist, the spaces between the wrist bones should be narrow and equal. If there is widening of the scapholunate joint, you should immobilize it in a short arm cast. If there is any angulated, displaced, or overriding wrist or forearm fracture, make sure the x-ray films cover both elbow and wrist.

Radial and ulnar fractures can be associated with dislocations of the accompanying bone. Suspect this type of injury in a patient with wrist and elbow pain after trauma. A Galeazzi fracture is a fracture of the radius and dislocation of the distal ulna. A Monteggia fracture is a fracture of the ulna and dislocation of the proximal radius. Use a lateral wrist film to assess for lunate or perilunate dislocations. These often can be reduced by pulling on the hand and pushing directly over the displaced lunate.

A common wrist injury is the Colles fracture (fracture of the distal radius with dorsal displacement of the distal fracture fragments) from falling on an outstretched hand. These injuries should be reduced with local or regional anesthesia. Traction on the hand with volarly directed digital pressure usually leads to successful reduction (Fig. 15-12). A sugar-tong forearm splint or short arm cast should then be applied for immobilization.

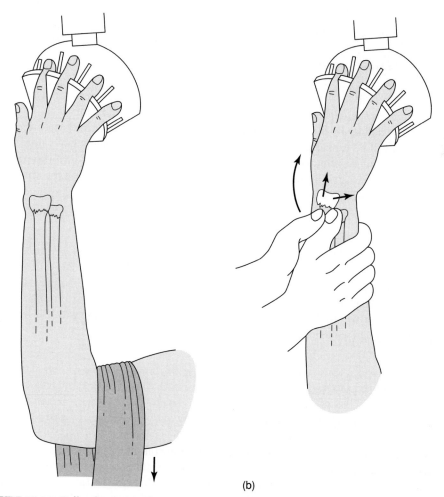

(a)   (b)

FIGURE 15-12 Colles fracture reduction. A: Place hand in fingertraps and apply longitudinal pressure to the humerus. B: Apply digital pressure (after anesthesia) over the distal radius to reduce the fracture.

ELBOW INJURIES

ELBOW FRACTURES

Elbow fractures may present with no evidence of bone fracture on radiography, but more subtle signs may indicate a fracture. If a patient is tender to supination and pronation (check by shaking hands with the patient, then twist the hand back and forth), suspect a radial fracture. Even if the radiograph is negative, check the lateral film for fat pad signs. The anterior fat pad will be bowed forward (sail sign) and the posterior fat pad will appear (not seen normally) if an intraarticular fracture has occurred.

NURSEMAID'S ELBOW

Nursemaid's elbow is a radial head dislocation in a child under 4 years of age. Suspect this with any vague pain or decreased use of the limb. A typical history is that a parent pulls the child up by the hand, causing traction at the elbow. The child will protect the arm and will be unwilling to move it. The radiograph of the elbow looks normal. To reduce, extend the arm, then flex and supinate (turn the palms upward while flexing the elbow). Often a "click" of relocation is felt. Once the child starts moving the arm again, no further treatment is needed.

ELBOW DISLOCATIONS

For elbow dislocation (humeroulnar dislocation), check for vascular injury (brachial artery) by frequently checking the radial pulse. Usually sedation is required before reduction is attempted (see Chapter 18). Reduce by traction in-line with the humerus followed by elbow flexion (Fig. 15-13).

SHOULDER INJURIES

ROTATOR CUFF INJURIES

A common injury from a fall on the shoulder or arm is a tear of the rotator cuff muscles. The radiograph of a shoulder with a rotator cuff injury appears normal. The best and most subtle diagnostic test for a rotator cuff muscle tear is decreased strength of abduction against resistance with the arm at 10 to 20 degrees abduction. Rotator cuff tears often can be treated with a sling and progression of ROM. Occasionally, surgery is indicated.

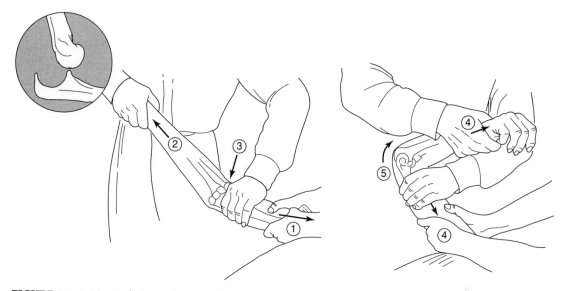

FIGURE 15-13 Manipulative reduction of posterior elbow dislocation (the olecranon is posterior to the humerus). While an assistant holds the arm and makes steady countertraction (1), grasp the wrist with one hand, and apply steady traction on the forearm in the position in which it lies (2). While traction is maintained, correct any lateral displacement with the other hand (3). While traction is maintained (4), gently flex the forearm (5). Note that with reduction, a click is usually felt and heard as the olecranon engages the articular surface of the humerus. (Reprinted from DePalma AF. *Management of fractures and dislocations: an atlas.* Philadelphia: WB Saunders, 1970: 793, 794; with permission.)

ACROMIOCLAVICULAR SEPARATION

Acromioclavicular (AC) separation (dislocation) presents as pain and swelling over the AC joint, usually from a direct fall on the shoulder. AC separation is categorized by three degrees. The first degree shows tenderness and swelling over the AC joint, but the shoulder radiograph is normal. In the second degree, the radiograph shows partial congruity of the clavicle and the acromion (clavicle is "popped-up" part way). In the third degree, the radiograph shows no AC joint congruity (end of clavicle is completely above the acromion). Treat all three types just with a sling and pain medications.

CLAVICLE (COLLAR BONE) FRACTURES

Clavicle fractures present with pain and swelling over the clavicle. If closed, treat with a sling and pain medications.

GLENOHUMERAL DISLOCATIONS

Shoulder (glenohumeral) dislocations are best diagnosed on scapular Y-view radiographs. The most common type are anterior dislocations. These can be reduced using the two-person traction-countertraction technique. If traction is applied gradually, usually you do not need to use sedation. After reducing the dislocation, treat by sling or by shoulder immobilizer for 6 weeks. Posterior dislocations may be caused by grand mal seizures and are reduced using the same technique as for anterior dislocations. Humerus fractures often can be treated with a sugar-tong or posterior arm splint, but may require surgery if displaced, involving the glenoid, or associated with radial nerve injury. A scapular fracture can be associated with other major chest injuries. If it is isolated, just treat with a sling and pain medications. The patient may need surgical fixation if the glenoid surface is displaced.

HIP AND FEMUR INJURIES

Hip fractures are common among elderly patients who fall or experience trauma. Most commonly, patients cannot walk, although the ability to walk does not rule out a hip fracture. Hip fractures are classified as subcapital, femoral neck, intertrochanteric, subtrochanteric, and trochanteric (avulsion). Almost all require surgical fixation. In children, hip injury pain may be referred to the knee and vice versa. A hip dislocation should always be reduced as quickly as possible (the longer the dislocation is unreduced, the greater the chance of ischemic necrosis of the femoral head). These always require general anesthesia for reduction. Most femoral shaft fractures will require surgery. Blood loss even from closed femoral shaft fractures can be enough to cause shock. Field treatment of femoral fractures is splinting, fluid resuscitation, and consultation with an orthopedic surgeon.

KNEE AND LEG INJURIES

Knee injuries are common. They are typically due to tendon or ligamentous injuries, but may indicate a fracture. For the knee examination, look for swelling, joint effusion, and tenderness. After knee examination and ligament assessment, obtain knee radiographs. Knee sprains in which there is not instability of the joint can be treated with a knee immobilizer or brace for 1 to 4 weeks. Ambulation on non–weight-bearing crutches for 3 to 7 days also is helpful. Unstable knee ligament injuries should be referred to an orthopedist.

Patellar dislocation can usually be reduced with just passive full extension of the knee (or lateral pressure on the patella) (Fig. 15-14). Knee (tibiofemoral) dislocation represents a true emergency. The knee is usually unstable. Check the neurovascular status of the limb. Apply a splint early and seek orthopedic assistance.

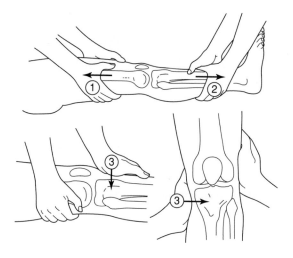

FIGURE 15-14 Manipulative reduction of a knee dislocation. 1: An assistant fixes and provides countertraction on the thigh. 2: Another assistant provides straight traction on the leg (this usually reduces the dislocation). 3: The physician puts direct pressure over the displaced bones. (Reprinted from DePalma AF. *Management of fractures and dislocations: an atlas.* Philadelphia: WB Saunders, 1970:1623; with permission.)

An acute knee joint effusion can be caused by a variety of problems. If the effusion is from trauma, the joint usually should not be tapped acutely because you may introduce infection. If the joint is red and warm with pain during ROM without trauma, the joint should be tapped to rule out the possibility of infection versus inflammation.

ANKLE INJURIES

The most common ankle injury is a sprain of the anterior talofibular ligament, with pain and swelling below the lateral malleolus. Ankle sprains should be treated with a firm brace (such as Air Cast brand) or firm taping with adhesive tape. Elastic (Ace) wrap only is an insufficient treatment. Crutches for 2 to 3 days also may be helpful.

In children under 12 years of age, pain and tenderness over the lateral malleolus may represent a fracture to the growth plate of the distal fibula. Although the radiograph may be normal, you should suspect a possible fracture and treat with a walking cast for 3 to 4 weeks.

Ankle dislocations are unusual, and may need emergent reduction to restore arterial circulation to the foot.

TOE INJURIES

Toe fractures and dislocations generally can be treated the same as finger injuries. If a toe is swollen after an injury but there is no deformity and joint motion is okay, then often radiography is not necessary. The patient could be treated by presumptively buddy-taping the toe to the adjacent toe and wearing a hard-soled shoe (Fig. 15-15)

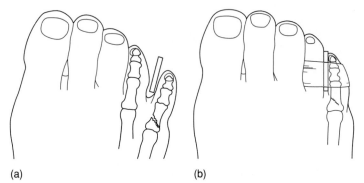

(a)   (b)

FIGURE 15-15 Buddy-taping of a fractured toe. A: The injured toe is folded toward an adjacent noninjured toe after placement of a soft corn pad between the toes. B: The toes are held together with an adherent wrap placed around both digits. (Courtesy of Kenneth R Walker, S.P.M.)

LUMBAR OR THORACIC SPINE FRACTURES

Suspect lumbar or thoracic fractures in severe direct trauma (i.e., from motor vehicle injuries) or jumping type falls. In all patients with a possible spinal fracture, keep them immobilized until you are able to examine the neurologic status and obtain radiographs. If there is any neurologic deficit, you should obtain emergent consult with a spine surgeon. Maintain back immobilization. If spinal cord injury is suspected, treat with methylprednisolone 30 mg/kg (if <8 hours from the time of injury), and emergently consult a spine surgeon.

PELVIC TRAUMA

Pelvic injuries often represent multisystem injuries. Sixty percent of pelvic fractures are due to vehicle accidents, 30% are due to falls. Immediate problems associated with pelvic trauma are massive hemorrhage, bony disruption of the pelvis, urologic injury, bowel and vaginal tears or perforations, and neurologic injury. Massive hemorrhage is the major cause of death from pelvic fracture. The degree of hemorrhage is dependent on the fracture type, and is truly massive in large posterior fractures.

To examine the pelvis, grasp the iliac crests on the supine patient and rock back and forth, checking for pain and instability. Examine the genital area by "milking" along the urethra. If there is blood at the urethral meatus, suspect a disruption of the urethra and do not pass a Foley catheter. Obtain a urethrogram and cystogram. The AP radiograph view of the pelvis shows most fractures, although other views may be helpful, such as inlet, outlet, and tangential views. Stable pelvic fractures may be treated by pain medication and rest. Unstable pelvic fractures usually require surgical fixation. Acetabular fractures may be associated with posterior hip dislocation. They often require surgery to prevent severe arthritis of the hip joint.

Coccygeal fractures are usually caused by a fall in a sitting position. They may also be caused by childbirth. Treatment of these involves analgesics, stool softeners, and a sacral pad to sit on.

SUMMARY

Bony injury may be associated with other life-threatening injuries. As always, check the ABCs. Stop hemorrhage as part of the primary survey. Identify all potential limb injury sites on the secondary survey, and radiograph all suspected fracture sites. Splint suspected and confirmed fractures. Rapidly assess and treat suspected vascular injuries or compartment syndrome. Decide if definitive repair should be performed in the emergency department or in the operating room, or transfer the patient to a higher level of care if needed. Arrange appropriate follow-up with an orthopedic specialist for most fractures and dislocations.

CHAPTER 16

Wound Management

C. James Holliman

The proper management of wounds in the field setting is one of the most basic and important practices, and yet is overlooked by many health providers. The objectives of wound care and repair are to lessen pain, prevent infection, enhance healing, and achieve the best cosmetic results. This chapter discusses the management of various wounds and how to promote healing through proper wound management.

EVALUATION OF WOUNDS

As discussed in prior chapters, the most important first step in any injured patient is to evaluate the ABCs. It is not unusual for a health-care worker to be distracted by a severe extremity injury and ignore the potentially disastrous occurrence of airway compromise or shock. After stabilizing the patient, the critical actions for wound management are as follows:

- Stop active bleeding.
- Identify injuries.
- Decide on type of repair needed.
- Consider tetanus immunization.
- Consider antibiotics.
- Provide instructions to patient.

TYPES OF WOUNDS: ABRASIONS, LACERATIONS, AVULSIONS, AND THERMAL INJURIES

- Abrasion: a surface injury to the epidermis only
- Superficial laceration: a short length break in epidermis
- Deep laceration: penetrates to dermis or deeper tissues
- Complex laceration: irregular edges (nonlinear) and involves deeper structures
- Skin avulsion: the complete removal of epidermal and/or dermal tissue
- Crush injury: compression to the tissue causing significant destruction
- Burns: thermal or chemical coagulation of the epidermis and dermis
- Frostbite: freezing injury to the epidermis and dermis
- Infected wound: wound with an established microbial invasion of tissue and local cellulitis
- Abscess: purulent collection under the skin with localized induration

STEPS IN WOUND EVALUATION, PREPARATION, AND CLOSURE

- Stop active bleeding.
- Adequately expose the wound area.
- Anesthetize the wound if indicated.
- Clean the wound and debride as necessary.
- Close the wound if indicated.

STOP THE BLEEDING

Bleeding from most external wounds can almost always be controlled with direct pressure. Simply place a dressing over the bleeding wound and hold firm, constant pressure to the area until the bleeding is controlled. If bleeding continues, such as with an arterial injury, it may be necessary to apply a tourniquet or a blood pressure cuff above the injury and temporarily cut off arterial circulation. This may be safely done for up to 15 minutes at a time, until you can either ligate or repair arterial bleeding.

EXPOSURE

Be sure to expose the entire wound so that you can see all margins and injuries. This may seem like obvious advice, but often wounds to the scalp or hard-to-reach areas may be difficult to adequately expose. Consider removing hair to expose the field, but usually this is not needed (the hair can just be slicked down with water, Betadine, or K-Y jelly). Shaving increases wound infection rates. Never shave an eyebrow (it might not grow back).

REMOVE FOREIGN BODIES

Most foreign bodies may be removed by simple extraction. Occasionally, extension of the wound is necessary for greater exposure. Often, a small foreign body such as a splinter or a piece of metal is too deeply imbedded and is best left in the tissue. Such is the case with bullet wounds, which usually heal well if there is no nerve or artery injury. Leave deeply imbedded objects in place for removal in the operating room if you suspect nerve or artery damage.

If faced with the problem of how to remove an imbedded fishhook, there are three techniques. First, try local anesthesia, then simply pull the hook out (suitable only if small barb hook), or insert an 18-gauge needle to cover the barb, and back the needle and hook out together. Alternatively, punch the barb through the skin, and then cut the barb off with wire cutters, and then back the shank out.

WOUND CLEANSING

Clean the wound thoroughly, clearing dirt and debris away with saline or sterile water, and then irrigate the wound. For irrigation, an 18- or 19-gauge needle and a 20- to 30-mL syringe provide the best irrigation pressure (Fig. 16-1). The best cleaning agent is sterile saline because it is cheap and isotonic; however, it is not bactericidal. Normal saline with iodine (2–3 cc's iodine per liter) is perhaps the best choice. It is bactericidal but not tissue toxic. Iodine-based solutions are effective for cleaning grossly contami-

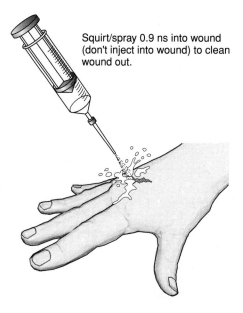

Squirt/spray 0.9 ns into wound (don't inject into wound) to clean wound out.

FIGURE 16-1 Wound irrigation.

nated wound margins, but most cleansing agents damage exposed tissues, so try to avoid getting the cleansing agent in the wound itself. Other cleaning solutions are more expensive and offer no advantage to saline. In the field setting, sterile (boiled) water may be used for dirty wounds, but it is hypotonic and can cause some tissue damage. Avoid using full-strength cleaning solutions and concentrated hydrogen peroxide, which may delay healing.

DEBRIDEMENT

Debridement is the removal of dead or dirty tissue, and can help convert a ragged and infection-prone wound into a cleaner wound. In general, remove as little tissue as possible when debriding (Fig. 16-2). Perform debridements parallel to the lines of least skin tension (the lines of Langer) if possible to minimize scarring. The lines of Langer generally run parallel to natural skin folds or perpendicular to the underlying muscle fibers. For example, they are horizontal on the forehead and circumferential on the forearm or leg.

WOUND PREPARATION

It is important to prepare a wide area to keep the wound area clean. For finger wounds, you should at least prepare the two adjacent fingers. For very dirty hands, consider placing a sterile surgical glove on the patient's hand, and then tear off a portion of the glove to expose the wound area. Use an agent with a broad antimicrobial spectrum (e.g.,

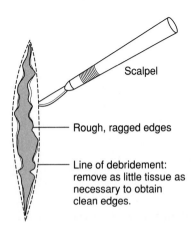

Scalpel

Rough, ragged edges

Line of debridement: remove as little tissue as necessary to obtain clean edges.

FIGURE 16-2 Wound debridement.

Betadine or Hibiclens). Most agents need to dry on the skin to achieve the best anti-microbial effect.

LOCAL ANESTHETIC AGENTS

Lidocaine (Xylocaine) in 0.5% to 2.0% concentrations is available with and without 1:100,000 epinephrine. Dose limits for subcutaneous infiltration are 5 mg/kg without epinephrine and 7 mg/kg with epinephrine. Buffering (1 mL of 1 mEq/mL or 7.5% $NaHCO_3$ added to 9 to 10 mL of lidocaine solution) and warming may decrease pain of infiltration. Buffered lidocaine is stable and may be used for at least 1 week.

Bupivacaine (Marcaine) in 0.25% to 0.75% concentrations is available with and without epinephrine. It is the same local anesthetic class (amide) as lidocaine. It can yield up to 6 to 8 hours of local anesthesia, and can be mixed as a 1:1 mixture of 0.5% Marcaine and 2% lidocaine for digital or intercostal or wrist blocks. Dose limit is usually quoted as 2.0 to 2.5 mg/kg.

Remember to never use anesthetics with epinephrine on distal appendages because of the risk of vascular compromise. As the saying goes, avoid epinephrine on "fingers, nose, penis, toes."

LOCAL ANESTHETIC INJECTION TECHNIQUE

It is best to use a 27-gauge or smaller needle, inject slowly, and inject through the wound surface (it is more painful to inject through intact skin next to the wound). If a 3-cm needle is used, gradually advance all along one side of the wound. You do not usually need to pull back on the syringe before injecting, just look for raising of a subcutaneous bleb. For digits, inject on the proximal side first, limiting the volume injected to 3 mL per digit. (For additional discussion on local and regional anesthesia, refer to Chapter 18.)

USE OF TAC

TAC stands for the combination of tetracaine (0.5%), adrenalin (1:2,000), and cocaine (11.8%) and is an excellent topical anesthetic for open wounds. It should not be used for wounds on or near mucosal surfaces (due to rapid absorption of cocaine), areas of the body served by end arteries (digits, penis, ear lobes, tip of nose), during pregnancy, or in patients with a history of high blood pressure. It is most useful for scalp or face lacerations in children. The dose limit is 2 mL for adults. For small wounds, soak cotton-tipped applicators in TAC and place directly in the wound. Apply gentle continuous pressure over the wound to facilitate TAC entry into tissue. It takes 10 to 15 minutes to work. Blanching of wound margins confirms effect. LET (4% lidocaine, 1:2,000 epinephrine, 0.5% tetracaine) can be used instead of TAC. It has the same effectiveness and it is safer (no cocaine). It is safe to use on mucus membranes, but not areas served by end arteries (as for TAC).

CHOICE OF SUTURES

First, choose the needle type. A cutting needle is triangular in cross-section, and can punch through tough skin. However, it can tear delicate tissues. Its main use is epidermis repair (outer layer). A taper needle is round or circular in cross-section. It does not puncture epidermis well. It is good for fascia and deep tissues. Next choose the suture type: Nonabsorbable suture is indicated for skin repair, fascia under tension, and vascular (blood vessel) repairs. Absorbable suture material is indicated for subcutaneous layers, intraoral mucosa (including tongue), and fascia not under tension.

Monofilament (single-strand) suture's advantages are that it is less reactive and less likely to become infected. Braided (multiple strands wound around each other) suture's advantages are greater tensile strength, ease of knot tying, and ability to hold knots better. For a comparison of sutures, see Tables 16-1 to 16-3.

BASIC SUTURING TECHNIQUE

Simple suture technique requires a little practice, but is relatively easy to learn and very useful in the field. The procedure for simple closure of wounds is illustrated in Fig. 16-3. Patients may return for removal of sutures, or may be instructed for self-removal. Table 16-4 gives guidelines for timelines for suture removal. Consider leaving sutures in longer for patients with insulin-dependent diabetes, chronic steroid use, immunosuppression, poor nutrition, and age over 70 years.

TABLE 16-1 COMPARISON OF NONABSORBABLE SUTURES

Nylon (Dermalon): inexpensive, best for most skin repairs
Polypropylene (Prolene): smoother and stronger than nylon, has a blue
   color that makes it easier to see on dark-haired scalp
Braided nylon (Surgilon): strength of nylon with the tying ease of silk,
   but expensive
Silk: more reactive, with more infection risk; has no advantages over
   other better sutures
Wire (stainless steel): the least reactive and strongest type of suture, but
   is difficult to tie and uncomfortable for the patient, and requires wire
   cutters for removal.

TABLE 16-2 COMPARISON OF ABSORBABLE SUTURES

Plain gut absorbs in 5–10 days (by inflammation).
Chromic gut absorbs in 10–14 days (by inflammation).
Polyglycolic acid/polyglactin (Vicryl, Dexon) absorbs in 30–90 days
    (by hydrolysis). These synthetics are braided; they are also stronger,
    less reactive, and last longer than gut sutures.
Polydioxanone (PDS) absorbs in 100–210 days; it is a monofilament
    and is minimally reactive and smooth to tie. The gut types of sutures
    have been shown in studies to cause more wound pain and can
    cause wound redness and swelling, simulating wound infection.

ALTERNATIVE TECHNIQUES FOR WOUND CLOSURE

Steri-strips (tape strips) are good if the wound edges are not under much tension, and
are appropriate if the patient won't get the wound wet for 3 days. Tincture of benzoin
helps hold the strips. Start at the center of the wound and bisect outward with each subsequent tape strip. Running subcuticular polypropylene is probably the best cosmetic
suture, although it is difficult to learn. It is often helpful to buttress this repair with tape
strips. Staples can be used for wound closure, especially for scalp wounds, and their
main advantage is speed. However, staples may be uncomfortable for the patient, require
a staple remover, and have a poorer cosmetic result.

MAIN SUTURING TECHNIQUES

The simple interrupted suture technique is appropriate for most wounds. It is quick to
place, easiest to learn, and usually causes wound edge eversion.

TABLE 16-3 SUTURE SIZE GUIDELINES

WOUND LOCATION	RECOMMENDED SUTURE SIZE
Scalp	3-0, 4-0
Face	6-0, 5-0
Chin	6-0, 5-0 (two layer)
Trunk	4-0
Arm	4-0
Hand	5-0
Leg	4-0
Foot	4-0, 3-0

General rule: 6-0 on face, 5-0 on hand, and 4-0 elsewhere
on body.

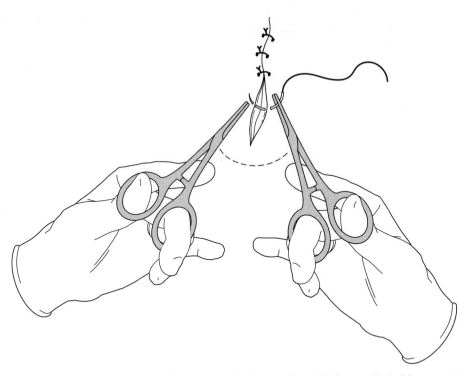

FIGURE 16-3 Basic suturing techniques. Grasp the needle with the needle holder at a 90 degree angle, about one third of the way up from the suture end of the needle. Hold the needle holder with thumb in one finger hole, fourth finger in the other finger hole, and second finger extended for stability. Never grasp the tip of the needle with the needle holder. Start to puncture the skin vertically with the needle. If using a small needle on a wide wound, transit the wound in two passes. Exit the needle on the other side the same distance from the wound edge. Usually you should make the needle pass deeper than wide to achieve eversion of wound edges. To instrument tie a suture knot, grasp the needle side of the suture with the left hand. Pull the suture part way through, leaving a 2-cm tail. Point the needle holder at the tail of the suture. Use the left hand to throw two loops around the end of the needle holder. Grasp the tail suture end with the needle holder. Pull the tail through the two loops (this actually creates the knot). Cinch the double throw knot down. Make sure the knot sets down flat (you may have to cross your hands 90 degrees). Use the left hand to throw a single loop around the needle holder. Then grasp the tail of the suture with the needle holder and pull the tail through the loop. Alternate subsequent throw loops above and below the needle holder (so that square, not granny, knots result). Space sutures the same distance apart and the same distance on either side of the wound (such as 1 mm apart and 1 mm from wound edges for delicate facial lacerations, or up to 1 cm apart and 1 cm from the wound edge for cruder repairs not under tension). Tie at least five to six knots (throws) for nylon. Tie at least seven to eight knots (throws) for prolene. Tie three knots for absorbable sutures.

TABLE 16-4 SUTURE REMOVAL GUIDELINES

WOUND LOCATION	SUTURE REMOVAL (DAYS)
Scalp	7
Face	3–5
Chin	7
Trunk	7–10
Arm	7–10
Hand	10–14
Leg	10–14
Sole of foot	14–21

Continuous running suturing is the fastest method. However, if the suture breaks at one point, the whole suture line will fall apart. Generally it is not recommended unless there is a large time-consuming laceration length to repair.

Interrupted vertical mattress sutures are the best to evert wide wound edges, but they take longer to place. You can start with this method at the center of the wound, and once eversion is achieved, finish with simple interrupted suturing.

Interrupted horizontal mattress suturing is good where the skin is thin (back of hand, etc.). It is equivalent to having two sutures per knot (so is a quick technique).

In the continuous interlocking suture (or baseball stitch), each loop is partially locked into the next loop. It can cause tissue necrosis, and is only useful occasionally in a patient with a coagulopathy who has continued bleeding from the initially placed interrupted suture sites.

CHOICES FOR WOUND DRESSINGS

Dry gauze is suitable for most wounds or if tape strips are used. Nonadherent dressings are preferred for abrasions, nailbed injuries, skin flaps, or the thin-skinned elderly: Vaseline gauze, Xeroform gauze, adaptic gauze (most expensive), and Telfa (not really nonadherent). Antibiotic ointments may be helpful to apply after closing the wound, but are not usually necessary.

In general, encouraging active motion of a wounded extremity is better than passive immobilization or splinting of the extremity. There is no increase in wound separation problems if sutures are left in for at least 14 days (as on the hand). Finger splints are usually unnecessary for properly repaired finger lacerations.

CUTANEOUS ABSCESSES

Cutaneous abscesses are a common form of skin infection. Predisposing factors to abscesses include puncture wounds, animal or human bites, follicular infections, and intravenous (IV) drug use. Patients with a cutaneous abscess present with localized pain, swelling, and warmth over the infected site. A careful examination should be performed to exclude involvement of deeper structures such as muscle or bone, or extension of the abscess along tissue planes or the formation of fistulous tracts.

Laboratory testing and radiographs are not required in uncomplicated abscesses. A needle aspiration may be used to confirm the presence of pus in the affected area. The most common and effective treatment for cutaneous abscess is incision and drainage (Fig. 16-4). After incision and drainage is performed, the wound should be irrigated, and packing should be placed to prevent the reaccumulation of pus and proper wound healing. Repack the wound every 2 to 3 days as necessary to encourage drainage of residual purulent material. Unless there is significant local cellulitis, antibiotics are not necessary.

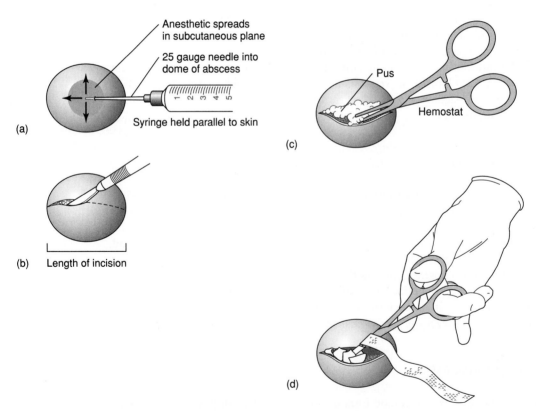

FIGURE 16-4 Incision and drainage of a simple cutaneous abscess.

INCISION AND DRAINAGE OF A SIMPLE CUTANEOUS ABSCESS

1. Prepare the site: scrub with antibacterial solution and drape with sterile drapes.
2. Anesthesia: Local or regional anesthesia may be sufficient, although larger abscesses may require conscious sedation (see Chapter 18).
3. Needle aspiration: Inject 16- to 18-gauge needle and aspirate for pus.
4. Incision: Use scalpel to make an adequate incision for exploration and eventual packing.
5. Drainage: Express pus and break up loculations with hemostat.
6. Packing: Pack the wound with sterile gauze packing to keep the wound open. Dress the wound and arrange for follow-up care.

TETANUS

Tetanus is a major cause of morbidity and mortality in less developed settings, particularly in injuries with substantial tissue damage. Always ask the patient when the last tetanus booster was administered, and give tetanus booster if more than 5 years have passed since the last immunization. (See Chapter 8 for recommendations on tetanus immune globulin.)

SKIN GRAFTS

Simple skin grafts may be accomplished in the field setting with relatively little difficulty. Wounds that require skin grafts include those that involve large (>2 cm) skin defects that have destroyed the dermis. Split-thickness grafts may be taken from the back, thigh, or buttocks and transplanted to the affected site. To obtain a split-thickness graft, use a dermatome or a simple sterile razor to remove the skin by dividing the dermis (Fig. 16-5). Place the graft on a clean, freshly debrided wound site and secure by simple sutures and tape strips.

FURTHER WOUND CARE

Consider antibiotics for bite wounds, contaminated wounds, hand or foot wounds, if there is delayed presentation (>6 hours for limb or trunk; >12 hours for head wounds), or if the wound is already infected. Risk factors for infection include diabetes, malnutrition, vascular disease, and age over 70 years. Antibiotics most commonly used are first-generation cephalosporins if available.

Lacerations may need to be referred to a specialist if associated anatomic injuries are present. You may need to consult a plastic surgeon for repair if facial nerve involvement is suspected, if a flap is required, if a large skin graft is needed, or if the wound involves a major cartilage injury or parotid duct laceration. Ophthalmologists should be

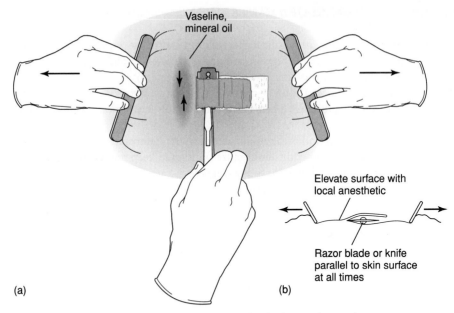

FIGURE 16-5 Obtaining and transplanting a split-thickness skin graft.

consulted for repair of lid margin lacerations, through-and-through lid lacerations, avulsions of the lid or periorbital tissue, ptosis, or suspected globe injury.

BURN INJURIES

ETIOLOGY

Stupidity is the major factor that leads to most burns. At least 75% of burns are preventable. Burns have many causes: flame (75%), scald (15%), chemical (5%), electrical (5%), and radiation (>1%). Many residential fires are caused by cigarette smoking (19%), heating system malfunction (14%), incendiary devices (16%), electrical devices (12%), and cooking devices (7%).

DIAGNOSIS AND ON-SCENE CARE

The most important aspect of on-scene care for burns is to not become a victim yourself. Turn off the gas/pump/electric power, etc. if possible. Remove the patient from the heat source by pushing with dry nonconductive material such as wood if in contact with electricity. Immediately move the patient from the vicinity if there is danger of explosion. Keep low to avoid smoke. Put the fire out, extinguish burning clothing by smothering or by using water or a fire extinguisher.

Once the fire is out, evaluate the patient. The ABCs of trauma care are the same for the burn patient as for any other trauma patient. Get off all potentially affected clothing and determine the burn wound extent and burn wound depth. Soak clothing or the burn area with water if heat transfer is still possible. Continue to copiously irrigate if there is a chemical burn. Arrange transport, and immobilize the neck or back if needed.

If the burn patient has early respiratory distress despite oxygenation, consider endotracheal intubation. All patients should receive 100% oxygen initially. The airway evaluation steps are the same as for other trauma patients (remember cervical spine precautions and immobilization). After evaluating the ABCs, address associated injuries from explosions, falls, car accidents with fire, and high voltage electrical. Treat the associated injuries first. Do not focus on just the burn. The burn patient initially should be treated as a trauma patient (not a dermatology patient). A major burn causes multiorgan dysfunction and is not just a skin injury.

Remember to obtain an "AMPLE" history

Allergies
Medications
Prior illnesses
Last meal (time)
Events preceding the injury

History to obtain about a burn patient is the type of burn (flame, chemical, electrical, or flash), substances involved, any associated trauma, if it occurred in a closed space, time of injury, and duration of contact with smoke.

SMOKE INHALATION INJURY

Smoke inhalation causes 80% of fire deaths. The main problems are carbon monoxide poisoning and smoke inhalation injury. Asphyxia also can occur with flame events because the air oxygen content may go to only 5% in a flash fire. Smoke inhalation injury should be suspected from the history if there are burns from explosions, burns indoors or in a closed space, clothing fires, or if the patient is unconscious after the burn.

Symptoms of smoke inhalation injury are hoarseness, sore throat, cough, and shortness of breath. Physical signs are burns of the face, mouth, neck, singed nasal hairs, carbon deposits on lips, nose, carbonaceous sputum, rales, rhonchi, wheezes, or stridor. Studies to consider on the smoke inhalation victim are arterial blood gases (ABGs) and carboxyhemoglobin levels if available. If there is hypoxemia or hypercapnia, consider early intubation. The chest radiograph is often normal, but may show fluffy infiltrates at 24 hours.

Treatment of smoke inhalation injury includes moist oxygen, pulmonary toilet (cough and deep breathing, incentive spirometry, suction), intubation (oral or nasal, if upper airway edema or impending respiratory failure), mechanical ventilation if available (may need positive end-expiratory pressure if severe respiratory failure), and bronchodilators (useful only for wheezing if present). Antibiotics are not useful prophylactically, and steroids increase mortality and are contraindicated.

CARBON MONOXIDE POISONING

This is probably the most common cause of death from fires. The carboxyhemoglobin level should be measured in all flame burn patients if available (venous values can be used, not just arterial).

Carboxyhemoglobin level half-life on room air is 4 hours, on 100% oxygen 40 minutes, and at 2 atmospheres pressure hyperbaric oxygen 25 minutes. Symptoms and treatment recommendations for carbon monoxide poisoning are listed in Table 16-5. Hyperbaric chambers are not commonly available in most clinical settings, so the mainstay of treatment for carbon monoxide poisoning is 100% oxygen. Complications of carbon monoxide poisoning are cerebral edema, cerebral infarcts, acute myocardial infarction, persistent learning deficit, personality changes, memory impairment, and death from progressive encephalopathy.

DETERMINING BURN WOUND EXTENT

The extent of a burn is expressed as percentage of total body surface area (TBSA). The area of the patient's hand is about 1% TBSA. The "rule of nines" also may be used (Fig. 16-6).

TABLE 16-5 SYMPTOMS AND TREATMENT
OF CARBON MONOXIDE POISONING

Carboxyhemoglobin levels
    <10% is usually asymptomatic (same as smokers)
    10%–20% (headache, nausea, irritability, dyspnea)
    20%–40% (arrhythmias, central nervous system, vomiting)
    40%–50% (seizures, coma, cardiovascular collapse)
    >60% (often is fatal)
Treatment of elevated carboxyhemoglobin levels
    <10%: 100% oxygen for 1 hour or until symptoms resolve
    10%–20%: 100% oxygen until symptoms resolve (usually 2 h)
    20%–40%: 100% oxygen; recheck levels; consider hyperbaric
        oxygen
    >40%: 100% oxygen; most should probably get hyperbaric oxygen

If patient is pregnant or has any neurologic symptoms, he or she should get hyperbaric treatment regardless of level.

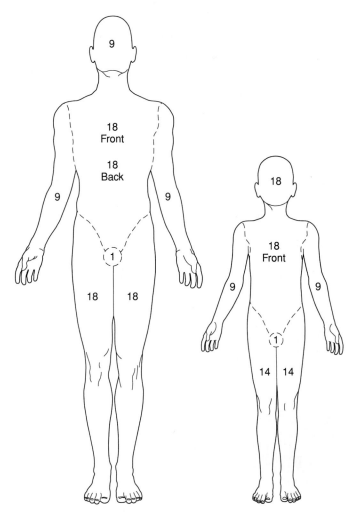

FIGURE 16-6
Rule of nines: head, 9% for an adult (18% for a baby); arm, 9% each; anterior trunk, 8%; posterior trunk, 18%; leg, 18% each (14% each in baby); and genitalia, 1%.

BURN WOUND DEPTH

Is it difficult to determine the depth of a burn from the initial appearance, especially in children. Two weeks of observation may be needed to accurately determine depth of injury. See Fig. 16-7 for classification of burns.

BURN SHOCK AND TREATMENT

Burn shock is due to large fluid losses in the interstitial space, is associated with a >25% TBSA burn, lasts 18 to 48 hours, then spontaneously resolves. The aim of early fluid

First degree: superficial

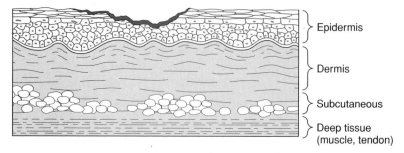

Epidermis

Dermis

Subcutaneous

Deep tissue
(muscle, tendon)

Second degree: partial thickness

Some dermal injury — — Bullae

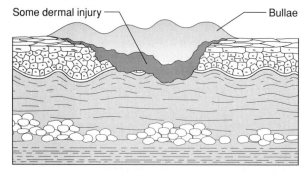

Third degree: full thickness

Burn through dermis, into
subcutaneous and deep tissue

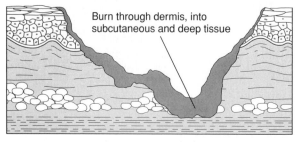

FIGURE 16-7 Burn classification. First degree is like sunburn (red, painful, no blisters). Do not count this area when determining burn surface area to calculate fluid therapy requirements. These heal in 3 to 7 days without scarring. Admit the patient only if a baby or dehydrated or hyperthermic. Second-degree burns (or partial thickness) are usually red but can be white, and are usually painful with blisters. These heal in 7 to 28 days, and may scar. These may need skin grafting. Third-degree (full-thickness) burns are usually white (may be red), leathery, and insensate, and usually have no blisters. Thrombosed subcutaneous vessels are the only definite sign of full-thickness injury. These will heal from the edges if less than 3 cm in diameter (otherwise they need skin grafting).

resuscitation is to treat burn shock and to maintain intravascular volume despite the body-wide loss of capillary seal. IV resuscitation is the mainstay of treatment for burn shock. Peripheral lines and femoral IV lines are adequate, although central monitoring for fluid balance is helpful if available. It is acceptable to place an IV line through burned tissue. You should change all IV catheters every 48 to 72 hours.

Isotonic crystalloid (0.9% normal saline) is the best fluid for resuscitation. The Parkland formula is the most commonly used. It is composed of 4 mL lactated Ringer's solution times × kg body weight × % TBSA burn. Give first half in first 8 hours (from time of the burn), and the second half over the next 16 hours (e.g., for a 50% TBSA burn in a 70-kg man, 4 × 70 × 50 equals 14,000 mL; give 7,000 mL over the first 8 hours, or about 1 L per hour). The Parkland formula for children involves adding 4 mL/kg/% burn to maintenance fluid requirement (100 mL/kg for children under 10 kg, 1,000 mL + 50 mL/kg for 10–20 kg, or 1,500 mL + 20 mL/kg for 20–30 kg). Use the formula only as a guide; adjust it up or down as needed.

The key criterion in monitoring fluid resuscitation is urine output. Target outputs are 30 mL/h in adults, 1 mL/kg/h in children, and 2 mL/kg/h for electrical burns. You should also monitor the patient's mental status and skin perfusion in nonburned areas.

ESCHAROTOMY

Circumferential full-thickness burns of a limb may cause ischemia of the distal limb, and full-thickness burns of the thorax may cause restriction of breathing. In the case of severe burns around the arms or legs, look for loss of tissue perfusion and consider early escharotomy, or surgical opening of the wound to allow expansion of the underlying tissues. The principle is the same for fasciotomy (Fig. 16-8).

ADMISSION CRITERIA FOR SEVERE BURNS

Patients with severe burns should be transferred to a burn center if available. Those with moderate burns should be admitted to a local hospital. Patients with minor burns may be treated on an outpatient basis.

Minor burns are defined as second degree of less than 15% TBSA in adults or less than 10% TBSA in children, third degree of less than 2% TBSA, no involvement of the face, hands, feet, or genitalia, no smoke inhalation, and no complicating factors.

Moderate burns are defined as second degree of 15% to 25% TBSA in adults or 10% to 20% TBSA in children, third degree of 2% to 10% TBSA (not involving hands, feet, face, or genitalia), circumferential limb burns, household current (110–220 volt) electrical injuries, smoke inhalation with minor (<2% TBSA) burns, possible child abuse, and injuries in patients not able to care for their burns as outpatients.

Severe burns are defined as second degree of greater than 25% TBSA in adults, second degree of greater than 20% TBSA in children, third degree of greater than 10% TBSA, high-voltage electrical burns, deep second- or third-degree burns of face, hands,

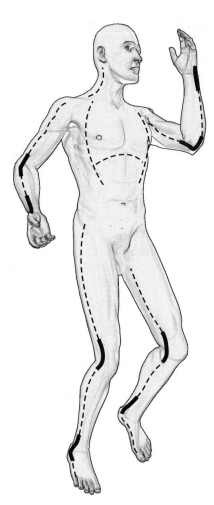

FIGURE 16-8 Performing an escharotomy: To perform an escharotomy, incise through burned tissue till deeper tissue gapes. No anesthesia is needed. Delay the procedure only up to 4 hours after the onset of restricted circulation. Have ointment and bandaging material ready. To perform escharotomy, incise along the medial and lateral limb, or incise along the anterior axillary line and transverse subcostal for thoracic burns.

feet, or genitalia, smoke inhalation with greater than 2% TBSA burn, burns with major trunk, head or orthopedic injury, and burns in poor-risk patients (elderly, diabetic, chronic obstructive pulmonary disease, etc.).

WOUND CARE FOR BURNS

Blisters should be debrided if they are large, already broken, already infected, or if unsure of the depth of the underlying burn. Do not debride thick palmar or plantar blisters.

Debridement eliminates dead tissue, lessens the risk of infection, allows better assessment of burn depth, and may permit better limb mobility. Have ointment and bandaging material ready, perform it as quickly as possible (limit exposure time to air), wipe the tissue loose with a dry 4 × 4 gauze, and dress the wound.

Topical agents to apply are silver sulfadiazine (Silvadene), which is painless, soothing on application, and bacteriostatic, although expensive and not always available. Gentian violet is good for mild to moderate burns, but should not be used on full-thickness burns.

OUTPATIENT BURN CARE

Carefully instruct the patient and family in the dressing change procedure. Change the ointment and dressing at least once a day (preferably twice a day). See the patient for a recheck in 2 to 3 days if he or she is reliable. Patients should be instructed to remove the bandage and dressing, wash off the old Silvadene ointment with warm soapy water (may soak the area first), peel off any loose or broken blisters and pat the area dry, reapply new Silvadene ointment 2 to 4 mm thick, and reapply a new bandage. The patient may take pain medicine 30 minutes before changing the ointment and bandage.

On recheck visits, look for redness and tenderness outside the original burned area. Thick drainage from the burn is usually just exudate and not a sign of infection. Determine whether the patient is maintaining satisfactory range of motion of the affected area. Advice to the patient after the burn heals is to keep the area moist with cold cream. Keep the area out of the sun for 6 months (to prevent unpredictable lightening or darkening of the affected skin). Treatment of hypertrophic scarring, if it occurs, involves intensive physical therapy and active range of motion exercises.

Delayed complications of burns are infections, burn wound sepsis, pulmonary infection, IV line infections, fungal infections, pulmonary emboli, deep venous thrombosis, multiple organ failure, anemia, hypothermia, and graft failure.

PREVENTION OF BURNS

Teach your patients about prevention. Keep very hot water out of reach of children, construct barriers around open fires, and keep cooking pots out of reach. Educate children about fires and matches. Familiarize yourself with building exits when on trips or in new buildings.

ELECTRICAL INJURIES

There are three main types of electrical injuries: household current (110–120 volts or 220–240 volts), high voltage (>1,000 volts), and lightning. Electrical line voltages are cross-country lines greater than 100,000 volts, residential and industrial area 7,620 volts, household heavy appliances 220 to 240 volts, and interior household lines 110 to 120 volts alternating current (AC; 60 cycles per second in United States).

AC AND DC INJURIES

Alternating current has a tetanizing effect on muscles. "Let-go current" (the current level at which the person is unable to release his or her grasp on the conductor) is 15 milliamps for men and 10 milliamps for women. Strong sustained muscle contraction can cause fractures. Direct current (DC) is felt as heat only and can cause a single violent muscle contraction that can throw the victim from the power source. Household current injuries in one series caused half of all electrical deaths. The major risk is ventricular fibrillation (caused by the AC feature of current). Deep tissue damage directly from the current is rare if voltage is under 1,000 volts. However, low voltage can cause fractures and dislocations. If the electrocardiogram is normal and there is no skin burn, admission to the hospital is not necessary for household current exposures.

Oral cavity electric burns can occur from children biting an electric cord. The temperature of the electric arc is 1,300°C, so usually these injuries represent more a thermal injury than electrical current injury. Most involve lower lips, and can involve the tongue. Complications are drooling, adhesions, impaired speech, tooth damage, and impaired mandible growth (rare). "Corner of mouth" burn (from biting an electrical cord) treatment is by a topical agent (Silvadene) and a mouth stretcher. No surgical treatment should be considered for at least 1 year. Warn parents about delayed bleeding from the labial eschar sloughing off.

HIGH-VOLTAGE ELECTRICAL INJURIES

People at risk are electric company linemen, roofers, agricultural workers (carrying irrigation pipes), parachutists, reckless teenagers (climbing towers), and car drivers (hitting power poles).

High-voltage current causes coagulation necrosis of tissue along the current path. The points of maximum destruction are at skin entrance and exit sites, and these may cause extensive muscle necrosis in limbs or the trunk beneath unburned skin.

Initial treatment for high-voltage electrical burns is to turn off the current, remove the patient from the electrical source (use nonconductive materials to push), and start cardiopulmonary resuscitation if necessary.

Immobilize the spine if there was an associated fall. Provide oxygen, airway, and respiratory support and assess for other injuries. Patients with significant muscle injury may develop compartment syndrome. Indications for fasciotomy are the same as described above for escharotomy.

High-voltage electrical injury complications include acute myocardial infarction, arrhythmias, renal failure (preventable if sufficient resuscitation fluid is given), infections, sepsis, peripheral neuropathy, amputations, and cataracts. Infectious complications are sepsis, pneumonia, and osteomyelitis.

PREVENTION OF ELECTRICAL INJURIES

Education is key. Instruct patients to turn power off at source before working on wiring or an appliance, and replace damaged electrical cords and appliances. Encourage the use of nonconductive electric plug fillers when children are present. Don't handle any electrical apparatus when hands or area are wet. Use ground fault interrupter type outlets wherever possible.

LIGHTNING

Lightning injuries impart a sudden massive DC shock (up to 1,000,000 volts and 200,000 amps). Lightning is defined as the natural atmospheric electric discharge that occurs between regions of net positive and net negative charge, and is usually associated with cumulonimbus clouds. It may occur with nimbostratus clouds, snowstorms, and volcano gas.

Lightning incidence is about 8 million lightning strikes per day (from the 50,000 thunderstorms per day in the world). Lightning causes several thousand deaths per year worldwide, more than any other type of weather-related death. Lightning (unlike the old wives' tale) can strike twice in the same place. A Virginia park ranger was hit seven times over a 30-year period (he later committed suicide). Tall buildings commonly receive multiple strikes each year.

CLINICAL FEATURES

Types of lightning injury are a direct strike (high morbidity because the head is hit), splash current (on outside of body and causes flamelike burns), and ground current (may cause mass casualties from one strike; arrhythmias or asystole predominate).

Types of injuries from lightning are

- Skin: superficial and deep skin burns
- Neurologic: loss of consciousness, respiratory paralysis, and limb weakness
- Cardiac: ventricular fibrillation and asystole
- Eye: cataracts are most common effect (may appear 6 weeks to 24 months afterward)
- Ear: current damage to inner ear or auditory nerve and tympanic membrane rupture (50%) due to the proximity of thunder noise generation
- Extremity: Muscle necrosis
- Gastrointestinal: bleeding and pancreatitis

TREATMENT

There are two different treatment regimens. For most victims (who have deep tissue damage or flame burns on skin), follow the same scheme as for high-voltage injuries (high-volume fluid resuscitation, fasciotomy, etc.). For victims who just have central nervous system stunning, treat the same as for head trauma.

PREVENTION

Risk factors for a direct strike are being outside, carrying a metal object, having a metal object (hairpin or helmet) on head, and having no taller objects in the vicinity. If outside, avoid being the tallest object in the vicinity. Avoid hilltops, poles, towers, and trees. If in a group, spread out. Avoid wet soil. Lie flat or curled up. Stay away from metal equipment. If your hair stands on end, run from the area right away. If inside, stay away from radiators, stoves, appliances, gas, and water pipes. Avoid showering or bathing until the storm is over. Do not use the phone and stay away from fireplaces.

SUMMARY

Wound management can be accomplished with basic materials and relatively simple procedures. It is important to assess the ABCs in all patients presenting with wounds, and to evaluate for underlying traumatic injuries, such as orthopedic injuries and neurovascular injuries.

CHAPTER 17
Dermatology

M. James Eliades and Edbert B. Hsu

Dermatologic problems are among the most common complaints encountered by the primary care provider in the field. A basic understanding of infectious and inflammatory skin manifestations can help any practitioner correctly diagnose most skin conditions.

DEFINITIONS

To properly characterize a rash or skin lesion, the following definitions may be used:

- Papule: a palpable raised, scaly, or crusted lesion of less than 1.5 cm. A plaque is a large papule (>1.5 cm).
- Nodule: a palpable, solid lesion that may involve the epidermis, dermis, or subcutaneous tissue; larger and deeper than a papule.
- Macule: a nonpalpable area of color change of less than 1.5 cm without any scaling or crusting. A patch is a large macule (>1.5 cm).
- Blister: a lesion filled with fluid. If it is less than 1 cm, it is called a vesicle; a large blister is called a bulla. A blister that is cloudy or filled with purulent fluid is called a pustule.
- Erosions: areas where the epidermis has been removed, whereas ulcers penetrate deeper, at least into the dermis.

BLISTERING DISEASES

VESICULAR DISEASES

SCABIES The scabies mite is a microscopic, arachnid-type pest spread typically by close contact.

RASH Scabies produces an extraordinarily itchy mite infestation, and is particularly common in children. The primary lesion is a linear papulovesicle, but generally there is widespread excoriations and erythema. A few oval, edematous 1- to 3-mm burrows may be seen that have not yet been removed by scratching. Scraping these with a no. 15 scalpel occasionally yields the mite, ova, or mite feces. Scratching can cause superimposed infection, producing purulent lesions, lymphadenopathy, and fever (Fig. 17-1).

DISTRIBUTION Scabies is generally limited to below the neck, in the skin folds of the digits, web spaces, axillae, groin, penis, and inframammary folds.

SPREAD Scabies is spread by close skin contact in the family, or by clothes and bedding.

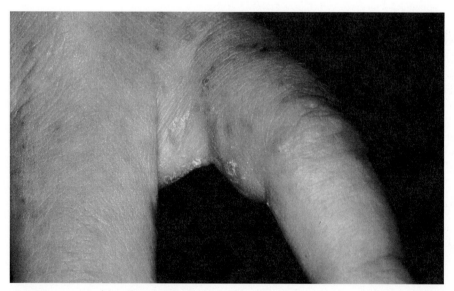

FIGURE 17-1 Scabies. (From Fitzpatrick TB et al. *Color Atlas & Synopsis of Clinical Dermatology: Common and Serious Diseases,* 4th ed. New York: McGraw-Hill, 2001; with permission.)

TREATMENT

- 5% permethrin cream, or benzyl benzoate lotion on the whole body except the face applied overnight
- All household members should be treated.
- Wash all clothes and bedding and hang them in the sun. Bathe and change clothes daily.
- Patient education
- Nighttime sedation if needed with diphenhydramine, hydroxyzine HCl, or similar agents

ALTERNATIVE TREATMENT Lindane may be mixed with body rubbing oil (1 part lindane in 15 parts oil). Apply and leave as above, then repeat in 1 week. Lindane has neurotoxic side effects and should not be used with young children, or in pregnant or breast-feeding women.

LICE Lice are tiny insects that are spread by close contact.

- Rash: Papules with itching. The lice are rarely seen, but their eggs are visible on the hair follicles. Scratching can cause infection and lymphadenopathy.
- Distribution: Areas of the body with hair
- Spread: By close contact, as well as by clothing and bedding
- Prevention: Bathe and wash hair often and put bedding and pillows in the sun every day.
- Treatment: A thorough washing followed by application of permethrin lotion. Leave for 10 minutes, then rinse.
- Alternative Treatment: Wash hair with a mixture of 1 part lindane and 10 parts water, leaving for 15 minutes before rinsing. Repeat this in 1 week. Nits remain on the hair, although they will be dead.

TICKS Ticks are blood-sucking parasites typically found in rural and forested regions.

- Rash: The tick should be visible in the burrow it has made.
- Distribution: Anywhere, but presumably more often on exposed parts of the body
- Prevention: Brush sulfur powder on exposed parts before going into a field.
- Treatment: Never pull on the body of the tick, because the mouth may break off and stay in the burrow. Put alcohol on the tick, or hold a cigarette near it (being careful not to burn skin).

TUMBU FLY

- Rash: Swelling on the scalp of children, which looks like a boil. The fly lays its eggs on the scalp, which then hatches; the insect burrows under the skin, causing the swelling.

■ Treatment: Apply petroleum jelly to the swelling, which will cause the insect to come out. Keep the area clean.

HERPES ZOSTER/SHINGLES

RASH The patient presents with red, nonscaling edematous papules and plaques, often preceded by a day or two of intense, burning pain (Fig 17-2).

DISTRIBUTION The rash occurs characteristically in a dermatomal pattern, most often on the torso, or on the face or upper scalp. The rash does not cross the midline.

SPREAD The disease is seen in people who have previously had varicella (chickenpox).

TREATMENT

■ Lightly bandage areas to prevent constant irritation by clothing.
■ For pain control, short-term narcotics are often needed.
■ If available, acyclovir (800 mg five times a day for 7–10 days), famciclovir, and valacyclovir have been shown to shorten the course of the disease when given in the first 72 hours of onset of the rash.

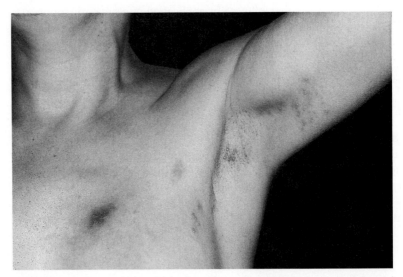

FIGURE 17-2 Herpes zoster/shingles. (From Fitzpatrick TB et al. *Color Atlas & Synopsis of Clinical Dermatology: Common and Serious Diseases,* 4th ed. New York: McGraw-Hill, 2001; with permission.)

VARICELLA (CHICKENPOX)

RASH Pruritic scattered papules, vesicles, pustules, and crusting in all stages of healing.

> **KEY POINT:**
>
> The hallmark of chickenpox is lesions in all stages of healing.

DISTRIBUTION All over, but most prominent on the torso, face, scalp, and genital area. The disease occurs most often in children. Mucous membranes also may be involved and appear as erosive lesions.

SPREAD Varicella is extremely contagious and sometimes preceded by signs of an upper respiratory infection or fever.

COMPLICATIONS Encephalitis and pneumonia (rare).

TREATMENT

- Nighttime sedation for itching with agents such as diphenhydramine
- Cool baths, especially with colloidal oatmeal
- Treatment of secondary infection with antibiotics with an oral antistaphylococcal medication such as cephalexin, dicloxacillin, or erythromycin
- Acyclovir 20 mg/kg/dose, up to 800 mg five times a day, can reduce the severity and duration of the disease if begun during the first 24 hours of rash development. It should be given to immunosuppressed and adult patients because of the increased risk of complications.

HAND, FOOT, AND MOUTH DISEASE

RASH/DISTRIBUTION Erosions of the oral mucosa, followed 1 to 2 days later by the appearance of oval vesicles over the palms and soles. Lesions in skin creases are common, as are papules over the buttocks and genitals. The disease is viral in origin, and most often caused by coxsackievirus or enterovirus.

TREATMENT

- Reassurance
- Pain control for oral lesions with cool liquids, and topical anesthetic such as diphenhydramine elixir

ACUTE ALLERGIC CONTACT DERMATITIS

RASH Hypersensitivity reaction causing coalescing, edematous papules and vesicles often producing a cobblestoned appearance. Rash is pruritic.

DISTRIBUTION Occurs over area exposed to the allergen, usually after 1 to 2 days. When the allergen is a plant such as poison ivy or sumac (*Rhus* dermatitis), the lesions often occur in a linear pattern where the plant brushed against the skin.

SPREAD Direct contact with an allergen.

TREATMENT

- Clean thoroughly to remove allergen.
- Nighttime sedation as needed, such as with diphenhydramine
- Topical triamcinolone ointment 0.1% twice a day until clear
- Moisturizing cream over corticosteroid twice daily as skin heals
- Prednisone orally may be added for more severe disease, 40 to 60 mg/day in adults, or 1 to 2 mg/kg in children for 7 to 10 days.

BULLOUS DISEASES

BULLOUS ERYTHEMA MULTIFORME (ERYTHEMA MULTIFORME MAJOR, STEVENS-JOHNSON SYNDROME, TOXIC EPIDERMAL NECROLYSIS)

RASH A hypersensitivity reaction known as erythema minor begins as red, non-scaling papules with a central dusky erythema that looks a bit like a bulls-eye or target lesion. This then blisters diffusely and is known by the names above. Toxic epidural necrolysis (TEN) occurs when blistering becomes extensive and coalesces with areas of detached epidermis.

DISTRIBUTION Diffuse

CAUSE Many, including infection and reaction to medication. Stevens-Johnson syndrome and TEN are usually caused by medication, and occur within 2 weeks of starting the medicine:

- Penicillins
- Sulfonamides
- Cephalosporins
- Nonsteroidal antiinflammatory drugs (NSAIDs)
- Phenytoin
- Barbiturates

- Allopurinol
- Carbamazepine
- Hydrochlorothiazide
- Furosemide
- Quinidine
- Procainamide

TREATMENT Patients with severe disease should be treated as if they have extensive burns.

- Stop offending medication.
- Fluid support and control of primary or secondary infection
- Debridement of necrotic tissue
- Pain control
- If available, consider transfer to a burn center.
- Care of mucous membranes, including the eyes
- Some clinicians recommend systemic corticosteroid use if begun in the first 48 hours (before extensive blistering) and continued for 2 to 3 days. Methylprednisone 1 g/day is one possible regimen.

BULLOUS PEMPHIGOID

RASH Diffuse blistering often preceded by itching. After the blisters rupture, erosions and crusting are evident. The Nikolsky sign (detachment of epidermis with lateral pressure on the skin) is negative.

> **DID YOU KNOW?**
>
> This disease can be distinguished from bullous erythema multiforme by the lack of mucous membrane involvement, blistering arising from noninflamed skin, slower onset of disease, and no history of new medication use.

DISTRIBUTION Starts on the torso and in body folds, but spreads to the remainder of the body.

CAUSE Autoimmune disease of the elderly

TREATMENT

- Local wound care and treatment of secondary infection
- Pain control
- Oral prednisone 40 to 80 mg/day, increased after 5 to 7 days if blistering is progressing

- Patients occasionally respond to topical corticosteroids
- Patients occasionally respond to dapsone and tetracycline with or without nicotinamide

PEMPHIGUS VULGARIS

RASH Erosions in the mouth followed by flaccid blisters with large, round erosions and a positive Nikolsky sign

---

DID YOU KNOW?

Pemphigus vulgaris can be identified by the presence of oral erosions and the absence of tense blisters.

KEY POINT:

Patients with pemphigus vulgaris and TEN both have mucous membrane involvement and flaccid blisters, but pemphigus vulgaris is characterized by slower onset, less inflammation of the skin, and less toxic appearance.

DISTRIBUTION Begins in mouth and other mucous membranes, then spreads diffusely to the skin.

CAUSE Autoimmune disease in the young and middle-aged adult

TREATMENT

- Local wound care and treatment of secondary infection
- Pain control
- If biopsy can be performed, or TEN can definitely be excluded by history, systemic corticosteroids can be given.
- Prednisone 60 to 80 mg/day with an increase in 4 to 5 days if blistering continues
- Patients sometimes need high doses of steroids or steroid-sparing immunosuppressive agents.

STAPHYLOCOCCAL SCALDED SKIN SYNDROME

RASH Diffuse areas of separation of the most superficial level of epidermis, usually not enough to cause fluid loss or secondary infection.

> **KEY POINT:**
>
> Staphylococcal scalded skin syndrome (SSSS) can be differentiated from TEN by the characteristic radial fissuring/crusting around the mouth and lack of mucous membrane involvement seen in SSSS. There is rarely a history or new medication use, and the child appears well.

DISTRIBUTION Diffuse

CAUSE Toxin from *Staphylococcus aureus*, occurring almost exclusively in children.

TREATMENT

- Local wound care
- Fluid replacement as needed
- Oral antistaphylococcal antibiotics such as cephalexin 50 mg/kg/day divided four times a day, or dicloxacillin 50 mg/kg/day divided four times a day.

NECROTIZING SUBCUTANEOUS INFECTIONS Gas gangrene, necrotizing fasciitis, hemolytic streptococcal gangrene, anaerobic gangrene

RASH

- Erythema, induration, and warmth characteristic of cellulitis
- Edema, intense pain, and pallor or grayish discoloration
- Anesthesia, purpura, and hemorrhagic bullae

Progression through these steps from mild to severe can be impressively rapid, often occurring in hours.

> **KEY POINT:**
>
> Patients become rapidly ill and can be hypo- or hyperthermic, hypotensive, and confused.

DISTRIBUTION Usually the extremities or groin region

CAUSE Bacterial infection

TREATMENT

- If available, radiography to detect gas

- Surgical debridement
- Antibiotics: Intravenous (IV) Penicillin G 1 to 2 million units with clindamycin 600 mg every 6 to 8 hours; an aminoglycoside, chloramphenicol, ciprofloxacin, or a third-generation cephalosporin can be added.

PUSTULAR DISEASES

FOLLICULITIS

RASH A pruritic or painful red papule that can progress to a pustule and finally crusting. This can occur on normal or eczematous skin with a surrounding ring of erythema. Fungal folliculitis normally occurs within a plaque of tinea, and sterile folliculitis usually has less-surrounding erythema.

> **TIPS AND TRICKS:**
>
> In differentiating folliculitis from acne, it is useful to note that acne is usually distributed over the face, back, and chest, and blackheads are usually present.

DISTRIBUTION

- *Staphylococcus:* more commonly associated with atopic dermatitis, but can occur anywhere on normal skin
- *Pseudomonas:* skin folds, and under the bathing suit (associated with spa use)
- Sterile: torso, especially over the back and under restrictive clothing
- Fungal: over tinea plaques, and over the lower legs of women with tinea pedis who shave their legs

CAUSE Inflammation of the follicle, either sterile or more often caused by infection (*Staphylococcus/Pseudomonas/*fungal)

TREATMENT

- *Staphylococcus:* Antistaphylococcal antibiotics such as cephalexin or dicloxacillin 500 mg twice a day for 2 weeks. If eczema is present or disease is prolonged, mupirocin ointment can be added four times a day for 5 days.
- *Pseudomonas:* Stop the source of the bacteria. Ciprofloxacin is indicated only for those with systemic symptoms; otherwise disease is self-limited.
- Sterile: Removal of irritant by wearing loose clothing. For resistant cases, tetracycline or erythromycin can be used.
- Fungal: Griseofulvin 500 mg twice a day (20–25 mg/kg/day for children) for 1 month. Fluconazole/itraconazole can be used for those who develop side effects.

ACNE

RASH Red papules/pustules/comedones (whiteheads and blackheads); scarring can occur.

DISTRIBUTION Usually over the back, chest, and face of teenagers, but all age groups are susceptible.

CAUSE Blockage of a hair follicle with subsequent cyst formation and rupture followed by inflammation

TREATMENT

- Frequent washing of the area with soap or benzoyl peroxide
- If available, a keratolytic agent such as topical tretinoin 0.025% cream applied overnight
- Sun protection
- If extensive inflammation or cyst formation is present, then tetracycline or erythromycin can be used.
- Occasionally acne responds to topical antibiotics.

RED SCALING DISEASES

PAPULOSQUAMOUS DISEASES

PSORIASIS

RASH Salmon pink papules and plaques with sharp margins and silvery white scales. Removal of scales may result in pinpoint bleeding.

DISTRIBUTION Typically involves the scalp, elbows, knees, and intertriginous areas.

CAUSE Triggering factors include physical trauma, infections (acute streptococcal infection), stress and/or drugs (corticosteroids, antimalarial drugs); strong genetic component.

COMPLICATIONS Compromised lifestyle, "heartbreak of psoriasis" often a source of embarrassment; psoriatic arthritis may affect 5% to 8% of patients.

TREATMENT Application of topical corticosteroids, topical anthralin, vitamin D analogues, or occlusive dressing for 24 to 48 hours. Avoid local trauma.

FUNGAL INFECTIONS

RASH Erythematous scaling plaques with sharply marginated lesions, some maceration.

DISTRIBUTION Affects the feet (athlete's foot or tinea pedis); groin or pubic region (jock itch or tinea cruris); trunk, legs, or arms (ringworm or tinea corporis); and scalp (tinea capitis) (Fig. 17-3).

CAUSE Dermatophytic infection

COMPLICATIONS Pruritus and pain with secondary bacterial infection

TREATMENT

- Prevention includes daily washing, use of shower shoes, antifungal powder, benzoyl peroxide wash.
- Apply topical antifungal agents to affected sites twice a day.
- Consider systemic treatment for extensive infection or treatment failure.

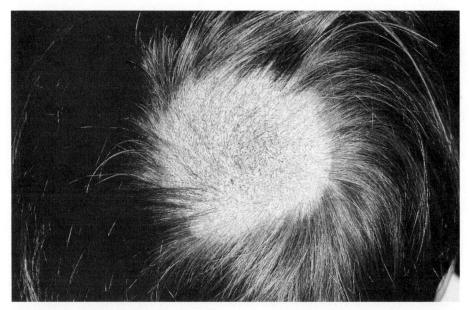

FIGURE 17-3 Ringworm (tinea capitis). (From Fitzpatrick TB et al. *Color Atlas & Synopsis of Clinical Dermatology: Common and Serious Diseases*, 4th ed. New York: McGraw-Hill, 2001; with permission.)

PITYRIASIS ROSEA

RASH Dull erythematous plaques with central scales

DISTRIBUTION Single herald patch, usually on the trunk followed by characteristic pattern of lesions. "Christmas tree" distribution on the trunk and proximal arms and legs

> **HELPFUL HINT:**
>
> Look for a single herald patch on the trunk, found in almost all patients. The secondary generalized rash, occurring 1 to 2 weeks later, may have the form of a Christmas tree.

CAUSE Inflammatory disorder

COMPLICATIONS Pruritus

TREATMENT Pruritus may be controlled by exposure to sunlight or ultraviolet B phototherapy. Spontaneous remission in 6 to 12 weeks

SECONDARY SYPHILIS

RASH Initial secondary eruption is macular, pink, and poorly defined. Subsequent secondary eruptions are brownish-red and pink papules and more localized (Fig. 17-4).

DISTRIBUTION Scattered discrete lesions. Generalized eruption occurs on the trunk, whereas localized eruptions may occur on the head, neck, palms, and soles. Condylomata lata frequently occur in the anogenital region and mouth.

CAUSE Sexually transmitted infection caused by *Treponema pallidum*

COMPLICATIONS May progress to tertiary syphilis.

TREATMENT Benzathine penicillin G, 2.4 million units intramuscularly (IM), in one dose. Alternative treatments include ceftriaxone 250 mg IM daily for 10 days, doxycycline 100 mg orally twice daily for 2 weeks, or erythromycin 500 mg orally four times daily for 2 weeks.

> **HELPFUL HINT:**
>
> Beware of the Jarisch-Herzheimer reaction, which is an acute febrile reaction that may occur after any treatment for syphilis. Treatment includes reassurance, bed rest, and aspirin.

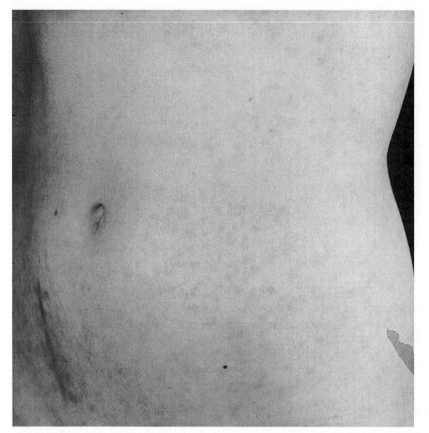

FIGURE 17-4 Secondary syphilis. (From Fitzpatrick TB et al. *Color Atlas & Synopsis of Clinical Dermatology: Common and Serious Diseases,* 4th ed. New York: McGraw-Hill, 2001; with permission.)

ECZEMATOUS DISEASES

SEBORRHEIC DERMATITIS

RASH Nonpruritic, red plaques with greasy, yellowish scales; poorly demarcated.

DISTRIBUTION Scalp, especially the hairline and behind and in the ears, which may extend onto the face; rarely on the upper chest or skin folds of the body.

CAUSE An inflammatory condition of unclear etiology occurring commonly in neonates, and in postpubertal and debilitated patients and patients with acquired immunodeficiency syndrome.

> **DID YOU KNOW?**
>
> In children this is called "cradle cap," and usually occurs before 2 months of age, whereas atopic dermatitis usually occurs after 5 months of age.

TREATMENT Mechanical removal of scalp scale with antiseborrheic shampoo. May use baby shampoo or mineral oil in children. Severe cases may require topical corticosteroids.

ALTERNATIVE TREATMENT Ketoconazole shampoo

ATOPIC DERMATITIS See section on Eczema.

RED NONSCALING DISEASES

INFECTIOUS

CELLULITIS

RASH Localized and painful erythema, induration, and warmth

DISTRIBUTION Anywhere, including orbital/periorbital area

CAUSE Bacterial infection of the dermis and subcutaneous tissue, usually incited by some type of trauma to the affected area (puncture wound, laceration, insect bite, etc.)

ASSOCIATED SYMPTOMS Fever, lymphadenopathy, and malaise

COMPLICATIONS Osteomyelitis, progression to deeper infection/necrotizing fasciitis

TREATMENT

- Antistaphylococcal/antistreptococcal antibiotics such as cephalexin or dicloxicillin
- In children, additional coverage of *Hemophilus influenzae* with an antibiotic such as ceftriaxone
- Elevate affected area.
- Pain control

ERYSIPELAS

RASH Sudden onset of deep red plaques with well-demarcated and raised borders and edema

DISTRIBUTION Usually over the cheeks and nose

CAUSE Bacterial infection of the dermis, usually streptococcal species

TREATMENT

- IV penicillin or an antistaphylococcal penicillin
- Pain control

FURUNCLES

RASH Erythematous, painful nodule with central necrosis that may progress to abscess formation

DISTRIBUTION Often found on the neck or in bearded areas.

CAUSE Staphylococcus aureus

TREATMENT

- Recommended prevention is with use of antibacterial soap.
- Incision and drainage of furuncle
- Systemic antibiotics recommended include cephalexin 250 to 500 mg four times daily for 10 days or dicloxacillin 250 to 500 mg four times daily for 10 days.

VASCULAR REACTIONS

URTICARIA

RASH Flat, pink, coalescing wheals (papules and plaques) that are intensely pruritic. Edema may be present, causing the center to be pale.

DISTRIBUTION Diffuse, but often highly concentrated over the back, abdomen, and upper extremities

CAUSE Usually a hypersensitivity reaction, but can be caused by other immunologic/nonimmunologic causes. Common allergens include the following:

- Medications: penicillins, sulfa drugs, aspirin, NSAIDs
- Infections
- Food: shellfish, peanuts
- Envenomations: insect bites

TREATMENT

- Removal of offending allergen
- Antihistamine such as diphenhydramine 25 to 50 mg or hydroxyzine HCl 25 mg every 6 hours
- Corticosteroids such as prednisone 40 to 60 mg/day orally for 3 to 4 days for severe cases
- May add histamine blockers such as cimetidine

ERYTHEMA NODOSUM

RASH Red, nonscaling plaques that are poorly demarcated, often with a target appearance

DISTRIBUTION Most often over the anterior portion of the lower legs.

CAUSE A vascular hypersensitivity reaction in the subcutaneous fat. Some of the more common causes include the following:

- Medications: sulfa drugs, oral contraceptives
- Infection: *Yersinia, Coccidioides, Histoplasma, Streptococcus,* tuberculosis
- Inflammatory diseases: inflammatory bowel disease, sarcoid

TREATMENT

- Treatment or removal of offending agent
- NSAIDs
- Elevation of limb
- Bandaging for comfort as needed

COLORED LESIONS

WHITE LESIONS

TINEA VERSICOLOR (PITYRIASIS)

RASH Tan color papules that initially are well demarcated and 5 to 10 mm in diameter and eventually coalesce into plaques with a characteristic arcuate border; mild scaling

DISTRIBUTION Upper chest, back, antecubital fossae

CAUSE Yeast infection caused by *Pityrosporum ovale;* most common in young men

TREATMENT

■ Severe disease: ketoconazole 200 mg orally in the morning for 3 to 5 days (fluconazole or itraconazole as alternatives)
■ Mild diseases: topical clotrimazole, miconazole, or ketoconazole twice daily
■ Prevention of recurrence: an equal propylene glycol and water mixture applied once a month

VITILIGO

RASH Depigmentation with white macules and sharply demarcated borders that sometimes coalesce into larger lesions. Occasionally, pink color over the patches due to mild inflammation or sunburn.

DISTRIBUTION Common over the extensor surface of joints and around orifices.

CAUSE Possibly autoimmune. Prevalence of 1% to 2% in the general population; more common in males and children.

COMPLICATIONS Slightly increased risk of other autoimmune diseases.

TREATMENT

■ Protection from the sun
■ Triamcinolone 0.1% cream has variable results given twice a day sparingly.
■ Hydrocortisone 1% or 2.5% can be used for the face or skin folds.

ALBINISM

RASH Hypopigmentation with a whitish color.

DISTRIBUTION Can be partial or complete, with blond/white hair and blue eyes producing an impressive red reflex.

CAUSE Genetic abnormality.

COMPLICATIONS Visual impairment and neurologic abnormalities.

TREATMENT

■ Protection from the sun
■ Genetic counseling where available
■ Management of visual abnormalities by a trained ophthalmologist where available

YELLOW LESIONS

IMPETIGO

RASH Shiny, golden yellow crusting lesions; most common in children

DISTRIBUTION Face is most often affected.

CAUSE Staphylococcus aureus, Streptococcus pyogenes; arises from minor skin breaks.

TREATMENT

- Maintain good hygiene. Wash affected area carefully with soap.
- Apply topical antibiotic ointment.
- Avoid contact with other children.
- For widespread infection, treat with penicillin VK 250 mg four times daily for 10 days or erythromycin 250 to 500 mg four times daily for 10 days.

COMPLICATIONS If left untreated, may progress to healing with scar, or invasive infection including cellulitis, bacteremia, septicemia, or lymphangitis.

KERATOTIC LESIONS

WARTS (VERRUCAE)

RASH Well-demarcated, skin colored, flat or hyperkeratotic papules and plaques; occasionally painful.

DISTRIBUTION Face, beard areas, hands, feet.

CAUSE Cutaneous human papillomavirus (HPV) infection.

TREATMENT

- Spontaneous resolution over months to years
- Apply podophyllin or biochloracetic acid for 3 to 4 days.
- Painful plantar warts can sometimes be removed, but may require cryosurgery or laser surgery.

CALLOUSES AND CORNS

APPEARANCE Areas of hardened or thick skin; corns can be painful.

DISTRIBUTION Occur on feet where footwear pushes against skin or on hands due to repetitive forces.

CAUSE Repetitive pressure or contact.

TREATMENT

■ Wear comfortable footwear.
■ Soak feet in warm water.
■ Use a file to trim down painful corns.

NONKERATOTIC LESIONS

INTRADERMAL NEVI

APPEARANCE Small, well-demarcated pigmented macules or papules; appear during childhood to adolescence and are commonly known as moles.

DISTRIBUTION Diffuse

TIPS AND TRICKS:

Dysplastic nevi are characterized by a nonuniform, raised, or rapidly enlarging or changing appearance.

TREATMENT

■ Most nevi are benign and do not cause symptoms.
■ Surgical removal is recommended for dysplastic nevi.

DID YOU KNOW?

Large numbers of nevi are associated with melanoma.

GENITAL WARTS

RASH Soft, fleshy, skin-colored papules found in young, sexually active adults.

DISTRIBUTION Anogenital mucosa or skin.

DID YOU KNOW?

Condom use reduces transmission to uninfected sex partners. Ninety to 100% of male sex partners of infected females become infected with HPV.

CAUSE HPV infection

COMPLICATIONS Associated with cervical dysplasia and cervical squamous cell carcinoma

TREATMENT

- Genital warts may spontaneously resolve in 20% to 30% of patients.
- Podophyllin or trichloroacetic acid may be applied to genital warts, with repeated weekly applications as necessary.
- Subclinical HPV infection is more common.

CANCERS OF THE SKIN

Cancers of the skin often occur in light-skinned individuals in areas of sun exposure. There are three predominant types.

BASAL CELL CARCINOMA

There are four variants, the most common being the nodular type. It is a pearly, skin-colored papule with well-demarcated borders that are elevated. There is a central area of depression, and telangiectasias are common. The superficial variant is also common, and appears as sharply demarcated, pink, flat papules or plaques. Less common are the pigmented and morpheaform types. These lesions can resemble intradermal nevi.

SQUAMOUS CELL CARCINOMA

These lesions appear as keratotic, infiltrated papules, plaques, or nodules. Unlike basal cell carcinoma, the borders may not be well demarcated, and the lesions are not pearly. They are often hard, and the surface may appear dome shaped or irregular. They often occur on a bald scalp, the face, dorsum of the hands, or the forearms.

MALIGNANT MELANOMA

The lesions can arise de novo, or from preexisting nevi. They occur commonly on the upper back of men, or the lower legs of women. The early lesions appear macular, and are often large with irregular/blurred borders. The color can vary from brown to black, blue, or gray with associated areas of erythema.

> **KEY POINT:**
>
> Most skin cancers are not dangerous if recognized and treated in time.

TREATMENT Surgery is required for removal.

CUTANEOUS SIGNS OF AIDS AND IMMUNOSUPPRESSION

VIRAL LESIONS

HERPES ZOSTER INFECTION See section on blistering lesions

MOLLUSCUM CONTAGIOSUM

RASH Whitish appearing, discrete, dome-shaped papules that can appear solid, or blisterlike

DISTRIBUTION

- Children: widespread
- Adults: genital area
- Immunosuppression/HIV: facial lesions in adults

CAUSE Viral, common in children, usually sexually transmitted in adults

TREATMENT

- Difficult in immunosuppressed individuals because lesions recur
- Application of cantharidin to the tip of each lesion (can cause dyspigmentation)
- Curettage
- Freezing with liquid nitrogen is available (can cause dyspigmentation).

FUNGAL LESIONS

CANDIDIASIS

RASH White papules and plaques that can be removed from the surface of the mucous membranes by scraping with a tongue blade.

DISTRIBUTION Oral mucous membranes, vagina, penis of uncircumcised men.

CAUSE Fungal infection caused by *Candida* species.

DID YOU KNOW?

Oral mucous membrane infection with *Candida albicans* is an AIDS-defining illness.

TREATMENT

- Fluconazole 100 mg/day until the lesions are clear
- Nystatin solution swish and swallow, or clotrimazole troches *orally*

MALIGNANCIES

KAPOSI'S SARCOMA

RASH Nontender plaques that appear red, brown, purple, or black. (Fig. 17-5)

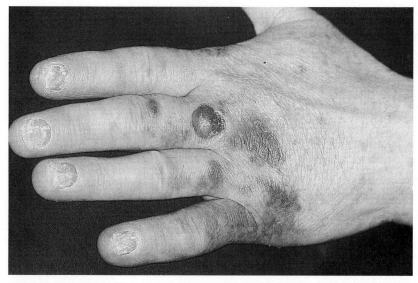

FIGURE 17-5 Kaposi's sarcoma. (From Fitzpatrick TB et al. *Color Atlas & Synopsis of Clinical Dermatology: Common and Serious Diseases,* 4th ed. New York: McGraw-Hill, 2001; with permission.)

DISTRIBUTION Anywhere over the skin or mucous membranes. Can also have visceral involvement of the respiratory and gastrointestinal tracts, and the lymph nodes.

CAUSE Immunosuppression of many causes, including medication and illnesses. The sarcoma often regresses with reversal of the condition. Human herpes virus 8 has been identified in many AIDS patients with Kaposi's sarcoma.

TREATMENT

- As above, often resolves spontaneously with reversal of immunosuppression.
- In the United States and Europe, radiation, chemotherapy, and cryotherapy have been used as treatment.

PEDIATRIC CONSIDERATIONS

CHILDHOOD EXANTHEMS: VIRAL

ROSEOLA (EXANTHEM SUBITUM)

RASH Pink, nonscaling, irregular macules and papules usually 2 to 3 mm in diameter

DISTRIBUTION Head and torso, with occasional involvement of the pharynx

CAUSE Herpes virus 6

COMMON AGE Children 6 months to 3 years

ASSOCIATED SYMPTOMS Preceded by high fever that resolves just before appearance of rash

TREATMENT Supportive, including acetaminophen for fever

ERYTHEMA INFECTIOSUM (FIFTH DISEASE)

RASH/DISTRIBUTION "Slapped cheek" appearance over face, bright red and non-scaling and reticular, non-scaling erythema over extremities

CAUSE Human parvovirus B19

COMMON AGE Children 5–15 years

ASSOCIATED SYMPTOMS Occasionally precedes low-grade fever

TREATMENT Reassurance

RUBELLA (GERMAN MEASLES)

RASH Nonscaling macules and papules that coalesce into a morbilliform-appearing rash. Forscheimer spots, discrete tiny red lesions, can appear over the posterior palate.

DISTRIBUTION Begins over the head and neck, then spreads to the extremities over the next couple of days.

COMMON AGE Usually occurs in preschool children, but can occur in adolescents and adults as well.

ASSOCIATED SYMPTOMS Prodrome can include fever, eye pain, sore throat, malaise.

COMPLICATIONS Congenital rubella in newborns

TREATMENT Reassurance

MEASLES (RUBEOLA)

RASH Pink macules that often become confluent, and sometimes purpuric (Fig. 17-6)

DISTRIBUTION Starts on the face, then spreads to the torso and extremities. Bluish gray macules with surrounding erythema on oral mucous membranes (Koplik spots) also may be seen.

COMMON AGE Preschool

ASSOCIATED SYMPTOMS Children may become seriously ill and commonly present with cough, coryza, conjunctivitis, fever, and lymphadenopathy.

COMPLICATIONS Bacterial pneumonia, encephalitis. Measles is a major cause of mortality in refugees and unimmunized populations.

TREATMENT

- Symptomatic
- Recognition and treatment of secondary infections
- Administration of measles vaccine should be an emergency health priority in vulnerable groups.
- Consider concomitant administration of vitamin A supplements.

CHILDHOOD EXANTHEMS: BACTERIAL

SCARLET FEVER

RASH A fine, lacy, "sandpaper" rash.

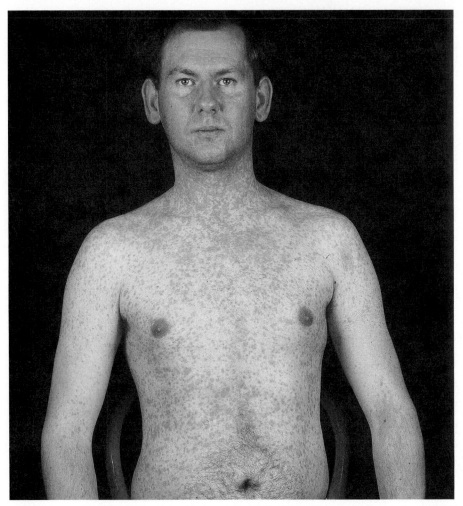

FIGURE 17-6 Measles (rubeola). (From Fitzpatrick TB et al. *Color Atlas & Synopsis of Clinical Dermatology: Common and Serious Diseases,* 4th ed. New York: McGraw-Hill, 2001; with permission.)

DISTRIBUTION Usually on the torso with linear petechiae in the skin folds of the upper extremities (Pastia lines). The face, while often flushed with circumoral pallor, is usually spared of the typical rash. Palatial petechiae and a red mucous membrane are typical, and the tongue often develops a white coating with prominent red papillae. Desquamation of the hands, feet, skin folds, and torso is common as the rash fades.

CAUSE Group A beta-hemolytic streptococcal toxin in children 2 to 10 years of age

ASSOCIATED SYMPTOMS Fever, sore throat, malaise, abdominal pain, vomiting, and headaches usually preceding the rash by 2 days

COMPLICATIONS Poststreptococcal rheumatic fever and glomerulonephritis, tonsillitis, otitis media

TREATMENT

- Oral penicillin
- Supportive care including control of fever with acetaminophen/paracetamol
- Alternative therapy is erythromycin or cephalosporins in penicillin-allergic patients.

ACUTE MENINGOCOCCEMIA

RASH Scattered pink papules that can become purpuric (Fig. 17-7). Petechiae may be the first sign of the serious nature of the illness and may be seen in the conjunctivae and on the palate. Palatal petechiae may be the earliest finding in dark-skinned individuals.

DISTRIBUTION Widespread, often in large numbers

CAUSE Infection with *Neisseria meningitidis.*

ASSOCIATED SYMPTOMS Fever, headache, and general malaise, often accompanied by severe diarrhea.

COMPLICATIONS Early complications include disseminated intravascular coagulation, pulmonary edema, renal failure in the hypotensive patient, and a persistently depressed level of consciousness. Those who survive the early phase may develop allergic complications such as arthritis, vasculitits and ulceration, episcleritis, and pericarditis.

TREATMENT Ceftriaxione 50mg/kg IV every 6 hours (may add ampicillin). Supportive therapy in an intensive care unit where possible

OTHER

KAWASAKI DISEASE

RASH Usually diffuse, red, nonscaling; may be morbiliform or resemble erythema multiforme; desquamation occurs.

DISTRIBUTION

- Red, nonscaling rash may be diffuse.

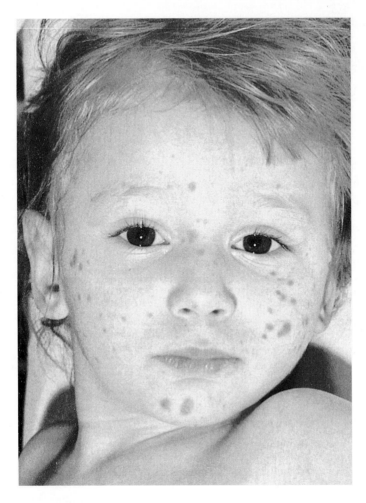

FIGURE 17-7
Acute meningococcemia. (From Fitzpatrick TB et al. *Color Atlas & Synopsis of Clinical Dermatology: Common and Serious Diseases,* 4th ed. New York: McGraw-Hill, 2001; with permission.)

■ Desquamation occurs early in the diaper region, and later on the hands and feet.

CAUSE Unknown. Usually occurs in children under 4 years of age, and is more common in Japanese and Korean children.

ASSOCIATED SYMPTOMS At least five of the six following symptoms are usually present:

■ Fever equal to or greater than 39°C
■ Erythema and edema of palms and soles with possible desquamation of distal digits
■ Polymorphous exanthem
■ Conjunctival injection

■ Oral mucous membrane injection, strawberry tongue, cracked lips
■ Nonpurulent lymphadenopathy

COMPLICATIONS Coronary artery aneurysm, myocardial infarction, valvular insufficiency, arrythmias, aseptic meningitis, hydrops of the gallbladder, arthralgias/arthritis

TREATMENT

■ Early therapy very effective
■ IV gamma globulin 2 g once
■ Aspirin 80 to 100 mg/kg/day divided four times a day for 2 weeks

DIAPER RASH/DERMATITIS

RASH Very common condition in infants that begins as pink plaques that become progressively erythematous and moist

DISTRIBUTION In the diaper region, mostly over skin in direct contact with the skin such as the scrotum and vulva; less common in the skin folds. Plaques in the skin folds, especially with papules and pustules, should raise suspicion for a superinfection with yeast.

CAUSE Irritation of the skin from urine, perspiration, and feces.

TREATMENT

■ Frequent diaper changes to keep the area dry
■ Hydrocortisone cream 1% or 2.5% applied sparingly twice a day
■ Superinfected: Add nystatin ointment, miconazole cream, or clotrimazole cream four times a day. Azole creams also can be used.
■ Severe disease with superinfection: Flucanozole 3-5 mg/kg/day orally for 3 to 5 days
■ Zinc oxide paste can be placed over the medication to protect the skin from urine or feces.

CRADLE CAP

RASH Yellow, oily crust that forms on the scalp of babies; local skin often red and irritated.

DISTRIBUTION Scalp

CAUSE Infrequent washing of the baby's head, or from keeping the head covered

TREATMENT

■ Wash head daily with medicated soap, if possible.
■ Clean off all the crust and dandruff gently. Wrapping the head with towels soaked in lukewarm water may loosen scales.
■ Keep the baby's head uncovered and open to air and light.

ECZEMA

RASH Red patches with little blisters

DISTRIBUTION Most commonly located on the backs of hands or wrists, or the upper surface of the feet; tends to occur on both hands or both feet.

CAUSE Due to a general body sensitivity. There is a genetic component (over two thirds of patients have a personal or family history of atopy), but many exacerbating factors. Some contributing factors include allergies, emotional stress, and hormonal or seasonal changes.

TREATMENT

■ Apply cold compresses to the rash.
■ With signs of infection, treat as for impetigo.
■ Allow sunlight exposure.
■ Apply a cortisone or corticosteroid cream.

CUTANEOUS SIGNS OF MALNUTRITION

The syndromes listed are classic presentations. Health practitioners may have difficulty distinguishing types of malnutrition. Protein emergency malnutrition leads to attributes of both marasmus and kwashiorkor, so skin findings may be mixed.

PELLAGRA

RASH Skin is dry and appears burnt, particularly in areas exposed to sun.

DISTRIBUTION Involves areas exposed to sun, mostly on the arms, backs of legs, and nape of the neck

CAUSE Dietary deficiency of niacin

ASSOCIATED SIGNS AND SYMPTOMS Often accompanied by other signs of malnutrition, including sores in the corners of the mouth; red, sore tongue; and a distended abdomen.

TREATMENT Eating a balanced, nutritious diet cures pellagra. Recommended foods include lentils, ground nuts, chicken, fish, eggs, meat, and cheese. Whole wheat is preferable to corn and maize. For severe pellagra, vitamin B supplementation may be helpful.

KWASHIORKOR

RASH Dark marks resembling bruises or peeling sores; glistening erythema with zones of hyperkeratosis, dryness, and hyperpigmentation.

TIPS AND TRICKS:

Children with kwashiorkor are usually edematous and lack protein in their diets.

DISTRIBUTION Often the skin of the legs and occasionally arms is involved. The feet may be swollen.

CAUSES Protein malnutrition associated with poor protein intake

ASSOCIATED SIGNS AND SYMPTOMS Pitting edema with brittle hair, apathy, irritability, and hepatomegaly

COMPLICATIONS Hypoglycemia, fluid and electrolyte disturbances, increase in infections, vitamin deficiencies, and anemia

TREATMENT Dietary therapy, supportive care, and treatment of complications

MARASMUS

RASH Dry, thin skin that wrinkles easily

TIPS AND TRICKS:

Children with marasmus are usually very wasted, with a skin-and-bones appearance and have a calorie-deficient diet.

DISTRIBUTION Diffuse

CAUSE Protein energy malnutrition due to an overall lack of calories.

ASSOCIATED SIGNS AND SYMPTOMS Muscle wasting, absence of subcutaneous fat, hair loss, apathy, and weakness, with the appearance of an old person.

COMPLICATIONS As above for kwashiorkor.

TREATMENT As above for kwashiorkor.

SPECIAL CONSIDERATIONS

DENGUE

RASH AND DISTRIBUTION In the first 24 to 48 hours of the disease there is a generalized erythematous rash. When the fever abates on the third to fifth day, a morbilliform rash appears on the trunk and spreads to the face and extremities centripetally, sometimes accompanied by a recrudescence in the fever.

CAUSE An acute, self-limited illness caused by a mosquito-borne *Flavivirus*

ASSOCIATED SIGNS AND SYMPTOMS Abrupt onset of fever, chills, headache, eye pain, myalgias, arthralgias, vomiting, lassitude, and low back pain. Bradycardia and lymphadenopathy may develop.

COMPLICATIONS Neutropenia, anemia, thrombocytopenia, and hemorrhage

TREATMENT Supportive care

TYPHOID FEVER

RASH Blanching, erythematous maculopapular lesions 2 to 4 mm in diameter

DISTRIBUTION Most frequently on the abdomen, chest, extremities, and back.

CAUSE Infection with the bacteria *Salmonella typhi*, most commonly by ingestion of contaminated food or water. In rare cases, it can be transmitted by direct finger-to-mouth contact.

ASSOCIATED SIGNS AND SYMPTOMS Fever, chills, dull frontal or diffuse headaches, anorexia, diffuse abdominal pain, abnormal bowel function, sore throat, occasional seizures in children under 5, apathy, relative bradycardia (<25% of patients), delirium, coated tongue, hepatosplenomegaly

COMPLICATIONS Intestinal perforation or hemorrhage, delirium, myocarditis, proteinuria, renal failure

TREATMENT Chloramphenicol

ALTERNATIVE TREATMENT In multidrug-resistant areas, fluoroquinolones and third-generation cephalosporins are the antibiotics of choice.

LEPROSY

RASH AND DISTRIBUTION There are a number of different classifications of leprosy, each with its own particular features. The earliest manifestations are often poorly differentiated macules that may appear hypopigmented in dark-skinned individuals or mildly erythematous in light-skinned individuals. At this stage there is mild diminution of sensation and sweating, and a change in skin texture. In tuberculoid leprosy, patients have one or more of these macules that are sharply demarcated with finely papulated edges (Fig. 17-8). These can be small, or cover large areas of the body and are characterized by a more profound loss of sensation, sweating, and hair. Enlarged cutaneous nerves can sometimes be palpated. Lepromatous leprosy is characterized by vague macules in children that can progress to larger ones, and often involve nodules on the face, ears, buttocks, and extremities. There is usually no alteration in sensation or sweating in the early childhood forms; however, this does develop as the disease progresses.

CAUSE Mycobaterium leprae. Routes of natural transmission are unknown.

ASSOCIATED SYMPTOMS Sensory loss, decrease in sweating and hair loss

COMPLICATIONS Testicular atrophy, thick nasal or oral mucosa with voice changes, punctate or interstitial keratitis. Neuritic leprosy affects a major nerve trunk, with resultant pain, parethesias, paresis, and muscular atrophy. Reversal reactions are observed with erythema/edema of the lesions and acute neuritis, leading at times to sensory loss and paralytic deformities.

TREATMENT Dapsone, clofazimine, rifampin (see World Health Organization recommendations—Appendix 1).

ONCHOCERCIASIS (RIVER BLINDNESS)

RASH Both acute and chronic skin changes may be seen:

■ Acute papular onchodermatitis consists of small scattered pruritic papules that can progress to vesicles or pustules with erythema and edema that can affect a single limb, the trunk, or face.

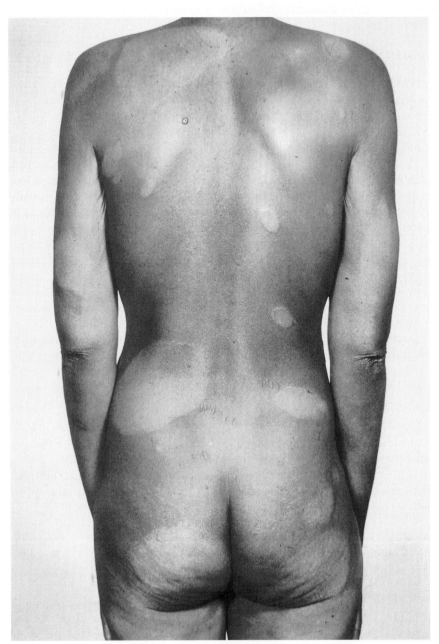

FIGURE 17-8 Leprosy: tuberculoid type. (From Fitzpatrick TB et al. *Color Atlas & Synopsis of Clinical Dermatology: Common and Serious Diseases,* 4th ed. New York: McGraw-Hill, 2001; with permission.)

■ Chronic papular onchodermatitis consists of flat-topped papules of different sizes with hyperpigmentation, and often accompanied by acute lesions.

■ Lichenified onchodermatitis consists of pruritic, hyperpigmented, hyperkeratotic plaques with associated lymphadenopathy, often limited to one limb.

KEY POINT:

A pattern resembling that of onchoderciasis is seen after treatment with microfilaricidal drugs.

DID YOU KNOW?

Lichenified onchodermatitis also referred to as sowda or leopard skin is classically seen in Yemen and the Sudan.

DISTRIBUTION In Africa, commonly over the lower extremities, buttocks, pelvis, and thighs

ASSOCIATED SYMPTOMS Itching (often the earliest symptom) and lymphadenopathy; atrophy and "hanging groin" later in the disease; onchocercomas, lymphadenitis, and eye changes

COMPLICATIONS Blindness and disfiguring skin changes

TREATMENT Ivermectin

LEISHMANIASIS

RASH Primary lesions occur at the site of a sand fly bite. Single or multiple cutaneous papules commonly evolve into ulcers and nodules at the bite, which eventually heal spontaneously with a depressed scar. Forms of leishmaniasis include Old and New World cutaneous leishmaniasis, mucocutaneous leishmaniasis, and diffuse cutaneous leishmaniasis. Old World cutaneous leishmaniasis may manifest as a single dry ulcer with a papule on the face that heals slowly, or multiple crusted papules and nodules resembling a volcano with a depressed center. New World cutaneous leishmaniasis presents as small, erythematous firm papules that become encrusted and ulcerate , which are also known as chiclero ulcers or bay sores. Mucocutaneous leishmaniasis presents as one or more lesions on the lower extremities that ulcerate and heal spontaneously. Metastatic lesions can appear in the nasopharynx or perineum. Diffuse cutaneous leishmaniasis resembles lepromatous leprosy.

DISTRIBUTION Exposed site, especially ankles and legs; the face is affected only in children. Mucocutaneous leishmaniasis affects the nasal mucosa, lips, and floor of mouth.

SPREAD Transmitted by *Leishmania* promastigotes deposited on skin of the host into blood drawn by probing sand fly vector.

TREATMENT No chemoprophylaxis for travelers exists. Lesional therapy includes topical 15% paromomycin sulfate, 12% methylbenzethonium chloride in white paraffin twice daily for 10 days. Sodium antimony gluconate IV or intramuscularly in a single daily dose of 10 mg/kg may be used. Amphotericin B or pentamidine or sodium antimony gluconate plus gamma interferon is used for refractory cases.

CHAPTER 18

Anesthesia and Pain Management

James Li and Steven M. Green

Health care in remote or poverty-stricken regions is frequently delivered under desperate circumstances. This is particularly true for patients whose injuries or illnesses require urgent surgery. In such cases, a needed procedure may be impossible due to the lack of proper anesthesia or a skilled anesthetist. This chapter was written for any medical caregiver, from nurse to medical student to surgeon, who must perform anesthesia in a remote locale, where someone more experienced is not available. Though no substitute for training and experience, it provides a basis for effective anesthetic practice where resources are limited, whether by poverty or disaster.

Physicians in the developing world must deal ingeniously with a lack of supplies, particularly in impoverished and remote areas. Standard care rarely includes capnography, pulse oximetry, or advanced cardiopulmonary monitoring. Typically, only one injectable anesthetic is available, inhalation anesthesia is limited to halothane or ether, manual suction and a bag-valve-mask assembly constitute the only advanced resuscitation equipment, and supplemental oxygen is scarce.

BE PREPARED: LEARN FROM EXPERIENCED CLINICIANS

No learning is as effective as that gained while working with an experienced mentor. For clinicians newly embarking upon practice in the developing world, we suggest first practicing with a group of more experienced physicians to learn and practice essential anesthetic techniques. For medical practitioners who plan to practice in the developing world, refer to the educational resources at the end of this chapter.

FOCUSING ON THE ESSENTIALS

Anesthesia encompasses an enormous field, and practitioners may feel overwhelmed at the prospect of mastering a new discipline. However, in the developing world certain simple skills learned well can suffice for almost all situations. For the purpose of field anesthesia, it is not necessary to have an exhaustive knowledge of all medications used in anesthesiology. We encourage practitioners to familiarize themselves with a small list of agents chosen to both serve a broad range of cases and perform well under harsh circumstances (Table 18-1).

TABLE 18-1 ESSENTIAL LIST FOR FIELD ANESTHESIA

ANESTHETIC DRUGS	DOSE/ AMOUNT	COMMENTS/ INSTRUCTIONS
Essential		
Ketamine	50 mg/mL and 100 mg/mL vials. 2–4 mg/kg IV	Higher-concentration vials reduce volume needed for pediatric IM injections.
Atropine	Multiuse vials	
Promethazine	25 mg IV/IM/PO/PR	This drug possesses not only antiemetic, but also antihistamine and sedative properties, making it more useful than agents having only one use.
Diazepam	2.5–5 mg IV/IM	May substitute alternatives such as lorazepam or midazolam if available; diazepam is the least expensive benzodiazepine.
Lidocaine (lignocaine)	4.5 mg/kg max	An all-purpose solution of plain 2% lidocaine can be diluted and mixed with epinephrine as needed for most types of infiltration anesthesia. Other local anesthetics such as bupivacaine and procaine can be substituted for lidocaine if available.
Lidocaine (lignocaine), hyperbaric	5% lidoccaine with 5% to 7.5% dextrose in single-use 2-mL vials	This is for spinal anesthesia and is also known as "heavy" lidocaine. Similar spinal agents are available (5% prilocaine in 5% dextrose, 4% mepivacaine in 10% dextrose, and 0.5% bupivacaine in 5% dextrose). Though duration of action varies between agents, the dose of these others is approximately the same as that of lidocaine.
Morphine	2–5 mg IV 5–10 mg IM	May substitute meperidine (pethidine) or other narcotics if available; meperidine is sometimes more easily available than morphine and can be used in its place.

TABLE 18-1 ESSENTIAL LIST FOR FIELD ANESTHESIA   *(continued)*

ANESTHETIC DRUGS	DOSE/ AMOUNT	COMMENTS/ INSTRUCTIONS
Essential		
Powdered succinylcholine (suxamethonium)	1.5 mg/kg IV	Once reconstituted, succinylcholine loses efficacy unless refrigerated. Many developing world practices lack refrigerated facilities, so powder is reconstituted as it is required.
Naloxone	Multiuse vials. 0.4–2 mg IV/IM	For reversal of opiate overdose.
Pressor agent: Ephedrine Dopamine	As directed	For hypotension due to spinal anesthesia Ephedrine is frequently available at low cost to developing world practices. Pressors chosen for use in spinal anesthesia should have predominantly alpha-agonistic effects. Alternative alpha agents include methoxamine, phenylephrine, and metaraminol.
Oxytocin (or ergotamine)	3–10 units IM 5–20 units in 500 cc NS	For uterine contraction following cesarean
Epinephrine	Adrenaline, in 1 mg/mL multiuse vials. .01 mg/kg/dose	In the developing world, this is probably least useful for resuscitation, because primary cardiac disease is virtually nonexistent. Nonetheless, epinephrine is useful as a supplement for local anesthetic solutions and for treatment of bronchospasm and anaphylaxis.
Optional		
Pancuronium	Multiuse vials 0.1 mg/kg IV	Pancuronium provides longer paralysis in abdominal operations. Other non-depolarizing neuromuscular blocking agents are also appropriate, but pancuronium is inexpensive and its duration is shorter than others, so that if reversal agents are missing, the patient does not require many hours of hand ventilation before regaining normal respiratory capacity. Alternative agents include tubocurarine, vecuronium, atracurium, mivacurium, and rocuronium.
Neostigmine	Multiuse vials	For reversing nondepolarizing neuromuscular blockade

This list may vary depending on the previous experience of the health-care provider. However, three anesthetic methods form the foundation of practice in the developing world:

■ Injectable ketamine
■ Spinal anesthesia
■ Local subcutaneous infiltration

These three are chosen for emphasis in this chapter because of their great utility under adverse conditions. In developing world practice, this utility is due to widespread use, low cost, ready availability, and well-understood side effect profiles that can be practically anticipated. Practitioners who are versed in the use of ketamine, spinal, and local anesthesia possess an indispensable skill, because most operations can be performed comfortably using one or more of these methods. None requires intubation, supplemental oxygen, or more monitoring than periodic measurement of heart rate, blood pressure, and respiratory effort.

EQUIPMENT AND SUPPLIES

The following list of equipment and supplies is recommended for a developing world anesthesia practice. These are chosen for use under many conditions, widespread and inexpensive availability, and minimization of wastable materials (Table 18-2).

TABLE 18-2 ESSENTIAL EQUIPMENT AND SUPPLIES

EQUIPMENT	DESCRIPTION
Stethoscope	Two stethoscopes are useful for field practice in anesthesia. The first is the standard clinician's stethoscope. The second is the anesthetist's, also known as a monaural stethoscope. The latter has a plug that is worn in one ear and is connected to a length of tubing that attaches to a diaphragm taped to the patient's chest. This is useful for continuous monitoring of a patient's pulse rate, pluse intensity, and breath sounds during an operation. A reusable monaural earplug can be procured from one's home anesthesia service. Under normal circumstances, the earplug is designed to be attached to disposable single-use chest prices. However, the diaphragm from a standard stethoscope can be used repeatedly with a monaural earplug if detached from the standard stethoscope and attached to a section of nasogastric tubing.
Blood pressure cuff	
Pulse oximeter	If available. These are not essential but are no longer prohibitively expensive and provide an extra margin of safety in patient monitoring.

TABLE 18-2 ESSENTIAL EQUIPMENT AND SUPPLIES *(continued)*

EQUIPMENT	DESCRIPTION
Recleanable supplies	
Foot-operated nonelectrical suction	Few manufacturers make such devices. One model is available from Ambu (800/262-8462).
Bag-valve mask	Both pediatric and adult sizes are needed. For children, facemasks, fitting neonates, infants, and older children are recommended.
Mouth-operated (De Lee) suction	
Three-way tracheostomy dilator (cricothyrotomy)	A hemostat may serve this purpose, but not as well. Some developing world practitioners carry a scalpel on a shortened handle and a small hemostat for the purpose of immediately performing emergency cricothyrotomy if necessary.
Nasal airways	
Oral airways	
Scalpel	
Universal adult/ pediatric laryngoscope handle and blades	An all-purpose adult laryngoscope blade is a curved size 4. This can easily be adapted to adults with smaller airways, but a smaller blade cannot be easily adapted for those with larger airways. For neonatal resuscitation following cesarean section, an assortment of pediatric straight blades (sizes 1–3) is recommended. The universal laryngoscope handle runs from AA batteries and fits both adult and pediatric blades.
Endotracheal tubes	For adults, a red rubber noncuffed 9-0 endotracheal tube can be easily recleaned and used repeatedly. For fasted patients, the large size usually fits snugly through the cords and obviates the need for a cuff. However, cuffed tubes are recommended for all adult emergency cases, and an assortment should be obtained. Most pediatric intubations will be neonatal resuscitation, so neonatal endotracheal tubes also should be obtained.
Nasogastric tubes	When possible, use "Luer-lok" syringes in order to prevent the needles from slipping during local infiltration. To reduce waste, obtain plastic syringes that are autoclavable.
IV tourniquet	
Syringes	
Spinal needles	
Needles for local anesthesia	The following assortment is recommended: short, fine gauge (0.45 x 16 mm) for intradermal injection; medium, fine gauge (0.65 x 30 mm) for subcutaneous injection; long, small gauge (0.8 x 100 mm) for infiltration anesthesia. Also recommended are standard needles for intramuscular injection.

TABLE 18-2 ESSENTIAL EQUIPMENT AND SUPPLIES *(continued)*

EQUIPMENT	DESCRIPTION
Headlamp or flashlight	For emergency operation at night
Gloves	
Restockable supplies	
Betadine	For spinal anesthesia preparation
Alcohol and cotton	For IV skin or local infiltration preparation
IV catheters	
Saline	
Tape	

SAFETY ISSUES: THE GOLDEN RULES OF ANESTHESIA

1. Perform a preoperative assessment. Patients with conditions such as sepsis, hypovolemia, anemia, heart disease, and diabetes have higher rates of operative morbidity. Most patients in the developing world do not have a well documented chart, nor are full chemistry and hematology panels always feasible. Therefore, the physical examination becomes the most important screening tool for detecting potential risk factors for high surgical morbidity. The risk of operation can often be lowered by treatment in preparation for anesthesia. If the patient is a particular anesthetic risk, try to ascertain this before induction.

2. When possible, operate on a fasted patient. Aspiration is always possible. However, the risk of not operating is sometimes worse than the risk of aspiration, so the fasting rule is not an absolute one. For patients who must undergo surgery with full stomachs, pretreatment with antacids can reduce the morbidity of aspiration because acid is worse than neutral aspiration. The American Society of Anesthesiologists makes the following recommendations for preoperative fasting durations (Table 18-3). Unless contraindicated, children should be offered clear liquids up until the recommended period of fasting to minimize the risk of volume depletion and hypoglycemia.

3. Keep the airway clear. Use a table that can be rapidly placed head down (Trendelenburg position). If a patient should vomit during anesthesia, dramatic and immediate measures should be taken to prevent aspiration. The patient should be quickly rolled onto one side and the head of the table tipped down, using gravity to facilitate exit of vomitus from the airway and pharynx. Have suction instantly ready to clear the airway of secretions and vomitus. Remember this three-part

TABLE 18-3 FASTING GUIDELINES FOR ANESTHESIA

AGE GROUP	SOLIDS AND NONCLEAR LIQUIDS (h)	CLEAR LIQUIDS (h)
Adults	6–8	2–3
Children >36 mo	6–8	2–3
Children 6–36 mo	6	2–3
Children <6 mo	4–6	2

sequence so that it is both instinctive and immediate. Patients who have received spinal anesthesia should never be placed head down, even if shocked. (For other patients, there is some debate whether the Trendelenburg position actually helps anyone who is hypotensive.) The reason is that further shock and respiratory failure may rapidly ensue if the spinal anesthetic agent is allowed to bathe the upper spinal cord during a head-down maneuver.

4. Check equipment before starting. Ensure that all of your equipment is in good working order. It could make the difference between life and death in the operative setting.

5. Have a vein open. This is normally done when intravenous (IV) anesthesia is used. It is vital in spinal anesthesia, due to commonly observed sympatholytically associated hypotension. It is less important in children undergoing intramuscular (IM) ketamine anesthesia. If IV access is warranted in a child, it can be performed after the anesthetic effect has begun to reduce their discomfort.

6. Monitor pulse and blood pressure. This is particularly important for children and patients undergoing spinal anesthesia because both groups may decompensate rapidly. The best monitor is a person dedicated to the task, who listens to the patient's heartbeat and respiration simultaneously by means of a monaural stethoscope taped over the patient's left chest.

7. Before intubating, always have someone who can apply cricoid pressure (Sellick's maneuver). When intubation is performed, cricoid pressure should begin when the first sedative is injected and should not be released until confirmation of proper tube placement has been completed. If a patient actively vomits, the roll/head drop/suction maneuver should be immediately performed, and cricoid pressure gently released simultaneously, in order to prevent esophageal rupture.

8. Recover in recovery position. When the operation is complete, place the patient in recovery position to avoid aspiration while wakening. Recovery position is essentially the same as the roll/head drop maneuver, but is performed prior to vomiting.

SIGNS OF GOOD ANESTHETIC PRACTICE

The following are some general characteristics:

■   Anesthetized patients are never left alone on the table but are always monitored by a competent person, before, during, and following operation.

■ A well-labeled resuscitation tray with a supply of medications is always available.

■ When a bottle or bag of IV fluid is empty, it is either replaced or removed. If there is a strip of paper down the bottle or bag marking where fluid should be each hour, care is likely very good. Empty drips hanging over a patient's bed are a sign that the management of fluid therapy is poor.

■ Anesthetic records are kept and mishaps discussed constructively in order to prevent future ones.

■ All anesthetics are given on a table that can be tilted head down in an area where suction is immediately available.

LOCAL AND REGIONAL ANESTHESIA

GENERAL METHODS

Two percent plain lidocaine is inexpensive and can be diluted to other strengths and supplemented with epinephrine for most needs. Multiuse vials also can be autoclaved if sterility after prolonged use is a concern. More concentrated solutions are needed for nerve blocks, whereas solutions as dilute as 0.25% are effective for infiltration anesthesia (Table 18-4).

Injection of lidocaine is painful. The nerves most sensitive to pain are located in the dermis, so intradermal injection is more painful than subcutaneous injection. Pain can be minimized by placement of the needle tip first rapidly through the skin surface, then moving the needle to a desired injection site. Finer needles, slower injection rates, and solutions buffered with bicarbonate (about 1 part standard 8.4% bicarbonate to 10 parts lidocaine) reduce the pain of injection.

When injecting local anesthesia, use the finest needle available that will not break during injection. The length of the needle should be chosen to minimize the need for repeated injections through the skin. For best control of the injection rate, needles should be fitted to the smallest syringe able to contain the desired volume for infiltration.

Inject while pushing the needle forward (as well as when withdrawing the needle) in a gentle fluid motion. Bending a longer needle so that it remains parallel to the skin during injection makes injection in the correct plane easier. Ideally, a patient should feel

---

TABLE 18-4 MIXING LIDOCAINE FOR INJECTION

To make 0.4% lidocaine with epinephrine (a solution favored by some hospitals for large-volume infiltration anesthesia), add 20 mL of 2% plain lidocaine to 80 mL sterile saline. Supplement this with 0.5 mL of 1:1,000 epinephrine solution (0.5 mg). This results in an epinephrine dilution of 1:200,000 in 100 mL of 0.4% lidocaine solution.

only a single needle prick per wheal. Whenever possible, subsequent injections should be performed through skin that has already been anesthetized (Fig. 18-1).

FIELD BLOCKS

An alternative to simple infiltration anesthesia is the field block. This is most useful for blocking sensation to a large patch of skin, where local infiltration would require multiple smaller injections. Field blocks work well for abscess incision and drainage, for excision of small skin lesions, and for repair of complex lacerations. If done properly, the patient feels only two pricks (Fig. 18-2).

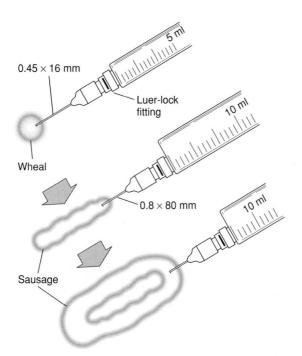

FIGURE 18-1 Local anesthesia. Swab the skin to be anesthetized with an antiseptic solution. Inject a small amount of lidocaine into the skin using the finest needle and smallest syringe necessary. Draw up a larger portion of solution and attach a needle long enough to inject, if possible, the entire length of the skin to be anesthetized. Bend the needle appropriately to allow injection to parallel the skin surface. Puncture the skin through the initial wheal, and direct the needle as close to the surface of the skin as possible. Inject the solution in a slow fluid motion while pushing the needle tip forward along the desired skin tract. Proper infiltration will give the skin an "orange peel and sausage" appearance. Withdraw the needle, injecting supplemental solution as needed to finish the sausage-like tract. Finally, and without withdrawing the needle from the skin, inject again in a slightly deeper subcutaneous plane. Properly done, this will create a second broader and deeper tract beneath the superficial one.

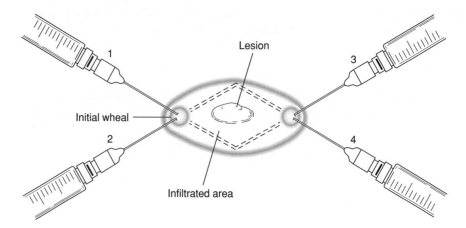

FIGURE 18-2 Field blocks. The field block consists of two intradermal wheals placed at opposite corners of an imaginary diamond surrounding the patch of skin to be anesthetized. Through one wheal, a longer needle is placed and a longer deeper wheal is raised to form one side of the diamond. The process is repeated by withdrawing the needle without exiting the skin, and redirecting it forward to form the second side of the diamond. Through the opposite intradermal wheal, the entire process is repeated, so that four sides of a diamond are obtained, each intersecting another, and a complete boundary of skin anesthesia is thus placed around the patch to be anesthetized

LOCAL INSTEAD OF GENERAL ANESTHESIA

Local anesthesia is always the safest technique, particularly when a patient's stomach is not empty. It requires little equipment and has no airway effects. However, its limitations include the finite amount of local agent that is safe to inject, the inability to inject through infected tissue, and the difficulty of its use on children and anxious patients. Supplement local anesthesia with oral or IV sedatives when necessary for the patient's comfort and surgeon's safety. These can be given before and supplemented intravenously during the operation as needed. Examples of premedication include oral or injectable promethazine, diazepam, morphine, and low-dose IV ketamine (0.25 mg/kg).

Although blocking cutaneous nerves through local infiltration eliminates most incisional pain, it does not provide muscle relaxation. Thus, regional intercostal blocks, rectus muscle blocks, or spinal anesthesia also may be required.

Several common operations can be performed under local anesthesia. These include cesarean section, ventral and inguinal herniorrhaphy, and abscess incision and drainage. Of these, local anesthesia for cesarean section should be avoided if the surgeon is just learning to perform the procedure, because muscle relaxation is more difficult when compared with spinal anesthesia. (See section on Special Considerations: Obstetrics at the end of this chapter for a more detailed discussion about cesarean section anesthesia.)

INTERCOSTAL BLOCKS

Block of the ninth through twelfth intercostal nerves is an alternative method for muscle relaxation in the patient dissociated with ketamine or undergoing abdominal operation with local infiltration. This procedure seems simple, but can be difficult for novices, and a detailed discussion of it is beyond the scope of this text. It cannot be done quickly, so it is not practical for emergency cesarean section. It also must be performed with great care, in order to prevent pneumothorax, a potentially fatal complication if unrecognized. Higher blocks using this method also can be used for other abdominal operations, but at the risk of respiratory compromise if too many intercostal muscles are paralyzed.

RECTUS MUSCLE BLOCK

See the later section on Special Considerations: Obstetrics.

INGUINAL HERNIORRHAPHY BLOCK

This involves infiltration of the skin over the site to be incised, followed by deeper infiltration of the parietal peritoneum and hernia sac once exposed. The technique uses up to 100 mL of 0.4% lidocaine (epinephrine-supplemented) and gives the surgeon an advantage because the hernia can be identified during the operation when the patient coughs.

SAFE DOSAGES

The maximum safe dose of plain lidocaine is 3 mg/kg, or 200 mg total for adults. This safety margin is roughly doubled if epinephrine-supplemented lidocaine is used instead of plain lidocaine. Lidocaine toxicity is rare and is usually preceded by a metallic taste. It causes central nervous system effects such as seizures. Treatment of toxicity consists of anticonvulsant therapy and support of vital functions. For adults, these considerations are only important when large doses of lidocaine are used, such as in local infiltration of the abdomen for cesarean section, when general or spinal anesthesia is contraindicated. Such infiltration may require 100 mL or more of local anesthesia solution.

Each percentage of solution equals 10 mg/mL of actual agent (or 1 g/100 mL). Thus, 1 mL of 1% solution contains 10 mg of lidocaine, and 1 mL of 2% solution contains 20 mg of lidocaine. For a 50-kg woman, 150 mg of lidocaine is the amount contained in only 7.5 mL of 2% of the solution. Injecting 100 mL of 2% solution would give the patient 2,000 mg of lidocaine, more than a dozen times the safe dose.

Such considerations now become obvious for children, who weigh much less than pregnant women. The maximum safe lidocaine dose for a 20-kg child needing repair of a large scalp laceration is 60 mg, the amount of lidocaine contained in only 3 mL of 2%

solution. This amount may not be enough to properly anesthetize an area for repair or incision. Thus, the solution must either be diluted, or epinephrine-supplemented solution used, or both. In the case of the 20-kg child, 60 mg of lidocaine is also contained in 12 mL of 0.5% solution, which for infiltration is as effective as 2%. If epinephrine-supplemented 0.5% solution is used, the maximum safe dose is doubled to 120 mg, and 24 mL of solution can be safely injected, provided that epinephrine can be safely used at the injection site.

PAIN MANAGEMENT

SIMPLE ORAL ANALGESICS

Despite a multitude of oral analgesics marketed in the developed world, acetaminophen and nonsteroidal agents are still standards. Both are inexpensive, well understood, and have wide safety margins. Outside the United States, acetaminophen is known as para-cetamol, and is widely marketed under the brand name Panadol. Of the nonsteroidal class, ibuprofen and diclofenac are the least expensive, are widely available, and have the least potential for causing gastrointestinal hemorrhage. Outside the United States, diclofenac is available over the counter, and is widely marketed under the trade name Voltaren. Both diclofenac and aspirin are available in many countries as IV agents, and can be used as antipyretic agents for febrile patients who are unable to take oral medications.

OPIATE ANALGESICS

The prototype opiate analgesic is morphine. The major distinction between opioid agents lies in relative potency rather than mechanism of action. Morphine is most commonly given by IM or IV injection. A starting IM dose is 0.1 mg/kg, about 7 mg in an average adult. Small but frequent IV doses titrated to effect are more effective than larger infrequent IM doses. The starting dose for IV morphine is roughly one fourth the IM dose, 0.03 mg/kg (2 mg in an average adult) titrated to effect. Maximum dose is 0.5 mg/kg, though some patients are tolerant and require more.

Meperidine is similar to morphine but has approximately ten times less potency. It is mentioned here as an alternative to morphine, due to broader availability in some regions. Outside the United States, meperidine is known as pethidine. A starting IM dose of meperidine is 1 mg/kg, about 70 mg in an average adult. The starting dose for IV meperidine is 0.25 mg/kg titrated to effect.

When combined with diazepam, both morphine and meperidine may cause apnea. Apnea is also possible if high doses of each agent are given alone, but is much more of a risk when used in combination with a benzodiazepine. To prevent such occurrences in anesthesia of this type, the minimum dose of opioid should be used, carefully titrated with diazepam to effect. In some centers, combination diazepam and meperidine sedation is used routinely for dilation and curettage procedures, and when this is done, appropriate monitoring of the patient is needed.

When performing combination sedation with diazepam and either morphine or meperidine, always give the opioid first through the IV line. Diazepam is painful to inject, and this pain can be moderated by injecting the analgesic agent first.

KETAMINE FOR ANALGESIA

In areas where morphine is expensive or not widely available, patients with severe pain, as from cancer or multiply fractured ribs, can receive ketamine by low-dose infusion. This method is identical to ketamine infusion for anesthesia, described later in this chapter, but is dosed at a rate low enough so only analgesic effects of ketamine are obtained.

To infuse ketamine for analgesia, first give a small bolus (0.25 mg/kg) of ketamine IV, titrated carefully to eliminate pain but not produce dissociation. Next, hang a solution of 0.5 mg/mL ketamine in saline to run at about 15 to 30 drips per minute, using a nonmicrodrip chamber (15 drops/mL). Titrate the solution to maintain analgesia.

GENERAL ANESTHESIA IN THE FIELD SETTING

There are times when local anesthesia is not appropriate for surgery. The operation may require muscle relaxation, the patient may be anxious, or the field of operation may be too large to safely anesthetize with local agents. In these situations, three methods are commonly used in resource-scarce regions: dissociative anesthesia with ketamine, spinal anesthesia by epidural or subarachnoid routes, and inhalational anesthesia. In certain cases, muscle paralysis is often added using long-acting IV nondepolarizing agents, or, in particularly resource-scarce regions, the short-acting depolarizing agent succinylcholine.

Epidural and inhalational anesthesia are beyond the scope of this discussion due to their increased complexity and equipment requirements. Both ketamine and spinal (subarachnoid) anesthesia are discussed in detail below. The use of neuromuscular blocking muscle relaxants is not complex but is unsafe for the inexperienced practitioner due to increased possibilities of aspiration and asphyxia. It is, however, within the scope of the practitioner experienced in advanced airway management, who is skilled in both intubation and rescue cricothyrotomy. Use of muscle relaxants makes fine operations (such as thyroidectomy) and all abdominal operations much easier for the surgeon. In a few cases, surgery would be impossible without such relaxation. Therefore, a brief discussion of use and methods follows the sections on ketamine and spinal anesthesia.

KETAMINE

The bulk of clinical experience with ketamine comes from the developing world. In such countries it is routinely and safely administered thousands of times daily by nonanesthetists operating in areas with few resources, such as described by King in *Primary Anaesthesia* (Oxford University Press, 1990:60).

Ketamine produces a most useful state of dissociative anaesthesia. The patient rapidly goes into a trance-like state, with widely open eyes and nystagmus. He is unconscious, amnesic and deeply analgesic. His airway is remarkably preserved, with his head in almost any position, far more so than with any other anaesthetic. Not surprisingly, this remarkable drug has made many operations possible that would otherwise have been impossible for lack of a trained anaesthetist. Ketamine is especially useful if you have no recovery ward and patients have to recover in their own beds. Ketamine is remarkably safe and is certainly the safest anaesthetic if you are inexperienced. Nevertheless, it is not absolutely safe, so be vigilant. In some hospitals without a trained anaesthetist, 90 percent of the operations are done with ketamine. IM ketamine acts rapidly. You also can give it IV as a bolus injection or as a drip, either alone or with relaxants.

Ketamine is an agent that represents the ideal for use in remote medical practice. It has the unique ability to safely provide anxiolysis, analgesia, and amnesia simultaneously. Its effects are potent: analgesia is roughly double that of morphine, and amnesia is on the same order as midazolam. Ketamine use obviates the need for local anesthetic infiltration during surgery or in wound repair. When given skillfully and in a calm environment, it is more often than not a pleasant experience for patients. It can be used safely without supplemental oxygen or intubation. It produces neither hypotension (except in severe states when catecholamine stores are totally depleted) nor respiratory depression (unless injected too rapidly), so it is ideal for use in emergency cases when patients are in mild to moderate shock.

Ketamine's therapeutic range makes it one of the safest sedative agents for most emergency clinical situations. Distinct and useful effects are obtained when administered at different doses. Low-dose ketamine infusion provides potent analgesia, making it useful in performing minor procedures such as wound debridement and painful dressing changes for burn victims. In higher doses, amnesia and complete cognitive-corporeal dissociation is added, making it useful as a single agent for more complex but brief emergency procedures. In yet higher doses, the combination of effects makes prolonged surgical anesthesia possible. As such, ketamine may be used as a single agent for emergency surgery of nearly all types.

INDICATIONS Ketamine provides effective sedation for a wide variety of clinical procedures, including

- Pain control for fractures or burns
- Debridement of wounds, dressing changes
- Incision and drainage of large abscesses
- Orthopedic reductions
- Emergency amputations
- Facial procedures

Other examples of use include operations on several sites at once where local anesthesia would exceed limits, face-down procedures, and emergency operations on hypotensive patients. Due to higher rates of laryngospasm with pharyngeal stimulation, it is not ideally suited for intraoral or airway operations, although in skilled hands it has been used successfully for dental procedures, tonsillectomy, esophagoscopy, and bronchoscopy.

Ketamine provides no muscle relaxation, so it may make an emergency abdominal operation such as appendectomy or cesarean section more difficult. Nonetheless, ketamine has made possible many operations that would be otherwise impossible with no anesthetic, and is considered the agent of choice by many for emergency abdominal operations where the surgeon must also perform as anesthetist.

PREMEDICATION BEFORE USING KETAMINE   Some clinicians routinely premedicate all patients with promethazine or a benzodiazepine to reduce postprocedure agitation, although this practice may prolong the recovery period. Promethazine is widely used in Africa for adult premedication, and may have some advantage over the benzodiazepines due to its additional antiemetic effects. Ketamine may be combined with an antisialogogue to reduce its stimulant effect on oral and respiratory secretions. Either glycopyrrolate, in a dose of 0.01 mg/kg (maximum dose 0.2 mg), or atropine, in a dose of 0.01 mg/kg (0.1 mg minimum to 0.5 mg maximum), is acceptable. Pretreatment 30 minutes prior to ketamine administration is best, but both glycopyrrolate and atropine may be mixed in the same syringe as ketamine if time is short. Some physicians forego the use of an antisialogogue (more often in adults), preferring ketamine-induced hypersalivation to the additional tachycardia caused by atropine or glycopyrrolate.

BASIC METHODS   For children, IM injection is usually the least traumatic method of obtaining effective sedation. Centers that mandate IV access for all sedative procedures may negate the benefit of ketamine's anxiolytic properties by requiring performance of a painful procedure (IV placement) before initiating sedation. IM injection alone has proven safe in large reviews. If IV access is mandatory, one technique that may preserve the goal of anxiolysis is to first administer IM ketamine at an anxiolytic or greater dosage. Following effect, an IV line can be established without patient distress and any remaining doses of ketamine needed can be given either by the IV or IM route.

For adults, IV infusion is usually the safest and most easily titratable to effect. Infusion via this method further prevents rare apnea and laryngospasm, most commonly observed with rapid and high IV bolus doses of ketamine. Dissociation by ketamine infusion usually requires less agent for longer procedures and greatly reduces recovery time.

INTRAMUSCULAR METHOD   Ketamine is usually dosed initially at 4 mg/kg (with a range of 0.5–17 mg/kg reported in the literature, depending on procedural requirements). Analgesia alone is usually obtained with a dose of 1 mg/kg IM. Complete dissociation is usually obtained with a dose of 4 to 10 mg/kg IM. (Veterinarians routinely give 15–50 mg/kg IM to anesthetize animals for surgery.) Onset of action (glazed eyes and nystagmus) usually occurs within 5 minutes and lasts for up to 30 minutes, depending on the dose used.

Before beginning any painful procedure, analgesic effect should be tested by pricking the patient with a needle. Booster doses of 2 to 5 mg/kg IM every 10 minutes (without additional antisialogogue) may be given if initial sedation is inadequate. The 100 mg/mL ketamine solution is preferred for IM administration to reduce the volume of injected solution.

INTRAVENOUS INFUSION METHOD Mix ketamine with saline or D5W to make a 1 mg ketamine to 1 mL solution (500 mg ketamine in 500 mL fluid). To prevent inadvertent overdosage, the total amount of ketamine mixed can be limited to the maximum safe dosage (3 mg/kg IV). Using a regular nonmicrodrip IV chamber (15 drops/mL), the IV is opened to flow at a rapid drop rate (about 2 drops/kg/min). Onset of action (glazed eyes and nystagmus) usually occurs within 2 minutes and lasts until 10 minutes after the infusion is terminated. Before beginning any painful procedure, analgesic effect should be tested by pricking the patient with a needle. Once sedation is deep enough, the drip is turned down to approximately half of the induction rate (1 drop/kg/min). It is stopped 10 minutes prior to the end of the procedure.

INTRAVENOUS BOLUS INJECTION METHOD This is the most commonly used alternative to the two methods described above. IV bolus ketamine is usually dosed initially at 1 to 2 mg/kg. If ketamine is the only anesthetic to be used, slightly more is required than would be used for induction alone. An average adult dose for routine anesthesia is 100 mg, although 50 mg may be sufficient for small adults, and 200 mg may be required for obese patients or chronic alcoholics. The dose should be given slowly, over a minute or two. Onset of action (glazed eyes and nystagmus) usually occurs within a minute. Surgical anesthesia lasts about 15 minutes, with full recovery in about 60 minutes. As above, before beginning any painful procedure, analgesic effect should be tested by pricking the patient with a needle. Booster doses of 1/2 to 1 mg/kg IV every 10 minutes (without additional antisialogogue) may be given if initial sedation is inadequate. The maximum dose for routine use, except in alcoholics, who may require much more, is 3 mg/kg. The more dilute 10 to 50 mg/mL ketamine solutions are preferred for IV administration. Injection should be performed slowly to avoid rarely observed ketamine-induced apnea.

RECOVERY The fear of the ketamine recovery experience should not preclude its use. Management of this period requires a certain finesse that separates the physician experienced in ketamine sedation from the novice. Because of the unique effects of dissociation, patients undergoing ketamine sedation experience a sense of semiconscious bodily detachment as they awaken. During this period, imagination can be confused with actual environmental stimuli. The physician has much control of the patient's recovery experience, and may positively direct this experience by simple and repeated suggestion, and by controlling the recovery environment. By the same mechanism, misinterpreted or noxious stimuli may cause patients to have a frightening recovery. During this period, physical contact, noise, and stimulation should be minimized and caretakers should not to try to awaken the patient prematurely. Blood pressure monitoring during this period has been discouraged by some anesthesiologists, who note undue disruption of recovery from cuff stimulation. Recovery reactions are less frequently dramatic in pediatric and elderly patients.

For patients who are recovering poorly, administration of any number of sleep-inducing agents during recovery is helpful. Patients at high risk for agitated recovery can be medicated prior to initiating the procedure. Such agents sedate the active but partially dissociated mind, blunting the confusion between imagination and reality. If such medication is used, promethazine is effective and provides antiemetic effects. Many developing world practitioners consider it the drug of choice. Benzodiazepines and haloperidol have demonstrated efficacy as well. Sedative agents are not essential for smooth recovery. Using reassurance alone, there were no unpleasant reactions in one series of adult ketamine sedation (Fig. 18-3).

SAFETY ISSUES Ketamine is suitable for most age groups provided the physician supervising its use is versed in its age-related effects and contraindications. Emergence phenomena are less common and less severe in pediatric and elderly patients. Apnea is more frequently observed in children under 3 months of age. Potential transient side effects of ketamine administration include hypersalivation, muscle hypertonicity, clonus, stridor, emesis, rash, and agitation. Ketamine's relative contraindications are listed in Table 18-5. These relative contraindications are mostly unconfirmed by formal studies. In cases necessitating emergency sedation, ketamine's benefits may outweigh the risks listed above, particularly if substituting other sedative agents will bring greater risks. The literature demonstrates that ketamine has a safety profile that outperforms many other sedative agents, making it the agent of choice for many potentially difficult emergency situations.

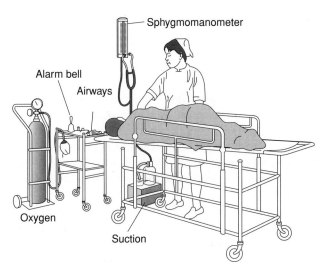

FIGURE 18-3 Quiet room recovery.

TABLE 18-5 RELATIVE CONTRAINDICATIONS FOR KETAMINE USE

Airway instability or tracheal pathology (unless used with endotracheal intubation)

High predisposition to laryngospasm or apnea (active pulmonary infection or age under 3 mo)

A full meal within 3 h (due to a higher aspiration risk)

Severe cardiovascular or disease (angina, heart failure, due to possible cardiostimulant effects)

Cerebrospinal fluid obstructive states (severe head injury, central congenital or mass lesions)

Intraocular pressure pathology (glaucoma or acute globe injury)

Previous psychotic illness (due to potential activation of psychoses)

Hyperthyroidism or thyroid medication use (due to the possibility of severe tachycardia or hypertension)

SPINAL ANESTHESIA

In many developing world hospitals, all abdominal operations are performed with spinal anesthesia. Spinal anesthesia involves injection of lidocaine (or similar agents) directly into the spinal canal to anesthetize the nerves passing through the subarachnoid space. Solutions of lidocaine mixed with dextrose are heavier than cerebrospinal fluid (CSF) and are therefore called hyperbaric solutions. This property allows control of the level of anesthesia, because gravity pulls the heavier anesthetic solution through the CSF toward the spinal nerves lying below the point of spinal injection. By positioning a patient properly (using a tilting table), choosing the level of injection into the spinal canal, and altering the amount of hyperbaric lidocaine injected, a skilled anesthetist can consistently provide anesthesia and muscle relaxation at predicted spinal levels.

Spinal anesthesia is reliable in experienced hands, but not as safe as ketamine. However, its risks are less than those of paralysis and intubation. In one common use, cesarean section, a proportion of patients will become hypotensive due to its sympatholytic effects. This can be avoided by preloading patients with saline prior to anesthesia. If this fails, hypotension can be treated with ephedrine or other alpha agonist agents. Rarely, a patient becomes both hypotensive and apneic if anesthesia ascends to block the intercostal high thoracic levels. If a high block is recognized early and steps are taken to support both vasodilation and respiratory depression, the patient is safe. However, this requires vigilance and preparation ahead of time; unrecognized, it will prove fatal. For these reasons, spinal anesthesia should never be used in patients who are in shock prior to operation or when IV fluid is unavailable.

Equipment for spinal anesthesia must be sterilized, by either autoclaving or boiling. Boiling, however, is not safe at elevations above a thousand meters. At these altitudes, if an autoclave is not available, another anesthetic method should be used instead. Chemical sterilization is dangerous due to inadequate removal of bacteria and previous cases of neurologic damage from inadvertent injection of the sterilizing fluid.

INDICATIONS

Spinal anesthesia with lidocaine provides paralysis and paresthesia for approximately an hour. If bupivacaine is used, anesthesia is prolonged to 3 hours. Use spinal anesthesia for operations of the lower abdomen, pelvis, or extremities. Spinal anesthesia is safer than inhalational anesthesia for patients who cannot be intubated, such as those with severe asthma, pneumonia, or contorted airway anatomy. It is also safer than general anesthesia for patients in renal or cardiac failure.

It is not safe for operations lasting beyond the duration of the anesthetic solution (e.g., 1 hour with lidocaine), in children, for thoracic operations, for patients in shock, or for patients with cellulitis overlying the skin injection site.

METHODS

Begin by starting an IV drip (18 gauge or larger) in the patient and preloading with a liter of saline solution, followed by a maintenance drip. Initial blood pressure and pulse should be recorded. Equipment for resuscitation, including extra IV fluid, ephedrine, intubation supplies, a bag-valve assembly, and suction, should be readied. If time allows, premedicate the patient with promethazine, diazepam, or a similar sedative.

For lumbar puncture, placement of the patient, the spinal needle, and the volume of injection each affect the highest level reached by the anesthetic solution. Recognizing that many methods are used, the two with the greatest utility, the low spinal block and the mid-spinal block, are described below (Fig. 18-4). For both methods, the patient should be lying laterally in preparation for lumbar puncture, with the table tilted exactly 5 degrees head down. If difficulty is encountered entering the dural space, these blocks also can be performed with the patient sitting upright initially, although slightly more solution must be used to reach the same level of anesthesia.

LOW SPINAL BLOCK (L1 AND BELOW) The low spinal block provides anesthesia from the L1 dermatome downward. It is useful for operations of the pelvis and legs. A dose of 1.5 mL hyperbaric lidocaine should be injected into the dural space and the patient immediately laid flat on his or her back, with the table returned to the 0 degree position.

LOW SPINAL FOR CESAREAN SECTION For women about to undergo cesarean section, a flat position may induce hypotension from uterine compression of the inferior vena cava. Therefore, they should receive spinal injections sitting up, while held by an assistant. Following injection, the mother should remain sitting up for 5 minutes, in order for the anesthesia to take effect. She should be supported during this time, or she may faint and fall off the table. After 5 minutes, she can be laid on the table, with a pillow placed under her right flank to tilt her uterus leftward off the vena cava. This method reliably provides anesthesia to the uterus, perineum, and abdominal wall but sometimes requires local anesthetic supplementation of the proposed skin incision site from the level of the umbilicus (T10) to the level of the inguinal ligaments (L1).

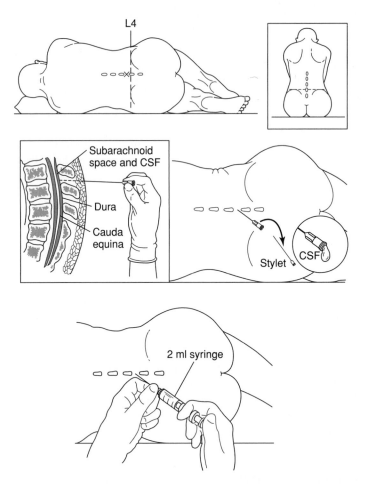

FIGURE 18-4 Lumbar puncture for spinal anesthetic. Lumbar puncture is performed using the standard sterile technique in the L3-4 interspinous space, the level of the iliac crests. (The L2-3 space also can be used.) To ensure sterility and prevent inadvertent injection of preservative, anesthetic solution for spinal injection should always come from a single-use ampule rather than a multidose vial. As mentioned, all equipment used for spinal anesthesia should be sterilized by autoclave, or by boiling if autoclave is unavailable. Entrance into the dural space should be confirmed by the flow of CSF before injecting anesthetic.

MID-SPINAL BLOCK (T7 AND BELOW) The second method, known as a mid-spinal block, provides anesthesia from T7 downward. For mid-spinal block, 2.0 mL of hyperbaric lidocaine should be injected into the dural space and the patient immediately placed on his or her back, leaving the table in the 5 degree head-down position. This method is not appropriate for cesarean section due to hypotensive effects of the supine position as well as from higher level sympathetic spinal blockade.

ONSET Spinal anesthesia requires approximately 10 minutes to take effect. Before beginning the operation, the anesthetic level should be tested by gently pinching the patient with forceps or checking for cold sensation paresthesia with a wet towel. If the block is above the T8 level, be prepared to treat complications of a high spinal blockade.

RECOVERY When the operation is complete, move the patient carefully to a recovery stretcher maintaining a supine position. Rapid movement, sitting upright in particular, often causes sudden hypotension and syncope. Allow the patient to recover while supine until the spinal block has completely disappeared.

COMPLICATIONS

If hypotension ensues, administer IV fluids at the maximal rate. If hypotension is associated with bradycardia, give atropine. Some anesthetists routinely use atropine to premedicate patients who are undergoing spinal anesthesia for cesarean section, due to the vagal effects of the gravid uterus on heart rate as well as bradycardia primarily caused by hyperbaric lidocaine. If the patient is bleeding heavily, consider giving blood if isotonic volume expansion does not immediately correct shock. This is particularly important for the woman with a ruptured ectopic pregnancy, or who is bleeding rapidly from a difficult cesarean section.

If hypotension is not corrected with fluid, give 10 to 20 mg of IV ephedrine, which will counter the vasodilatory effect of spinal anesthesia produced by sympathetic nerve blockade. This may be repeated as needed. Other alpha-agonistic agents may be used instead of ephedrine if available. Remember that hypotension should not be treated by placing the patient in a head-down position, because this may cause a high-level spinal block, resulting in worsening shock and apnea (Fig. 18-4).

If a patient has difficulty speaking or breathing, he or she probably has experienced high spinal blockade. Give supplemental oxygen and if necessary intubate the trachea in order to assist ventilation and prevent aspiration. Due to the hypotensive effects of high spinal anesthesia, sedation for intubation should be performed with ketamine or other agents that will not exacerbate shock.

MUSCLE RELAXANTS

Muscle relaxants should only be used by those who are skilled in intubation and who are experienced with both relaxant contraindications and measures needed in the event of paralysis-related complications. Mishaps with relaxant use lead rapidly to death for the patient. Patients who are paralyzed require continuous bedside monitoring by an anesthetist dedicated to this task, particularly in hospitals with little monitoring equipment. Because the paralyzed patient neither breathes nor moves, there is little outward change to indicate that a patient has died until the skin grows cold. Thus, at the first sign that something has gone wrong, the patient may already be past rescue. Muscle relaxants must be used with proper sedation, because the paralyzed patient may appear sedated even when wide awake.

INTUBATION

Patients who are paralyzed must be intubated so that they do not aspirate, and ventilation can be adequately assisted. In most hospitals in underdeveloped countries, ventilation after intubation must proceed by hand using a bag-valve assembly. Automatic ventilators and inhalational anesthetic machines are uncommon and, when present, require some expertise in their operation. Before paralysis, a plan for prolonged sedation with relays of bag ventilation should be made in the event that paralytic reversal fails. With such a plan, all patients will recover eventually.

SUCCINYLCHOLINE

Brief operations requiring muscle relaxation can be performed using a sedative and succinylcholine paralysis alone. Because succinylcholine effects last only minutes, either a continuous infusion or intermittent supplemental boluses of this agent are needed to maintain longer paralysis. The dose of succinylcholine should never exceed 4 mg/kg, or 300 mg total for an average adult. Ideally, use should be reserved for operations that can be completed within 20 minutes but use for up to 60 minutes is permitted provided the maximum dose is not exceeded.

The principal danger of using succinylcholine for prolonged paralysis is the conversion from a short-lived depolarizing to a long-lasting nondepolarizing blockade that does not reverse immediately once the infusion is stopped. Furthermore, about 1 patient in 2,000 lacks the enzyme, pseudocholinesterase, needed to break down succinylcholine for reversal of paralysis, and will have prolonged paralysis even after a single dose for rapid-sequence intubation. Patients at particular risk for this complication include those on antimalarial drugs; those with liver disease, anemia, or malnutrition; those poisoned by organophosphates (or who have received neostigmine on purpose); and pregnant women.

Succinylcholine should be used with atropine, particularly in children in whom profound vagal effects of paralysis may lead to frank asystole. The dose is 0.02 mg/kg for children, with a usual adult dose of 0.6 mg. For prolonged succinylcholine use, atropine should be redosed at 0.2 to 0.6 mg IV every 20 minutes as needed when the patient's pulse decreases to 60 or below.

To use succinylcholine by infusion, mix 150 mg of succinylcholine in 500 mL saline or dextrose in water to make a 0.03% solution. Intubate using a rapid-sequence technique that minimizes the bolus dose of succinylcholine (25-75 mg for adults), so that the overall dose used during the operation is also minimized. After intubation, run the drip at 2.5 mg/min, about 140 drops/min using a nonmicrodrip (15 drops/mL) IV set. Keep a clock nearby and periodically inform the surgeon about the period left before the drip must be stopped. Succinylcholine also may be administered in intermittent boluses of 10 to 20 mg. This may be mixed in the same syringe with atropine, to give 0.2 to 0.6 mg with each intermittent dose. Without it, the second or third dose usually causes bradycardia.

In the setting of resource-scarce practices, succinylcholine is often combined with ketamine infusion to provide sedation with paralysis. This combination has advantages over inhalation anesthesia with paralysis, because neither supplemental oxygen nor a vaporizing apparatus is needed. In practices using ether inhalational anesthesia, the combination has advantages when electrical or heated cautery is required, due to the explosive potential of ether.

PANCURONIUM

When available, nondepolarizing paralyzing agents are safer and easier to use than succinylcholine for prolonged paralysis. Many agents are available, and principles of use are similar for them all. Pancuronium is chosen as a prototypical agent, and has advantages for use in underdeveloped countries, due to availability, affordability, and medium duration (about 30 minutes).

To use pancuronium, intubate the patient using a rapid-sequence technique with succinylcholine. Wait until the succinylcholine begins to wear off before giving a longer-acting paralyzing agent. Next, administer pancuronium in a dose of 0.05 mg/kg (about 5 mg in average adults). This can be supplemented as needed with boluses at half the initial dose. Note that time to effect for all nondepolarizing agents is much longer than for succinylcholine, so be patient before giving additional doses. As soon as a long-acting agent is given, sedate the patient again if induction was performed with a short-acting sedative. Be prepared to redose sedative agents if a patient gives any sign of waking. If paralyzed, the only indication of a wakeful state may be an increase in the patient's blood pressure, pulse, or degree of skin diaphoresis. For most operations, ketamine by infusion is an ideal sedative for combination with longer-acting muscle relaxants.

When the operation is complete, nondepolarizing paralysis must be reversed with neostigmine and atropine. This should not be performed until at least 20 minutes following the initial dose, or 10 minutes following the last dose, of pancuronium. Reversal is necessary even if a patient appears to be breathing normally, because he or she still may be unable to cough. Peak effect of neostigmine takes approximately 5 minutes.

Give neostigmine mixed with atropine in the same syringe, in doses of 0.04 mg/kg and 0.02 mg/kg, respectively. Standard adult doses are 2.5 mg and 0.6 mg, respectively. Atropine is necessary to counter bradycardia due to direct vagal effects of neostigmine. Both agents should be given slowly, and atropine should be repeated if the patient has persistent bradycardia. If reversal is ineffective, do not give more neostigmine.

A patient should remain intubated until paralysis has completely worn off. The endotracheal tube is ready to be removed once the patient can lift his head off the pillow, open his eyes, and breathe normally. Have the patient inspire deeply and cough as the tube is rapidly removed. Suction his airway immediately following extubation.

SPECIAL CONSIDERATIONS: PEDIATRICS

METABOLISM, ENERGY, AND HEAT

Glycogen is more rapidly depleted in children than in adults. Thus, children should be allowed to drink milk until 6 hours prior and 3% dextrose in water until 2 hours prior to surgery. IV fluids during surgery should contain dextrose, and children should be allowed to feed immediately on waking. Moreover, if respiration fails during surgery, a child's high metabolic rate results in hypoxia much more rapidly than in an adult. Children also lose heat more rapidly than adults, and may therefore become hypothermic during surgery, particularly if paralyzed.

FALSELY SECURE VITAL SIGNS

Children with life-threatening bleeding often do not exhibit hypotension and other signs of hemorrhagic shock until they are nearly dead. Pay attention to children with declining vital signs who are undergoing surgery. Once vital signs decline, full shock rapidly ensues unless immediate therapy is undertaken. For this reason, all children undergoing major operations should be monitored with a monaural stethoscope taped to the left chest, by which breath sounds, pulse, and pulse intensity can be continuously monitored.

VAGAL EFFECTS OF MEDICATION

Children have more sudden swings in heart rate due to vagal sensitivity. Atropine, for example, should always be used as premedication for succinylcholine paralysis in children 10 years of age and younger due to the possibility of cardiac standstill due to vagal effects of depolarizing paralysis. (It should also be considered for older children, and kept on hand for potential resuscitation of any patient undergoing rapid paralysis.) Atropine, however, is dangerous if the ambient temperature is over 30°C, because it may raise a child's core temperature, producing hyperpyrexia and seizures.

INTUBATION CONCERNS

Airway anatomy in children is different than in adults. Intubation in small children can be facilitated by placement of towels under the neck and shoulders simultaneously to lift these anteriorly without hyperflexion of the neck.

SPECIAL CONSIDERATIONS: OBSTETRICS

DILATION AND CURETTAGE

Dilation and curettage can be performed safely with conscious sedation, using a benzodiazepine and opiate combination such as morphine and diazepam. Be cautious, however, not to oversedate the patient, which may result in respiratory depression and hypoxia. The procedure also can be performed with ketamine, but the patient should be placed in position for surgery first, because she will be unable to cooperate once dissociated.

CESAREAN SECTION

SPINAL ANESTHESIA Several methods have already been discussed briefly. The simplest and perhaps most commonly used method is spinal anesthesia. This reliably provides anesthesia and muscle relaxation, is simple to perform, and allows the mother to stay awake following delivery if desired, in order for her to immediately bond with her newborn. The major disadvantage is the possibility of hypotension from blockade of the spinal sympathetic nerves. However, this is both avoidable and treatable with saline preloading and alpha agonist pressor agents.

KETAMINE ANESTHESIA Ketamine is also simple, particularly in the event that the patient will die without surgery and the only available surgeon has little experience with anesthesia or cesarean section. The major difficulty with ketamine, however, is complete lack of muscle relaxation. In fact, abdominal muscles are often contracted as the patient moves during the dissociative state, making it more difficult to deliver or replace the uterus through the rectus incision.

RECTUS MUSCLE INFILTRATION ASSISTS MUSCLE RELAXATION Muscle contraction from the rectus segments accounts for most of the difficulty in performing cesarean section in unrelaxed patients. Such contraction can be relieved by directly injecting the rectus muscle in eight segments (four on each side of the incision) once the skin is incised and the rectus is directly visualized. When each segment is visualized, inject in the center of each segment with 5 mL of 0.4% epinephrine-supplemented lidocaine. After pushing the needle through the anterior rectus sheath, use the needle tip to feel for the posterior sheath. Once this is felt, raise the needle slightly so that the injection occurs in the body of the muscle toward the middle part of the sheath. Recall that the posterior sheath ends halfway between the umbilicus and symphysis pubis at the arcuate line, so this applies only to the upper two thirds of the rectus muscles.

LOCAL ANESTHESIA This method is the safest for mothers, but is more difficult for inexperienced surgeons due to the increase in patient discomfort and lack of adequate muscle relaxation. Approximately 100 mL of 0.4% epinephrine-supplemented lidocaine is used to anesthetize the skin.

This solution is then used to paralyze the rectus muscles, as described above. It is also necessary to anesthetize the parietal and visceral peritoneal membranes, to prevent further pain and discomfort when incised and manipulated. The advantage to this method is in its safety. However, local anesthesia is usually incomplete, particularly when intraabdominal structures are manipulated.

When possible, premedicate a mother with promethazine and keep her tilted to the left to prevent uterine pressure on her inferior vena cava. If available, supplemental oxygen should be administered until the delivery is complete.

Prepare 100 mL of epinephrine-supplemented 0.4% lidocaine. (Preparation of 0.4% lidocaine solution is discussed in the earlier section on Local and Regional Anesthesia: General Methods.) Using a long infiltration needle (100 mm), inject two large intradermal and subcutaneous bands of the solution from the pubis to a point 5 cm above the umbilicus, on either side of the pending incision. (Alternatively, some surgeons inject one wide band in the midline and cut directly through it.). The injection must always be parallel to the skin, otherwise it may pass through the thin abdominal wall and puncture the uterus. The needle may be bent to facilitate this method. As with field blocks, the solution should be injected continuously without the need to check for intravascular needle placement, while the needle is both pushed forward and withdrawn through the skin (Fig. 18-5).

After the skin incision is performed, inject 10 mL of solution immediately beneath the linea alba, in order to anesthetize the parietal peritoneum. Then inject the rectus segments as described. Remember to wait for the anesthetic solution to take effect. On reaching the uterus, inject another 5 mL of the solution under the loose visceral peritoneum where the lower uterine segment will be incised. This only anesthetizes the visceral peritoneum in the region of the uterine incision, so be careful not to disturb the rest of the abdominal cavity during the remainder of the operation.

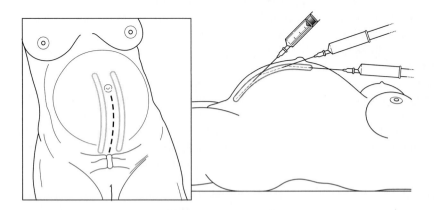

FIGURE 18-5 Local infiltration for anesthesia for cesarean section.

Supplemental IV agents are best avoided until the cord is clamped, to reduce transfer to the baby. However, be generous with them once delivery is complete. If the operation cannot be continued due to patient discomfort, use ketamine to supplement local anesthesia.

CONCLUSION

The physician who practices in a remote or resource-scarce region is frequently a generalist but must perform a variety of specialist duties simultaneously, acting at once as internist, pediatrician, obstetrician, parasitologist, intensivist, surgeon, and anesthetist. For the health worker practicing in a remote setting, learning a few straightforward anesthesia techniques can provide the skills necessary to perform a wide range of procedures in the field setting.

SELECTED READINGS

American Society of Anesthesiologists. Practice guidelines for sedation and analgesia by non-anesthesiologists. *Anesthesiology* 1996;84:459–471.

Ankcorn C, Casey WF. Spinal anaesthesia—a practical guide. *Update Anaesthesia* 1993;3:2–15.

Bewes P. *Surgery: a manual for rural health care workers.* Nairobi: African Medical and Research Foundation, 1984.

Collins C, Gurung A. Anaesthesia for caesarean section. *Update Anaesthesia* 1998;9:7–22.

Dobson M. *Anaesthesia at the district hospital.* Geneva, Switzerland: World Health Organization, 1993.

Green SM. Dissociative agents. In: Krauss BS, Brustowicz R, eds. *The practice of pediatric sedation in the outpatient setting.* Baltimore: Williams & Wilkins, 1999.

King M, ed. *Primary surgery [Trauma (Vol. 2) and Nontrauma (Vol. 1)].* Oxford, UK: Oxford University Press, 1987 and 1990.

King M, ed. *Primary anaesthesia.* Oxford, UK: Oxford University Press, 1990.

Li J. Ketamine: emergency applications. In: Plantz SH, Adler J, eds. *Emergency medicine, 1st ed.* Boston: Boston Medical Publishing, 1998. www.emedicine.com/emerg/topic802.htm

Sewell J, Robinson G, eds. World Anaesthesia Online. www.nda.ox.ac.uk/wfsa/

Vanstrum G. *Anesthesia in emergency medicine.* Boston: Little, Brown, 1989.

CHAPTER 19
Toxicology

Timothy B. Erickson

The poisoned patient may present with a variety of clinical symptoms, including gastroenteritis, altered mental status, seizures, cardiac dysrhythmias, and respiratory distress. In many cases, during the initial management, the offending agent is unknown. To complicate matters, a large percentage of overdoses involve multiple drugs, making identification of the primary causal agent more challenging (See Fig. 19-1).

In the international setting, familiarization of commonly prescribed and abused drugs available to a specific region or group of people is paramount. In developing countries, access to medicinal agents is limited. However, this may quickly change with the influx of medical relief following natural disasters and war. In addition, expanded urbanization worldwide has increased illegal drug trafficking exponentially.

Advanced treatments commonly available in industrialized nations (e.g., antidotes, ventilators, dialysis equipment) are often unavailable in less-developed countries. Therefore, the health-care provider must be resourceful and, at times, creative.

KEY POINT:

The majority of poisonings can be treated by removing the patient from the source of exposure, and by using general decontamination measures and providing supportive care.

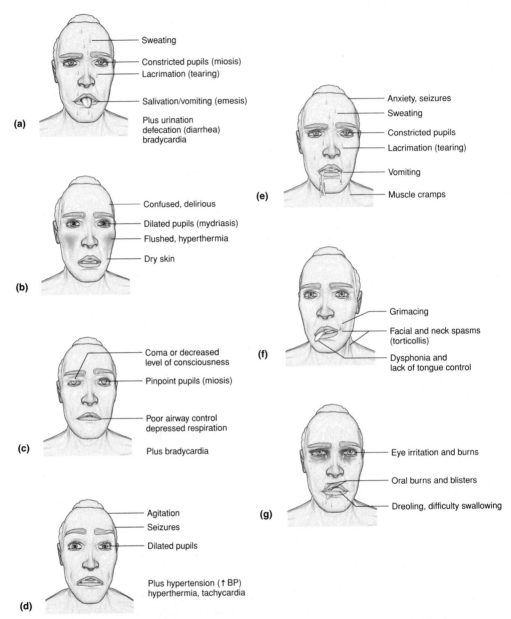

FIGURE 19-1 Toxic syndromes (toxidromes). A: Symptoms and physical findings in poisoning with cholinergics. B: Symptoms and physical findings in poisoning with anticholinergics. C: Symptoms and physical findings in poisoning with opioids. D: Symptoms and physical findings in poisoning with sympathomimetics. E: Symptoms and physical findings of anticholinesterase inhibition (organophosphate poisoning). F: Extrapyramidal symptoms of organophosphate poisoning. G: Signs of caustic ingestions.

EVALUATION OF THE ACUTELY POISONED PATIENT

CRITICAL ACTION:

As with any acutely ill patient, attention to the ABCs (airway, breathing, and circulation) is the critical first priority.

After addressing the ABCs, it is important to look for signs and symptoms of serious poisonings and life-threatening conditions that may be associated with a toxic exposure. Look for these presenting symptoms:

- Coma and decreased level of consciousness: consider alcohols, sedatives such as benzodiazepines, opioids (heroin), carbon monoxide exposure, and antidepressants.
- Shortness of breath: insecticides such as organophosphates, hydrocarbon aspiration, herbicides (paraquat), and salicylates
- Severe vomiting and diarrhea: acetaminophen, salicylates, iron, lead, organophosphates, caustics, digitalis, plants, and mushrooms
- Status epilepticus and tetany: cocaine, antidepressants, insecticides, carbon monoxide, lead, isoniazid (INH), salicylates
- Cardiac dysrhythmias: antidepressants, antimalarials, digitalis, cocaine, amphetamines, and volatile substance abuse

KEY POINT:

High-Risk Patients: Be particularly concerned about the potential for toxic exposure or drug-related problems in the following high risk patients:

- History of depression, mental illness, or prior suicide attempts
- Chronic medical conditions or those using multiple medications
- Young children; farmers and industrial workers; and patients with a history of illicit drug use

DIFFERENTIATING TOXIC EXPOSURES

In the field setting, resources are limited and the health-care provider needs to rely more heavily on a thorough history and physical examination. Important historical questions should address the time of exposure, the route of exposure [oral, intravenous (IV), inhalational], reason for poisoning (accidental, suicidal), amount of drug ingested, whether the patient has vomited, the patient's significant past medical history, and whether other victims in the community or surrounding area were affected (vital information particularly with environmental toxins).

Certain classes of drugs present with specific symptoms or characteristic physical findings. These clinical presentations are termed toxic syndromes or toxidromes. Some of the more common toxidromes and the agents that cause them are listed below.

Cholinergic agents (Fig. 19-1A) include organophosphate insecticides and betel nut (chewed worldwide, common in India). Think of the mnemonic *DUMBELS:*

*D*iarrhea, defecation, diaphoresis
*U*rination
*M*iosis
*B*ronchosecretions, bradycardia
*E*mesis
*L*acrimation
*S*alivation

Anticholinergic agents (Fig. 19-1B) include antihistamines (diphenhydramine), atropine, tricyclic antidepressants (TCAs), and jimson weed. The toxic syndromes are characterized as follows:

- Dry as a bone (dry skin)
- Blind as a bat (dilated pupils)
- Hot as hell (hyperthermic)
- Red as a beet (flushed skin)
- Mad as a hatter (delirium)

Opioid agents (Fig. 19-1C) include heroin, codeine, morphine, poppies, and methadone. The toxic syndromes are characterized as follows:

- Miosis
- Coma
- Respiratory depression
- Decreased bowel sounds
- Bradycardia
- Hypothermia

Sympathomimetic agents (Fig. 19-1D) include cocaine, amphetamines, pentachlorophenol (PCP), nicotine, and caffeine. The toxic syndromes are characterized as follows:

- Tachycardia
- Hyperthermia
- Dilated pupils
- Hypertension
- Seizures

■ Tachypnea
■ Agitation

In the international setting, laboratory facilities are often limited. As a result, qualitative urine toxicology screens or quantitative blood levels for specific toxins may not be available for diagnostic purposes. If available, baseline laboratory evaluations can be performed and the results used to narrow the differential diagnosis. However, shot-gunning with general laboratory tests using scarce resources is not necessary.

THE ANION GAP

The anion gap equation may be valuable and is calculated by taking the patient's serum sodium reading minus the sum of the chloride and bicarbonate readings: $Na - (Cl + HCO_3)$ (normal = 8–12). Several toxins cause an elevated anion gap metabolic acidosis in the overdose setting. The mnemonic *METAL ACID GAP* may be helpful:

Methanol, metformin
Ethylene glycol
Toluene
ASA (acetylsalicylic acid; aspirin)
Lactic acidosis
Aminoglycosides (uremia-inducing agents)
Carbon monoxide, cyanide
INH, iron
Diabetic Ketoacidosis (DKA)
Generalized seizures (toxin induced)
Alcohol ketoacidosis
Paraldehyde

If cardiotoxic agents are suspected, the patient should be placed on a cardiac monitor if possible and a 12-lead electrocardiogram (ECG) obtained if available. If the medical facility has radiographic capabilities, a chest radiograph should be obtained on patients with respiratory compromise or acute dyspnea.

DID YOU KNOW?

An abdominal radiograph may be diagnostic with certain radiopaque toxins such as the heavy metals (iron, lead, mercury, arsenic) or in "body packers" smuggling illegal contraband across international borders.

DECONTAMINATION MEASURES

ACTIVATED CHARCOAL If the patient presents with a recent toxic ingestion, gastric decontamination is usually warranted. The most efficacious decontamination method with the fewest side effects is administration of oral activated charcoal (AC). AC possesses a high surface area that will absorb the majority of toxic agents when given in doses of 1 to 2 g/kg prepared in a slurry of water. For several drugs, such as aspirin, theophylline, phenobarbital, digitoxin, and carbamazepine, multiple dosing of AC (every 2–4 hours) may enhance elimination due to enterohepatic or enteroenteric recirculation of the drug. AC is relatively ineffective against pesticides, hydrocarbons, caustic agents, alcohols, and small ionic compounds such as iron and lithium. In some Asian countries and Australia, where AC is unavailable, a similar claylike substance called Fuller's earth is commonly used. In some charcoal preparations, cathartics (e.g., magnesium citrate and sorbitol) are added in order to induce diarrhea. Administration of a cathartic with the first dose of charcoal in older children and adults is usually recommended. However, overzealous use of cathartics can result in patient dehydration and electrolyte imbalance if not used cautiously.

EMETIC AGENTS The emetic agent syrup of ipecac is harvested from Cephaelis ipecacuanha in Brazil and Central America. In the average patient, it induces vomiting within 20 minutes after oral administration. It is contraindicated in patients with active seizures and depressed mental status due to its aspiration potential. It is also contraindicated following caustic and hydrocarbon ingestions due to the potential for reintroduction of the agent to the esophagus and lung, respectively. When effective, syrup of ipecac may delay administration of AC. Ipecac may have a limited role in children who have recently ingested plants, berries, and mushrooms or agents not well absorbed by charcoal (e.g., iron).

> **KEY POINT:**
>
> Gastric lavage is indicated only in patients who present within 1 hour after ingestion of a potentially lethal poison and who are alert or have a protected airway.

GASTRIC LAVAGE The procedure uses a large-bore orogastric tube. The patient's stomach is irrigated and suctioned with several liters of water or normal saline until the gastric effluent is clear of pill fragments or gastric debris. Like ipecac, it is contraindicated in caustic and hydrocarbon ingestions. If the patient is lethargic, comatose, or experiencing airway difficulties, oral intubation should be performed prior to lavage in order to protect the airway from aspiration.

WHOLE-BOWEL IRRIGATION Whole-bowel irrigation with high molecular weight polyethylene glycol solution (commonly used for presurgical bowel preparations and radiologic procedures) is osmotically and electrolyte safe. This Go-Lytely solution can be used following ingestions of iron, lead, and international drug smugglers (intestinal body packers of cocaine and heroin). The typical dosage is 1 to 2 L/h administered via a nasogastric tube or by drinking one large cup every 10 minutes.

ENHANCED ELIMINATION

Urinary alkalinization with bicarbonate may be efficacious in promoting renal excretion following overdoses of weak acids (e.g., salicylates and phenobarbital). The goal is to maintain a urinary pH of 7.0 to 8.0.

If available, hemodialysis may be indicated following life-threatening doses of agents with low molecular weights, low volumes of distribution, and water-soluble properties. Ingestions that may require hemodialysis are listed in the mnemonic *I STUMBLE:*

*I*sopropanol
*S*alicylates

TABLE 19-1 ANTIDOTES TO SPECIFIC TOXINS

TOXIN	ANTIDOTE
Acetaminophen/paracetamol	N-acetylcysteine
Carbon monoxide	Oxygen
Cyanide	Cyanide antidote kit (sodium nitrite, sodium thiosulfate)
Arsenic	BAL
Lead	BAL, CaEDTA, Succimer
TCAs	Sodium bicarbonate
Opiates	Naloxone
Anticholinergics	Physostigmine
Organophosphates	Atropine, pralidoxime (2-PAM)
Digitalis, digoxin	FAB fragments
Beta blockers, calcium channel blockers	Glucagon
Calcium channel blockers, hydrofluoric acid	Calcium
Iron	Deferoxamine
Methemoglobinemia	Methylene blue
INH	Pyridoxine
Methanol/ethylene glycol	Ethanol/4-methylpyrazole (4-MP)
Benzodiazepines	Flumazenil

Theophylline
Uremia-inducing agents
Methanol
Barbiturates
Lithium
Ethylene glycol

ANTIDOTES

A small number of poisons have a direct antagonist or antidote to counteract its toxic properties. However, in developing countries, these tend to be undersupplied and too expensive to stock. Common toxins and their specific antidote are listed in Table 19-1.

ENVIRONMENTAL/HOUSEHOLD TOXINS

INSECTICIDES (ORGANOPHOSPHATES)

BACKGROUND Pesticide overuse, poisoning, and improper storage is a worldwide concern. Additionally, chemical warfare agents typically contain insecticide-type nerve agents (e.g., Sarin, Tabin VX). The most commonly used insecticides include organophosphates, carbamates, and pyrethrums.

Some organochlorine agents such as DDT, although prohibited in the United States and other industrial nations, are still used in many developing countries where federal and environmental regulation is lacking. Look for this in industrial or farm workers who use insecticides.

CLINICAL FEATURES Due to cholinergic excess, initial signs and symptoms of organophosphate and carbamate toxicity are muscarinic in nature (see Fig. 19-1A). These are best remembered by the mnemonic DUMBELS:

Diarrhea, defecation, diaphoresis
Urination
Miosis
Bronchosecretion, bradycardia
Emesis
Lacrimation
Salivation

Unlike carbamates, organophosphates also affect nicotinic receptors, causing muscle twitching, weakness, tachycardia, and areflexia. Central nervous system (CNS) effects of organophosphates include confusion, seizures, coma, and respiratory depression.

DIAGNOSIS In acute poisonings, no tests can identify organophosphate toxicity; therefore, the initial diagnosis is based on a history of exposure and clinical features. A laboratory finding of low cholinesterase enzyme activity may confirm the diagnosis, but most health-care facilities worldwide do not have access to this test.

> **KEY POINT:**
>
> When caring for a patient exposed to organophosphates, be sure to use gloves and protective clothing to decrease your own exposure.

TREATMENT The patient should be removed or evacuated from the source of insecticide exposure. If skin exposure has occurred, the patient's clothing should be removed and the skin irrigated with copious amounts of water. The health-care provider must be careful in this setting to wear protective gowns and gloves because insecticides can be rapidly absorbed by skin contact, causing systemic toxicity.

Once in the health-care facility, the patient's airway must be assessed. With severe organophosphate poisoning, the patient often has copious bronchosecretions, which may require intubation and frequent suctioning. Once the airway is protected, the patient should be lavaged if a significant amount of insecticide was recently ingested. If the patient is exhibiting muscarinic signs and symptoms of poisoning, atropine at 2 to 4 mg every 15 minutes should be administered IV (or via the endotracheal tube if IV access is not possible). The end point of therapy is the drying of secretions; historically, many milligrams of atropine have been required. The antidote pralidoxime (2-PAM) is indicated if the patient is exhibiting nicotinic toxicity or if the patient is requiring multiple doses of atropine. The dose is 1 to 2 g IV in adults and 25 to 50 mg/kg in children.

PREVENTION Prevention of insecticide poisoning includes public health education, proper storage, and use of safer agents with less human toxicity, such as pyrithroid agents. International, federal and environmental regulatory agencies have a role in controlling the overuse of the more dangerous pesticides.

HERBICIDES (PARAQUAT)

BACKGROUND Paraquat is a herbicide that is widely used in Central America, Australia, Asia, and the Orient. In these countries, it is also a common suicidal agent with an extremely high mortality rate (up the 50%) if a significant exposure is left unrecognized or untreated.

CLINICAL FEATURES The patient typically presents with oropharyngeal burns that resemble those of a caustic ingestion. Several hours after ingestion, the patient develops a pulmonary fibrosis because of pulmonic cell damage. As a result, the patient may become tachypneic or develop respiratory distress and hypoxia. Within 48 to 72 hours, the patient can develop oliguria, anuria, and renal failure.

DIAGNOSIS Diagnosis of paraquat poisoning is made by history of ingestion or exposure. The clinical syndrome of oral caustic-appearing burns, respiratory distress, and renal failure should lead the health-care provider to suspect paraquat poisoning.

TREATMENT Treatment includes airway protection with intubation, and decontamination with gastric lavage followed by administration of AC or Fuller's earth. High-flow oxygen is contraindicated with paraquat poisoning because it worsens the patient's pulmonary fibrosis. Renal failure is best treated with emergent hemodialysis if available. Unfortunately, the mortality rate of paraquat poisoning is very high, particularly in suicidal victims who ingest significant quantities.

HYDROCARBONS

BACKGROUND Hydrocarbon-containing agents are widely available internationally and are found in almost every household, whether used as a heating or light source, fuel, or lubricant. As a result, these compounds are commonly ingested accidentally by children, and are accessible to adults with suicidal intent. Several classes exist, including aliphatic, straight chained, chlorinated, and aromatic hydrocarbons. The toxicity of hydrocarbons is based on the particular compound's aspiration potential. The lower the viscosity and higher the volatility, the greater the aspiration risk.

CLINICAL FEATURES Patients who ingest hydrocarbons typically present with gastrointestinal (GI) distress, including vomiting and diarrhea. A characteristic gasoline-like odor will be noted on the breath. If aspirated, the patient will exhibit coughing, gagging, tachypnea, respiratory distress, fever, and hypoxia. With significant overdoses, the patient may present with CNS depression.

DIAGNOSIS Hydrocarbon toxicity should be suspected in any pediatric patient with coughing or respiratory distress with access to these household agents. A chest radiograph may show signs of aspiration pneumonitis if taken within 6 to 24 hours postingestion. Arterial blood gas analysis or pulse oximetry will usually demonstrate signs of hypoxia. There are no blood level titers diagnostic of hydrocarbon poisoning in the typical clinical setting.

TREATMENT With the majority of hydrocarbon ingestions, administration of ipecac or gastric lavage is contraindicated because it will reintroduce the agent to the trachea, thereby worsening aspiration. However, if the patient has ingested more than 5 mL/kg or the hydrocarbon contains a dangerous additive such as an organophosphate or heavy metal (leaded gasoline), or is an aromatic hydrocarbon (benzene, toluene), gastric lavage may be indicated, as long as the patient's airway is protected. Corticosteroid administration is not recommended.

PREVENTION Prevention of hydrocarbon poisoning includes patient education, proper storage, and regulation of the more dangerous additives accessible to the public. The availability of safer fuel and heating sources decreases the need for the more deadly compounds.

CARBON MONOXIDE

BACKGROUND Carbon monoxide (CO) is the leading cause of poisoning deaths in industrialized nations. It is an odorless, tasteless, invisible gas that binds to hemoglobin 250 times more readily than oxygen, thus resulting in cellular hypoxia. Sources of CO poisoning include automotive exhaust, heavy cigarette smoking, industrial furnaces with poor ventilation systems, faulty methane and propane heaters, as well as open household fires, whether ignited accidentally or used purposefully for cooking and heating.

DID YOU KNOW?

Household and cooking fires are an extremely common and underestimated source of CO poisoning in rural, underdeveloped countries.

CLINICAL FEATURES Patients exposed to CO present with a wide variety of symptoms, including flulike symptoms, headache, dizziness, vomiting, ataxia, syncope, dyspnea, chest pain, seizures, and coma. The classic cherry red skin is a rare finding, and only seen in severe, fatal cases.

DIAGNOSIS The diagnosis is made on clinical suspicion in a patient presenting with any of the above signs and symptoms. In countries with cold seasons, CO poisoning epidemics result when furnaces are lighted for the first time. CO poisoning typically affects an entire household, making it imperative that the health-care provider inquire about other members of the family.

If available, a CO level can be measured using the same laboratory equipment that analyzes arterial blood gases. A venous blood sample also can be measured for CO. Although levels do not correlate well with the degree of toxicity and clinical signs, patients are generally symptomatic with levels over 35% to 40%, and severely poisoned at levels over 60%.

Pregnant patients with CO poisoning are a great concern because the fetal hemoglobin has a much higher affinity for CO and, therefore, lower threshold for toxicity.

> **CRITICAL ACTION:**
>
> Treatment for CO poisoning includes:
> 1. removal from source of exposure
> 2. 100% O_2 if available, especially if the patient is pregnant
> 3. Consider hyperbaric chamber if available.

TREATMENT Treatment of CO poisoning includes removing the victim from the source of exposure into the open air and ventilating the enclosed area. If the patient is symptomatic, the antidote for CO is high-flow oxygen therapy. The half-life of CO is approximately 5 hours on room air and decreases to 90 minutes with 100% oxygen mask delivery. The patient should be given oxygen therapy until asymptomatic, or, if blood can be measured, when the CO level decreases to less than 10%. The exception to this rule is if the patient is pregnant. In this scenario, the mother should be given oxygen therapy for an additional five times the length of time it took for her to be completely symptom free or for her CO level to decrease to zero. In this way, the fetal hemoglobin can be completely cleared of CO poisoning. If available, hyperbaric oxygen is indicated in patients with CO levels over 35% (if pregnant, levels over 15%) or in patients with significant CNS symptoms (i.e., syncope, seizures, coma).

PREVENTION Prevention includes public education regarding the dangers of CO poisoning and advice on proper heating and cooking systems as well as improved occupational regulation of potential CO sources.

LEAD

> **DID YOU KNOW?**
>
> Lead poisoning or plumbism has been long recorded historically, including theories that it may have contributed to the fall of the Roman Empire because the aqueducts delivering fresh water to the political leaders were lined with lead.

BACKGROUND Lead poisoning remains a significant environmental problem in industrialized nations and its impact is vastly underestimated in developing countries. Sources of lead poisoning include old paint chips accidentally ingested by children, aerosolized lead dust in urban settings, house and building renovations, leaded gasoline (still readily available in many countries), lead-lined ceramics used in cooking and drinking, retained lead bullets in war-torn regions, occupational exposures (e.g., bridge painters), and lead-containing cosmetic products (popular in the Middle East and India). Lead poisoning inhibits heme synthesis in the bone marrow, resulting in hematologic and CNS toxicity.

CLINICAL FEATURES In the acute setting, lead poisoning presents with colicky abdominal pain and vomiting, weakness, and dizziness. Chronically it can result in microcytic, iron deficiency anemia. With severe poisoning, the patient can present with mental status changes, cognitive dysfunction, motor abnormalities, and encephalopathy.

DIAGNOSIS The diagnosis of lead poisoning can be made on clinical suspicion with a history of exposure along with presenting signs and symptoms. If possible, blood lead levels should be analyzed. Although levels do not always correlate clinically, levels of over 40 μg/dL are considered consistent with mild toxicity (weakness, abdominal complaints, anemia) and levels of over 70 μg/dL can result in CNS toxicity and encephalopathy. Hemoglobin or complete blood count should be assessed periodically. Abdominal radiographs may detect radiopaque lead paint chips in children with pica. Radiographic skeletal lead lines can be detected in children chronically poisoned with lead, representing growth plate arrest.

TREATMENT Management of lead poisoning begins with recognition and removal of the patient from the source of exposure. If a child has ingested multiple lead paint chips as demonstrated on abdominal radiography, whole-bowel irrigation with poly-ethylene glycol solution can be instituted. If lead poisoning has resulted from retained lead bullets or shrapnel, surgical removal is indicated.

If elevated lead levels are documented and the patient is symptomatic, chelation therapy is recommended. With mild to moderate toxicity, oral chelation with Suc-cimer (DMSA) has proven efficacious. Because Succimer is a newly approved anti-dote, it may not be available in most international settings. If the patient is demonstrating severe toxicity with CNS dysfunction, chelation with IV calcium EDTA (ethylenediaminetetraacetic acid) and intramuscular (IM) BAL (British Anti-Lewisite) is recommended.

PREVENTION Prevention of lead poisoning begins with public awareness, especially in light of the exponential growth of urbanization worldwide. Once recognized, the most important preventive therapy is to remove the patient from the source of exposure, coupled with environmental lead abatement.

CAUSTICS

BACKGROUND Caustic agents are compounds that cause tissue destruction on contact. They are generally categorized as either acids or alkali (basic). Common acids include sulfuric and hydrochloric acids, which are found in car batteries and toilet bowl cleaners. Upon ingestion, acids generally cause a coagulation necrosis on the gastric mucosa. Alkalis such as sodium hydroxide are found in drain cleaners and lyes. Ingested alkalis generally cause liquefaction necrosis, leading to deep penetrating damage to esophageal tissue.

CLINICAL FEATURES Patients who ingest caustics typically present with oropharyngeal blisters, dysphagia, drooling, throat pain, stomach pain, and vomiting. Patients with dermal or ocular exposure complain of severe pain, with evidence of irritation, burns, or ulceration (Fig. 19-1G).

DIAGNOSIS Diagnosis of caustic burns is based on a history of exposure along with the clinical features described above. No practical laboratory tests exist to measure specific acid or base levels.

Arterial blood gas can be analyzed if systemic toxicity is suspected, although the damage is typically limited to a localized area, thus not affecting total body pH. An upright chest and abdominal radiograph should be obtained to rule out perforation as demonstrated by free air.

Regardless of the specific agent, if the patient is symptomatic an endoscopic examination should be performed to assess the degree of caustic damage to the GI mucosa.

KEY POINT:

Do not induce vomiting in patients who have ingested caustic substances. The chemical will do more harm if reexposed to the esophagus or if aspirated.

TREATMENT Dilution with small aliquots of milk or water may lessen the degree of tissue damage. A base should never be used in an attempt to neutralize an acid or vice versa. With dermal or ocular exposure, the skin or eyes should be irrigated with copious amounts of normal saline or tap water on site, prior to transportation to the health-care facility. Once at the medical facility, syrup of ipecac or gastric lavage is generally contraindicated with caustic ingestions because the procedure may reintroduce the offending agent to the esophagus. If endoscopic examination of the GI tract demonstrates first-degree burns, no treatment is necessary. If a second degree or circumferential burn results, treatment with corticosteroids and antibiotics is recommended. If third-degree burns or perforation has occurred, steroids are contraindicated because they will exacerbate the resultant mediastinitis or peritonitis.

HYDROFLUORIC ACID

Hydrofluoric acid deserves special consideration. Although a weak acid, it behaves like a base, causing liquefaction and deep tissue damage on contact. It is a common compound used in cleaning masonry and in glass etching. Typically, the patient's degree of pain is out of proportion to the appearance of the burn on physical examination. Treatment of dermal burns include copious irrigation and application of calcium gluconate gel or IM injections around the burn's circumference.

PREVENTION Proper storage and labeling of acids and alkali are essential to prevent accidental ingestion, particularly in children. Improved occupational safety measures will lessen severity of dermal and ocular burns in the work setting.

TOXIC ALCOHOLS

BACKGROUND The toxic alcohols include methanol (windshield washer fluid, gasohol, moonshine), ethylene glycol (antifreeze, coolant), and isopropanol (rubbing alcohol). With each toxin, it is not the parent compound but rather the resultant metabolites formed by the enzymatic pathway via alcohol dehydrogenase that are poisonous. The toxic metabolites of methanol are formaldehyde and formic acid; ethylene glycol produces glycolic and oxalic acid; and isopropanol produces acetone. Internationally, epidemics of ethylene glycol poisoning have been described in Russia and Scandinavia, and methanol poisoning has been reported in India and Europe when it is used as a substitute for ethanol-based liquor.

> **TIPS AND TRICKS:**
>
> Suspect toxic alcohol ingestion in alcoholics who present with a severely depressed mental state, respiratory failure, or renal failure.

CLINICAL FEATURES

Patients poisoned by the toxic alcohols, whether intentionally or accidentally, typically present with a depressed mental status and respiratory drive. All three compounds cause some form of GI distress. Significant methanol toxicity eventually results in ocular damage and blindness. Ethylene glycol poisoning results in renal failure and pulmonary edema. Isopropanol can cause gastric bleeding.

DIAGNOSIS Diagnosis is based on a history of ingestion and clinical features. Additionally, unlike ethanol and isopropanol toxicity, methanol and ethylene glycol result in a metabolic acidosis with elevated anion gap: anion gap = $Na - (Cl + HCO_3)$; normal = 8 to 12.

Methanol, ethylene glycol, and isopropanol all exhibit an elevated osmolal gap calculated by the following equation: $2(Na) + glucose/18 + BUN/2.8 + EtOH/4.6$, where EtOH is ethyl alcohol. The osmol gap is the difference of the measured osmol minus the calculated osmol (normal 10).

If available, serum methanol, ethylene glycol, and isopropanol can be measured. However, the turn-around time for laboratory results is often too long to withhold therapy. Because fluorescein is present in antifreeze products, fluorescence of the patient's urine under a Woods lamp may be another diagnostic clue.

TREATMENT Toxic alcohol poisoning, particularly with ethylene glycol and methanol, is life threatening. Therefore, management should never be withheld while awaiting definitive laboratory results.

Gastric lavage and AC is rarely efficacious because the alcohols are rapidly absorbed through the gastric mucosa. Ipecac should not be used because of the patient's lethargic state and aspiration potential.

> **DID YOU KNOW?**
>
> Toxic alcohol ingestion is treated with ethanol (hard liquor of most varieties is inexpensive and readily available worldwide). Four shot glasses of whiskey, four glasses of wine, or six beers should be enough to inhibit the formation of the toxic metabolites.

Toxic alcohol ingestion is treated with ethanol in the form of liquor, such as vodka or whiskey. Ethanol competitively inhibits the alcohol dehydrogenase enzyme-induced pathway described above. It can be administered IV as a drip, or given orally. Four shot glasses of whiskey, four glasses of wine, or six beers should be enough to induce a level of 100 to 150 mg%, the level necessary to inhibit the formation of the toxic metabolites. However, this level of inebriation needs to be maintained until the toxic alcohol is excreted through the kidneys.

If the patient is severely poisoned or acidotic, or has elevated serum level or evidence of end-organ damage, therapy with hemodialysis (if available) should be instituted. In the United States and Europe, the new antidote 4-methylpyrazole (4-MP) has been approved for the management of ethylene glycol and methanol poisoning, although it is often too expensive to be adequately stocked.

PREVENTION Prevention of toxic alcohol poisoning includes proper storage and labeling to keep these agents away from children and suicidal adults. The development of less toxic additives to engine coolants, such as propylene glycol and the addition of bittering agents to make the sweet taste of these toxic alcohols less palatable, are other preventive measures.

PHARMACEUTICAL AGENTS

ANTIMALARIALS

BACKGROUND Antimalarial agents are commonly prescribed in tropic and equatorial regions for prophylaxis against and treatment of malaria. Agents include chloroquine (developed during World War II), quinine (obtained from the bark of the cinchoma tree), and mefloquine. These drugs have arrhythmic properties and may be cardiotoxic. Large overdoses of chloroquine can cause myocardial depression, vasodilatation, and hypotension. With quinine overuse or poisoning, a clinical syndrome called cinchonism may result, producing vision loss, tinnitus, palpitations, and mental status changes.

> **DID YOU KNOW?**
>
> Chloroquine is one of the most commonly used drugs for suicide attempts in malaria-prone regions.

CLINICAL FEATURES A patient with malaria may already have chills, diaphoresis, high fever, headache, and mental status changes (cerebral malaria). Onset of action in an overdose setting with the more common antimalarials is rapid (within 2 hours). Initially the patient may have abdominal pain, nausea, and vomiting due to the irritation of the esophageal and gastric mucosa. Patients often complain of palpitations, drowsiness, headache, tinnitus, vision changes, and irregular heart beat. If the overdose has been chronic from misuse of the medication, the patient also may report insomnia and nightmares.

DIAGNOSIS Diagnosis is based on a history of ingestion or IV administration along with the above clinical features. If malaria is suspected in the patient, a malaria smear can confirm this. ECG may demonstrate sinus bradycardia, widened QRS, T-wave changes, ST segment depression, prolonged QT intervals, complete heart block, and ventricular tachycardia and fibrillation.

TREATMENT Treatment is largely supportive. Be prepared to treat cardiorespiratory arrest in cases of large overdose. Hypotension can be managed with IV fluids and pressor agents. Because the patient may become rapidly unstable, syrup of ipecac should be avoided. With recent potentially life-threatening ingestions, gastric lavage may be helpful. Activated charcoal should be administered. Extensive clinical experience in Africa has demonstrated successful use of early mechanical ventilation, high-dose benzodiazepines, and epinephrine in cases of severe chloroquine poisoning.

PREVENTION Prevention includes keeping these agents out of the reach of children and public education regarding their potential toxicity. Other measures to prevent malaria also may be recommended, including mosquito netting, insecticides, and antimalarials with fewer side effects, such as tetracycline.

ACETAMINOPHEN (PARACETAMOL)

BACKGROUND Acetaminophen or paracetamol is available worldwide as a pain reliever and fever reducer and is found in many over-the-counter cold and flu preparations. In an overdose setting, it is potentially lethal. Large doses of acetaminophen deplete glutathione stores in the liver, resulting in the accumulation of toxic metabolites. Acute doses of 7 to 8 g of acetaminophen in an adult or 140 mg/kg in children are considered toxic. Chronic ingestion of alcohol or other drugs that are metabolized through the liver (e.g., INH) may exacerbate acetaminophen's hepatotoxicity at lesser doses.

CLINICAL FEATURES Patients with acetaminophen toxicity typically present with nausea, vomiting, and abdominal pain during the first 24 hours after ingestion. At 36 to 48 hours, the patient usually experiences resolution of GI symptoms or enters a quiescent phase. From 72 to 96 hours postingestion, the patient experiences renewed nausea, vomiting, and right upper quadrant pain, along with jaundice, bleeding, and mental status changes consistent with hepatic encephalopathy.

DIAGNOSIS The diagnosis is made based on a history of ingestion along with laboratory data consistent with liver damage. As a result, serum glutamic oxaloacetic transaminase (aspartate transaminase), serum glutamic pyruvic transaminase, and bilirubin levels, as well as prothrombin time should be assessed, if possible, and followed in a serial manner. However, liver function test results may not be abnormal until 48 to 72 hours after ingestion. In the first 4 to 24 hours following an acute, single ingestion, a serum acetaminophen level can be measured and plotted on a nomogram (Fig. 19-2). Optimally, the level is drawn at 4 hours postingestion and plotted on the nomogram. If the level falls within the potential hepatotoxic range, antidote therapy is indicated as discussed below.

TREATMENT Initial treatment consists of gastric decontamination with lavage if the patient presents within 1 hour of ingestion and has not already vomited. AC also can be administered orally to adsorb excess drug in the gut. The mainstay of therapy is the antidote N-acetylcysteine, which acts to replenish depleted glutathione stores in the liver. Indications for use include a 4- to 24-hour hepatoxic acetaminophen level as plotted on the nomogram, a single acute ingestion of 7 to 8 g in an adult (140 mg/kg in a child), or late presentation of a patient already demonstrating liver toxicity. The antidote is given orally in the United States (140 mg/kg single loading dose, followed by 70 mg/kg maintenance dose every 4 hours for 17 doses). In Europe, the antidote is also given IV. If levels are unavailable in the international setting, and a significant overdose is suspected, it is best to administer the full course of antidote because the benefits greatly outweigh the risks.

KEY POINT:

If the antidote for acetaminophen ingestion, -N-acetylcysteine is not available for a patient with a potentially toxic ingestion, transfer them to the nearest facility with access to it.

PREVENTION Prevention includes keeping acetaminophen products away from children or suicidal adults as well as public education as to the potential danger of this seemingly benign medication.

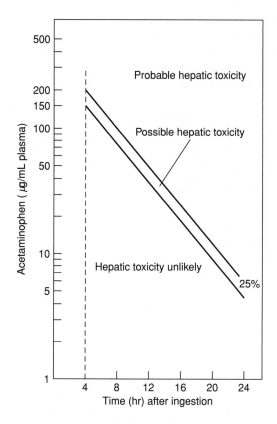

FIGURE 19-2 Rumack-Mathew nomogram for acetaminophen poisoning. (Reprinted from Rumack BH, Mathew H. *Pediatrics* 1975;55:871; with permission.)

ASPIRIN (SALICYLATES)

BACKGROUND Like acetaminophen, aspirin is available worldwide, and used as a pain reliever, fever reducer, and prophylaxis against cardiac disease. Acetylsalicylate acid (ASA) uncouples oxidative pathways, resulting in anaerobic metabolism and acidosis. It also directly stimulates respiratory centers, causing tachypnea and respiratory alkalosis. Aspirin overdose can result in significant morbidity and mortality if not recognized and managed aggressively.

CLINICAL FEATURES Patients typically present with nausea, vomiting, tinnitus, and abdominal distress. Because of the irritating effect of ASA on the gastric mucosa, the patient also may present with melanotic stools. Patient are usually tachypneic, tachycardic, and hyperthermic. In severe overdoses the patient may experience generalized seizure activity and noncardiogenic pulmonary edema.

DIAGNOSIS Diagnosis is based on a history of acute ingestion or the fact that the patient is chronically taking aspirin on a daily basis. If available, serum ASA levels should be followed in a serial fashion to assure a declining level. Levels above 100 mg/dL in the acute setting are considered severe and life threatening. Patients chronically on ASA are severely poisoned at lower levels (>70 mg/dL) because of the resultant long-term CNS exposure. Like acetaminophen, there does exist a salicylate nomogram, but it has little practical use and does not correlate well clinically.

> **KEY POINT:**
>
> Because aspirin can form concretions (hard lumps) in the gut, multiple doses of activated charcoal may be indicated with larger ingestions.

TREATMENT Management of acute aspirin poisoning consists of gastric deconta-mination with lavage for recent ingestions, followed by oral AC. Because ASA is a weak base, elimination can be enhanced by urinary alkalinization with sodium bicarbonate. In severe overdoses, consider dialysis.

PREVENTION Prevention includes keeping aspirin products away from children and suicidal adults. Public education as to the dangers of this commonly ingested drug in an overdose setting also is necessary.

BENZODIAZEPINES

BACKGROUND Benzodiazepines are widely prescribed all over the world. They are used for anxiolytic and sedative properties as well as for muscle relaxation. Of great concern is their addictive properties in the chronic setting. Benzodiazepines such as diazepam (Valium) and lorazepam (Ativan) are first-line medications for seizure control.

CLINICAL PROPERTIES As with other sedative hypnotics (e.g., barbiturates), patients who overdose on benzodiazepines typically present with respiratory depression, brady-cardia, and lethargy or coma. Rarely do they suffer from cardiovascular collapse.

DIAGNOSIS Diagnosis of benzodiazepine overdose is based on a history of inges-tion or chronic use, along with the clinical features described above. Specific serum ben-zodiazepine levels are usually unavailable and have poor clinical correlation.

TREATMENT Treatment is mainly supportive and targeted at airway control. Because these patients present with CNS and respiratory depression, intubation and mechanical ventilation are often required with larger overdoses. Once the airway is con-trolled, if the ingestion is recent (within 1 hour) the patient may be lavaged or given AC via an orogastric tube. The benzodiazepine antagonist flumazenil will rapidly reverse the sedative effects of benzodiazepines, but is not often available. It should be reserved for acute, isolated benzodiazepine overdoses with airway complications because mixed ingestions and reversal of patients who use benzodiazepines chronically may result in withdrawal seizures.

ANTIDEPRESSANTS

BACKGROUND Antidepressants are prescribed worldwide. The most common agents are cyclic antidepressants (e.g., TCAs, amytriptyline, doxepine) and selective serotonin reuptake inhibitors (SSRIs; e.g., fluoxetine, sertraline, St. John's wort). The toxic potential of the cyclic antidepressants is more severe and is the focus of our discussion here. TCAs have anticholinergic properties and powerful alpha blockade abilities (resulting in hypotension), along with sodium channel interaction at the myocardium, causing cardiotoxicity.

CLINICAL FEATURES Following TCA overdose, the patient can present with an anticholinergic toxidrome (hyperthermic, dry, flushed skin, dilated pupils, and mental status changes or delirium). In addition they are tachycardic and hypotensive. In severe overdoses, lethargy, coma and generalized seizure activity can result.

DIAGNOSIS Diagnosis is based on a history of ingestion or history of depression and access to antidepressants. In addition, a patient with depressed mental status, seizures, and anticholinergic properties should be treated as a TCA overdose until proven otherwise. ECG often demonstrates QRS widening (>100 msec) along with tachydysrhythmias and ventricular tachycardia/fibrillation.

Urine and blood toxicology screens to detect TCAs are available, but are often inaccurate with poor clinical correlation.

TREATMENT

> **CRITICAL ACTION:**
>
> Carefully watch the airway in patients with a TCA overdose. They can decompensate quickly and often need ventilatory support.

Treatment of the patient with a TCA overdose includes rapid control of the airway because patients develop acute mental status changes within the first 2 hours of ingestion. Cardiac dysrhythmias and widening of the QRS are best controlled with administration of sodium bicarbonate (one to two ampules IV in order to stabilize the sodium channels in the myocardium, and to alkalinize the serum, thereby enhancing TCA protein binding. The goal is to maintain a serum pH of 7.45 to 7.55. In addition to IV fluids, alpha agonists such as levofed may be required for refractory hypotension. Gastric lavage followed by AC administration is indicated in recent ingestions after the patient's airway is protected with intubation. The antidote physostigmine, although indicated with severe poisonings of pure anticholinergic agents such as diphenhydramine and atropine, is contraindicated in TCA overdoses.

Poisoning with SSRIs is less severe than with TCAs, and patients generally do well with supportive care along with gastric decontamination.

PREVENTION Prevention of TCA poisoning includes keeping these medications away from children and suicidal adults. Unfortunately, many depressed patients on TCAs have suicidal ideations, and safer agents with fewer side effects such as SSRIs may be more appropriate.

IRON

> **TIPS AND TRICKS:**
>
> Suspect iron overdose in any young child with GI bleeding, especially if the mother is pregnant and taking prenatal vitamins with iron.

BACKGROUND Iron is commonly found in prenatal vitamins and multivitamins, and prescribed for patients with iron deficiency anemia. It is a common overdose among pregnant patients because of accessibility and in children because of the sweet-tasting outer coating. In fact, in the United States, it is responsible for nearly one third of all pediatric poisoning deaths. Iron is a direct mucosal irritant causing GI bleeding, and in the overdose setting can also cause metabolic acidosis and hepatic failure.

CLINICAL FEATURES In the overdose setting, patients typically present with vomiting and abdominal pain along with hematemesis and hematochezia. Like acetaminophen, the initial GI phase is followed by a quiescent phase 12 to 24 hours after ingestion. Within 24 to 48 hours, the patient experiences liver damage and may present with jaundice and bleeding abnormalities. With severe poisoning the patient may develop hepatic encephalopathy.

DIAGNOSIS The diagnosis of iron poisoning is based on a history of ingestion and accessibility to iron-containing products. If a child presents with a history of vomiting blood, ask if the mother is pregnant and taking iron tablets. Patients typically develop hyperglycemia, leukocytosis, and metabolic acidosis with elevated anion gap, and have elevated liver function test results. Abdominal radiography will demonstrate radiopaque iron tablets, if the ingestion was recent. If possible, the serum iron level also should be monitored. Serum iron levels of over 350 mg/dL denote moderate toxicity, and levels of over 500 mg/dL are consistent with severe or potentially life-threatening poisoning.

TREATMENT Treatment of patients with iron poisoning consists of gastric lavage (or ipecac in children) if the ingestion has occurred within 1 hour and the patient has not already vomited. AC does not bind iron well due to its small ionic size. If the abdominal radiograph is positive for pill fragments, therapy with whole-bowel irrigation (polyethylene glycol solution) is indicated at 1 to 2 L/h (25 mL/kg in children) until the radiograph is clear of radiopaque fragments.

If available, chelation therapy with the antidote deferoxamine is indicated (15 mg/kg/h IV), not to exceed 6 to 8 g in the first 24 hours). If administered too rapidly, hypotension can ensue. Following chelation therapy, if body iron binding sites are saturated (as in the overdose setting), the patient's urine will change to a vin rosé color. This color change may be subtle, so the decision to chelate should not be based solely on this criterion.

PREVENTION Prevention includes informing parents and pregnant mothers to keep these products in safety-capped containers and out of the reach of children.

ISONIAZID

BACKGROUND Isoniazid (INH) is widely prescribed for antituberculosis therapy. With the incidence of tuberculosis (TB) increasing rapidly worldwide, many patients are on INH. INH causes a severe metabolic acidosis and generalized seizure activity refractory to most conventional therapies. Patients who are slow acetylators (African Americans, white Americans) are more prone to toxicity. Fast acetylators include Japanese, Thai, Korean, Chinese, and Eskimo individuals.

DID YOU KNOW?

Because of the sweet-tasting elixir preparation used for children, INH is a common pediatric poisoning in Asian countries.

CLINICAL FEATURES Patients with INH poisoning may present with a history of ingestion or history of being treated for TB. Clinically they may have nausea, vomiting, altered mental status and generalized seizure activity.

DIAGNOSIS Diagnosis of INH poisoning is based on a history of ingestion or TB therapy. The combination of severe metabolic acidosis and elevated anion with refractory seizures is treated as INH toxicity until proven otherwise. The patient also may have radiographic evidence of TB (cavitary lesions) on chest radiographs. Patients chronically on INH may have signs of hepatic damage on liver function testing. Serum INH levels can be measured, but the turnaround time is too long to impact clinical management.

TREATMENT Management consists of supportive care and gastric decontamination with lavage and charcoal administration if the ingestion was recent. Ipecac is contraindicated because of potential seizure activity. Severe acidosis should be corrected with sodium bicarbonate administration. Seizure activity is often refractory to benzodiazepines, barbiturates, and phenytoin. The antidote of choice for INH poisoning is pyridoxime (vitamin B6). It interacts with the GABA receptors, counteracting seizure activity. The dose is 1 g of vitamin B6 for every gram of INH ingested. If the amount of INH ingested is unknown, a starting dose of 5 to 10 g is recommended. If IV pyridoxime is unavailable, vitamin B6 tablets can be crushed and mixed into a slurry and administered via a nasogastric tube.

PREVENTION Prevention of INH poisoning includes keeping these preparations away from children and suicidal adults as well as the concomitant administration of pyridoxime on a daily basis. Newer generation anti-TB drugs may have fewer side effects in the overdose setting.

DIGITALIS

BACKGROUND Digitalis (Europe) or digoxin (United States) is a common cardiac glycoside that is used worldwide for the treatment of atrial fibrillation and congestive heart failure. Digitalis toxicity results in the poisoning of the sodium potassium adenosine triphosphatase pump of the myocardial cell, resulting in hyperkalemia, as manifested by brady- and tachydysrhythmias. Without aggressive therapy, digitalis poisoning carries a high mortality rate.

KEY POINTS:

Types of cardiac dysrhythmias in digitalis ingestions

- Bradycardia
- AV nodal blocks
- Atrial tachycardias
- Ventricular tachycardia

CLINICAL FEATURES Patients presenting with a digitalis overdose initially experience nausea and vomiting. The patient also may describe dizziness, vertigo, and altered color perception. Classically, the patient experiences hypotension and bradydysrhythmias, particularly atrioventricular nodal blocks. The patient also may present with any type of atrial and ventricular tachydysrhythmia. With severe poisoning, the patient may experience CNS toxicity ranging from subtle mental status changes to seizures and coma.

DIAGNOSIS Diagnosis of digitalis poisoning is based on a history of ingestion or access to cardiac drugs in a patient presenting with the above clinical features. In addition, cardiac monitoring and ECG can demonstrate dysrhythmias consistent with digitalis poisoning. Potassium levels with acute poisoning are usually elevated. With chronic poisoning, patients may be eukalemic or hypokalemic depending on whether they are concomitantly on a diuretic. If available, serum digoxin or digitalis levels can be obtained. Therapeutic digoxin levels range from 0.8 to 1.8 ng/mL. Acute toxicity levels of over 5.0 ng/mL denote moderate poisoning, and those over 10.0 ng/mL denote severe poisoning.

TREATMENT Management of acute digitalis overdose consists of gastric lavage followed by AC if following a recent ingestion. Bradycardia and hypotension can be treated with atropine and pressors, respectively, although both are usually refractory. The mainstay of digitalis poisoning consists of administration of the IV FAB fragment antidote Digibind. Indications include the presence of digitalis or digoxin poisoning and a potentially unstable dysrhythmia, potassium levels of over 5.5 ng/mL, and digoxin levels of over 10.0 ng/mL. Unfortunately, Digibind is expensive and rarely available in developing countries. Dosing is 10 vials IV if the digoxin level is unknown or pending and the patient is too unstable to await levels. Otherwise, the number of vials can be calculated using the specific formula available in the FAB package insert.

PREVENTION Prevention includes proper education of cardiac patients taking digitalis or digoxin. In addition, this dangerous medication should be kept out of the reach of children.

DRUGS OF ABUSE

HEROIN

BACKGROUND Heroin is an opioid narcotic harvested from poppy seeds. Although traditionally smuggled across international borders from regions surrounding Southeast Asia, Nigeria, and Afghanistan, most recently the Colombian cocaine cartels have dramatically increased trafficking of heroin throughout North America. Whereas adulterated heroin is usually abused IV (i.e., mainlining), a more pure form is snorted, much like cocaine. Because heroin is highly addictive, infiltration of narcotics into a country can have a major impact on the health of urban populations.

CLINICAL FEATURES Patients presenting following a heroin overdose have CNS and respiratory depression, along with miotic or pinpoint pupils. They also experience hypothermia and bradycardia. If heroin has been abused IV, the patient may have needle track marks on examination of the extremities.

DIAGNOSIS Diagnosis of a heroin overdose is based on a history of abuse or a patient presenting with the classic triad of miotic pupils, coma and respiratory depression. Urine toxicology screens will also quantitatively test positive for opiates if heroin has been abused within the last 72 hours. Finally, a dramatic response to IV administration of the pure opioid antagonist naloxone, also confirms the diagnosis. Diagnosis of heroin body packers may be established by noting several radiopaque densities on an abdominal radiograph or KUB.

TREATMENT

> **DID YOU KNOW?**
>
> Body packers smuggle heroin by ingesting many (up to 100) packets of latex-wrapped pure heroin. Treatment includes whole bowel irrigation, AC administration, and if ineffective, emergent surgical removal.

The mainstay of treatment is recognition and administration of the antidote naloxone. The patient should be placed in restraints prior to administration since it will precipitate acute withdrawal in chronic abusers. An initial dose of 2 mg can be given IV. If no response, up to 10 mg can be given. Since the effect of heroin lasts up to 4 hours, and the response to naloxone is no more than 1 hour, repeated doses may be necessary. If naloxone administration does not resuscitate the patient, the airway should be protected with intubation, and the other etiologies for altered mental status should be considered.

PREVENTION Prevention includes tougher drug trafficking laws and control at international borders as well as improved narcotic detoxification programs to treat addicted individuals.

COCAINE

BACKGROUND Cocaine is a highly addictive sympathomimetic drug which stimulates both alpha and beta receptors. It is abused and smuggled across international borders worldwide but is primarily harvested in South American countries such as Colombia and Bolivia. Cocaine powder is typically snorted nasally, but is commonly smoked in rock or crack form.

CLINICAL FEATURES Patients under the influence of cocaine experience a euphoric high that is short lived and highly addictive. Patients typically present with tachycardia, hypertension, tachypnea, diaphoresis, anxiety, and dilated pupils (mydriasis). If severely intoxicated, the patient can suffer chest pain from cardiac ischemia, seizures, profound hyperthermia, rhabdomyolysis, cerebral vascular accidents, intracranial bleeds, and death.

DIAGNOSIS The diagnosis of acute cocaine toxicity is based on a history of abuse or access to the drug. If the history is unobtainable, a patient presenting with the above sympathomimetic signs and symptoms is treated as having cocaine intoxication until proven otherwise. Urine toxicology screens can quantitatively test positive for cocaine metabolites if the drug was abused within the 72 hours of sampling. If the patient presents with chest pain, serial ECGs and cardiac enzymes should be monitored. If the patient experiences seizure activity, a computed tomography scan of the head should be ordered if the health-care facility has radiologic capabilities. As with heroin body packers, an abdominal radiograph of an alleged cocaine smuggler may be diagnostic if the patient has ingested several latex-wrapped packets.

TREATMENT Treatment of the patient with cocaine toxicity includes supportive care and immediate attention to abnormal vital signs. If the patient is hyperthermic, rapid cooling measures with spray/mist, circulating fans, and strategic ice packs should be applied. If there is evidence of myoglobinuria and rhabdomyolysis, the patient should be given fluids, alkalinized, and given mannitol. If the patient is tachycardic, anxious, hyperactive, and experiencing chest pain, benzodiazepines in liberal doses are required. If the chest pain is truly ischemic in nature, nitroglycerin can be administered. However, beta blockers are discouraged because the patient will experience the resultant effects of unopposed alpha receptor stimulation. Seizure also can be managed with high doses of benzodiazepines.

PREVENTION Prevention of cocaine trafficking includes stricter international laws against drug smuggling and abuse. Addiction treatment programs are also necessary in order to treat those individuals addicted to this potentially devastating drug.

AMPHETAMINES

BACKGROUND Amphetamines (or speed), commonly abused in the 1960s, have regained popularity with newer designer forms. Drugs such as Ecstacy, Adam, Eve, Ice, and Crank are abused worldwide and are easier to manufacture and distribute than cocaine or heroin. In Europe, Ecstacy has overtaken heroin as the most commonly abused drug. In Yemen, Ethiopia, and Eastern Africa, a plant with amphetamine-like properties called khat is commonly chewed and abused. As with cocaine, amphetamines are sympathomimetic agents with powerful alpha- and beta-receptor stimulation. Amphetamines can be abused orally, nasally, and IV.

CLINICAL FEATURES Patients high on amphetamines typically present with tachycardia, tachypnea, anxiousness, and dilated pupils. Severely intoxicated individuals experience chest pain, seizures, hyperthermia, and intracranial bleeds.

DIAGNOSIS Diagnosis of intoxicated patients includes a history of abuse or access to drugs. In any patient presenting with the above sympathomimetic signs and symptoms, amphetamine abuse should be considered. Urinary toxicology screens can quantitatively screen for amphetamines if used within 72 hours of sampling. However, several of the newer designer drugs will test negative on typical amphetamine screens. If the patient experiences chest pain, an ECG should be obtained. If seizures occur, a CT scan of the head should be ordered, if available.

TREATMENT Treatment of patients high on amphetamines includes supportive care and immediate attention to abnormal vital signs. If hyperthermic, the patient should be aggressively cooled with mist/sprays, fans, and strategic ice packs. If there is evidence of rhabdomyolysis and myoglobinuria, the patient should be given fluids, alkalinized, and given mannitol to force diuresis. If hyperactive, anxious, tachycardic, and tachypneic, as with cocaine, liberal doses of benzodiazepine can be administered. Seizure activity also can be treated with benzodiazepines. If the amphetamine was recently ingested, standard doses of AC should be given.

PREVENTION Similar to cocaine and heroin abuse, stricter drug laws may lessen abuse of amphetamines. Public education as to the potential dangers of these drugs is also essential.

HALLUCINOGENICS

BACKGROUND Hallucinogenic agents include many drugs such as LSD, marijuana, PCP, peyote, mescaline, anticholinergic plants, morning glory seeds, nutmeg, and mushrooms. Hallucinogenic agents alter one's perception and reality through visual and auditory changes. These drugs are commonly abused worldwide. In some parts of the world, many of these agents are legal for use.

CLINICAL FEATURES Patients under the mild influence of a hallucinogenic agent typically present with mellowing and loss of inhibitions. Patients with moderate toxicity may present with altered mental status, tachycardia, tachypnea, and dilated pupils (mydriasis). Patients with severe intoxication can present with violent behavior, traumatic injuries (PCP), profound hyperthermia, and evidence of rhabdomyolysis.

DIAGNOSIS Diagnosis includes a history of use and access to drugs. In addition, patients who present with altered mental status and visual and auditory hallucinations should be considered under the influence of any of these agents. Urine toxicology screens do exist for drugs such as marijuana, but if positive, may not indicate recent use because this drug is fat soluble and remains in the system for several weeks with heavy, chronic use. PCP also may test positive if abused within 72 hours of sampling. LSD levels are usually not available in the clinical setting.

TREATMENT Treatment of the majority of patients under the influence of hallucinogenic drugs includes supportive care, reassurance, and placing them in an environment with minimal external stimulus until the effect of the drug wears off. Patients with severe intoxication and violent behavior (high-dose LSD and PCP) often need physical restraints and chemical sedation with either benzodiazepines or haloperidol. In addition, they need to be rapidly cooled if hyperthermic and alkalinized with bicarbonate, along with mannitol diuresis if in rhabdomyolysis.

PREVENTION Prevention of severe intoxication with hallucinogenic agents includes public education as to the potential dangers of these mood-altering drugs.

INHALANTS/VOLATILE SUBSTANCES

BACKGROUND Inhalants or volatile substances deserve special mention. These agents have become popular in many cities around the world because of their easy access, low cost, addictive properties, and the fact that most of these products are not considered illegal substances. Commonly abused agents include model glue, spray paints, typewriter correction fluid, gasoline, butyl ethers, and cleaning solvents. Routes of administration include direct sniffing, huffing (rag saturated, then inhaled), and bagging (product sprayed into a plastic bag then inhaled). Chronic use of these agents can have a profound effect on the cardiac, renal, and central nervous systems.

DID YOU KNOW?

Inhalants are fast becoming some of the more commonly abused drugs by children and adolescents in industrialized and developing countries worldwide.

CLINICAL FEATURES Adolescents under the influence of volatiles may have mental status changes, behavior abnormalities (as noted by parents and teachers), tachycardia, tachypnea, and a characteristic hydrocarbon odor on the breath or skin. Profound intoxication can result in pulmonary aspiration, seizures, cardiac dysrhythmias, and death.

DIAGNOSIS Diagnosis is based on a history of exposure, access to these products, and the presence of the clinical features described above. There are no standard tests to detect these individual agents.

TREATMENT Treatment of the majority of patients under the influence of an inhalant includes supportive care and reassurance alone. If in respiratory distress, the patient's oxygen status should be assessed and the airway protected because these agents have high aspiration potential. Due to the fact that many of the volatile substances can sensitize or irritate the myocardium, the patient should be monitored for cardiac dysrhythmias and treated appropriately. Liberal use of epinephrine is discouraged because it may overstimulate the already sensitized myocardium. Beta blockers and lidocaine may be indicated if the patient has tachydysrhythmias.

PREVENTION Prevention of volatile substance abuse includes widespread public awareness as to the high prevalence and dangers of these substances. Parents and community leaders need to be made aware and take an active part in curtailing access of these products to children and adolescents.

MUSHROOMS Mushroom collection and ingestion is extremely popular worldwide, particularly in Europe. Each mushroom group varies from region to region and should be considered poisonous until proven otherwise.

> **TIPS AND TRICKS:**
>
> There are old mushroom pickers, and there are bold mushroom pickers, but there are no old, bold mushroom pickers.

A complete description of mushroom types and toxicities is beyond the scope of this book. If a patient presents with GI irritation, vomiting, and headaches, and has a recent history of ingesting mushrooms, consider mushroom toxicity. The cyclopeptide group is the most dangerous, and accounts for 95% of mushroom poisoning fatalities in North America and Europe. The general treatment for mushroom ingestions is decontamination, supportive care, and identifying possible life-threatening varieties, such as Amanita galerina (death cap or destroying angel).

PLANTS

As with mushroom ingestions, if you have an acutely ill patient, ask whether he or she has ingested some unusual food or plant. Here are some of the common types of plant-related ingestions and problems:

- Castor bean *(Ricinus)*. Brown/white speckled seeds. Clinical presentation: mimics septic shock, leukocytosis, hypotension, dehydration. Treatment: supportive care, fluids, lavage, AC.
- Foxglove *(Digitalis)*. Ornamental, tubular pink, purple, or white flowers. Clinical presentation: gastritis, cardiac conduction disturbances. Treatment: supportive care, lavage, AC, Digibind.
- Hemlock (water cicuta, poison conium). Fernlike leaves with white umbrella-like flowers. Clinical presentation: salivation, vomiting, seizures, bradycardia, hypotension, death. Treatment: supportive care, AC, lavage, atropine, intubation, control seizures.
- Holly *(Ilex)*. Green leaves with barbs and bright red berries. Clinical presentation: gastritis. Treatment: supportive care.
- Jimsonweed *(Datura)*. Funnel-shaped white or purple flower many seeds in star-shaped fruit. Clinical presentation: anticholinergic effect (dry skin, tachycardia, dilated pupils, delirium, flushed skin). Treatment: supportive care, lavage, AC, physostigmine if severe toxicity.

- Lily of the Valley *(Convallaria)*. Long green leaves, white bell-shaped flowers. Clinical presentation: gastritis, cardiac disturbances. Treatment: supportive care, lavage, AC, Digibind.
- Mandrake *(Mandraora)*. Green leaves resembling lettuce. Clinical presentation: anticholinergic. Treatment: supportive care, lavage, AC, physostigmine.
- Mistletoe *(Phroradendron)*. Green leaves with white berries. Clinical presentation: gastroenteritis, potential cardiotoxicity. Treatment: supportive care, lavage with ipecac, AC.
- Nightshades *(Solanum species)*. Potato shrublike, small flowers (yellow purple, white) with red or black berries. Clinical presentation: nausea, vomiting, abdominal pain, hallucinations. Treatment: supportive care, lavage with ipecac, AC.
- Oleander *(Nerium)*. Ornamental shrub, white, pink, yellow flowers in clusters. Clinical presentation: gastroenteritis, conduction disturbances. Treatment: supportive care, lavage, AC, Digibind.
- Pitted fruits such as apricots, peaches, cherries, and apples (amygdalin, cyanide-like). Clinical presentation: dyspnea, cyanosis, seizure, vomiting, cardiovascular collapse. Treatment: supportive care, lavage, AC, cyanide antidote kit.
- Pokeweed *(Phytolacca)*. Shrublike clusters of dark purple berries, made into poke salad when properly cooked. Clinical presentation: abdominal cramping, nausea, vomiting, may cause convulsions with large ingestions. Treatment: supportive care, lavage, AC.
- Rhubarb. Large green leaves with edible reddish/pink stalks, calcium oxalate crystals. Clinical presentation: oral burns, gastritis, renal compromise. Treatment: lavage, AC, oral calcium gluconate.
- Rosary or jequirity pea *(Abrus)*. Popular with beaded jewelry, bright scarlet seed with black hilum. Clinical presentation: severe gastritis, bloody diarrhea. Treatment: supportive care, fluids, lavage, AC.
- Tobacco *(Nicotinia)*. Yellow, white tubular flowers. Clinical presentation: salivation, GI distress, confusion, convulsions, tachycardia, hypertension. Treatment: supportive care, AC.
- Yew *(Taxus* species) (Chinese, Japanese, and Western). Evergreen tree, seed waxy red with open end. Clinical presentation: nausea, vomiting, abdominal pain, with severe overdose causing convulsions and cardiac conduction disturbances. Treatment: supportive care, lavage, AC, monitor cardiac activity.

HERBAL MEDICATIONS

Herbal treatments have become increasingly popular worldwide. Many individuals mistakenly assume that herbal remedies are safer, but there have been increasing reports of adverse reactions and deaths. Lack of strict governmental regulations make it difficult to regulate quality. Here are a few of the most common herbal remedies:

- Ginkgo. 5 million prescriptions in Germany alone. Used to treat peripheral vascular disease, free radical scavenger, increase cerebral circulation.
- St. John's wort (Herbal Prozac). Used in Europe to treat depression and sleep disorders. Better than placebo, similar to standard antidepressants (6-week onset).
- Ephedra (Chinese Ma Huang). Marketed as an alternative to Ecstacy. Weight reducer, increase stamina (promises euphoria/hallucinogenic effect with no health risks). Deaths reported.
- Feverfew. European antipyretic, for migraines, contains parthenolide (serotonin antagonist).
- Ginseng. Used for centuries in China as an aphrodisiac. Builds up general viability, increased physical capacity. (Most products do not contain enough to make a difference.)
- Ginger (Chinese rhizome). For motion sickness, indigestion.
- Pennyroyal (Hispanic). Used to treat colic in adults and infants. Also used as an abortifacient. Can cause hepatotoxity and liver failure.
- Echinacea (Native American). Acts as an immunostimulant, increases phagocytosis, promotes activity of lymphocytes, used to prevent the common cold.
- Saw palmetto (Native American). Used to treat prostatic hypertrophy, increases urinary flow, reduces conversion of testosterone to dihydrotestosterone (DHT).
- Kava. Root of the tropical black pepper, South Pacific psychoactive drug, sleep aid, relaxant, benzodiazepine-like effect, made into a tea.
- Yohimbine. Bark of the West African yohimbe tree, alpha$_2$ antagonist, aphrodisiac properties, priapism.

CHAPTER 20

Environmental Illnesses

C. James Holliman and Chayan C. Dey

Illnesses and injuries caused by environmental exposure can lead to serious health threats. This chapter reviews the diagnosis and management of illnesses related to exposure to factors in the environment, including high and low temperatures and potentially dangerous animals.

HEAT-RELATED ILLNESSES

DEFINITION

Heat-related illnesses result when the core body temperature exceeds 38°C. Heat-related illnesses are sometimes referred to as hyperthermia. Heat-related illness can be divided into three different types: mild heat-related illness, heat exhaustion, and heatstroke.

CAUSES

The general causes of heat-related illnesses are listed in Table 20-1 and described below:

- Heat edema: pooling of fluid in the extremities that occurs in the first few days of exposure to hot weather
- Heat cramps: spasmotic cramping of extremities from mild electrolyte imbalance, frequently due to replacing lost body fluids with nonsodium fluid or water only.

TABLE 20-1 GENERAL CAUSES OF HEAT-RELATED ILLNESSES

Infections	Environmental exposure
Drug reactions	Overexertion
Neuroleptic malignant syndrome	Alcohol withdrawal
Malignant hyperthermia	

- Heat syncope: lightheadedness and syncope during the early stage of heat exposure where one is slightly volume depleted and not acclimated to the heat
- Heat exhaustion (sodium depletion): mildly inadequate fluid with inadequate salt intake. This typically occurs in young people exercising in a hot environment and not being used to the hot weather.
- Heat exhaustion (water depletion): elderly people with inadequate free water intake. This is more dangerous and can lead to heatstroke.
- Heatstroke: severe, life-threatening heat-induced emergency. Heatstroke is associated with metabolic acidosis, electrolyte imbalance, and mental status changes.

ACCLIMATIZATION

Acclimatization to heat exposure is the process by which the body autoadapts to better tolerate environmental heat. The effects are gradual over several weeks. Most important are increased sweating (from 1 L/h to 3 L/h) and decreased sodium content of sweat. When newly exposed to a hot environment, it is important to allow this acclimatization process to occur before attempting significant physical exertion; otherwise nonacclimatized individuals are at risk for heat-related illness.

DRUG REACTIONS

Examples of drug reactions causing heat-related illnesses are listed in Table 20-2. Predisposing factors to heat-related illness (excluding drugs) can be divided into three categories, which are listed in Table 20-3. Often, it may be due to a combination of these factors.

CLINICAL FEATURES

Patients with heat stroke can present with confusion, lethargy, or coma. Although heatstroke is most common in very hot weather, it can occur in normal climates in high-risk patients. Be sure to address the possibility of a heat-related emergency in elderly patients presenting with mental status changes.

TABLE 20-2 EXAMPLES OF DRUG REACTIONS THAT CAN CAUSE
HEAT-RELATED ILLNESSES

Hypersensitivity
  Antibiotics
  Phenytoin
  Alphamethyldopa
  Procainamide
  NSAIDs

Hypermetabolism
  Thryoid hormone
  Cocaine
  Amphetamines
  Phencyclidine (PCP)
  Monoamine oxidase inhibitors
  Salicylates

Impaired thermoregulation
  Ethanol
  Phenothiazines
  Cimetidine

Malignant hyperthermia
  Halogenated general anesthetics
  Succinylcholine

Impaired heat dissipation
  Anticholinergics
  Tricyclic antidepressants
  Phenothiazines

Impaired cardiovascular compensation
  Diuretics
  Laxatives
  Beta blockers

Direct pyrogens
  Cancer chemotherapy agents
  Amphotericin
  Metal fumes
  Injection of cotton fragments

Immunizations

Neuroleptic malignant syndrome
  Antipsychotics
  Lithium
  Levodopa withdrawal
  Metoclopramide

CRITICAL ACTION:

  Heatstroke is a true medical emergency. It requires rapid identification and treatment with cooling and fluid resuscitation.

Other diagnoses to consider are listed in Table 20-4.

TABLE 20-3 PREDISPOSING FACTORS TO HEAT-RELATED ILLNESS

EXOGENOUS HEAT GAIN	ENDOGENOUS HEAT GAIN	IMPAIRED HEAT DISSIPATION
Being in a closed space	Exercise	High environmental
Lack of air conditioning	Agitation	temperature/humidity
Prolonged contact with hot	Fever	Lack of acclimatization
water such as in hot tubs	Infection	Excessive clothing
	Hyperthyroidism	Diabetes
		Sweat gland dysfunction
		Previous heatstroke

TABLE 20-4 DIFFERENTIAL DIAGNOSIS OF HEATSTROKE

Meningitis/encephalitis
Cerebral falciparum malaria
Cerebrovascular accident/traumatic intracranial bleed
Diabetic ketoacidosis with infection
Thyroid storm
Neuroleptic malignant syndrome
Malignant hyperthermia

TREATMENT

Treatment should focus on the ABCs: airway, breathing, and circulation. The most important intervention in heatstroke is rapid cooling and adequate hydration (Table 20-5). External cooling is best accomplished using cool mist and fans. Circulating cooling blankets are also effective. In rare cases, internal cooling with iced lavage might have to be performed via Foley catheter and nasogastric tubes. The core temperature should be measured using the most accurate method available, and external cooling should be stopped when temperature goes below 38.5°C.

TABLE 20-5 TREATMENT OF HEAT-RELATED ILLNESSES

ILLNESS	CAUSE	TREATMENT
Heat edema	Pooling of fluid in the extremities that occurs in the first few days in hot weather	No special treatment is needed Elevation Support hose
Heat cramps	Replacing of lost body fluids with non-sodium fluid or water only	Rest in a cool area Fluids containing sodium chloride [IVF or oral rehydration solution (ORS)]
Heat syncope	Occurs during the early stage of heat exposure where one is slightly volume depleted and not used to the heat	Removal from heat source Fluids Rest Hospitalization is not usually necessary
Heat exhaustion (sodium depletion)	Mildly inadequate fluid with inadequate salt intake Young person exercising in a hot environment and not being used to the hot weather	Rest Cooling Fluids with sodium (IVF or ORS)
Heat exhaustion	In elderly people inadequate free water intake can lead to to heat stroke	Cooling Rest Fluids without salt (D_5W or oral water)

NEUROLEPTIC MALIGNANT SYNDROME

DEFINITION

Neuroleptic malignant syndrome is a rare and potentially fatal reaction most commonly associated with the use of antipsychotic agents or withdrawal from dopamine agonists, such as amantadine or levodopa. It occurs with therapeutic doses of antipsychotic agents and is not related to duration of therapy. It usually develops over 1 to 3 days and lasts 1 to 2 weeks after stopping oral antipsychotic agents but may last several weeks after using intramuscular (IM) antipsychotic agents. Think of this when a patient presents with delirium and unexplained high temperature.

CLINICAL FEATURES

Fever, tremor, rigidity, mental status changes, increased heart and respiratory rates, sweating, elevated liver enzymes, dark urine, and muscle breakdown may be observed.

TREATMENT

The most important part of treatment is supportive care, with rapid cooling, fluid and electrolyte repletion, and critical care management (Table 20-6). Be sure to address other potential and more common causes of high temperature, including infection.

MALIGNANT HYPERTHERMIA

DEFINITION

Malignant hyperthermia is an inherited condition that is similar in presentation to neuroleptic malignant syndrome. It is suspected to be due to excessive release of intracellular

TABLE 20-6 TREATMENT OF NEUROLEPTIC MALIGNANT SYNDROME

Airway, breathing, IV access, and cardiac monitor
Relax skeletal muscle quickly with IV benzodiazepines.
Cool patient with ice packs, mist, fan, or any means possible.
Give IV fluids.
Stop the antipsychotic agent or restart the dopamine agent.
For restoration of CNS dopamine levels consider
   Bromocriptine 2.5–20 mg orally three times daily
   Amantadine 100 mg orally twice daily
   Levodopa 100–250 mg orally three times daily
For significant muscle rigidity use dantrolene 1–10 mg/kg/day IV or orally.

calcium during the administration of halogenated general anesthesia and depolarizing neuromuscular blockers (succinylcholine).

CLINICAL FEATURES

Fever, tachycardia, muscle rigidity (possible masseter spasm), disseminated intravascular coagulation (DIC), acidosis, irregular heart rate, hypotension, rhabdomyolysis, and myoglobinuria may be observed.

TREATMENT

PREVENTION Because this is an inherited condition, it is important to take a family history of problems with general anesthesia (Table 20-7). If a risk of malignant hyperthermia is suspected because of a positive family history or prior occurrence, choose another anesthetic. If general anesthesia is needed, pretreat with 1 mg/kg dantrolene orally for 8 hours (four doses) prior to surgery or 2.5 mg/kg intravenously (IV) 30 minutes before surgery. Have cooling materials and adequate dantrolene in the operating room prior to inducing anesthesia.

HYPOTHERMIA

DEFINITION

Hypothermia occurs when the body temperature dips below 35°C (95°F). Severe hypothermia is a body temperature of less than 28°C. Although this occurs mostly in colder

TABLE 20-7 TREATMENT OF MALIGNANT HYPERTHERMIA

1. Stop the anesthetic and use new tubing or anesthesia machine.
2. Ventilate with 100% O_2.
3. Discontinue the surgery if possible and close the wound quickly.
4. Call for help.
5. Start external cooling with ice and cold packs and hypothermic blanket.
6. Give dantrolene 1 mg/kg IV every 3–5 minutes until symptoms subside or dose of 10 mg/kg reached.
7. Draw blood (CBC, lytes, BUN, glucose, creat, PT, PTT, LFTs, CPK, ABGs, and calcium).
8. Insert NG and Foley and start NG iced lavage.
9. Start IV bicarb ± mannitol if acidosis or myoglobinuria present.

CBC, complete blood count, BUN, blood urea nitrogen;
PT, prothrombin time; PTT, partial thromboplastin time; LFT, liver function tests; CPK, creatine phosphokinase; ABG, arterial blood gases; NG, nasogastric.

climates, it may develop without exposure to cold environments. Hypothermia is not uncommon in warm months and can develop indoors during the summer. There are many causes of hypothermia:

■ Hypothalamic and central nervous system (CNS) disease
■ Metabolic diseases
■ Drug-induced (alcohol or any CNS depressant)
■ Sepsis
■ Environmental conditions
■ Extremes of age
■ Dermal disease
■ Major incapacitating illness (acute myocardial infarction, congestive heart failure, cerebrovascular accident)

CLINICAL FEATURES

See Table 20-8.

FIELD CARE If an individual is found unconscious out in the environment, begin cardiopulmonary resuscitation (CPR) if there are multiple rescuers. If there are two or fewer rescuers, cover the patient with clothing or a blanket and seek help. Gentle handling of the patient is important so as not to induce cardiac dysrhythmias. CPR should be started if the temperature is greater than 32°C and the patient is in cardiorespiratory arrest, or if ventricular fibrillation or asystole is seen on the cardiac monitor. Chest compressions should be performed at half the normal rate for severely hypothermic patients. Rewarming is best done in a hospital setting.

REWARMING The objective is to increase the core temperature by more than 1.0°C per hour. Passive rewarming is suitable if the body temperature is over 32°C. Try to put

TABLE 20-8 CLINICAL FEATURES OF HYPOTHERMIA

TEMPERATURE (C°)	CLINICAL FINDINGS	TYPICAL CARDIAC RESPONSE
>35	Mild confusion, lethargy, shivering	Sinus tachycardia
33–35	Amnesia	Sinus bradycardia, Osborne J waves
28–32	Semiconscious, muscle rigidity, pupils dilated	Atrial fibrillation
<28	Unconscious, tendon reflexes absent	Ventricular fibrillation
<26		Asystole

the patient in a heated area and cover the body and scalp with warm material. A warm-water bath and axillary and groin hot packs may be used.

Disadvantages of external rewarming alone are as follows:

■ May cause core temperature afterdrop and resultant ventricular fibrillation
■ May cause increased hypoxia and acidosis if there is sudden increased metabolism peripherally, but the cold heart is unable to compensate
■ May cause hypotension from peripheral vasodilation

If the core temperature does not increase at least 1°C/h, then start more aggressive techniques (Table 20-9). Bretylium may be given if ventricular fibrillation occurs, but defibrillation may not be successful until core temperature is greater than 30°C. If the patient is rewarmed to over 33°C and there is still no sign of life, then the patient should be pronounced dead.

PREVENTION

■ Adequate clothing (wool retains heat when wet whereas cotton garments do not)
■ Trip planning
■ Avoid alcohol/sedatives in cold climates
■ Change wet clothes promptly
■ Limit wind exposure
■ Maintain fluid intake

TABLE 20-9   CORE REWARMING TECHNIQUES (IN ORDER OF INVASIVENESS)

1. Warmed O_2 (42°C) by mask or ETT (suitable for every patient)
2. Warmed IV fluid (42°C); only limited heat exchange possible with this
3. Nasogastric tube lavage (good safe technique)
4. Rectal tube lavage
5. Peritoneal dialysis catheter lavage
6. Chest tube lavage (very effective)
7. Thoracotomy/mediastinal lavage
8. Cardiopulmonary bypass (fem-fem); quickest rewarming techniques and probably the best if it can be quickly instituted

ETT, endotracheal tube.

FROSTBITE

DEFINITIONS

Frostbite is tissue injury caused by exposure to freezing temperatures. Frostnip is the initial clinical response to cold and is reversible. The skin becomes blanched and numb, followed by sudden cessation of cold and discomfort. If treated quickly at this point with rewarming it will not progress to frostbite. There are two types of nonfreezing cold injury.

Trench foot (immersion foot) results from exposure to wet cold and temperatures above freezing for 1 to 2 days, and is characterized by skin damage resembling partial-thickness burns. Deep damage is rare. The affected part should be treated by drying, rewarming, and no weight bearing.

Chilbain (pernio), due to intermittent exposure of bare skin, especially on the lower extremities, to cool windy weather, is characterized by reddish blue, warm, swollen patchy areas on the skin, as well as itching and burning. Treatment consists of warm soaking, pain control, and soothing skin ointment.

CLASSIFICATION

The two types of frostbite, superficial and deep, can only be differentiated prior to thawing. In the superficial type, the affected part is cold, pale, gray, and bloodless, but is pliable and soft. In the deep type, the affected part feels woody or stoney.

Usual progression of signs with frostbite are redness, burning, blanching, numbness, "clumsy" feeling of extremities, and firm, tense involved tissue.

Progression of signs after rewarming of superficial frostbite are as follows:

- 24 hours: large clear blisters.
- 2 to 7 days: skin blackens, demarcates (dry gangrene).
- Months later: the outer layers peel off, revealing sensitive new skin.

In deep frostbite, if the distal limb portions remain cold and cyanotic after rewarming, risk of progression to wet gangrene (infected necrosis) is greater.

TREATMENT

1. Rapid rewarming in 42°C water (do not thaw in the field if refreezing might occur—refreezing is more damaging than allowing prolonged freezing)
2. Pain control with narcotics
3. Tetanus prophylaxis
4. Topical antibiotics (Silvadene, etc.) for second-degree burns
5. No weight bearing
6. No debridement, surgery, or amputation should be considered for at least several months unless wet gangrene or infection occurs.
7. If large amounts of tissue are involved, watch for rhabdomyolysis and renal failure.
8. Start physical therapy early but do not put any direct shear stress on the damaged tissue.

DROWNING

DEFINITIONS

Drowning, like other accidental deaths, often strikes young healthy individuals. Prevention is the key to avoid unnecessary deaths. The patient's prognosis after near drowning depends on the speed of rescue and resuscitation. There are many ways to classify drowning (Table 20-10).

TABLE 20-10 CLASSIFICATION OF DROWNING

TYPES OF DROWNING	DEFINITION	DEATH TIME FRAME
Drowning	Death from suffocation after submersion	< 24 h
Secondary drowning	Death from complications related to submersion (pulmonary injury, sepsis, renal failure)	> 24 h
Near drowning	Survival following suffocation after submersion	Temporary survival

TABLE 20-11 PROGNOSIS ASSOCIATED WITH OXYGEN DEPRIVATION AFTER SUBMERSION

IMPORTANT ASPECT OF HISTORY	POSSIBLE PROGNOSIS OUTCOMES
Estimated time of submersion	Longer time results in worse prognosis
Type and temperature of the water	Freshwater drowning destroys lung tissue properties Colder water may provide better outcome
Amount and type of water contamination	The more water aspirated, the worse the outcome Contaminated water ingestion can cause lung damage and infection
How soon and type of resuscitative measures	Quicker rescue results in better prognosis
Whether vomiting occurred	Vomiting can lead to aspiration pneumonia
How soon after the victim first gasped	If <30 min after rescue, <10% have mental retardation or spastic quadriplegia If not till 60–120 min after rescue, 50%–80% have serious neurologic problems
How soon patient transported	Earlier transport results in better outcome
History of drug or alcohol use	Results in worse prognosis

CLINICAL FEATURES

The threats to life after submersion are due to respiratory failure and neurologic injury because of lack of oxygen to the brain. There are many mechanisms of injury, including water aspiration, aspiration of other substances (sand, algae, vomit, etc.), and laryngospasm of the trachea. Whatever the mechanism, the final common pathway is profound lack of oxygen. Patients at risk have undergone a "significant" episode and display symptoms such as coughing and shortness of breath, or have a history of factors (Table 20-11). The patients generally can be classified into four categories, and the appropriate treatment is described in Table 20-12.

PROGNOSIS

Several parts of the history of the drowning influence the prognosis of the patient (Tables 20-11 and 20-12). Remember to ask these questions so as not to miss the sicker patients.

TABLE 20-12 CLASSIFICATION AND TREATMENT OF PATIENTS AFTER SUBMERSION

PATIENT GROUPS	HOSPITAL TREATMENT	DISPOSITION
Group A: awake and with no history of significant submersion	Do ABC Clear spine Monitor/give oxygen Look for other injuries	Discharge
Group B: awake but with history of significant submersion	As above, as well as laboratory studies (chest radiograph, complete blood count, electrolyte, urinalysis) and pulse oximetry if available	Discharge after observation in emergency room for several hours Admit overnight if needed Discharge if stable next day
Group C: conscious but obtunded	As above, as well as arterial blood gases if available Patient may need intubation if becoming worse Restrict fluids to prevent cerebral edema	Admit to intensive care unit or send to higher care facility Observe for a length of time patient gets better Discharge only if no delayed deterioration
Group D: comatose	As above, as well as intubation/hyperventilation Restrict fluid Diuretics Temperature control	Admit to intensive care unit or send to higher care facility

Prognosis worsens from groups A to D.

When a drowning patient comes to the hospital, another prognosis tool that can be used is the Orlowski scale, which consists of five factors:

1. Patient is under 3 years of age.
2. Submersion was for more than 5 minutes.
3. No CPR was performed in the first 10 minutes after rescue.
4. Coma on hospital admission.
5. pH is less than 7.1 on hospital admission.

ALTITUDE ILLNESS

Altitude illnesses occur when one ascends above 2,500 meters after having been at a lower altitude for at least 10 days. Males and females are affected equally. Altitude illnesses can recur, or may occur in patients who previously had no type of problem with altitude exposure. Exacerbating factors are sudden ascent, sudden exertion before acclimating to higher altitude, alcohol, and sleeping pills. Being young or being in good physical condition does not appear to be a protective factor.

There are four forms of altitude-related illness: acute mountain sickness (AMS), high-altitude peripheral edema, high-altitude pulmonary edema (HAPE), high-altitude cerebral edema (HACE), and high-altitude retinopathy. AMS can rapidly proceed to the worsening conditions of HACE and HAPE (Table 20-13). The differential diagnosis includes dehydration, hypothermia, exhaustion, respiratory infection, hyperventilation syndrome, psychiatric disorders, and carbon monoxide poisoning.

HIGH-ALTITUDE RETINAL HEMORRHAGE

Above 4,500 m, 20% to 40% of individuals develop this type of hemorrhage. It usually does not affect vision unless bleeding occurs across the macula. No therapy is needed and descent is unnecessary.

MAMMAL BITES

CLINICAL FEATURES

Complications of the bite injuries are cosmetic deformities, fractures, tetanus/rabies, and infections. Many diseases can be transmitted from mammals to humans (by bite, scratch, or lick). The average infection rates from mammal bites, possible bacteria involvement, and increased infection risk factors are listed in Table 20-14. General treatment of animal bite wounds is described in Tables 20-15 and 20-16.

TABLE 20-13 ONSET, SYMPTOMS, AND TREATMENT OF TYPES OF ALTITUDE ILLNESS

ALTITUDE ILLNESS	ONSET	SYMPTOMS	TREATMENT
Acute mountain sickness (AMS)	Occurs within 8–24 h after ascent	Headache Nausea/anorexia "Hangover" feeling Insomnia Reduced urine output	Usually does not require descent and resolves in 1–3 days if ascent is delayed If severe, descend 300 m and reascend If severe, give oxygen, acetazolamide 250 mg PO twice daily, and/or dexamethasone 8 mg orally then 4 mg every 6 h *Prophylaxis:* (a) staging of ascent, with 1–2 days at 2,000 m before proceeding; (b) take either acetazolamide 250 mg twice daily starting 24 h before ascent or dexamethasone orally 4 mg every 6 h for several days
High-altitude pulmonary edema (HAPE; noncardiogenic pulmonary edema) *(Can be fatal)*	Occurs 24–72 h after arrival at altitude, usually >4,000 m Most common on second night.	Cough → Shortness of breath at rest → Chest ache → Worsening cough→ Increased breathing rates → Frothy sputum or hemoptysis → Pulmonary rales	Rapid descent, at least 600 m, is most important High flow oxygen Rest and keep patient warm Avoid exertion on descent Medications that may be helpful: Nifedipine 10 mg orally right away, follow by 20 mg twice daily (drug of choice if oxygen or descent unavailable) Acetazolamide 5 mg/kg/day Furosemide 40 mg once if not dehydrated Morphine
High-Altitude Cerebral Edema (HACE) *Can be fatal or permanent neurologic disability*	Occurs usually 2–3 days Onset more gradual than HAPE	Severe headache Confusion Ataxia Nausea/vomiting Visual changes Hallucinations Seizures Coma	Only effective treatment is descent of at least 1,000 m Oxygen Treat symptoms with analgesics and antiemetics May try acetazolamide and dexamethasone Diuretics to reduce brain edema

HUMAN BITE WOUNDS

Even though a human bite wound can occur anywhere in the body, the most common area of injury is usually in the knuckle of the hand. The injury happens when one uses a closed fist to strike another person in the mouth and instead ends up cutting their hand on the other person's teeth. This can be a serious problem since the human mouth has many bacteria that can easily infect the hand. Thus, important steps must be taken

TABLE 20-14 INFECTION AGENTS AND RISK FACTORS ASSOCIATED WITH MAMMAL BITES

AVERAGE MAMMAL BITES INFECTION RATES		SPECIFIC BACTERIA IN BITE INFECTION	INCREASED INFECTION RISK FACTORS
Dogs	2%–5%	*Staphylococcus* (30% in dog bites)	Age <2 or >50 years
Cats	30%–50%	*Pasteurella multocida* (75% in cat bites)	Diabetes
			Immunosuppressive illness
Rats	2%–10%	Streptococci (10%–20% of all bites)	Chronic alcoholism
			Puncture wounds
Monkey	25%	Bacteroids and other anerobes	Large wounds
Humans	13%–50%	*Clostridium tetani* (rare)	Extremity wounds
		Mycobacteria (rare)	Delayed (>4 to 24 h) presentation.

TABLE 20-15 GENERAL TREATMENT OF MAMMAL BITES

Wound irrigation with sterile saline or cool boiled water (use several liters) and soap is the most important step.
Tooth puncture wounds should always be cleaned.
Remove all the dirt in the wound and clean the area.
Severely damaged tissue may have to be debrided.
Always suture face and scalp bite wounds.
Always suture rodent bites.
Dog bites can sometimes be sutured.
Never suture a human bite on the hand.
Never suture a cat bite or deep puncture wounds.
Dog bites can sometimes be sutured.
Antibiotics are indicated for all bites of the hand and other parts of the body with skin penetration (see Table 20–16).
Admit to hospital if patient has deep established infection.
Initial culture is not helpful. Late infection presentation should be cultured.
Do not forget tetanus or rabies prevention.
Recheck bite wounds in 1–2 days.

TABLE 20-16 ANTIBIOTIC CHOICES FOR ANIMAL BITE WOUNDS

ANIMAL BITE	PREFERRED ANTIBIOTIC
Cat	Penicillin VK 500 mg four times daily for 7 days **or** Azithromycin 500 mg orally for 1 day, then 250 mg orally daily for 4 day **or** Tetracycline 500 mg four times daily 7 days
Dog	Dicloxacillin 500 mg orally four times daily for 5–7 days **or** Cefalexin 500 mg orally four tmes daily for 5–7 days
Human	Cefalexin 500 mg orally four times daily for 5–7 days **or** Penicillin VK 500 mg four times daily for 7 days
Rodent	Penicillin VK 500 mg four times daily for 7 days

TABLE 20-17 TREATMENT OF HUMAN BITES

General Treatment
Clean wound by clearing dirt and washing well with cool boiled water.
If the wound is an abrasion and not deep, just clean and give tetanus
   prophylaxis.
Give antibiotic for 7 days.
Splint/elevate limb.
Do suture except if the bite is to the face.
Closed-fist injury
Obtain radiograph for broken bones and foreign body (bone chip).
Wash well with IV fluid or with boiled warm water.
Give IV antibiotic (penicillin or cephalosporin).
Splint.
Possible admission to the hospital
Admit to hospital
Human bites of the hand more than 24 h after injury
Infection beyond local cellulites
Purulent discharge
Pain when finger is moved (possible joint infection)
Tendon or joint injury
Open fracture

to clean the hand properly and make sure that the patient does not need to be admitted to the hospital (Table 20-17).

There have been no documented cases yet of AIDS transmission from human bites. Two other animal bite conditions that should be specifically mentioned are cat scratch fever and rat bite fever (Table 20-18).

TABLE 20-18 INFECTIONS TRANSMITTED BY CATS AND RATS

CAT SCRATCH FEVER	RAT BITE FEVER
May be due to a scratch or bite	Red petechial rash on the limbs, often palms and soles
Enlargement of local and regional lymph nodes	Fever
Red raised lesion that becomes filled with pus and heals in 1–4 weeks	Arthritis of large joints
Weakness	Treatment with penicillin VK 500 mg four times daily for 7 days or erythromycin shortens the course
Fever up to 3 months	
Usually improves without treatment	
Ciprofloxacin or gentamicin may improve symptoms.	

RABIES

CLINICAL FEATURES

Rabies is transmitted by inoculation with infectious saliva and can be transmitted by inhalation (rare) in caves or laboratories (Table 20-19). It causes severe fatal encephalitis. Patients with a recent animal bite present with mental status changes, hydrophobia, and dehydration (Table 20-20).

TREATMENT

Supportive care only. Do not suture a rabies-prone wound. Rabies is almost always fatal, so supportive care is best.

TABLE 20-19 RISK OF RABIES TRANSMISSION FROM ANIMAL BITES

HIGH RISK	LOW RISK
Bats	Rodents
Raccoons	Lagomorphs (hares and rabbits)
Skunks	Farm animals
Foxes/wolves	Indoor cats and dogs
Coyotes/bobcats	
Other carnivores	

TABLE 20-20 CLINICAL PROGRESSION OF RABIES

EVENT	TIME PERIOD	SYMPTOMS
Bite	First day	Local wound reaction or injury
Incubation period	Weeks to months	No symptoms
Prodromal Phase	2 days to 2 weeks[a]	Fever, malaise, headaches, sore throat
Neurologic Phase	One week to several weeks[a]	Anxiety, restlessness, spasms, numbness, swallowing problems, afraid of water, spasms
Paralytic Phase	Several weeks to months[a]	Paralysis, confusion
Death		

[a] refers to after incuation period is finished.

PROPHYLAXIS

The rabies prophylaxis protocol is as follows:

1. Rabies immune globulin (RIG): 20 IU/kg with half the dose IM and half the dose infiltrated around the wound (given on first day) AND
2. Human diploid cell vaccine (HDCV): 1 mL IM on days 0 (the day of the bite), 3, 7, 14, and 90. See also Table 20-21.

No follow-up antibody titer is usually needed. Don't forget usual wound care, tetanus prophylaxis, antibiotics, etc. Pregnancy is not a contraindication to prophylaxis. Countries without animal rabies are the Pacific Islands, Caribbean Islands, United Kingdom, Iceland, Singapore, Australia, Portugal, Spain, Sweden, Japan, and Taiwan.

TABLE 20-21 PROTOCOL FOR STARTING RABIES PROPHYLAXIS

| **HIGH-RISK BITES** | | **LOW-RISK BITES** | |
ANIMAL CAPTURED	**ANIMAL ESCAPED**	**ANIMAL CAPTURED**	**ANIMAL ESCAPED**
Send animal's head to public health laboratory for pathology examination. Treat only if laboratory confirms rabid animal.	Give prophylaxis.	Watch animal for 1 week. If animal gets sick, kill and send head to pathology laboratory. If animal stays well, no treatment is needed.	Consider prophylaxis, if attack was clearly unprovoked.

TETANUS

ETIOLOGY

See Table 20-22 for wounds that are likely to cause tetanus.

EPIDEMIOLOGY

It is possible that there are 1,000,000 deaths/year worldwide; 90% are due to neonatal tetanus. Other causes include acute injuries with a break in the skin surface (70%); ulcers, abscesses, IV drug use (20%); and no apparent source or wound (7%–20%).

TABLE 20-22 WOUNDS LIKELY TO CAUSE TETANUS

Animal bites
Stab or gunshot wounds
Holes made by dirty needles (such as in ear piercing)
Puncture wounds from metal nails
Improperly cleaned wounds; tetanus immunization not up to date
Clostridium tetani spores enter wound, reproduce, and produce
    toxin in the anerobic environment.

CLINICAL FEATURES

See Table 20-23 for the clinical features and four types of tetanus. The incubation period is time from inoculation to appearance of first symptoms. The period of onset is from first symptom to time of first reflex spasm. All cases are severe and progress rapidly. There is a 10% to 20% overall mortality rate even with intensive medical care. Patients over 60 years of age have a 52% mortality rate, whereas neonatal patients have a greater than 90% mortality rate. Tetanus severity (Table 20-24) can be used to judge how quickly the patient will need to be sent to a more advanced health facility.

TABLE 20-23 FOUR TYPES OF TETANUS

1. Generalized
    Jaw and neck stiff
    Body arched with legs and feet bent backward
    Abdomen rigid
    Severe muscle spasms
    Respiratory problems
    Blood pressure both increased and decreased with sweating
    Recovery with supportive care after second or third week
2. Localized
    Rigidity, spasm, pain in localized muscle group
    May progress to generalized tetanus infection
3. Cephalic
    Source of infection is in head or neck
    May progress to generalized tetanus infection
4. Neonatal
    Cause
        Umbilical cord is cut with a dirty instrument
        Umbilical cord is cut too close to the body
        Newly cut umbilical cord is tightly covered or not kept dry
    Symptoms
        Infant will not suck
        Infant cannot open mouth
        Muscle spasms
        Head bent back

TABLE 20-24 TETANUS SEVERITY CLASSIFICATION

SEVERITY	INCUBATION PERIOD (DAYS)	PERIOD OF ONSET (DAYS)	FINDINGS
Mild	10 or more	4–7	Local rigidity, mild trismus
Moderate	7–10	3–6	Severe trismus, difficulty swallowing, spasms
Severe	<7	<3	Severe spasms, diffuse rigidity, autonomic dysfunction

DIAGNOSIS

Try to send the patient to an intensive medical care facility if tetanus is even suspected. A prior episode of tetanus does not confer immunity (toxin dose is too low to stimulate antibodies). Reliable recent immunization history or documented antitetanus antibody excludes the diagnosis. Tetanus cannot be excluded just because no wound is present. The differential diagnoses for tetanus are many and include meningitis, rabies, hypocalcemia, and adverse reaction to antipsychotic medication reaction. A trial dose of 25 to 50 mg IV of diphenhydramine may help exclude a dystonic reaction to antipsychotic medication.

TREATMENT

See Table 20-25 for the treatment of tetanus.

PROPHYLAXIS The recommended immunization schedule is as follows:

- DPT IM at 2, 4, 6, and 18 months and at age 6 years
- Only DT (*not* DPT) after age 6
- Hypertet 250 units to any patient with tetanus-prone wound and 10 years since last immunization

HAZARDOUS MARINE ORGANISMS

There are many marine organisms throughout the world that can injure humans (Table 20-26). The success of treatment for stings depends on rapid initiation. Most injuries are instantly painful and require local wound care, removal of any foreign bodies, pain control, tetanus, and infection prevention. If the wound becomes infected, prompt debridement is needed, and antibiotic should be started. The antibiotic therapy should have coverage against *Vibrio* species. Some examples are tetracycline, trimethoprim-sulfamethoxazole, third-generation cephalosporin, and ciprofloxacin.

TABLE 20-25 TREATMENT OF TETANUS

PLAN	MEDICAL MANAGEMENT
1. Admit to intensive medical care setting	Limit examinations on patients (they can trigger spasms)
2. Respiratory management	May need assistance with respiration If available, consider intubation and mechanical ventilation
3. Antibiotic therapy	First choice: Metronidazole 500 mg IV every 6 hours for 7–10 days Second choice: Penicillin 1.5 million units every 6 h
4. Muscle relaxation (high-dose benzodiazepines or methocarbamol)	Diazepam 5 mg IV every 1–3 h to effect or Lorazepam 2 mg IV to effect or Midazolam 5–15 mg/h continuous IV infusion or Methocarbamol 3–4 g IV every 6 h
5. Muscle relaxation (for severe spasms)	Pancuronium 2 mg IV to effect
6. Management of autonomic dysfunction (control sympathetic overactivity)	Labetolol 0.25–1 mg/min continuous IV or Magnesium sulfate 70 mg/kg IV loading then 1–4 g/h infusion and morphine 0.5–1 mg/kg/h and clonidine 0.3 mg every 8 h
7. Wound management	Abscess drainage Debridement
8. Immunotherapy	Human tetanus immune globulin (Hypertet) 500–5,000 units IM Tetanus toxoid 0.5 mL IM at presentation, 6 weeks, and 6 months after presentation
9. Nutritional support	

SNAKEBITES

EPIDEMIOLOGY

There are about 3,000 species of snakes and 375 medically important species of venomous snakes worldwide. Annually there are possibly 1 million venomous bites and possibly 30,000 to 60,000 deaths worldwide. Factors determining relative risks of human envenomation by different snakes are venom toxicity/potency, effectiveness of the bite (at injecting venom), innate aggressiveness of the snake, and likelihood of human contact.

The risk of snakebite in most field situations is very low. Many bites occur owing to poor handling of pet snakes. Most accidental bites are to the lower extremity and occur in the summer.

TABLE 20-26 HAZARDOUS MARINE ORGANISMS

TITLE	CAUSES	SYMPTOMS	TREATMENT	SPECIAL HINTS
Sponge diver's disease	Contact with horny elastic skeleton body of sponges	Itchy dermatitis anaphylactoid reaction and large involvement (fever, nausea, cramps)	Remove spicules with tape, vinegar, rubbing alcohol Steroids by mouth for severe reaction	Use gloves to handle sponges Never break sponges with bare hands Dried sponges may still be toxic
Coelenterate toxicity	Contact with organism causes stinging organelles to be released into patient skin. The organelles release chemicals that are toxic.	Skin irritation, itching, throbbing pain, scar, usually usually resolves in 1–2 weeks	Evaluate ABCs Treat systemic symptoms if severe allergy reaction Pain control and tetanus To remove: (a) wear gloves and rinse with sea water only; (b) Soak the area with vinegar or rubbing alcohol for 30 min (c) scrape off the "fixed" organelles with razor blade	Do not use fresh water, hot water, or abrasion for they will cause more toxins to be released Antibiotics are usually not needed For box jellyfish, found in Australia (very dangerous): (a) use vinegar; (b) give IV antivenin IV antivenin 1–3 ampules; (c) IV steroids; monitor (d) Monitor respiration status
Sea urchin and crown-of-thorns sea star	Contact with the sharp venom-filled spines	Intense burning pain, redness, edema, deep pain, multiple punctures, abdominal pain, nausea, hypotension, respiratory problems	Immerse the area in nonscalding hot water for 30–90 min or until pain relief Remove the spines Treat systemic symptoms Pain control Antibiotics: ciprofloxacin or trimetho/sulfa	For sea cucumber contact, vinegar and rubbing alcohol may may help Radiography may be helpful in locating spines Watch for systemic infection

SNAKE VENOM TOXICITY

The purposes of snake venom are to immobilize prey, assist in or start the digestive process, and deter other predators. Neurotoxins with paralytic effects are the main toxins in cobras and sea snakes. Myotoxins cause tissue necrosis, and hemotoxins cause coagulopathies—these are the main toxins in pit vipers. Locally active toxins cause tissue necrosis, blistering, and local pain, and are common in many snake types. The clinical effects may vary within the same genus, and even in the same species in different countries.

TABLE 20-26 HAZARDOUS MARINE ORGANISMS *(continued)*

TITLE	CAUSES	SYMPTOMS	TREATMENT	SPECIAL HINTS
Mollusca (cone shells and octopuses)	Venom injected via long tooth.	Mild stings resemble bee stings. Severe stings can cause intense pain, paresthesias, and, respiratory problems.	No antivenin available. Supportive treatment only Treat systemic problems.	Local reactions are often absent, and generalized paresthesias may be the first sign of envenomation. Excising the bite area has been considered to remove venom.
Annelida worm	Bristles penetrate skin.	Intense pain, redness, and inflammation Untreated, the pain lasts 3–4 h, redness for 3–4 days.	Remove larger bristles with forceps; smaller bristles with tape. Vinegar or rubbing alcohol soak	Steroids may be helpful.
Stingrays	Contact with venomous spines at the tail	Intense local pain, edema, and bleeding Systemic symptoms of seizures, hypotension, paralysis, death	Explore the wound. Remove any stinger fragment. Immerse in hot water for 30–90 min. Pain control Antibiotics Observe for 4 h. Leave wound open.	Wound can become necrotic. Pain may last for 2 days.
Scorpionfish	Contact with venom spines and gland	Intense pain, edema, redness, and vesicles Systemic signs	Treatment same as for stingrays.	Most injuries come from handling in aquarium.
Catfish stings	Contact with venom from spines and pectoral fins	Local pain Systemic signs	Hot water soaks Wound care Antibiotics/tetanus	Marine catfish are more dangerous than freshwater catfish.

SNAKE IDENTIFICATION CHARACTERISTICS

The medically important venomous snakes all have fangs at the front of the upper jaw and may be classified as follows (Table 20-27). Become familiar with the poisonous snakes in your region and available treatment options.

CLINICAL FEATURES AND TREATMENT

Diagnostic confirmation of a venomous snakebite involves a history of a confirmed strike. If a strike is only suspected, this could be just an injury from thorns or a branch. Fang puncture marks may be one to four in number per strike (if the snake strikes more than once, these can be multiple).

Snakebites can cause a variety of symptoms, including local swelling, tissue necrosis, disturbed hemostasis, acute cardiotoxicity, acute renal failure, and muscle paralysis. Local signs with or without systemic envenomation signs confirm a venomous strike. Where the snake is available and can safely be killed without serious damage to its head, it can be taken to the hospital for identification.

Immediate management of snakebite is as follows:

1. Reassure victim that severe envenomation is well below 50% in bites by most snakes.
2. Immobilize and rest the bitten part to delay venom absorption.
3. The patient should lie on his or her side to maintain a clear airway and prevent inhalation of vomit.
4. Wipe wound clean with cloth to remove superficial venom and apply large firm dressing proximal to bite site.
5. Do not use tourniquet, suction, or wound incision.
6. Venom in the eye caused by the spitting cobra requires washing with water or any available fluid.

TABLE 20-27 CLASSIFICATION OF VENOMOUS SNAKES

TYPE	PHYSICAL CHARACTERISTICS	EXAMPLES	VENOM EFFECTS	SYSTEMIC SIGNS
Vipers (land snakes)	Long erectile fangs and distinct division between head and neck	Pit vipers Bothrops vipers, Echis saw-scaled vipers	Usually contains components that can cause bleeding and coagulopathies.	Perioral numbness, scalp numbness, metallic taste, nausea and vomiting, weakness, bleeding, paralysis, seizure
Elapids (land snakes)	Short fixed front fangs with no distinct division between head and neck	Cobras, mamba, kraits, coral snakes	Usually contain neurotoxic components that can cause respiratory and less-severe paralysis.	Bite site pain and numbness, muscle weakness, blurred vision, hypersalivation shortness of breath, respiratory failure
Sea snakes	Small heads and long thin bodies and prominent flattened tails	Multiple varieties	Usually contains neurotoxins and myotoxic component that can break down muscle.	Rhabdomyolysis and myoglobinuria
Colubrids		Keelback, boomslang, tree snakes	Similar to vipers but milder reactions	Similar to vipers

Once at the hospital, the management for snakebite includes evaluation and medical treatment for any symptoms (Table 20-28).

An IV line should be established at once. For elapid bites with evidence of paralysis, treatment with anticholinesterases (neostigmine, with atropine) is given if results of an IV Tensilon test are positive. Suitable antivenom should then be given in a dose of at least 100 mL IV, with medication available to counter any anaphylactic reactions. In serious cases, artificial ventilation may be needed for some hours.

Viper bite victims may suffer early shock, requiring aggressive resuscitation. Hemostatic defects are treated with infusions of blood, plasma, platelets, or fibrinogen as needed. If available, appropriate antivenom should be used. The classification of degree of envenomation by pit vipers and antivenin is listed in Table 20-29.

Antivenoms used should be as specific to the snake as possible, and preferably made in the country in question from the local species. Pretreatment prior to antivenin use is recommended and should consist of IV steroids (100 mg hydrocortisone or methylprednisolone), IV diphenhydramine 50 mg, and at least 500 mL IV fluids. Give each antivenin vial dose over half an hour to 2 hours IV (do not IV push the vials); for the first 10 minutes, give at slow rate. Stop or slow infusion (and consider epinephrine 0.1 mg boluses or drip IV) if patient manifests any signs of anaphylaxis (hypotension, wheezing, edema, hives).

The incidence of major allergic reactions is low with pretreatment. Serum sickness after antivenin administration occurs in 75% of patients receiving more than five vials of antivenin. It is manifested by fever, malaise, rash, arthralgias, and lymphadenopathy.

TABLE 20-28 MANAGEMENT OF SNAKEBITE IN HOSPITAL

Confirm the diagnosis.	Presence and severity of envenomation Timing and evolution of symptoms should be established.
Clinical evaluation of envenomation	Local inflammation, systemic bleeding, coagulation status, hypovolemic shock, myocardial damage, renal failure, neuromuscular paralysis, tender draining lymph nodes
Where available, laboratory evaluation of envenomaton should be performed.	Complete blood count Platelet Prothrombin time/partial thromboplastin time Electrolytes Liver function test Urinalysis Electrocardiogram
Local wound care	Tetanus toxoid immunization Wound cleansing/irrigation Consider antibiotics. Consider antivenin if systemic symptoms.

Patients with no signs of envenomation on admission should still be observed for up to 24 hours. If no signs develop within this period, they may be discharged.

TABLE 20-29 PIT VIPER ENVENOMATION CLASSIFICATIONS AND ANTIVENIN DOSAGE

DEGREE OF ENVENOMATION	SYMPTOMS	DOSE (NO. OF VIALS)
None	Struck but no venom injected and puncture marks only	None
Minimal	Mild bite site pain and local swelling and no progression by 60 min	0–5
Moderate	Swelling progresses beyond the bite site. Patient may get eccymosis, skin blebs, and numbness.	6–15
Severe	Swelling or pain involves entire extremity. Systemic signs (metallic taste, bleeding problems) Any major laboratory changes	15–30

Usually symptoms develop at a 7- to 21-day delay. Treat with systemic steroids (prednisone 1–2 mg/kg/day) for 7 to 10 days with antihistamines. Reevaluate extremity circumference, pain, prothrombin time, and platelet count every 2 to 4 hours until stable. Infuse an additional one to five vials as needed for any progression of above signs.

Additional therapy for snake envenomation is opiate analgesics, constant elevation of limb above the heart once antivenin is started, splinting of affected joints, IV hydration to lessen possible rhabdomyolysis, and initial physical therapy once pain and edema decrease.

In summary, determine the type of snake involved if possible, assess for envenomation, draw blood work early (especially type and crossmatch), monitor for complications, and decide if antivenin is needed. If antivenin is used, dilute and administer slowly. Usually pretreatment should be done to avoid an allergic reaction.

INSECT STINGS

BACKGROUND

The most common insect stings are from hymenoptera (bees, wasps, ants), diptera (flies), bed bugs, kissing bugs, lice, fleas, and midges. Other biting arthropods are mites, ticks, scorpions, centipedes, spiders, most particularly the brown recluse (*Loxosceles reclusa*), and tarantulas.

Types of reaction to insect stings are local allergic, generalized allergic or anaphylactic, toxic reaction (mostly gastrointestinal symptoms), delayed (resembles serum sickness), and local infection.

Dangerous local reactions may occur when there is:

■ Direct ocular sting, which may cause abscess of the lens, perforation of the globe, or atrophy of the iris.
■ Pharyngeal sting, in which local edema may cause airway compromise.

TREATMENT

See Table 20-30 for local and severe allergic reactions.

Brown recluse spider bites are often misdiagnosed. They usually just cause local tissue necrosis with surrounding erythema, which may progress to a slowly healing ulcer. Patients may have systemic symptoms, including fever, chills, malaise, weakness, nausea, and rash, and rarely hemolytic anemia and thrombocytopenia. Treatment involves local wound care and sometimes wound excision. Systemic antibiotics are not needed unless secondary infection develops.

ANAPHYLAXIS

DEFINITIONS

Anaphylaxis is a rapid generalized immunologic reaction after exposure to antigens in a sensitized person, with involvement of at least two of the following systems:

■ Respiratory: airway compromise from swelling or wheezing

TABLE 20-30 TREATMENT OF ALLERGIC REACTIONS TO INSECT STINGS

LOCAL	SEVERE
Remove embedded stinger.	Airway management (give oxygen)
Apply ice, give antihistamines.	Give IV fluids.
Give tetanus immunization if needed.	Medication:
Apply steroid cream.	Epinephrine 0.01 mg (0.3–0.5 mg in adults)
	Diphenhydramine 50 mg IV in adults
	Steroids IV (100–250 mg methylprednisone)
	or oral steroids
	Consider dopamine if blood pressure low.
	Remove stinger.
	Apply ice.
	Give tetanus immunization if needed.
	Observe 4–6 h.
	Discharge if no problems after 3–5 days on
	antihistamines and 3–5 days on steroids.

■ Cardiovascular: hypotension or cardiovascular collapse
■ Skin: diffuse cutaneous findings (urticaria, angioedema, or both)

Anaphylactoid reaction is a syndrome with presentation similar to that of anaphylaxis, expressed by similar mediators, but not triggered by immunoglobulin E (IgE) and not necessarily due to prior exposure to the inciting agent. Urticaria is a diffuse patchy erythematous pruritic rash with raised borders. Angioedema is a nonpitting subcutaneous tissue swelling (often of the face, mouth, or peri-airway tissue).

CLINICAL FEATURES

The mast cell is the final common pathway of all allergic reactions and is present in most tissues. When activated, mast cells release mediators that cause the clinical effects of allergic reactions (Table 20-31).

Causes of anaphylactic and anaphylactoid reactions are many, including IgE-mediated allergies, medications, hymenoptera stings, foods, and contact with latex. Penicillin is the most common medication allergy. It can occur from topical exposure (such as a mother preparing antibiotic suspension for a child). Angioedema due to acetylcholinesterase (ACE) inhibitors occurs in 0.2% of patients on ACE inhibitors. Allergic reactions to foods are most commonly due to legume vegetables (peanuts, soybeans, peas, beans), crustaceans, mollusks, cow's milk, and nitrites or sulfite preservatives in foods. It is important to differentiate true seafood allergy from scombroid poisoning (due to ingestion of spoiled fish containing histamine).

Latex allergy is an increasingly recognized problem. It can result in fatal anaphylaxis. Be careful to select nonlatex gloves and catheters for patients with this allergy. Allergic reactions to radiocontrast media occur in 1% of cases; 10% of occurrences are severe. Risk factors are prior reaction (30% recurrence rate), advanced age, renal or hepatic dysfunction, and asthma. Pretreatment reduces the recurrent allergic reaction rate from contrast agents to less than 1%. One suggested regimen is hydrocortisone 200 mg IV just

TABLE 20-31 CLINICAL MANIFESTATIONS OF
SYSTEMIC ALLERGIC REACTIONS

Anxiety with a sense of doom
Altered mental status
Difficulty in speaking or swallowing
Shortness of breath and wheezing
Abdominal cramps
Incontinence and diarrhea
Severe itching
Red skin color
Extremely itchy raised skin lesions (hives)
Hypotension
Bradycardia

TABLE 20-32 TREATMENT OF ALLERGIC REACTIONS

Manage breathing with oxygen
Epinephrine subcutaneously or IM (0.01 mg/kg or max 0.3 mg in adults)
IV fluids—rapid if there is low blood pressure
IV or oral diphenhydramine and steroids
Remove source of infection if possible
Oropharyngeal swelling can lead to loss of airway. Early intubation is
    recommended. Use one size smaller tube than usual.

prior to and 4 hours after contrast, and cimetidine 300 mg IV and diphenhydramine 50 mg IV just prior to contrast. Epinephrine and resuscitation equipment should be available. Pretreatment is indicated for patients requiring a contrast study with prior history of reaction or renal dysfunction.

Differential diagnosis of a severe allergic reaction includes sudden loss of consciousness, vasovagal syncope, seizures, dysrhythmias, stroke, acute respiratory distress, status asthmaticus, upper airway infection, foreign body aspiration, pulmonary embolus, cardiovascular collapse from intraabdominal bleed, or acute myocardial infarction.

TREATMENT

Because allergic reactions may progress rapidly and unpredictably, all patients with a possible systemic reaction should be rapidly triaged to an acute care room and continuously monitored (Tables 20-32 and 20-33). See Table 20-34 for drugs used in anaphylaxis.

TABLE 20-33 GENERAL CLINICAL EFFECTS OF THE ALLERGIC
            MEDIATORS

Skin	Itching, flushing, redness, hives, skin swelling
Respiratory	Upper airway swelling, bronchoconstriction, pulmonary hyperinflation ± pulmonary edema
Cardiovascular	Vasodilation, increased vascular permeability, volume depletion, shock, myocardial contractile dysfunction
Gastrointestinal	Cramping, vomiting, diarrhea

TABLE 20-34 DRUGS USED IN ANAPHYLAXIS

NAME	ACTION	FUNCTION	DOSAGE	SPECIAL HINTS
Epinephrine	Alpha and Beta agonist	Constricts blood vessels. Decreases vascular leaking. Resolution of swelling Opens up lung vessels. Increases cardiac pumping.	If hypotensive: give IV 0.1 mg of 1 mL cc of 1:10,000. IM/SC. 0.01 mL/kg of 1:1,000 MDI: 10–20 puffs	Heart rate increases Hypertension Irregular heart rhythm Consider need carefully in pregnancy, stroke, and heart patients.
Antihistamines	Block H_1 and H_2 receptors.	Lessens cell mediators. Effective for itching.	Diphenhydramine 50 mg orally for mild reaction and IV/IM for severe reaction	Should give 300 mg cimetidine or 50 mg ranitidine for better effect.
Steroids	Antiinflammatory effects	Stabilize cell mediators. Blunts delayed recurrence of symptoms.	Give to all patients with systemic reaction: hydrocortisone 100 mg IV/orally.	2–4 days follow-on oral use (prednisone 40 mg/day) may be needed depending on the reaction.
Glucagon	Beta agonist	Useful for cases refractory to initial treatments. Useful in patients on beta blockers.	1 mg IV dose to be repeated as needed.	May cause emesis.

Patients with mild local reactions should be observed for 30 minutes, then sent home on oral diphenhydramine if there is no symptom progression. Patients with systemic reactions that respond to initial treatment should be observed 2 to 4 hours for recurrence. Patients manifesting airway compromise or hypotension, even if they respond to treatment, probably should be admitted overnight. Patients on beta blockers, the elderly, and those with asthma or other comorbid diseases should be admitted.

Discharge medications for patients with allergic reactions include the following:

- Diphenhydramine 25 to 50 mg orally four times daily for 2 days
- Cimetidine 300 mg orally four times daily for 2 days
- Prednisone 40 to 50 mg orally (1–2 mg/kg) daily for 4–5 days
- Consider an epinephrine self-injection kit (Epi-Pen or Ana-Kit).
- Consider stand-by albuterol inhaler.

■ Consider nonsedating antihistamine.

■ Other discharge considerations for patients with systemic allergic reactions are education about preventive or avoidance measures.

In summary, evaluate all patients with allergic reactions immediately and assess the ABCs first. Epinephrine is the mainstay of treatment, but consider the use of additional medication. Observe to determine if relapse occurs or if there is a need for admission. Discharged patients should be instructed carefully about follow-up and prevention.

CHAPTER 21

Ophthalmology and Ear, Nose, and Throat

C. James Holliman

OPHTHALMOLOGY

Eye complaints are some of the most common and most easily treated illnesses seen in the field. With relatively few materials and medications, most eye problems can be effectively treated. It is important to recognize early signs of serious eye problems and begin proper treatment or seek a higher level of specialized care.

ESSENTIAL COMPONENTS OF THE EYE EXAMINATION

Proper diagnosis of eye problems begins with a good eye examination. The first thing to measure in almost all circumstances is visual acuity. The exception to this is in a chemical burn to the eye which requires immediate irrigation.

> **CRITICAL ACTION:**
>
> If the patient presents with a chemical exposure to the eye, examination should be delayed until the eye is adequately irrigated and as much of the remaining chemical is flushed out as possible.

A simple test of visual acuity is recommended before continuing with the rest of the examination. Test each eye individually by covering one eye and then the other. Test for visual acuity by counting fingers and checking light perception. Examine the external area by examining the periorbital area, lids, conjunctivae, cornea, anterior chamber depth, and pupillary light reaction. Be sure to evert the upper lid and lower lid to inspect the conjunctival area. For extraocular movements, check all directions of gaze. For the retinal examination, check disc, vessels, macula, and ocular media (Fig. 21-1).

If a patient has an eye injury or irritating infection, anesthetic drops may be needed to complete the examination. Proparacaine (Ophthaine) 0.5% has rapid onset and lasts 15 to 30 minutes. Tetracaine 1% also may be used, although it is a little more irritating initially, with a duration of 15 to 45 minutes.

BASIC OPHTHALMIC TECHNIQUES

INSTILLING EYE DROPS To instill eye drops (e.g., antibiotics, topical anesthetics, etc.), generally use one to two drops per eye. It is usually best to place the drop on the conjunctiva with the lower lid retracted downward. In uncooperative children, place the drops on the medial canthus and they will flow into the eye when the child finally opens it.

LID EVERSION Lid eversion is usually only needed for the upper lid. Grasp the lashes and fold the upper lid over a cotton-tipped swab as the patient looks downward. You should do this for all cases involving a possible conjunctival foreign body.

APPLYING OINTMENT For ointment application apply a strip of ointment along the lower conjunctiva. Do not touch the conjunctiva with the tip of the tube. Using excess ointment is alright. For patching, apply the ointment first, then make sure the patient's eyelid is closed. Fold one patch in half and apply over the closed lid. Apply a second unfolded patch and tape in place. Do not get tape on the eyebrow.

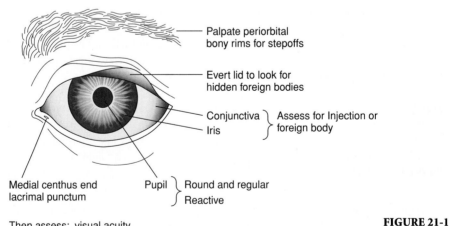

FIGURE 21-1
Basic eye examination.

DILATING FOR EXAMINATION Cycloplegics (red top bottles) paralyze the ciliary muscle and cause mydriasis (dilation). A variety of medications can be used. The best for initial examination is tropicamide (Mydriacil, 1%). It has a duration of a few hours. Cyclopentolate (Cyclogyl, 0.5%–2%) has a duration of 24 hours. Do not use atropine or homatropine in the outpatient setting because the duration of action is too long (the patient will have blurred vision and light sensitivity after the original problem has resolved).

ANTIBIOTICS The common ophthalmic antibiotics used as drops are 10% sulfacetamide (Sulamyd), gentamicin, and tobramycin. Chloramphenicol also may be used. Neosporin can be used but may cause neomycin-induced allergic sensitization. For ointments, erythromycin, gentamicin, sulfacetamide, and polysporin are available.

SPECIFIC CLINICAL PROBLEMS

CHEMICAL BURNS Chemical burns constitute an ophthalmologic emergency. Patients who work routinely with chemicals should be instructed ahead of time to be prepared for eye exposures, and to immediately flush all chemical exposures to the eye with large amounts of water. Although sterile isotonic solution is preferred, tap water or drinking water is a good alternative. The main concern is immediate irrigation of the exposed eye to minimize the irritation and damage (Fig. 21-2).

Irrigation can be accomplished by simply holding open the lid and flushing fluid in the eye. Irrigation lenses assist in this process, but usually require topical anesthesia and patient cooperation. Flush with at least 1 to 2 L of fluid per eye. If the patient complains of continued burning or irritation, continue to flush the eye.

Most chemical burns to the eye cause corneal irritation and abrasions. These are best treated with pain medicine (oral) and prophylactic antibiotics. Instruct the patient to return for a recheck in 1 to 2 days. If extensive involvement beyond the cornea exists, such as blistering to the lids, loss of visual acuity, or globe perforation, contact an ophthalmologist immediately.

CORNEAL ABRASIONS AND LACERATIONS Corneal abrasions are common in domestic and industrial workers. The patient most commonly complains of a foreign body sensation to the eye, and feels irritation to eye movement and blinking. Examine the eye by looking in all fields for an obvious foreign body. Often, the foreign body is gone, but the patient complains of a sensation of a foreign body due to a residual corneal abrasion.

Fluorescein examination with a ultraviolet (UV) light Wood's lamp is useful for identifying corneal injuries and abrasions. To use fluorescein stain, place a drop of buffered saline (Dacriose) solution or local anesthetic on the fluorescein paper strip and allow the drop to run onto the conjunctiva. Apply to the lateral conjunctiva (have the patient "look at his nose"). With UV light, abrasions and lacerations show up as areas of fluorescein uptake and appear bright green. After the examination, always irrigate the

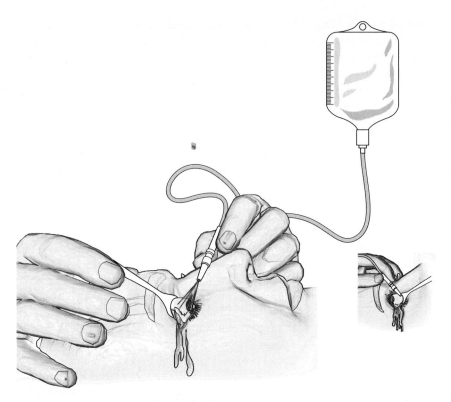

FIGURE 21-2 Irrigation of the eye for chemical exposures.

fluorescein from the eye with saline or Dacriose (because fluorescein is a conjunctival irritant).

If there is an "ice rink sign," be sure to evert the upper lid and check for a foreign body. Treat with topical anesthetic, ophthalmic ointment, and patch, and recheck in 12 to 24 hours. The patient may need a short course of oral pain medication for discomfort. Remember tetanus prophylaxis if the patient is not up to date. Instill an antibiotic to prevent infection. Use a patch for 1 to 2 days for comfort. To apply an eye patch, place one vertically folded patch in the orbital recess and then place a second patch horizontally and tape to the forehead and cheek.

REMOVING A CONJUNCTIVAL FOREIGN BODY Conjunctival foreign bodies can often be removed easily. For any corneal foreign body, be sure to rule out anterior chamber penetration before applying any drops or trying to remove the foreign body. Injuries with a high risk of globe penetration include high-speed grinders and industrial accidents. If the visual acuity is impaired, be sure to refer to an ophthalmologist. To remove a foreign body, first apply a topical anesthetic. Try irrigating the foreign body out with drops or irrigation solution. A moistened cotton-tipped applicator can be used to dab off the foreign body. If this does not work, you may carefully use fine forceps or a 25-gauge needle to remove some objects. The patient may need antibiotic drops for 2 days (four times daily) if there is significant residual conjunctival irritation. All patients with an embedded corneal foreign body that is successfully removed will have a residual corneal abrasion and should be treated with antibiotic ointment or drops.

ULTRAVIOLET KERATITIS Ultraviolet keratitis (or snow blindness or welder's arc keratitis) is described as superficial burns to the cornea, characterized by fine scattered punctate corneal defects. Treat these with topical anesthetic, antibiotic ointment, and patch, and recheck in 1 to 2 days.

ORBITAL TRAUMA

SUBCONJUNCTIVAL HEMORRHAGE Subconjunctival hemorrhage, or bleeding within the sclera, can occur from trauma, or may occur spontaneously from coughing or sneezing. Although it looks impressive, it resolves spontaneously and requires no treatment (Fig. 21-3).

TRAUMATIC IRITIS Traumatic iritis is usually caused by direct trauma to the eye, causing ciliary spasm and photophobia. Iritis causes a deep aching pain and ciliary flush (injected conjunctival vessels next to the iris). Treat with cycloplegics, and consider using steroid drops to minimize inflammation. Traumatic mydriasis (dilatation) also may accompany trauma. This is usually a temporary condition, and no additional treatment is needed.

TRAUMATIC HYPHEMA AND HYPOPYON Hyphema is blood in the anterior chamber caused by direct trauma. The eye examination may reveal pooling blood in the anterior chamber. Treat this with bedrest with the head elevated, pain control, and an immediate ophthalmology consult (Fig. 21-4). Hypopyon is an infection of the anterior chamber with a demonstrated pus collection (Fig. 21-5). This is an ophthalmologic emergency, and requires immediate drainage.

SUBCONJUNCTIVAL HEMORRHAGE

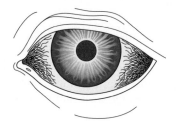

FIGURE 21-3 Subconjunctival hemorrhage.

HYPHEMA

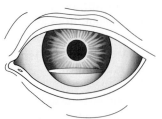

Blood layering in anterior
chamber with patient upright

FIGURE 21-4 Hyphema.

HYPOPYON

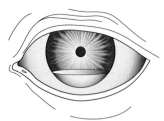

Purulent fluid layering
in the anterior chamber

FIGURE 21-5 Hypopyon.

GLOBE RUPTURE If you detect pupillary irregularity or an asymmetric-appearing iris after trauma, the patient may have a ruptured globe (Fig. 21-6). Place a protective eye shield (with no pressure on the eye) and arrange for ophthalmologist referral immediately.

RETINAL DETACHMENT Detachment or hemorrhage of the retina presents as a "veil or curtain across the eye" and causes decreased visual acuity. Treatment is bedrest, and immediate ophthalmology consult should be arranged.

LACERATIONS Lacerations of the eyelid margins or medial canthus that may involve the lacrimal canaliculus, and lacerations possibly involving the extraocular muscles should be referred to an ophthalmologist for repair. If there is no available ophthalmologist, or transportation is not immediately available, close external injuries carefully with 6.0 or 7.0 nylon suture as a temporary measure, and arrange for definitive surgical evaluation.

GLOBE PERFORATION

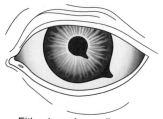

Either irregular pupil
or prolapsed iris
(beyond normal edge of iris)

FIGURE 21-6 Globe perforation.

OCULAR INFECTIONS

BACTERIAL CONJUNCTIVITIS Bacterial conjunctivitis can be caused by a variety of organisms, including *Staphylococcus aureus, Haemophilus influenzae, Streptococcus pyogenes,* or *Pseudomonas.* Patients present with irritative conjunctivitis and redness with thick, purulent discharge (Fig. 21-7). Treatment is with topical antibiotics (gentamicin or sulfacetamide) every 2 to 4 hours for 2 to 3 days. Conjunctivitis caused by gonococci results in severe inflammation and thick discharge and needs to be treated with topical and systemic antibiotics. If chlamydia conjunctivitis is suspected, treat with topical sulfacetamide plus oral erythromycin, tetracycline, or azithromycin.

ACUTE CONJUNCTIVITIS

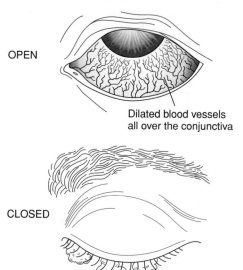

OPEN

Dilated blood vessels
all over the conjunctiva

CLOSED

Pus

FIGURE 21-7 Acute bacterial conjunctivitis.

VIRAL CONJUNCTIVITIS Viral conjunctivitis (pink eye) is very common. The eye discharge is usually thinner than for bacterial conjunctivitis. It may be very contagious, and strict instructions for hand washing must be given to the patient and family. Typical treatment for viral conjunctivitis is to treat with topical antibiotics, because bacterial and viral infections are difficult to distinguish.

ALLERGIC CONJUNCTIVITIS A patient presenting with red, itchy eyes in response to pollen or an allergic exposure may have allergic conjunctivitis. Patients typically have more itching and nasal symptoms compared with viral conjunctivitis, and symptoms are usually bilateral. Treatment is with topical or oral antihistamines.

TRACHOMA Trachoma is a chronic infection found most often in malnourished populations. It is transmitted by person-to-person contact and by flies. Trachoma leads to chronic inflammation and scarring of the cornea and eyelids, as well as bacterial superinfection (Fig. 21-8). Treatment is by careful cleaning and long-term antibiotics until infection is resolved. Trachoma can be prevented by face and hand washing and good general hygiene.

VITAMIN A DEFICIENCY Vitamin A deficiency is common among malnourished and mobile (refugee) populations, especially in children 6 months to 5 years of age. Vitamin A deficiency is a preventable cause of blindness, and begins with night blindness, followed by xerophthalmia, and finally keratomalacia or corneal degeneration (Fig. 21-9). On initial presentation, a mother may complain that the child "trips over things in the dark." Providing supplemental vitamin A can reverse night blindness. Xerophthalmia occurs when the tear ducts are dysfunctional and the cornea becomes dry. Bitot's spots may form on the outer sides of the conjunctiva and are associated with dry areas of the conjunctiva. These may lead to corneal ulcers and keratomalacia. In keratomalacia, the cornea becomes soft and opaque. The eye forms ulcerations that can proceed rapidly to blindness. The best treatment for blindness related to vitamin A deficiency is prevention. Foods rich in vitamin A should be encouraged, and supplements should be considered in high-risk populations.

HERPES SIMPLEX KERATITIS Herpes simplex keratitis should be suspected if there is corneal pain and herpes lesions involve the tip of the nose. Herpes simplex causes a dendritic corneal epithelial defect on fluorescein stain (Fig. 21-10). Be careful not to

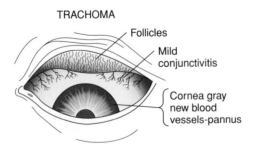

TRACHOMA

Follicles

Mild conjunctivitis

Cornea gray new blood vessels-pannus

FIGURE 21-8 Trachoma.

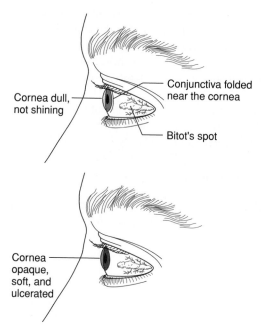

Cornea dull, not shining

Conjunctiva folded near the cornea

Bitot's spot

Cornea opaque, soft, and ulcerated

FIGURE 21-9 A: Xerophthalmia.
B: Keratomalacia.

treat with topical steroids, which will worsen the infection. Treat with antibiotic drops to prevent bacterial superinfection.

STYE (HORDEOLUM) A stye is a pustule at the lid margin, and it is usually caused by an infection of a hair follicle. The lid has a red, tender, nodular swelling. Treatment for a stye is hot compresses, antibiotic drops, or ointment. If the lid appears to be cellulitic, add oral antibiotics. A chalazion is a nontender mass on the mid-portion of the upper lid, and is usually a chronic inflamed cyst. Treatment is by incision and debridement, usually by an ophthalmologist.

HERPES SIMPLEX KERATITIS
(seen with fluorescein stain)

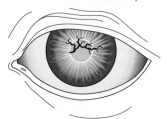

Dendritic corneal defect pattern

FIGURE 21-10 Herpes simplex keratitis.

ACUTE ANGLE CLOSURE GLAUCOMA   Acute angle closure glaucoma is caused by a blockage of the canal of Schlem and a build-up of aqueous fluid in the anterior chamber. Symptoms of this are severe eye pain, blurred vision, halos around lights, nausea, and vomiting. On examination, the conjunctiva is injected, the cornea is hazy or cloudy, and the pupil is in mid-position and nonreactive. Visual acuity is decreased, and intraocular pressure (IOP) is markedly increased (usually >50 mm Hg). Acute glaucoma requires an immediate ophthalmology consult and constriction of the pupil with 2% pilocarpine drops every 15 minutes for five doses, then one drop every 2 to 3 hours. Also, acute conditions may be treated with acetazolamide 500 mg intravenously (IV), then 250 mg IV every 4 hours; mannitol 1 to 1.5 g/kg IV is administered to dehydrate the eye. Definitive treatment is iridotomy or surgical peripheral iridectomy.

SUDDEN BLINDNESS   Sudden blindness can be caused by an acute central retinal artery occlusion. This is a true emergency but with dismal prognosis for sight recovery despite treatment. Acute central retinal vein occlusion causes a "blood-splashed" appearance of the fundus, engorged and tortuous retinal veins, and retinal hemorrhage. Treatment is the same as for central retinal artery occlusion, but the prognosis for visual acuity recovery is better.

EAR, NOSE, AND THROAT EMERGENCIES

EAR INFECTIONS

The differential diagnosis for ear pain includes acute otitis media, external otitis, or pain referred from neoplasm, dental source, temporomandibular joint (TMJ) syndrome, herpes zoster, mastoiditis, or chondritis.

ACUTE OTITIS MEDIA   Otitis media is a common infection of the middle ear. Patients present with pain in one ear more than the other, and often referred pain to the jaw. The tympanic membrane appears dull and red, with loss of landmarks, and the mobility of the membrane is decreased. Treatment for otitis media is with antibiotics, such as amoxicillin, second-generation cephalosporins, or trimethoprim-sulfamethaxazole. Decongestants are helpful for some patients. Acute bullous myringitis occurs with painful blebs on the tympanic membrane and a purplish membrane hue, and usually is caused by viruses or mycoplasma. Patients often have fever and hearing loss. Treatment is with oral erythromycin.

Acute otitis media may occur with perforation of the tympanic membrane. Patients complain of pain, and sudden relief with ear discharge otorrhea, indicating spontaneous perforation. The tympanic membrane is red and dull, and the canal has purulent fluid. Treatment is with systemic antibiotics. Most perforations resolve spontaneously.

EXTERNAL OTITIS   External otitis is an infection of the ear canal wall. The patient complains of itching and pain to the ear. Hearing is usually normal, unless cerumen or debris is plugging the canal. On examination, the patient has pain to movement of the outside of the ear, and the canal wall is red, scaly, and edematous. Treatment consists of topical antibiotic drops (cortisporin) or a diluted acetic acid (vinegar) solution. Treat with oral antibiotics if the ear appears red and cellulitic. Instruct the patient to avoid swimming, clean the canal of debris, and give pain medication.

MASTOIDITIS AND CHONDRITIS Mastoiditis and chondritis are infections over the mastoid and pinna area of the ear, respectively. There is local redness, tenderness, and swelling over the affected area. Treatment is typically IV antibiotics and evaluation for possible abscess.

HEARING LOSS Common causes of hearing loss include serous otitis media, severe external otitis, and cerumen impaction. Serous otitis media features include a dull, gray, bulging tympanic membrane and a history of recent upper respiratory infection or allergy. Treatment includes antihistamines if the patient also has allergic symptoms, because antibiotics and decongestants are not always helpful.

The diagnosis of cerumen impaction is obvious if the canal is blocked by cerumen. Often there is a history of hearing loss after showering. Treatment includes irrigation if there is no history of underlying pathology, mechanical removal carefully (plastic spuds are best), and chemical softeners (Debrox, Cerumenex, or hydrogen peroxide).

EAR TRAUMA

Ear trauma is generally limited to external structures, although loud noises may cause tympanic perforation. This should be considered if the patient has a history of sudden hearing loss and inner ear pain from a loud noise or slap on the ear. The perforation can usually be seen on examination. Most perforations heal spontaneously.

If the external ear is lacerated, you should perform a careful skin closure. It is usually not necessary to close lacerated cartilage. Simply approximate the cartilage and close the overlying skin. Apply a pressure dressing and ensure close follow-up. An auricular hematoma can cause erosion of the cartilage and permanent deformity. It is important to incise and drain auricular hematomas and apply a pressure dressing to prevent re-accumulation. Note that needle aspiration alone is rarely successful.

Foreign bodies in the ear usually do not require emergent removal. Evaluate for damage to the tympanic membrane and hearing loss. Insects may be removed by first immobilizing them by instilling xylocaine liquid, then extracting them with forceps. Vegetable matter (if soft) can be removed with suction or simple flushing with water. Antibiotic ear drops should be given after removal if the canal wall is inflamed. Consider using sedation for removing a foreign body from an uncooperative child.

SINUSITIS

Acute sinusitis is an infection of the frontal or maxillary sinuses. It is usually diagnosed by the presence of purulent nasal drainage, pain, or tenderness over the sinuses, and some patients may have maxillary dental pain. A wide variety of bacteria can cause acute sinusitis: *Streptococcus, Haemophilus, Staphylococcus, Moraxella,* and *Mycoplasma* are common offenders. The diagnosis can usually be made clinically by eliciting pain to tapping of sinuses. Radiography usually is not necessary.

Treatment involves:

1. Antibiotics (ampicillin, trimethoprim-sulfamethoxazole, second-generation cephalosporin) for 10 to 14 days
2. Topical decongestants (Afrin nasal spray)
3. Oral decongestants such as pseudoephedrine.

EPISTAXIS (NOSEBLEEDS)

Common causes of epistaxis include nose picking (most common), trauma, blood dyscrasias, nasal or sinus infections, vitamin deficiency, dry mucosa (common during winter), septal deformity, or hypertension (only if acutely severe).

To evaluate epistaxis, determine site of bleeding if possible. Most bleeding comes from the nasal septum. Apply constant, firm pressure to the nose to control bleeding. Swab or suction the nasal vault. Usually laboratory tests are not needed, unless there is prolonged or excessive bleeding.

Treatment of epistaxis involves the following:

1. Apply firm nasal pinch pressure for 10 minutes.
2. Suction with a small-caliber firm suction tip, removing all clot present.
3. Identify the bleeding site or mucosal lesion that was the source of the bleed.
4. Use silver nitrate cautery sticks and cauterize the area around the bleeding site first, then cauterize the bleeding site directly.
5. If the cautery does not stop the bleeding, then place an anterior nasal pack (vaseline gauze with extra antibiotic ointment; start layering along the bottom of the nose and pack each layer of gauze upward).
6. If no anterior bleeding site is seen, or if the bleeding persists after placement of an anterior pack, you should place a posterior pack or place a nasostat balloon catheter and inflate both balloons.

Consider hospitalization for epistaxis patients who are unreliable, recurrent bleeders, on anticoagulants, or who have severe concurrent medical conditions. Patients with nasal packing should always be placed on antibiotics to prevent sinusitis and possible toxic shock syndrome, and they may need pain medications. Nasal packs should be left in place 48 hours. Patients with posterior packs or balloon packs should always be admitted.

OROPHARYNGEAL INFECTIONS

Sore throat can be caused by pharyngitis, tonsillitis, or peritonsillar abscess. Bacterial causes of acute pharyngitis/tonsillitis include streptococci (most common), *Neisseria gonorrhoeae*, and *Corynebacterium diphtheriae* (which causes severe symptoms and is life threatening; its main feature is presence of a shaggy pseudomembrane in the pharynx). Viral causes include herpangina, mononucleosis (usually associated with prominent enlarged posterior cervical nodes), measles, varicella, parainfluenza, rhinovirus, herpes simplex, and adenovirus.

The triad of fever, exudative pharyngitis, and tender anterior cervical lymph nodes are likely to be caused by infection by streptococcal bacteria. Antibiotic treatment of streptococcal pharyngitis prevents rheumatic fever and rheumatic heart disease, so compliance with treatment is important. Treat with penicillin, amoxicillin, or erythromycin. Admission and IV antibiotics are indicated if diphtheria is suspected. Throat cultures are usually not necessary.

STRIDOR Stridor is difficulty breathing due to upper airway obstruction. It is important to differentiate stridor from wheezing, because stridor may be an indicator of impending respiratory compromise. Treatment of stridor depends on the cause of illness. While you are determining the cause of stridor, assess the patient's airway and prepare for intubation if necessary. Position the patient upright, supply oxygen, and keep him calm.

CROUP Acute laryngotracheobronchitis, or croup, is a viral infection that typically occurs in children 3 months to 3 years of age. Croup is slow in onset and associated with a low-grade fever, "croupy" (barking) cough, hoarseness, and stridor. Lateral neck radiography is performed to rule out epiglottitis, and anteroposterior (AP) radiographs may show the "steeple sign" of the tracheal air column (the tracheal shadow appears angled instead of forming a "shoulder" at the level of the cords). Treatment of croup involves giving dexamethasone 0.6 mg/kg orally or IM, and moist oxygen by mask for more severe cases; consider inhaled racemic epinephrine aerosol (0.5–1 mL) for severe cases. Occasionally airway management with intubation or admission is necessary.

EPIGLOTTITIS Acute epiglottitis (supraglottitis) is another dangerous cause of stridor. It occurs most commonly in children 3 to 7 years of age who have not been immunized against *Haemophilus influenzae* type B. The incidence has decreased dramatically since introduction of the *Haemophilus* type B vaccine. Acute epiglottitis is usually of sudden onset and causes a sore throat, stridor, high fever, muffled voice, and drooling. Patients appear ill. Lateral neck radiographs show the "thumbprint" sign of an enlarged epiglottis. Treatment involves minimal disturbance of the child (to prevent sudden worsening of the partial airway occlusion). Arrange for a controlled endotracheal intubation in the operating room. A second-generation cephalosporin (cefuroxime) should be given IV after the airway is secured. If there is difficulty getting the patient intubated, often bag-valve-mask ventilation is temporizing enough to allow time for arrival of a physician more skilled in intubation.

NECK ABSCESSES Head and neck abscesses also can cause stridor. These abscesses include peritonsillar, retropharyngeal, prevertebral, and parapharyngeal types. Patients may present with stridor, a muffled voice, and drooling. Radiography may be useful to define the area of swelling, but other studies such as computed tomography (CT) are more helpful. Once a head and neck abscess is identified, antistaphylococcal antibiotics should be given and plans for emergent surgical drainage made.

PERITONSILLAR ABSCESS Peritonsillar abscess is fairly common, and the affected patient presents with a "hot potato" or muffled voice and with a severe sore throat. Pharyngeal examination shows swelling adjacent to and displacing the inflamed tonsil; usually the uvula is displaced also (Fig. 21-11). Treatment involves needle aspiration to confirm abscess location and incision and drainage. Antibiotics should also be given, and they may need to be hospitalized for IV antibiotics and observation. Hospitalization often is indicated, and antibiotics should always be given. Most patients should have tonsillectomy after the infection resolves.

FACIAL TRAUMA

Facial trauma may occur as a result of a blunt blow to the face, such as from an assault or motor vehicle accident, or a penetrating injury. Causes of mortality from facial trauma include airway compromise, intracranial injury, or cervical spine injury. Delayed problems can result in meningitis or oropharyngeal infections.

Priorities in managing facial trauma are the same as for any other emergency and include immediate assessment for airway compromise and care to protect the cervical spine. Bleeding may be a major concern if it compromises the airway. It may be necessary to keep the patient sitting upright to keep the airway clear. If intubation is necessary, orotracheal intubation is preferred over nasotracheal intubation if there is a possible mid-facial fracture.

Causes of airway compromise with facial trauma include blood in the airway, debris in the airway (vomitus, avulsed tissue, teeth/dentures, foreign bodies), pharyngeal or retropharyngeal tissue swelling, and posterior tongue displacement from mandible fractures.

The secondary survey examination sequence for facial trauma involves the following:

1. Scalp: Check for lacerations, hematomas, stepoffs, and tenderness. Brisk bleeding may continue until sutured, so hurry the examination.
2. Ears: Check the pinnae, canal walls, and tympanic membranes. Suction gently under direct vision if there is blood in the canal. Check a drop of canal fluid on filter paper for the "ring sign," indicating cerebrospinal fluid leak. Assess hearing.
3. Overall facial appearance: Assess for symmetry, deformity, discoloration, and nasal alignment. Palpate the forehead and malar areas. Feel the external face for areas of tenderness. Be sure to feel over the zygoma and periorbital areas.

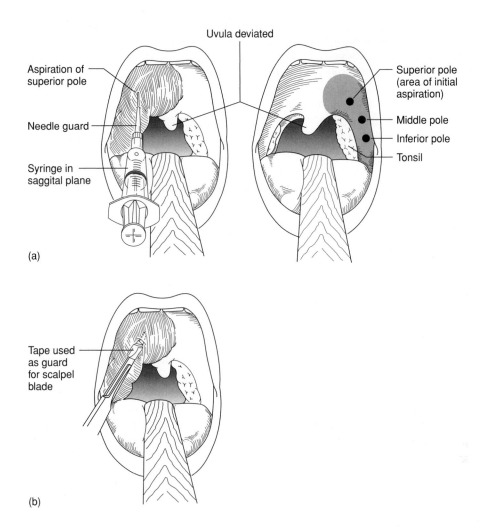

FIGURE 21-11 A: Needle aspiration of a peritonsillar abscess. Anesthetize the posterior pharynx with topical lidocaine spray. Advance an 18- or 20-gauge needle with needle guard into the area of greatest fluctuance. Aspirate as you advance the needle. Advance the needle in the sagittal plane. Do not direct the needle laterally toward the carotid artery or jugular vein. The superior pole is aspirated first, but the middle and inferior poles should be aspirated if pus is not obtained initially. Note that the tonsil itself is not aspirated. The peritonsillar space contains the abscess. B: Incision and drainage of a peritonsillar abscess. Normal-appearing oropharynx. Peritonsillar abscess on the right side of the throat. Incision of the abscess at the area of greatest fluctuance. Notice that the scalpel is taped to prevent deep penetration. Loculations are removed by gentle probing with hemostats.

4. Eyes: Check pupils, anterior chamber, fundi, and extraocular movements. Check the conjunctivae carefully for foreign bodies. Palpate the orbital rims. Avoid palpation of the globe if there is possible globe penetration.
5. Nose: Check the septum for hematoma and position. Check airflow in both nares. Palpate the nasal bridge for crepitus.
6. Mouth: Check dental occlusion. Reflect the upper and lower gingiva. Feel along mandibular and maxillary teeth to check for instability. Palpate along the exterior of the mandible. Pull forward on the maxillary teeth.
7. Neurologic: Check for movement and sensation on the face, mouth, tongue, and gag reflex.

Radiography of the face can include the following views to assess for injuries:

- Posteroanterior skull: This shows an undistorted frontal projection.
- Lateral skull: This shows a side view of the sinuses and facial bones.
- Caldwell view (posteroanterior 15 degrees caudally): This visualizes the orbital structures without petrous bone overlap.
- Towne's view (AP 30 degrees caudally): This shows the mandibular condyles and orbital floor.
- Water's view (posteroanterior of the face): This is the best single film for the maxillary sinuses, orbital floors, and zygoma.
- Axial view (submentovertex): This shows the zygomatic arch and the body of the zygoma.
- Mandible (AP, lateral, and obliques): A panorex view is best if available; TMJ films (for suspected condylar or subcondylar fractures or unexplained malocclusion); nasal film (lateral and AP; AP seldom adds information). CT is best for complex or multiple fractures if available.

FACIAL FRACTURES

The Lefort I fracture (nasomaxillary fracture) is a horizontal fracture extending through the maxilla between the floor of the maxillary sinus and the orbital floor. Its signs and symptoms are crepitus over the maxilla, malocclusion, and mobility of the maxilla. Treatment involves surgical fixation and antibiotics.

The Lefort II fracture (pyramidal fracture) is a subzygomatic mid-facial fracture with a pyramidal-shaped fragment separated from the cranium. Signs and symptoms are crepitus over the mid-face, lengthening of the face, malocclusion, infraorbital paresthesia, and facial/oral bruising. Treatment is by surgical fixation.

A Lefort III fracture (craniofacial dissociation) results in a floating fragment of the mid-facial bones, which are totally separated from the cranial base. Its signs and symptoms are lengthening of face (often "caved-in" or "donkey face" appearance), malocclusion, lateral orbital rim defect, ecchymosis, and often unequal pupil height. These fractures may require emergent surgery for bleeding control, and will eventually require operative fixation.

A simple scheme to differentiate the types of Lefort fractures is as follows: Pull forward on the maxillary teeth. If just the maxilla moves, it's a Lefort I. If the maxilla and base of nose move, it's a Lefort II. If the whole face moves, it's a Lefort III.

Mandibular fractures are commonly associated with other injuries, including facial fractures. Signs and symptoms include malocclusion, decreased jaw range of motion, chin numbness, and a palpable step deformity. Ask patients if their teeth "fit" as usual. Test for malocclusion by having patients bite and hold a tongue depressor. If they can hold it against your pull, the mandible is probably intact. Treatment involves surgical fixation.

Temporomandibular joint dislocation can occur from a direct blow to the mandible, but also can occur "spontaneously" (from yawning or laughing). The mandible dislocates forward and superiorly, causing masseter and pterygoid muscle spasm. Patients present with the mouth open, and the patient cannot close the mouth or talk well. It can be misdiagnosed as a psychiatric or dystonic reaction. Treatment involves manual reduction (place wrapped thumbs on molars and push firmly downward, then backward—be careful not to get bitten), and usually may require sedation or muscle relaxants. Follow-up treatment includes soft diet and pain medication.

Nasal bone fractures often can be diagnosed clinically, and radiographs are not needed. They do not need emergent reduction except to control persistent epistaxis, and usually do not need antibiotics. Early reduction (under local anesthesia) is useful if the nares is obstructed. If there is a nasal septal hematoma, incise and drain, place an anterior pack, start antibiotics, and follow up at 24 hours.

Zygomatic fractures are a common type of facial fracture, usually caused by a direct blow. Tripod fractures show depression of the malar eminence, and there may be fracture lines at the temporal, frontal, and maxillary suture lines. Symptoms and signs of a tripod fracture include facial pain, depression of the malar prominence, a fracture to the orbital rim and facial ecchymosis, and subconjuctival hemorrhage. Treatment is typically surgical.

Orbital fractures can be isolated ("blow out" fracture of floor) or associated with other major fractures. A complete examination to rule out globe injury is very important. Symptoms and signs of orbital fractures include diplopia (double vision), enophthalmos (sunken eyeball), impaired ocular movement, infraorbital numbness, and clouding of the maxillary sinus on radiography.

The inferior wall of the orbit is the most likely fracture site. Diplopia with orbital fractures if occurring on upward gaze suggests inferior blowout with entrapment of the inferior rectus muscle and inferior oblique muscles. Extraocular muscle dysfunction may be due to edema and will correct without surgery, but persistent muscle entrapment from an orbital fracture requires surgery to repair the orbital floor.

REPAIRING FACIAL LACERATIONS

Before repair of a facial soft tissue injury, be sure to rule out injury to the facial nerve, trigeminal nerve, parotid duct, and lacrimal duct. Remove any embedded foreign material such as dirt or gravel from in the skin to prevent "tattooing."

Because of the generous blood flow to the face, facial injuries may be closed up to 24 hours after they occur, and most bite marks can be cleaned thoroughly and closed. Refer to wound section for a discussion of wound closure.

CHAPTER 22

Dental Emergencies

Daniel J. Ross and Thomas D. Kirsch

Primary care physicians commonly see patients presenting with a dental complaint or injury, but are often poorly prepared to provide care. In order to successfully diagnose and treat these conditions, the field practitioner needs a thorough understanding of oral anatomy, dental anesthesia/analgesia, dental disease, mucosal conditions, traumatic dental emergencies, and minor dental procedures.

All patients (even those without dental problems) should be counseled on the importance of proper dental hygiene and good nutrition. Teach them to brush and to avoid sweets. *Where There Is No Dentist* by Murray Dickson is an excellent resource for prevention tips and techniques, patient education, and basic dental care.

GENERAL COMMENTS REGARDING DENTAL MEDICATIONS

The guidelines for prescribing found throughout this chapter are intended for providers working in less than ideal circumstances, and where follow-up may not be readily available. In addition to standard rules for prescribing medications, below are some general guidelines for dental prescriptions:

- Acceptable duration of antibiotic therapy for any dental infection is 7 to 10 days.
- Penicillin is the drug of choice for any dental infection, unless otherwise indicated. Erythromycin is an acceptable alternative.
- Amoxicillin is a well-tolerated alternative to penicillin in children.

TABLE 22-1 SUGGESTED DOSES FOR MEDICATIONS COMMONLY USED IN DENTISTRY

	ADULT DOSAGE	PEDIATRIC DOSAGE
Penicillin V	500 mg every 6 h	<12 yr 50 mg/kg/day divided into four doses
Erythromycin	400 mg every 6 h	30–50 mg/kg/day divided into four doses
Clindamycin	400 mg every 6 h	8–20 mg/kg/day divided into four doses
Amoxicillin	500 mg every 8 h	40 mg/kg/day divided into three doses
Tetracycline	500 mg every 6 h	Not recommended for children
Cephalexin	500 mg every 6 h	25–50 mg/kg/day divided into four doses
Nystatin	4–6 mL every 6 h (swish and swallow)	1 mL to each cheek four times daily
Clotrimazole oral	1 troche every 4 h	Not recommended for children
Acyclovir	400 mg every 8 h	10–20 mg/kg every 6 h
Acetaminophen	325–650 mg every 4 h	15 mg/kg/day divided into four doses
Ibuprofen	200–800 mg every 6 h	6 mo 5–10 mg/kg/day divided into four doses
Tylenol with codeine (#3 = acetaminophen 300 mg + codeine 30/mg)	1–2 tablets every 4 h	See below
Tylenol with codeine pediatric (5 mL = acetaminophen 120 mg + codeine 12 mg)		3–6 yr 5 mL; 7–12 yr 10 mL
Vicodin	1–2 tablets every 4 h	Not recommended for children
Diphenhydramine	25–50 mg every 6 h	5 mg/kg/day
Viscous lidocaine	10 mL	
BMX	5 mL liquid Benadryl/ 10 mL Maalox/10/mL viscous lidocaine	5 mL liquid Benadryl/ 10 mL Maalox/10/mL viscous lidocaine

Always consult a dosing reference prior to dispensing any medication. The above doses are merely suggestions.

Consult a drug reference such as *Physician's Desk Reference* or *Pocket Pharmacopia* prior to dispensing any medication to a woman who is pregnant or lactating.

Acceptable duration of antibiotic therapy for any dental infection is 7–10 days.

Penicillin is the drug of choice for any dental infection, unless otherwise indicated in the text. Erythromycin is an acceptable alternative.

Amoxicillin is a well-tolerated alternative to penicillin in children if available.

Children over 12 years of age can take the adult dose of penicillin.

Clindamycin is useful for severe infections, or as second-line therapy.

It is acceptable to give oral loading doses of antibiotics. An appropriate adult loading dose of penicillin is 2 g, erythromycin 1 g.

- Clindamycin is useful for severe infections, or as second-line therapy.
- It is acceptable to give oral loading doses of antibiotics. An appropriate adult loading dose of penicillin is 2 g, erythromycin 1 g.
- Dental-related pain can be quite severe. Most patients will require a narcotic analgesic combination for dental-related pain.

Table 22-1 lists suggested doses for medications commonly used in dentistry.

NOMENCLATURE

Normally, people have 32 teeth. From back to front there are 6 molars, 4 premolars, 2 canines, and 4 incisors in both the maxillary (upper) and mandibular (lower) dental arches. Third molars (wisdom teeth) are often congenitally missing. Teeth may be referred to by their type and location, or by their number. Teeth are numbered from 1 through 16 starting in the patient's upper right posterior and proceeding around to the left. The numbering then continues in the lower left, starting with 17, and proceeding through 32 on the right (Fig. 22-1).

The outside of the tooth or gums is called buccal or labial, whereas the inside is referred to as palatal or lingual. For example, the inner, upper gum is called the maxillary palatal mucosa.

TOOTH ANATOMY

Teeth are composed of three layers. From the outside these are the enamel, dentin, and pulp. Both the dentin and the pulp are living, and sensitive to noxious stimuli. The crown is covered with hard enamel, whereas the root is covered with cementum and may be exquisitely sensitive when exposed. Figure 22-2 shows useful tooth and periodontal nomenclature.

PERIODONTAL ANATOMY

The periodontium refers to the structures surrounding the teeth:

- The gingiva is keratinized epithelium that covers the gum tissue immediately surrounding the teeth and the maxillary hard palate. It is somewhat resistant to local trauma. The gum tissue apical to the gingiva is the alveolar mucosa, which is nonkeratinized and easily friable.
- The periodontal ligament anchors the apex of the tooth to its bony socket.
- The bones encasing the teeth are the mandible (jaw) and maxilla (upper).

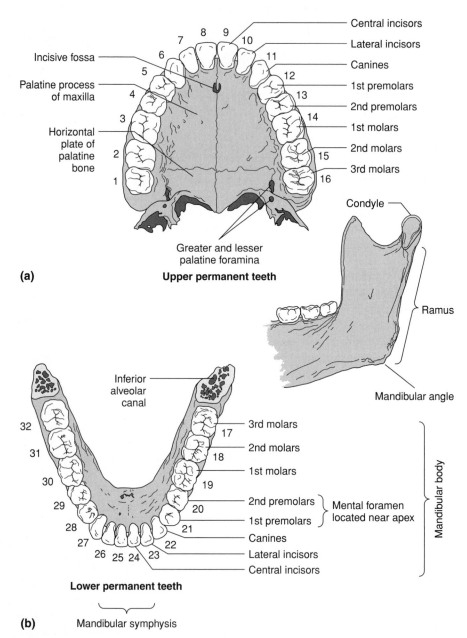

(a)   **Upper permanent teeth**

Central incisors
Lateral incisors
Canines
1st premolars
2nd premolars
1st molars
2nd molars
3rd molars

Incisive fossa
Palatine process of maxilla
Horizontal plate of palatine bone
Greater and lesser palatine foramina

Condyle
Ramus
Mandibular angle

Inferior alveolar canal

3rd molars
2nd molars
1st molars
2nd premolars
1st premolars
Canines
Lateral incisors
Central incisors

Mental foramen located near apex

Mandibular body

Lower permanent teeth

(b)   Mandibular symphysis

FIGURE 22-1 A: Upper permanent teeth. B: Lower permanent teeth.

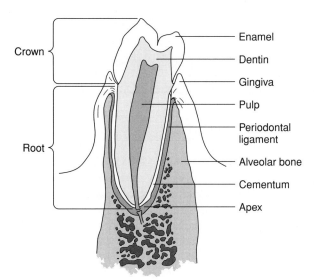

Crown

Root

Enamel

Dentin

Gingiva

Pulp

Periodontal
ligament

Alveolar bone

Cementum

Apex

FIGURE 22-2 Tooth and
alveolar anatomy.

INNERVATION

MAXILLARY NERVES

The maxillary (upper) teeth and contiguous structures are entirely innervated by
branches from the maxillary division of the trigeminal nerve, a purely sensory nerve.

MANDIBULAR NERVES

The primarily sensory mandibular nerve innervates the mandibular teeth and gives off
motor branches for the muscles of mastication. There are four important branches:

- The main innervation for the lower jaw is the inferior alveolar nerve. This nerve
  passes along the inside of the mandible and terminates as the mental nerve.
- The mental nerve innervates the buccal gingiva between the midline and the
  second premolar, as well as the skin of the lower lip and chin.
- The buccal nerve passes along the anterior border of the mandible and innervates
  the buccal gingiva between the second premolar and second molar.
- The lingual nerve initially travels with the inferior alveolar nerve, but then turns
  medially to innervate the lingual gingiva, the floor of the mouth, and the tongue.

BLOOD SUPPLY

The blood supply to the dentition and oral structures is entirely derived from branches
of the external carotid artery. These vessels roughly parallel the nerve supply and generally have the same name.

> **DID YOU KNOW?**
>
> Because of the dense collateral blood supply, arteries can be safely ligated to stop bleeding in an emergency.

PRIMARY DENTITION AND TOOTH ERUPTION

The first set of human teeth is referred to as primary teeth, or baby teeth, which erupt from about 6 months to 3 years of age. A full set of primary teeth consists of 10 mandibular and 10 maxillary teeth. There are no primary premolars. Lack of full primary dentition by 3–4 years of age warrants an evaluation for possible growth disturbances.

As teeth erupt through the gums, they may become painful, commonly known as teething in infants. Infants also can develop low-grade fever, refusal to feed, drooling, and occasionally diarrhea. Soft tissue in the area of the erupting tooth will appear inflamed. Temperature above 37.9°C (100.6°F) should point to a systemic process.

Treatment includes pain control and adequate hydration.

- Use topical anesthetic agents and pediatric acetaminophen or ibuprofen.
- Giving the child something hard to chew on also helps relieve the pain.
- Encourage oral fluids to prevent the rare need for intravenous (IV) hydration.

ERUPTION

The secondary (permanent) teeth begin to replace the primary dentition at approximately 6 years of age. As the adult dentition erupts, the roots of the primary teeth resorb, and they fall out (exfoliation). Then after 1 to 2 months the permanent tooth erupts, usually beginning with the first molar (6th year molars) and ending with the second molars (12th year molars). The third molars (wisdom teeth) typically erupt at 16 to 22 years of age if they are not congenitally absent. Wisdom teeth often enter the oral cavity at angles that prevent their complete eruption (impaction).

PERICORONITIS

Pericoronitis is inflammation that occurs around the crown of an erupting tooth and is especially common around impacted teeth. It is made worse by the impaction of food under the tissue.

Treatment is as follows:

- Saline irrigation with a large syringe and a 16- to 20-gauge angiocatheter or needle.
- Have the patient swish and spit with warm saltwater or dilute peroxide rinses four to five times a day, especially after meals.

■ Provide oral analgesics (Table 22-1).
■ Occasionally the inflammation may be severe enough to warrant oral antibiotics.
■ The definitive treatment is completed eruption or extraction of the tooth.

ANESTHESIA AND ANALGESIA

Good anesthesia is the key to successful dental procedures. Table 22-2 lists commonly used dental local anesthetics (all in the amide class), as well as maximal safe dosages.

To obtain profound anesthesia, sensation must be eliminated from the tooth pulp, the periodontal ligament, and buccal and lingual soft tissues. Table 22-3 outlines the nerves to achieve anesthesia for procedures in any particular region of the mouth.

Key points for good anesthesia include the following:

■ Remember that local anesthesia blocks sensation of pain, temperature, and touch, but not proprioception. Warn patients that they will feel pressure.
■ Marcaine (bupivicaine) has the advantage of longer duration of action, but has slower onset. The addition of a vasoconstrictor (epinephrine) lengthens the duration of action, and provides some hemostasis.

PROCEDURE FOR LOCAL ANESTHESIA

■ Always aspirate the syringe to ensure that the needle tip has not penetrated a vessel. If a flash of blood is found, withdraw a few millimeters, redirect, and reaspirate.
■ Local anesthetic solutions should be injected slowly and in minimal volumes to avoid pain and the risk of tissue necrosis.
■ Direct injection into an infected area should be avoided. Adjacent infiltration and proximal regional blocks are acceptable alternatives.

TABLE 22-2 COMMON DENTAL ANESTHETICS AND RECOMMENDED MAXIMAL DOSES

LOCAL ANESTHETIC AGENT	DURATION PULPAL ANESTHESIA	DURATION SOFT TISSUE ANESTHESIA	MAXIMAL DOSE (MG/KG)[a]
Lidocaine 1%	—	—	3–5
Lidocaine 1% with epinephrine	1/h	3–5/h	5–7
Lidocaine 2% with epinephrine	1–2/h	3–4/h	4.4
Bupivacaine 0.5%	—	—	2.5
Bupivacaine 0.5% with epinephrine	1–3/h	4–9/h	1.3

[a] Based on average adult = 70 kg.

TABLE 22-3 RECOMMENDED INJECTIONS FOR EXTRACTION OF SPECIFIC TEETH

TOOTH	PULPAL ANESTHETIC	BUCCAL SOFT TISSUE	LINGUAL SOFT TISSUE
Maxilla			
Central incisor	Infiltration at apex	Infiltration	Nasopalatine nerve block
Lateral incisor	Infiltration at apex	Infiltration	Nasopalatine nerve block
Canine	Infiltration at apex	Infiltration	Nasopalatine nerve block
First premolar	Infiltration at apex	Infiltration	Anterior palatine nerve block
Second premolar	Infiltration at apex	Infiltration	Anterior palatine nerve block
First molar	Infiltration over mesial root and infiltration over second molar apex	Infiltration over mesial root and infiltration over second molar apex	Anterior palatine nerve block
Second molar	Infiltration at apex	Infiltration	Anterior palatine nerve block
Third molar	Infiltration at apex	Infiltration	Anterior palatine nerve block
Mandible			
Central incisor	Inferior alveolar nerve block	Inferior alveolar nerve block	Lingual nerve block
Lateral incisor	Inferior alveolar nerve block	Inferior alveolar nerve block	Lingual nerve block
Canine	Inferior alveolar nerve block	Inferior alveolar nerve block	Lingual nerve block
First premolar	Inferior alveolar nerve block	Inferior alveolar nerve block	Lingual nerve block
Second premolar	Inferior alveolar nerve block	Inferior alveolar nerve block	Lingual nerve block
First molar	Inferior alveolar nerve block	Long buccal nerve block	Lingual nerve block
Second molar	Inferior alveolar nerve block	Long buccal nerve block	Lingual nerve block
Third molar	Inferior alveolar nerve block	Long buccal nerve block	Lingual nerve block

For teeth that border transitional areas innervated by two different nerves, additional infiltration injections may be required.

Reprinted from Peterson LJ, et al. *Contemporary Oral and Maxillofacial Surgery.* St. Louis: CV Mosby; permission pending.

- Direct injection into muscle tissue also should be avoided. This provides little anesthesia and may result in trismus.
- Neurovascular structures risk laceration when blocks are performed. If the patient reports paresthesias, or hematoma formation occurs upon needle insertion, injection should not be performed and the needle should be immediately withdrawn and pressure applied.

The onset of local infiltrative anesthesia is approximately 2 minutes. Regional blocks take about 5 minutes. Adequate anesthesia should be confirmed before any manipulation.

TOPICAL ANESTHETICS

Topical anesthesia is effective only for surface tissues, but it allows for painless needle penetration and temporary relief of local pain. It is very useful as a first step to reduce or eliminate the pain from injections. Because topical anesthesia requires higher concentrations of agent, there is greater potential for toxicity.

Topical agents include the following:

- Esters: benzocaine (most common), cocaine, tetracaine
- Amides: butacaine, lidocaine
- Ketone: dyclonine hydrochloride
- There are commercially available preparations of 20% benzocaine that are useful for minor oral pain secondary to toothaches, canker sores, injury, and irritation. Weaker preparations of 7.5% benzocaine treat the pain associated with teething in children under 2 years of age. These should not be used for infants under 4 months of age.
- Ethyl chloride also may be useful prior to injection or manipulation but has a very brief duration of action.

The following warnings should be heeded:

- Do not exceed a concentration of 4% for topical cocaine.
- Butacaine is twice as potent as cocaine topically and four times as toxic. Do not exceed 5 mL of 4% solution.
- Tetracaine has a great potential for systemic toxicity.
- Lidocaine is the only common agent that is useful in both topical and injected forms.

ANESTHESIA TECHNIQUES FOR MAXILLARY TEETH

There are three common methods for anesthesia of maxillary teeth: local infiltration, greater palatine nerve block, and incisive nerve block.

LOCAL INFILTRATION TECHNIQUES Unlike mandibular teeth, the maxillary teeth can be easily anesthetized with local infiltration on each side of the tooth. This is technically the least difficult of all infiltrative techniques (Fig. 22-3).

The procedure is as follows:

- Insert a 27-gauge needle 2 to 3 cm into the depth of the labial (buccal) sulcus, aiming for the apex (tip) of the tooth. Lightly touch the bone to facilitate diffusion of the anesthetic agent. Slowly inject 2 to 3 mL of solution.

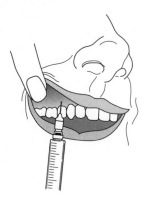

FIGURE 22-3 Maxillary local infiltration.

- To anesthetize the palatal (inner) side, insert only the needle tip (3–5 mm), about 1 cm apical to the gum line. Very slowly inject 2 to 3 mL of anesthetic solution. These injections are uncomfortable because the palatal mucosa is nondistensible, which also makes considerable injection pressure necessary.
- A useful clinical clue to the adequacy of infiltration is the blanching of the mucosal tissues immediately surrounding the injection site.

GREATER PALATINE NERVE BLOCK TECHNIQUES   An alternative, but more difficult technique to anesthetize the palatal side of the maxillary teeth is to block either the greater palatine or incisive nerves (Fig. 22-4).

- The greater palatine nerves are roughly located just anterior to the junction of the hard and soft palate, and about 1 cm medial from the gum line of the maxillary second molar. There are no other landmarks to help you.
- Inject about 2 mL of anesthetic solution near (but never into) the foramina.
- Wait 5 minutes and test for adequacy of anesthesia.

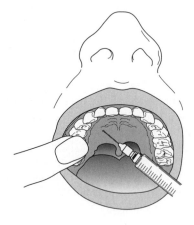

FIGURE 22-4 Greater palatine block.

INCISIVE NERVE BLOCK TECHNIQUES

■ The incisive nerves are located at the incisive papilla, just palatal to the backs of the maxillary central incisors. It is a small ovoid bump of keratinized tissue that is easy to locate.

■ The needle tip should be inserted 3 to 5 mm at the base of the papilla, and enough anesthetic solution should be injected to blanche the surrounding tissues (2 mL).

■ These injections may sting. Warn your patients in advance, and use topical anesthetic or distraction techniques if available.

ANESTHESIA TECHNIQUES FOR MANDIBULAR TEETH

The mandible (jaw) is hard, thick bone; therefore, it is more difficult to anesthetize the lower teeth by local infiltration. The exception to this rule is the area of the incisors, where anesthesia can be obtained via local lingual and buccal infiltration. The good news is that a regional block of the inferior alveolar nerve can anesthetize the entire side of the mandible.

ANTERIOR MANDIBULAR ANESTHESIA Local infiltration is effective in this area, but there is a great deal of overlap of innervation in the anterior mandible. This means that local infiltration is needed on both sides of the midline to achieve profound analgesia in the area. The lingual mucosa also must be anesthetized.

■ Local infiltrative anesthesia is performed in this area as described above, on both the buccal and lingual aspects. On the lingual aspect, the needle should enter the mucosa just below the level of the attached gingiva.

■ The floor of the mouth is highly vascular, and caution should be used to avoid inadvertent damage to vascular structures when performing lingual infiltration.

INFERIOR ALVEOLAR NERVE BLOCK Blockade of the inferior alveolar nerve provides profound analgesia to all tissues (including the intraoral soft and hard tissues) from approximately midline to the posteriormost tooth. Depending on the situation, additional consideration may need to be given to the buccal nerve.

■ The injection site for the inferior alveolar and lingual blocks is located about 1 cm above the upper (occlusal) surface of the mandibular molar teeth and just medial to the tip of an index finger placed on the coronoid notch. Note that the pterygomandibular raphe is medial to the fingertip in this position. The soft tissues in the area will make a V when the cheek is gently retracted. The needle should penetrate the soft tissue within this V (Fig. 22-5).

■ A long, small-gauge (25-gauge or smaller) needle is angled over the premolars on the opposite side of the mouth to the target area of the mandibular foramen described above.

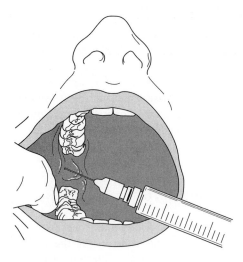

FIGURE 22-5 Inferior alveolar injection technique. Inject local anesthetic just behind the coronoid process 1 cm from the molar occlusal surface.

■ The needle tip is inserted 1 to 2 cm along the inner (medial) side of the mandibular ramus just lateral to the pterygomandibular raphe. The needle should always be in contact with the bone of the ramus and the syringe held in the original occlusal plane.

■ Once the long needle is inserted almost to the hub, aspiration is performed, and approximately 2 mL of anesthetic agent is slowly injected.

LINGUAL NERVE BLOCK To provide anesthesia to the lingual aspect of the mandible, lingual gingiva, and floor of the mouth, a block of the lingual nerve is needed. This is accomplished during the same inferior alveolar injection by withdrawing the needle

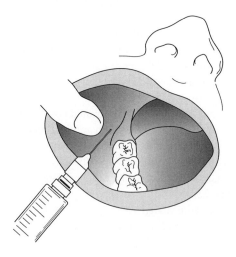

FIGURE 22-6 Buccal nerve block.

about 1 to 1.5 cm along the same path of insertion and depositing an additional 1 mL of anesthetic solution. The tongue itself also may be anesthetized via local infiltration for procedures isolated to the substance of the tongue (laceration, biopsy).

BUCCAL NERVE BLOCK A buccal nerve block (Fig. 22-6) provides anesthesia to the buccal gingiva between the second premolar and the second molar. The buccal nerve can be blocked by infiltrating 1 mL in the buccal fold just behind and lateral to the third (last) molar at the level of the occlusal plain (top of the tooth).

OTHER TECHNIQUES

MENTAL NERVE BLOCK A mental nerve block (Fig. 22-7) is best for anesthesia to the soft tissues of the lower lip, but is also useful when working on the lower front teeth anterior to the foramen. The mental nerve is the terminal branch of the inferior alveolar nerve. It is blocked by targeting the mental foramen:

- ■ Insert the needle approximately 5 to 6 mm at the buccal aspect of the apex of the first or second premolar.
- ■ Infiltrate 1 to 2 mL of solution.

The needle tip should never be inserted directly into the canal because it risks needle breakage and possible neurovascular injury.

INFRAORBITAL NERVE BLOCK Infraorbital block is not for the teeth but for repairing lacerations in the lateral aspect of the nose, philtrum, and upper lip.

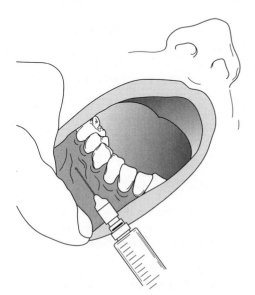

FIGURE 22-7 Mental nerve block. An injection of local anesthetic is being directed toward the root apex of the first premolar tooth through the mucobuccal fold.

■ Palpate the infraorbital foramen (about 1 cm below the inferior orbital rim in the midline of the eye) with the index finger, while elevating the upper lip with the thumb of the same hand.

■ Insert the needle in the depth of the labial sulcus at the center of the canine tooth and advance slowly up toward the index finger, and the underlying infraorbital foramina. The needle should follow an imaginary line that bisects the pupil.

■ After a negative aspiration, 2 to 3 mL of solution is injected.

KEY POINT:

Needles should never be introduced into foramina because of damage to vessels, nerves, and needle breakage.

PERIODONTAL LIGAMENT BLOCK A useful adjunct to providing pure dental anesthesia is the periodontal ligament block. Insert the needle directly into the periodontal space (space between the tooth and surrounding soft tissue) and slowly but firmly inject the anesthetic solution circumferentially around the tooth. Considerable injection pressure may be required (therefore, it hurts).

COMPLICATIONS OF INFILTRATIVE ANESTHESIA

■ Permanent paresthesias can result from injection into a neurovascular structure with hematoma formation.

■ Transient paralysis of the facial nerve can occur when anesthetic solution infiltrates beyond the intended areas and reaches the branches of cranial nerve VII.

■ Rare toxic complications include seizures, respiratory depression, loss of consciousness, and cardiovascular collapse.

■ When epinephrine is added, intravascular complications can include angina, hypertension, palpitations, and dysrhythmias.

■ Allergic reactions are rare with the amide class.

■ The long duration of action of bupivicaine can lead to increased risk of soft tissue injury from burns or accidental self-mutilation (lip biting), especially in the young, very old, or mentally/physically impaired.

DENTAL DISEASE

DENTAL CARIES

Dental caries (cavities) may strike any tooth or tooth surface but is most commonly found on the occlusal (chewing) surface and between the teeth. Caries are the result of destruction of tooth substance by the acid products of normal oral flora.

CLINICAL FEATURES A carious tooth may not be painful until the inflammation reaches the pulp. This is known as pulpitis and usually presents with sensitivity (pain) to liquids, cold air, or food. Symptoms are typically intermittent until the infection actually reaches the pulp, then the pain becomes constant, severe, and throbbing.

DIAGNOSIS   A carious lesion will appear as a hole or a black spot on the tooth surface, or around the margins of a filling. Find the cavities by probing with a sharp tip—the decay is soft and the needle sticks.

TREATMENT

■ Immediate treatment is often unnecessary unless the pain is severe and definitive dental care is not readily available.
■ All patients should be provided with oral or topical analgesia.
■ Temporary treatment includes removing food debris and loose filling material, then filling the defect with a temporary filling made of zinc oxide powder and eugenol liquid (oil of cloves) or commercial preparations such as Cavit or I.R.M.
■ To make the filling add small amounts of zinc oxide powder to one to two drops of eugenol liquid on a glass mixing slab until the mixture has reached a doughy consistency and can be rolled between the fingers without sticking. This ball is then packed into the defect with pressure. Excess material should be trimmed or scraped away, and any occlusal (biting) interferences should be scraped away until the patient feels a normal bite.
■ The cavity will still require definitive treatment by a dental professional in the near future.

PREVENTION   Patients should be taught about basic good oral hygiene, including brushing, flossing, observing a proper diet, and planning routine cleanings/examinations. Dietary items that are high in refined sugars or fructose should be avoided or consumed in moderation. A soft-bristle toothbrush should be used after each meal. A hard toothbrush can injure the gingiva and lead to tooth loss. The alternative is to use a 5- to 10-mm diameter stick from a soft, still green wood. One end can be sharpened to be used to clean between the teeth, and the other can be chewed until frayed to be used as a toothbrush.

Toothpaste is not necessary, but is helpful if it contains fluoride. If possible, patients should floss daily with a proper technique to avoid injury to the gums. When available, fluoride can be added to toothpaste or drinking water, or taken as a mouth rinse or vitamin supplement.

NURSING BOTTLE CARIES

Nursing bottle caries is a term applied to rampant carious lesions of the primary teeth caused by frequent bottle feedings or putting a baby to bed with a bottle. This is much worse when the bottle solutions contain sugar. The constant supply of bacterial substrate results in uncontrolled decay that is completely preventable.

TREATMENT AND PREVENTION Encourage breast-feeding. Teach parents to not leave bottles in their infants' mouths for long periods of time, or at bedtime. Children should use cups as soon as they are old enough. Baby teeth should be wiped clean with a soft cloth after feedings. In addition to treating the immediate condition, education is imperative to avoid further disease.

DENTAL ABSCESSES AND DENTAL INFECTIONS

Once a carious lesion reaches the soft tissues of the pulp, it can progress rapidly to involve the tissues at the root apex, which leads to constant, severe pain. This condition is known as periapical periodontitis. At this point the tooth is only salvageable by advanced endodontic therapy (a root canal). The purulence at the apex of the root compromises the tooth's attachment and leads to mobility. This is known as a dental abscess.

As the infection erodes through the alveolar bone, the location it spreads to is determined by muscle attachments and fascial planes. The most common dental infection is a vestibular supreme abscess. Patients complain of painful intraoral swelling and possibly intermittent drainage of purulent material. There is typically minimal extraoral facial asymmetry. There may be an obvious draining sinus tract. Localized palatal and sublingual space infections present in the same fashion. Canine space infections present with obliteration of the nasolabial fold. In general, these infections can be treated by field personnel with a simple intraoral incision and drainage. But it is critical to recognize when an infection has spread.

Other more serious fascial infections include those of the mandibular, submandibular, and cervical spaces. Suspected infection in any of these spaces requires urgent referral to a surgical specialist. General clinical factors can be used as criteria for referral:

- Infection progressing rapidly over 1 to 2 days
- Fascial space involvement
- Temperature greater than 101°F
- Toxic appearance
- Immunocompromised host
- Difficulty swallowing or tolerating oral secretions
- Difficulty breathing
- Severe trismus (inability to open the mandible more than 15 mm)
- Ocular involvement

KEY POINT:

Concurrent bilateral submandibular, sublingual, and submental space infections is a condition commonly known as Ludwig's Angina and is a true surgical emergency. Start IV antibiotics, and refer early.

CLINICAL FEATURES Abscessed teeth are exquisitely sensitive to pressure, and local cellulitis may be present. The patient also may develop trismus and there is often a foul odor. Patients may develop a reactive or infectious maxillary sinusitis due to the proximity of the maxillary root apices. As long as the infection remains enclosed within the tissues, it will be exquisitely painful. Purulence will follow the path of least resistance to drain. Eventually a sinus tract may form, allowing purulence to drain either through the tooth, the intraoral soft tissues, or extraorally. In chronic dental abscesses, patients often complain of swelling, purulence, and foul odor and taste, but not pain.

DIAGNOSIS Gently tapping on the teeth will cause marked pain and readily localize the affected tooth. There may be a soft spot in the alveolar process near the tooth apex or focal swelling palpable inside the mouth.

TREATMENT If there is mild tenderness, minimal mobility, and no signs of extension into the soft tissue, the diagnosis is a simple periapical periodontitis. In general, extraction of the tooth is indicated where advanced dental care and endodontic therapy are not readily available.

ANTIBIOTIC THERAPY

- Without a radiograph, any tooth that is sensitive to percussion should be presumed to be abscessed and an empiric course of antibiotics is warranted.
- If radiography shows evidence of extension of the infection beyond the root apex, treat with antibiotics.
- Penicillin (or erythromycin for penicillin-allergic patients) is the empiric dental antibiotic of choice.

ANALGESIA

- Ibuprofen or acetaminophen may suffice. However, most patients require a mild narcotic, such as acetaminophen with codeine or oxycodone (which can be combined with ibuprofen).
- Local anesthetic does not work well in the face of an abscess due alterations in tissue pH, but regional blocks do.

INCISION AND DRAINAGE

- If an abscess is fluctulant and pointing, perform incision and drainage (I&D).
- Be more aggressive with intraoral I&Ds. The mucosa heals well and the risk to vital structures is minimal. Extraoral I&D should be reserved for only the most obvious cases because there are numerous vital structures within the subcutaneous tissues.
- Antibiotics and analgesia should be given after this procedure. Once resolution of cellulitis and drainage of purulence is achieved, the tooth may be safely extracted.

PERIODONTAL DISEASE

Poor dental hygiene and poor nutrition lead to local inflammation of the tissues surrounding and attaching the tooth, allowing bacterial penetration. Early periodontal disease is isolated to the gingiva and is known as gingivitis. As the disease progresses, alveolar bone may be destroyed, leading to gingival pockets and tooth mobility. Food debris or plaque may become trapped in these pockets and create a localized infection known as a periodontal abscess. Periodontal disease is common in pregnant women.

CLINICAL FEATURES AND DIAGNOSIS Patients may complain of bleeding gums, foul odor, bad taste, loose teeth, pain, and swelling. The physical examination reveals gingival tissue that may be erythematous or necrotic and bleeds easily. An abscess may present as focal swelling, tooth mobility, pain on percussion, and purulence that is expressible from the gingival sulcus. With concurrent dental caries, it may be impossible to differentiate a dental abscess from a periodontal abscess without radiographs. Regardless, a periodontally diseased tooth may be so mobile that it cannot be salvaged and requires extraction.

TREATMENT An isolated periodontal abscess can be treated as follows:

- Incision and drainage
- Dilute peroxide rinses (1:5 dilution or 5%) four to five times daily
- Antibiotic therapy with either penicillin or erythromycin

These patients should be referred to a dentist for definitive follow-up care.

ACUTE NECROTIZING ULCERATIVE GINGIVITIS

Commonly called Vincent's infection or trench mouth, acute necrotizing ulcerative gingivitis (ANUG) is a rapidly progressing, disseminated form of periodontal disease typically seen in young adults. It is associated with diabetic and immunocompromised hosts. The risk for tooth loss is great.

CLINICAL FEATURES AND DIAGNOSIS Patients are in obvious discomfort and may be unable to eat. The gingival tissues are fiery red with obvious necrosis and pseudomembrane formation. The breath is fetid. Onset and progression are rapid even to the point of airway compromise.

TREATMENT

- These patients require admission and a course of IV tetracycline to cover for anaerobes and gram-negative results.
- Close monitoring is needed for signs of airway compromise.

- Diluted peroxide rinses and oral and topical analgesics may provide some relief.
- The patient's nutritional status should be addressed and supplementation, especially vitamin C, should be given if available.
- These patients require follow-up care with a dental professional.

MUCOSAL CONDITIONS

HERPES

Primary oral herpes infections usually first present in children 1 to 5 years of age. The pain can lead to poor oral intake, so an evaluation of hydration status is essential.

CLINICAL FEATURES AND DIAGNOSIS Complaints include pain, fever, sore throat, and poor oral intake. Patients, especially children, may be significantly dehydrated. Oral lesions are characterized by multiple small, shallow, painful ulcerations with a brightly erythematous border. Lymphadenopathy may be present. Yellow-crusted lesions may appear on the patient's lips and at the corners of the mouth. Recurrence is frequent. Patients with active ulcerations are infective by contact. Resolution typically occurs within 7 to 14 days.

To differentiate from other oral lesions, apthous ulcers or canker sores do not occur on attached gingiva. Herpetic ulcers do not typically occur between the teeth, thus distinguishing it from ANUG. Herpangina is distinguished by systemic viral symptoms and small, ulcerative lesions isolated to the soft palate and tonsillar pillars. This entity is caused by the coxsackie virus, occurs in children, and is self-limited. Complaints include pain, fever, sore throat, and poor oral intake.

TREATMENT AND PREVENTION

- Treatment is symptomatic with topical and systemic analgesics. A solution of BMX [Benadryl (diphenhydramine), Maalox, and viscous xylocaine (lidocaine)] is ideal in these patients who can rinse and spit.
- Patients should avoid spicy foods. Sucking on ice chips and adhering to a soft diet may be helpful.
- Painting extraoral lesions with gentian violet, tincture of benzoin, or petroleum jelly may help avoid superinfection.
- The duration of symptoms may be reduced if oral acyclovir is started during the prodrome, but this is extremely expensive and not curative.

APHTHOUS STOMATITIS

These lesions (commonly known as canker sores) are found almost exclusively on nonkeratinized, moveable mucosa. The etiology is unknown. Lesions typically resolve spontaneously in 10 to 14 days.

CLINICAL FEATURES AND DIAGNOSIS This condition is manifested by recurrent, small, shallow, painful ulcerations with erythematous borders. With an isolated ulcerative lesion, it is wise to rule out local trauma from a carious tooth, defective restoration, or poorly fitting appliance.

TREATMENT AND PREVENTION

■ Symptomatic treatment (BMX, ice chips, no spicy food, etc.) is the same as for herpetic lesions.
■ If available, topical steroids in an oral preparation have had success in hastening healing by 3 to 4 days in some patients.
■ Systemic (oral) analgesics are not usually needed.

OTHER ULCERS AND SORES

Dental trauma (caused by rubbing dentures, braces, broken teeth, etc.) is a common cause of oral ulcers. When dental trauma is suspected, the appliance (dentures, etc.) should be left out of the mouth for 2 to 3 days, and the patient should be placed on a soft diet and warm saltwater rinses. If a lesion persists for more than 10 days, a super-infection may be present and patients should be treated with a course of penicillin. Lesions that do not heal after antibiotics may be cancerous and should be evaluated by a dental professional. The same holds true for any unresolved swelling.

> **KEY POINT:**
>
> Ulcerative lesions that do not heal after treatment with a course of antibiotics should be considered cancerous until proven otherwise.

ORAL CANDIDIASIS (THRUSH)

Thrush is often seen in immunocompromised patients, in patients on concurrent antibiotics, and in infants. It can be painful, and may result in poor feeding and hydration.

CLINICAL FEATURES/DIAGNOSIS Thrush classically presents as numerous white, cheesy plaques that can be rubbed off (with some persistence) to reveal mucosal erythema or bleeding. Lesions may be present in any intraoral site. Make sure that plaques are not simply dried milk or formula.

TREATMENT AND PREVENTION Treatment consists of any one of many topical antifungal agents, including nystatin and ketoconazole, used directly on the lesion or by swishing and spitting.

ANGULAR CHELITIS

Angular chelitis is cracks or fissures at the corner of the mouth that may be painful, bleed, or crust. It has been associated with poor dentition, ill-fitting dentures, lip licking (perleche), and nutritional deficiencies (particularly pyridoxine and riboflavin). Superinfection with *Candida* or *Staphylococcus* is common.

TREATMENT AND PREVENTION Lesions may respond to steroid, antibacterial, and antifungal ointments. Consideration should be given to a nutritional supplement.

PELLAGRA

The clinical syndrome produced by niacin (vitamin B_6) deficiency is called pellagra. Oral manifestations are common and easily recognizable.

CLINICAL FEATURES AND DIAGNOSIS Glossitis and stomatitis typically present with an oral mucosa that is erythematous, swollen, tender, and atrophic. The pain is often described as burning, and the appearance of the tongue is often characterized as bald. Ulceration may occur in advanced stages.

TREATMENT AND PREVENTION

- Treatment is with dietary niacin supplementation.
- Topical agents, such as BMX, may provide symptomatic relief.

OTHER DENTAL-RELATED PROBLEMS

TEMPOROMANDIBULAR JOINT SYNDROME

The TMJ is an extremely complex and sensitive structure. The causes of TMJ syndrome include referred pain, muscle spasm, bruxism, and occlusal discrepancies of less than a millimeter (a filling that is left too high).

CLINICAL FEATURES AND DIAGNOSIS Patients may complain of pain with chewing, as well as clicking, popping, or locking sensations. Physical examination may reveal tenderness and crepitation of the TMJ, trigger points, heavy occlusal or incisal wear, and abnormal range of motion. TMJ disorders can be truly debilitating and require a complete evaluation, including radiography, by a dental professional.

TREATMENT

- Soft diet, analgesics such as nonsteroidal antiinflammatory drugs, and moist heat are the mainstays of immediate treatment.

■ Look for an occlusal discrepancy from a new filling that is too high. It can be filed down until the patient no longer senses an abnormal bite.

TRAUMATIC DENTAL EMERGENCIES

GENERAL ASSESSMENT AND TREATMENT OF DENTAL TRAUMA

Rapid and correct treatment following dental trauma can help to preserve teeth.

DIAGNOSIS

■ The entire oral cavity must first be irrigated and cleansed of blood, debris, and clots.
■ Evaluate the intraoral soft tissue injuries for foreign body contamination and adequacy of blood supply. Active bleeding should be controlled with direct pressure.
■ Each tooth or portion of tooth the patient had prior to the incident should be accounted for. If it cannot be found by physical examination, then radiography of perioral soft tissue as well as the abdomen and chest should be undertaken to look for aspiration of a tooth or fragment.
■ Bleeding from the floor of the mouth or the labial/buccal vestibule may indicate a fracture.
■ All bony prominences should be palpated for step deformities and crepitation.
■ Individual teeth should be evaluated for fractures, displacement, pain, and mobility.

> **TIPS AND TRICKS:**
>
> Ask the patient if the bite feels normal. If not, or if there is a tooth displaced, a dentoalveolar arch or jaw fracture should be sought.

Teeth may be displaced buccolingually (inward), intruded (pushed into the socket), extruded (partially pulled out of the socket), or completely avulsed (completely out of the socket). Teeth should be assessed for mobility in both horizontal and vertical directions.

TREATMENT Time is crucial for the treatment of lacerations, avulsions, and tooth fractures. The patient's tetanus immunization status should always be addressed. Specific treatments for each type of trauma are discussed below.

TOOTH FRACTURES

A crack in a tooth crown is an incomplete fracture of enamel without loss of tooth structure. A darkened, painful tooth with a history of a crack needs root canal therapy or extraction. The treatment of crown fractures is determined by the type of fracture. A type I fracture is of the enamel only. A type II fracture goes through the enamel and into the dentin. Dentin is yellow and sensitive to temperature as well as abrasion. A class III fracture penetrates to the pulp at the center of the tooth. A pinkish blush at the fracture line or droplets of blood emanating from the inside of the tooth is evidence of pulp involvement.

TREATMENT For class I fractures, no acute treatment is necessary, although any sharp edges of the cracked enamel can be smoothed with a dental file or emery board. Follow-up dental evaluation and periodic observation is recommended.

Class II fractures involve dentin, a living, sensitive tooth substance that requires coverage:

■ Calcium hydroxide paste (Dycal) should be applied to the exposed dentin as a "band aid." This can be covered with dry aluminum foil, but this is uncomfortable for the patient and cumbersome for the provider.
■ A simpler technique is to paint the fractured portion of tooth with Copalite (a clear tooth varnish), or clear acrylic nail polish after applying calcium hydroxide.
■ The tooth may require anesthesia with a long-acting anesthetic for patient comfort. Oral analgesics may be necessary.
■ The patient should be evaluated by a dental professional, including radiography, in 24 to 48 hours.

Class III fractures are characterized by exposure of the pulp, which is exquisitely painful. These injuries represent true dental emergencies.

■ These fractures require a long-acting local anesthetic, preferably prior to any manipulation of the tooth. Because these teeth may remain somewhat sensitive after local infiltration anesthesia, direct intrapulpal injection of anesthetic may be used (slowly inject directly into the dark pulp at the center of the fractured tooth). Oral analgesics will be necessary, and narcotic-containing compounds are recommended.
■ If a definitive treatment facility is less than 24 hours away and the pulpal exposure is small (<2 mm), the exposed pulp and dentin should be covered with Dycal, followed by Copalite.
■ If definitive treatment will be delayed by more than 24 hours, a small portion of the remaining pulp tissue should be amputated, and a cotton pledget moistened with anesthetic (lidocaine, etc.) solution should be placed over the exposed pulp tissue. A small amount of temporary filling material can be used to fill the remaining defect. Exposed dentin should then be covered with calcium hydroxide and followed by Copalite or clear acrylic nail polish.
■ Patients should avoid temperature extremes and biting in that area.
■ If follow-up with dental personnel for root canal therapy is not available, the tooth should be promptly extracted to avoid undue suffering and possible infectious sequelae.

CRITICAL ACTION:

Ellis class III fractures represent true dental emergencies. Patients should be seen immediately by a dental professional able to perform a root canal if available.

ROOT FRACTURES

Patients with root fractures may present acutely or later with a chronic toothache. The trauma may have been minimal, with some patients stating that they "bit down on something hard."

DIAGNOSIS This can be an extremely challenging diagnosis. Fractures are rarely visible on dental radiographs. The diagnosis is made by a history of trauma, pain on occlusion (have the patient bite on a tongue blade), or from removing a filling to directly examine the cavity floor.

TREATMENT In general, root fractures require extraction. Heroic and expensive measures can sometimes salvage a tooth with a fractured root.

SUBLUXATION AND CONCUSSION

A concussed tooth has been traumatized, but is not crooked or fractured, and there is no evidence of mobility. The only treatment needed is symptomatic relief with oral analgesics and a soft diet.

A tooth that has been loosened within its socket by trauma is called subluxed. These teeth usually have small fractures of the surrounding alveolar bone. They may be intruded (pushed into the socket), extruded (pulled out of the socket), or laterally displaced.

CLINICAL FEATURES AND DIAGNOSIS Assess for tooth mobility by gentle pressure from a tongue blade. The surrounding alveolar bone also should be palpated while the tooth is gently manipulated to look for a mobile bony fragment. There is typically a small amount of bleeding from the gingival sulcus, and there may be associated gingival lacerations. Ideally, dental radiographs are taken of the injured tooth before and after splinting.

TREATMENT The treatment of intruded teeth is controversial. In general, they should be left alone and treated symptomatically. The patient should be seen by a dentist as soon as possible, preferably within 24 hours, but after no more than 4 or 5 days.

Intruded primary teeth may injure the permanent tooth buds. If deeply intruded they should be extracted as carefully as possible. Subluxed, extruded, or laterally displaced teeth should be manually repositioned with finger pressure, then the tooth should be stabilized.

There are three methods to splint the teeth in place:

■ If available, cold curing periodontal packing material (such as Coe-Pak or Perio-Pack) is ideal splint material for practitioners without dental experience. To use this material, a catalyst and base are mixed together to form a puttylike consistency. This is then rolled into a log and framed around the front and back of the injured tooth as well as 2 or 3 adjacent stable teeth. The material needs to be kept dry and uncontaminated during the few minutes needed to cure.

■ If necessary softened bee's wax can be used in a similar fashion, but this splint is not nearly as stable.

■ Alternative and advanced techniques include acid-etched composite resin, direct interdental wiring, and resin-wire combinations. These are excellent materials in experienced hands; however, it is unlikely that they will be available in the field.

■ Anesthetic should be administered before any manipulation, and significant gingival lacerations should be closed with an appropriate suture material prior to splinting.

■ All patients should receive oral analgesics. Antibiotics are indicated for large soft tissue lacerations or large portions of fractured alveolar buccal/lingual cortex.

■ A soft diet with instructions to chew on the opposite side will aid patient comfort.

AVULSION

Avulsion is an injury in which a tooth has been completely dislocated from its socket. Time is a critical factor—the sooner the tooth can be reimplanted, the better the prognosis. After 2 hours the tooth is generally considered nonsalvageable. Primary teeth and severely carious teeth are never reimplanted.

CLINICAL FEATURES AND DIAGNOSIS Assess for the presence of a surrounding alveolar bone fracture. The time course and manner in which an avulsed tooth is handled and preserved from the time of injury is critically important. An avulsed tooth that is soiled should be gently irrigated with saline or saliva prior to reimplantation (do not rub the tooth clean). The best to worst transport media for avulsed teeth are Hanks' solution (commercially available), saliva (the tooth should be transported inside the patient's or caregiver's mouth), milk, saline, or tap water. The worst situation is transporting a dry tooth. An avulsed tooth should not be transported in the mouth if aspiration is a concern.

TREATMENT

■ It may be necessary to administer local anesthesia. Dental radiographs should be taken if available.

■ Gently irrigate the tooth in either Hanks' solution or saline.

■ The socket should be cleansed of blood and debris with suction and/or gentle irrigation.

- Gently replace the tooth in proper anatomic position.
- Occlusion with adjacent and opposing teeth should be checked.
- The tooth should be splinted and the patient should be placed on oral analgesics and antibiotics.
- Tetanus status should be addressed.
- Prescribe a soft or liquid diet.
- Follow-up should be arranged within 24 hours. Reimplanted teeth often require additional advanced dental procedures and close follow-up.
- Extraction may be the eventual outcome.

KEY POINT:

Replace avulsed teeth as soon as possible. In general, if an avulsed tooth has not been reimplanted within 2 hours, it is considered nonsalvageable.

ALVEOLAR FRACTURES

Alveolar fractures are fractures of the bones surrounding the upper teeth. They may be associated with several of the previously discussed injuries. Alveolar bone usually heals well, but once it is lost it does not grow back. Therefore, handle with care. The alveolar blood supply depends on the overlying mucosa, so these tissues should be handled with equal care. Fracture fragments often contain one or more teeth.

CLINICAL FEATURES/DIAGNOSIS The clinical diagnosis of these injuries has been previously discussed (gentle manipulation of injured teeth and their surrounding bone).

TREATMENT

- Fragments can often simply be manually manipulated back into appropriate position. Occasionally, this requires a surgical approach that is beyond the scope of field medical personnel.
- If the teeth are intact they can be splinted (as described above) to stabilize the fracture.
- Gingival (gum) lacerations should be appropriately closed and antibiotics prescribed.

ORAL LACERATIONS

Soft tissue injuries of the oral or perioral structures may occur in isolation, or in combination with any of the previously described dental injuries.

CLINICAL FEATURES AND DIAGNOSIS In general, intraoral lacerations of 1 cm or less may be left to heal unless they are gaping, or if there is exposed bone. When a laceration crosses the path of a vital structure (i.e., the facial or labial artery, the parotid or submandibular gland duct, the facial or inferior alveolar nerve or maxillary sinus), the patient should be immediately referred to a professional with a background or knowledge of facial surgery, if one is available.

TREATMENT

- Irrigation should be performed for all soft tissue injuries, whether they will be closed or not. Debridement also may be necessary.
- Use no. 4-0 chromic or black silk sutures for intraoral lacerations.
- No. 6-0 nylon is an excellent suture material for facial skin.
- Through-and-through lip lacerations should be closed in three layers from inside the mouth to outside the mouth.
- When closing lip lacerations, the vermilion border should be approximated first.
- Once past the wet line of the lip (closer to the outside), use nylon suture material.
- Oral antibiotics, analgesics, warm saltwater rinses, avoidance of spicy foods, and a wound check in 24 to 48 hours are all standards of care.
- Tetanus status should always be addressed.
- If absolutely necessary, closure can be delayed for up to 12 hours.

> **TIPS AND TRICKS:**
>
> When closing lip lacerations, the vermillion border should always be approximated first.

MINOR DENTAL PROCEDURES

UNCOMPLICATED EXODONTIA (TOOTH EXTRACTIONS)

Unfortunately, extraction (exodontia) is often the mainstay of dental therapy in developing countries. Tooth extraction is often compared to pulling a post out of the ground or pulling a nail out of a board. Actually, exodontia is an art and very much a procedure for which you need to develop a "feel." Complications can have serious sequelae and cause undue patient suffering. It is advised that field personnel should have some supervised experience prior to attempting extractions on their own. Exodontia should be as atraumatic as possible. All of the movements required for tooth extractions are intentional, controlled, and involve pressure, not force directly.

Basic equipment is essential for the procedure. There are many types of specialized dental forceps, but the no. 150 (maxillary) and no. 151 (mandibular) forceps are considered universal and can be used to extract any tooth in the mouth in a pinch situation. The addition of an English right angle for any anterior tooth and a cow horn for mandibular molars will facilitate extractions for the beginner. (Table 22-4).

TABLE 22-4 BASIC DENTAL EQUIPMENT
FOR MINOR DENTAL PROCEDURES

Elevators: small straight elevator, large straight elevator
Forceps: no. 150 (upper universal), no. 151 lower universal,
  no. 82 (cow horn), English right angle, no. 88 right and left
Scalpel handle with no. 15 blades
Woodsen periosteal elevator or dental spoon
Minnesota retractor
Weider retractor (tongue)
Fraser tip suction
Needle holder
Hemostat
Blumenthal rongeurs
Bone rasp
Suture material
Gelfoam

GENERAL CONSIDERATIONS AND CAUTIONS Prior to any extraction make certain that the tooth really needs to come out. Indications include the following:

- Constant throbbing pain with no hope for root canal therapy
- Pain with mobility
- An unrepairable fracture, fractured restoration, or root fracture

In general, do not perform extractions if a dental abscess is present unless the pain cannot be adequately controlled with oral analgesics. A course of antibiotics prior to extraction will improve anesthesia and overall outcome. Contraindications to simple extractions (i.e., leave it to the experts) include the following:

- A malpositioned tooth
- A tooth with a bulbous root
- Possible inferior alveolar nerve involvement
- If the apex of the tooth is involved with the maxillary sinus
- Tumor involvement
- Previous radiation therapy to the area
- If the buccal cortical plate is unduly thick secondary to exostosis

It is always wise to obtain a dental radiograph to look for the above problem before attempting an extraction.

TREATMENT

- Make sure that the patient does not have a bleeding disorder.
- Pretreat appropriately with antibiotics for bacterial endocarditis before starting (Table 22-5). Consideration for treatment should be given to any patient with a history of a heart murmur.

TABLE 22-5 PROPHYLACTIC REGIMENS FOR ENDOCARDITIS IN PATIENTS UNDERGOING DENTAL OR ORAL SURGICAL PROCEDURES (RECOMMENDATIONS OF THE AMERICAN HEART ASSOCIATION 1997)

Standard general prophylaxis:
  Amoxicillin: adults, 2.0 g (children, 50 mg/kg) given orally 1 h prior to procedure
Unable to take oral meds:
  Ampicillin: adults, 2.0 g (children, 50 mg/kg) given IM/IV within 30 min before procedure
Amoxicillin/ampicillin allergic patients:
  Clindamycin: adults, 600 mg (children, 20 mg/kg) given orally 1 h before procedure, or
  Cephalexin or cefadroxil: adults, 2.0 g (children, 50 mg/kg) orally 1 h before procedure, or
  Azithromycin or clarithromycin: adults, 500 mg (children, 15 mg/kg) orally 1 h before procedure
Amoxicillin/ampicillin/penicillin–allergic patient unable to take oral meds:
  Clindamycin: adults, 600 mg (children, 20 mg/kg) IV within 30 min before procedure, or
  Cefazolin: adults, 1.0 g (children, 25 mg/kg) IM/IV within 30 min before procedure

■ Make certain your anesthesia is adequate before beginning. Warn patients that they will feel pressure, but should not feel anything sharp.

THE EXODONTIA PROCEDURE In general, the technique and instrumentation is the same for all teeth. There are three basic steps (after good anesthesia): elevation, luxation, and extraction.

Step 1: Elevation
This step begins the expansion of the socket in the alveolar bone and the tearing of periodontal ligament fibers. In effect, it gets the tooth moving. Use the Woodsen periosteal elevator or small dental spoon to separate the attached gingiva away from the tooth on the buccal and lingual (or palatal) sides. Take care not to tear the gingiva, and do not penetrate much below the level of attached gingiva (Fig. 22-8). This is an important step, and will allow the extraction of the tooth without tearing the gingiva. It also allows for a more apical purchase with subsequent instruments that will prevent root fracture.
Continue elevation in the following fashion:

■ The straight-handled elevator is inserted into the interdental space, perpendicular to the long axis of the tooth (Fig. 22-9).
■ The inferior portion of the blade should be resting on an exposed alveolar bone. The superior portion of the blade is then turned toward the tooth being extracted.
■ Strong, slow, controlled pressure gradually expands the alveolar bone, and the tooth will begin to move.
■ Elevators are turned, not used as pry bars.
■ Elevation may be attempted on both interdental spaces.

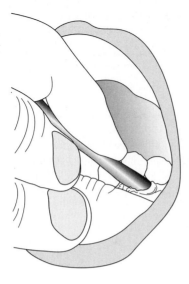

FIGURE 22-8 Separating attached gingiva with a Woodsen periosteal elevator.

- Great care must be taken not to loosen or injure the adjacent teeth. Do not rest against or lever against the adjacent tooth.
- Elevation is completed when the tooth is mobile. If there are adjacent, fully intact teeth, this step may be only minimally effective in loosening the tooth.

Step 2: Luxation

This step accomplishes complete expansion of the alveolar bone encasing the tooth and complete tearing of the periodontal ligament fibers. A tooth should never be torn

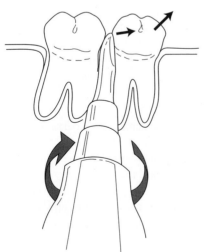

FIGURE 22-9 The handle of the small straight elevator is turned so that the occlusal side of the elevator blade is turned toward the tooth.

from its socket. The forceps are the major instrument of tooth luxation. At the completion of this step, the tooth is easily extracted.

- Correctly positioning the beaks of the forceps on the tooth is the key to successful luxation. The beaks should be applied as apically as possible (far down the tooth toward the root). After good elevation the forceps beaks should be able to wiggle slightly between the alveolar crest and the tooth. "Choking up" on the tooth in this way will lessen the possibility of root fracture (Fig. 22-10).
- Once the forceps beaks are in good position, hold the handles firmly, but do not squeeze too hard. You can easily fracture a tooth (especially a carious or previously restored tooth) with too much pressure to the handles. Occasionally this is unavoidable, and should be anticipated. Warn patients in advance so that they are not frightened.
- The beaks of the cow horn forceps are designed to fit between the roots of the mandibular molars. Apply them as apically as possible, then squeeze the handle firmly to engage the tooth. Pump the handle slightly up and down, then repeat this procedure once or twice to improve your purchase.

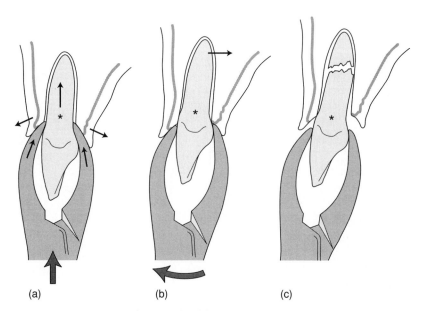

(a)   (b)   (c)

FIGURE 22-10. A: Extraction forceps should be seated with strong apical pressure to expand creatal bone and to displace the center of rotation as far apically as possible. B: If the center of rotation is not far enough apically, it is too far occlusally, resulting in excessive movement of the tooth apex. C: Excessive motion of the tooth apex caused by high center of rotation results in fracture of the root apex.

- The initial movement is always buccolingually. Slow, firm, sustained pressure gradually expands the socket and allows the tooth to "slip" out. Think of the mechanics involved in pulling a post from the ground.
- Use the fingers of your opposite hand to palpate the alveolar crest surrounding the tooth. Feel it expand as you luxate with slow, firm pressure. This also can provide a small amount of support for the bone to avoid fracture.

Step 3: Extraction

This step accomplishes the complete removal of an intact tooth. Some teeth are easier to get out than others, depending on their roots.

- Teeth with a single root are easily luxated and extracted with an unscrewing motion. Simply turn the tooth within its socket (Fig. 22-11).
- Teeth that have more than one root must be moved in a buccolingual direction only. Maxillary posterior teeth typically come out buccally.
- Mandibular posterior teeth usually come out buccally. Very rarely will they come out lingually, although this does not bode well for healing.

Once the tooth has been extracted it should be thoroughly inspected to be sure that it is intact and no part of the root has been left behind.

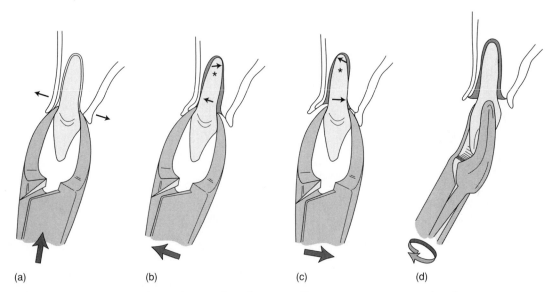

FIGURE 22-11 Extraction of a single rooted tooth. A: Maxillary incisors are extracted with a no. 150 forceps. The left hand grasps the alveolar process. The assistant helps to reflect and protect soft tissue. B: Forceps are seated as far apically as possible. C: Luxation is begun with labial force. D: Slight lingual force is used. E: The tooth is delivered to the labial incisor with rotational traction movement.

(a)   (b)   (c)   (d)

- The socket should be gently irrigated with sterile saline and inspected as well. A mouth mirror may be necessary.
- The expanded alveolar tissues should be compressed with firm digital pressure for several minutes. This will help control any bleeding.
- Sharply protruding segments of the alveolar bone, particularly in the posterior segments, may preclude adequate gingival coverage and healing. These should be gently filed smooth with the bone rasp before attempting to close the gingiva. Always irrigate and suction after using this instrument.

If extraction was atraumatic, the gingiva may not need suturing, but usually it does:

- Closure is best obtained with a simple figure-of-eight stitch around the socket, taking care to incorporate both interdental papilla (Fig. 22-12). Complete closure of the soft tissues is helpful, but not necessary, and often impossible in the maxillary posterior segments.
- Cotton gauze should be rolled and place directly over the extraction site. The patient is instructed to bite firmly against the roll to facilitate hemostasis. The roll should be left in place for approximately 20 minutes.
- It is normal for an extraction site to ooze slightly for up to 24 hours. Small amounts of heme inside the mouth can mix with saliva and appear to be large amounts of blood to the patient or to unsavvy health-care workers.

DISCHARGE INSTRUCTIONS

- Patients should be provided with extra cotton gauze and instructions to repeat the rolling and biting process if bleeding recurs. They should continue the pressure for 20- to 30-minute intervals. They should return if the bleeding is not controlled.
- Analgesics should be prescribed, and consideration should be given to a postoperative nerve block with a long-acting local anesthetic.

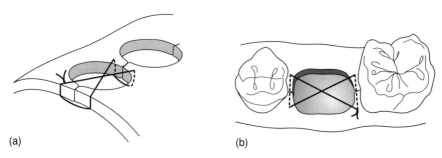

(a) (b)

FIGURE 22-12 A: Figure-of-eight stitch, which is occasionally placed over the top of the socket to aid in hemostasis. B: This is usually performed to help maintain a piece of oxidized cellulose in the tooth socket.

■ It is wise for the unskilled practitioner, whose technique may be less than atraumatic, to prescribe an empiric course of antibiotic therapy to all postoperative patients. Although the academics may argue about this point, a pinch of prevention is worth a pound of cure.

■ All diabetics or other immunocompromised individuals should receive postoperative antibiotics.

■ Patients should be instructed not to rinse their mouth for 48 hours. This may dislodge the clot and lead to a dry socket. They should avoid smoking, spitting, using straws, and drinking carbonated beverages for similar reasons. They should be instructed to avoid extremely hot or cold liquids, which may burn their lips or tongue after local anesthesia. A soft diet should be prescribed and they should be encouraged to continue eating.

■ Patients should be instructed to use ice packs to control swelling for 24 hours following dental extraction.

■ Patients should begin warm salt-water rinses four to six times per day after 48 hours. They also may resume brushing at this time, avoiding the area of the surgery.

WARNINGS

■ When an extraction involves grossly carious teeth or teeth with large restorations, anticipate tooth fracture. Choke up on the root with the forceps to get a good apical position.

■ Beware the cow horn and no. 88 forceps. These forceps are extremely useful, but can be dangerous if not used with a gentle hand. Never apply forceps to a tooth that has not been adequately luxated.

■ Extra care should be taken when extracting a primary tooth so that the permanent tooth bud is not injured. Never extract a primary tooth with a cow horn or no. 88 forceps.

■ Beware the right angle forceps in the maxillary anterior dentition. Maxillary teeth unscrew and come straight out. Never fulcrum off the palate with these forceps, or the buccal alveolar plate will fracture.

■ Expect minor soft tissue bleeding.

> **KEY POINT:**
>
> Minor bleeding, ecchymosis, edema, trismus, and discomfort are normal sequelae of uncomplicated dental extraction.

COMPLICATIONS   The best way to handle complications is to prevent them. Make an assessment about the potential for complications before you start. If you are not prepared to deal with the potential complications, do not extract the tooth.

PREVENTING COMPLICATIONS

■ Obtain a radiograph (if available) before extracting a tooth.
■ Adequately controlling and stabilizing instruments can prevent soft tissue injuries. Provide a stable support in case your instrument slips.
■ Don't attempt difficult extractions.

ALVEOLAR FRACTURE

■ Usually you can feel, and sometimes hear a cortical plate (surrounding bone) fracture when it occurs.
■ If the bone remains attached to periosteum, it will survive. Gently dissect the partially extracted tooth free of the bony segment. The soft tissue should always be sutured over a potential alveolar arch fracture.
■ If a large segment of the alveolus is mobile due to the fracture, stop trying to extricate the tooth. The mucosa should be closed, dental radiographs should be taken, and the tooth should be splinted to the adjacent teeth. The patient should be referred for immediate dental evaluation.
■ Small portions of alveolar bone occasionally come out along with the intended tooth. If this occurs at the apical tip of a maxillary molar, assume that there is an oroantral communication and treat accordingly. For other teeth, simply smooth the remaining alveolar process with the bone rasp and irrigate well. Antibiotics should probably be prescribed any time there is direct instrumentation of bone.

OROANTRAL COMMUNICATION

■ Extraction of a tooth whose roots appear to be involved with the maxillary sinus can lead to a maxillary sinusitis, or a chronic oroantral fistula.
■ If you suspect that the socket communicates with the sinus, have the patient blow against occluded nostrils. If a communication exists, air will bubble through the tooth socket into the mouth. Never probe the socket.
■ If a communication exists, the socket should be closed with a figure-of-eight suture, antibiotics should be prescribed, and the patient should be placed on sinus precautions.
■ Sinus precautions include no nose blowing or violent sneezing; no straws, cigarettes, or sucking; and no spitting or carbonated beverages.
■ A referral for dental evaluation should be made immediately.

MANDIBULAR FRACTURE Mandibular fractures occur when excessive force is applied when working in the posterior mandible, or when working with a mandible that is weakened by a large abscess or tumor.

■ A loud cracking sound, pain, and a suddenly uneven occlusion are the keys to diagnosis.

- Stop the extraction immediately.
- Inject a long-acting anesthetic and give antibiotics and analgesics.
- The patient's jaw should be gently guided into normal occlusion. Gentle force may be required to attain full occlusion of the fractured segment. This may be painful; you are reducing a fracture.
- This should be temporarily stabilized with a Barton bandage (head and chin bandage) (Fig. 22-13).
- Techniques for interdental wiring of fractures are described in many texts, but are probably impractical for field practitioners. These techniques can be exceedingly difficult, even in skilled hands under ideal conditions.

ROOT FRACTURE AND ROOT FRAGMENTS A root fracture is not an uncommon problem (but try to avoid it). It results from inadequate grasp with the forceps down toward the apex of the tooth, inadequate luxation, and excessive force.

- A reasonable attempt should be made by field personnel to remove fractured root tips. It may be necessary to raise a small soft tissue flap, and remove a small amount of buccal bone with the ronguers. There are many specialized instruments and techniques for root tip removal, whose description is beyond the scope of this text.
- If root tips cannot be successfully extracted, the soft tissue should be sutured closed, antibiotics and analgesics should be prescribed, and an x-ray should be taken if available. The patient should be immediately referred to a dental professional.

BLEEDING Soft tissue bleeding of the gums can be managed with direct pressure, injection of an epinephrine-containing local anesthetic, and closing the wound with sutures. Bleeding from an extraction site should be managed in a step-wise approach:

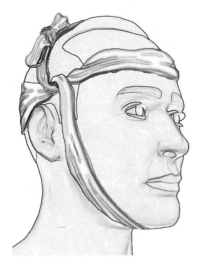

FIGURE 22-13 Barton bandage.

- After obtaining adequate anesthesia, apply direct pressure with moistened cotton gauze for 20 to 30 minutes. If bleeding continues, try this again.
- If available, Gelfoam or Surgicel can be packed into a continually bleeding socket. This material is secured with a soft tissue figure-of-eight stitch over the top of the socket.
- Occasionally, Gelfoam soaked in topical thrombin, or direct application of a microfibrillar collagen preparation, like Avitene, may be necessary.
- If these products are not available, try oversuturing.

NUMBNESS Direct or indirect nerve trauma from retraction, manipulation, or injection can lead to protracted anesthesia or dysesthesia. Symptoms generally resolve within 6 months, but can be permanent. The most typical nerve injury occurs in the distribution of the inferior alveolar or lingual nerves. If the symptoms do not resolve within a few weeks, these patients should be referred to a dental specialist.

ALVEOLAR OSTEITIS (DRY SOCKET) This is a common postextraction complication that presents with moderate to severe, dull, aching pain 2 to 4 days after an extraction. Examination reveals an open socket devoid of clot, and thus dry. Exposed bone will be visible in the socket base, and there will be a fetid odor. This is not an infection and does not require antibiotics.

- Treatment involves gentle warm, saline irrigation of the socket followed by equally gentle suction. A small piece of iodoform gauze impregnated with eugenol (oil of cloves) is then placed directly into the socket base. Topical benzocaine and a carrying medium such as balsam of Peru can be added to this if available. The combination of agents makes a nicely adherent and soothing paste, which is not readily diluted by saliva. Relief should be obtained within minutes. These ingredients are commonly available. However, if they are not, try any topical anesthetic and some form of carrying medium, such as petroleum jelly.
- This dressing needs to be changed daily until the pain is completely relieved. Patients will need oral analgesics. Resolution typically occurs within 3 to 5 days.

INCISION AND DRAINAGE

GENERAL CONSIDERATIONS Always remember that definitive treatment for an oral soft tissue infection of dental origin is either endodontic therapy or extraction. Extractions are difficult in the face of an abscess, and it is better to try to resolve the complicating soft tissue infection prior to extracting the tooth.

- Have suction ready before starting. If no suction is available, perform I&D with the patient sitting upright and be prepared to have them expectorate.
- It is never wrong to intraorally aspirate a simple, localized dental infection. This maneuver alone may provide a patient a day or so of relief and aid in clinically differentiating an abscess from a purely cellulitic process. Many seasoned dental

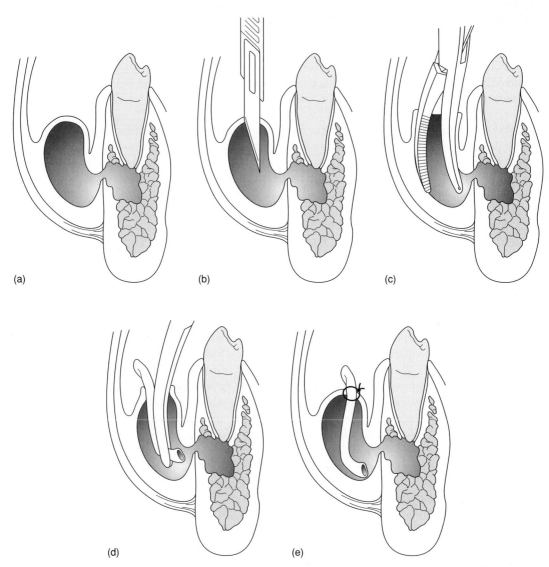

FIGURE 22-14 Small stab incision for irrigation and drainage. A: Periapical infection of lower bicuspid extending through the buccal plate and creating a sizable vestibular abscess. B: Abscess is incised with a no. 11 blade. C: The beaks of the hemostat are inserted through the incision and opened so that the beaks spread to break up any loculations of pus that may exist in abscessed tissue. D: A small rubber drain is inserted to the depths of the abscess cavity with the hemostat. E: A small rubber drain is sutured in place with a single black silk suture.

professionals advocate I&D for cellulitic processes as well. The thinking is that opening these mixed infections to the air will help kill anaerobes and prevent abscess formation.

METHOD There are two techniques for intraoral incision and drainage. Both are predicated by appropriate, proximal anesthesia (blocks are the preferred technique) and a radiograph. In addition, endocarditis prophylaxis should be addressed where appropriate.

- A simple stab incision can be made with a no. 11 blade in the area of greatest fluctulance, or that which best facilitates dependent drainage. Incision length should be no more than 1 cm.
- After the incision is made, a closed curved hemostat is inserted and spread in several directions to break up any loculations. Any remaining purulence should be expressed and suctioned.
- A sterile rubber drain (¼-inch Penrose or a strip of sterile surgical glove) should then be inserted to the depth of the abscess cavity (Fig. 22-14).
- The drain is then sutured in place to healthy mucosa (preferably attached gingiva) with a single silk suture.
- Remember that a large needle facilitates suturing intraorally. Take a big bite—mucosa is very forgiving,
- An intraoral drain should remain in place until the swelling has resolved and purulent drainage has ceased. This is typically achieved in 2 to 5 days. Patients should be placed on antibiotics and analgesics during this time.

The second technique for simple intraoral I&D differs only in the location of the incision.

- In this technique a no. 15 blade is used to make an incision at the alveolar crest within the gingival sulcus, scalloping around the teeth. The incision should extend one tooth medial and distal to the tooth in question or the area of abscess.
- The attached gingiva is then gently elevated from the bone with a blunt instrument. This blunt dissection is continued until the abscess cavity is penetrated. This typically occurs just with the level of unattached gingiva.
- The remainder of the procedure is as described above.
- This technique affords some mechanical advantages to the operator and is well tolerated postoperatively. It can be performed in both arches, buccally, palatally, and lingually.

SELECTED READING

Dickson M. *Where there is no dentist.* Berkeley, CA: Hesperian Foundation, 1983.
Holroyd SV, et al. *Clinical pharmacology in dental practice,* 4th ed. St. Louis: CV Mosby, 1988.

Regezzi JA, Sciubba JJ. *Oral pathology: Clinical pathologic correlations.* Philadelphia: WB Saunders, 1989.

Evers H, Haegerstam G. *Introduction to dental local anesthesia.* Fribourg, Switzerland: Mediglobe SA, 1990.

Malamed SF. *Handbook of local anesthesia,* 3rd ed. St. Louis: Mosby-Year Book, 1990.

Levine GN. *Pocket guide to commonly prescribed drugs.* Norwalk, CT: Appleton & Lange, 1993.

Simon RR, Brenner BE. *Emergency procedures and techniques,* 3rd ed. Baltimore: Williams & Wilkins, 1987.

CHAPTER 23

The Field Laboratory

Lynda Daniel-Underwood and Tamara L. Thomas

THE NEED FOR A FIELD LABORATORY

The practice of medicine in the field challenges the diagnostic skills of the clinician. The availability of electricity, running water, medications, laboratory studies, and radiographic equipment all affect the practice of medicine. In the urban, developed setting, medical practice often is largely dependent on extensive laboratory and radiographic testing. When practicing medicine in the field, you will be unable to rely on many of these laboratory or radiographic tests. The purpose of this chapter is to familiarize the clinician with the set-up and function of a basic field laboratory.

NEEDS ASSESSMENT

When working in a field setting, an important first step is to assess the diagnostic capabilities of the facility where you will be working. A simple needs assessment can be initiated with some basic questions.

ASSESS NEEDS AND MEDICAL CARE

- What setting are you practicing in—bush clinic, health-care clinic, regional hospital, or tertiary referral hospital?
- What types of medical conditions are common?

757

■ What are the routine standards of care? For example, do you have the ability to diagnose malaria? If not, do you have the resources to treat everyone with a fever with antimalarial medication? These basic decisions are important to address before establishing a new local standard of care.

ASSESS RESOURCES

■ What facilities are available? Are trained laboratory personnel available?
■ What are the laboratory capabilities? Do laboratory resources allow you to distinguish between different types of infectious diseases?
■ What are the radiographic capabilities?
■ Identify treatment resources (e.g., medical and surgical capabilities, inpatient care vs. outpatient care, medications available).
■ What do you need to help you practice?

KEY POINT:

Focus resources on most common local disease conditions seen; such as malaria, dysentery, respiratory infections, anemia.

SET-UP AND OPERATION OF A FIELD LABORATORY

LABORATORY DESIGN

Laboratory design may be challenging in rural, underdeveloped settings. Essential components include access to electricity, running water, and light. Ideally, there should be an area designated for processing specimens, located close to the entrance. The counter workspace should be at a comfortable height to accommodate sitting on a stool or standing. There also should be storage areas for chemicals and other supplies to decrease risk of contamination. All equipment necessary for specific testing should be located in the designated area, space permitting (e.g., chemical strips for urinalysis located in the area designated for urine testing). The area should be well ventilated with at least one window. If no electricity is available, the window may provide ambient lighting for microscope and reading tests with color changes.

LABORATORY EQUIPMENT AND SUPPLIES

The equipment necessary for a laboratory depends on its intended use. Basic equipment would include the following:

- Glucose monitor
- Centrifuge (if electricity available)
- Hemocytometer [white blood cell (WBC), red blood cell (RBC), platelet counts]
- Microscope
- Tally counter (for counting cells)
- Flame or heat source
- Containers for sharps disposal, chemical disposal

Basic supplies would include the following:

- Chemistry strips
- Urinalysis kit
- Glucose
- Diluting pipettes for WBC, RBC, platelet counts
- Chemicals
- Diluents
- Stains
- Capillary tubes (spin hematocrit)
- Slides (for stains)
- Tubes (for drawing blood and testing)
- Tourniquets (for drawing blood)
- Gloves
- Alcohol and/or betadine pads
- Cotton balls or 2 × 2 gauze pads
- Needles, syringes, or vacutainer blood-draw system

SANITATION AND BODY FLUID PRECAUTIONS

Sanitation issues arise in all hospitals and laboratories and are particularly difficult to address in many areas of the developing world. Blood and body-fluid precautions continue to be a challenge when practicing with limited resources. In addition, many areas of the developing world must reuse severely limited supplies. Disposable gloves and medical items often are cleaned and reused. Review of simple precaution principles in such areas can be helpful.

- Hand washing
- Gloves/masks
- Eye protection
- Patient care equipment cleaning
- Environmental control
- Cleaning/disinfection
- Handling and disposal of used needles

> ### KEY POINT: START WITH THE BASICS—HAND WASHING
>
> Hand washing is essential. Address these system issues in remote hospitals and clinics. Make it easy for health-care workers to wash their hands. Provide soap, water, and a sanitary drying system. This small cost easily pays for itself by decreasing the spread of infectious disease.

QUALITY CONTROL

Quality control is a challenge in the remote setting. Although there may be limited supplies, equipment, and staff, it is essential to be able to depend on your results. Develop simple guidelines for regular quality checks including simple methods for record keeping and equipment and material checks. The key is to keep it simple.

TESTS OF CHOICE IN THE FIELD SETTING

There are a number of simple tests that can be useful in remote settings to confirm the presence of organisms in suspected infectious diseases. The laboratory approach to some of the major infectious diseases in less-developed settings is described below and in Table 23-1.

CHOLERA Diagnosis of cholera is clinical in most cases. Confirmatory tests and cultures are important to confirm suspicions of an epidemic. These are usually performed at a regional reference laboratory.

ENTERIC FEVERS Typhoid and paratyphoid fevers are relatively uncommon, and most field laboratories do not have access to culture diagnosis or rapid diagnostic studies.

SHIGELLOSIS *Shigella* infestation is typically made by the presence of blood and polymorphonuclear cells (PMNs) in the stool. Culture confirmation is not useful in the field setting.

AMEBIC DYSENTERY Microscopy of fresh stool sample is sufficient for diagnosis.

BACTERIAL MENINGITIS Cerebrospinal fluid (CSF) gram stain or antigen detection may be accomplished in the field setting.

TUBERCULOSIS Microscopic examination of sputum (Ziehl-Neelsen) or acid-fast staining can be accomplished in the field laboratory. Cultures are usually available at the reference laboratory level.

TABLE 23-1 DIAGNOSTIC STUDIES IN THE FIELD LABORATORY

DISEASE	SPECIMEN TYPE	DIAGNOSTIC TEST	FIELD LABORATORY OR OR REFERENCE LABORATORY	CONFIRMATION TEST AT REFERENCE LABORATORY
AIDs/HIV	Serum	ELISA	Field	Serology
		Fluorescent antibody		
		Latex agglutination		
Anthrax	Lesion, sputum	Gram stain	Field	Culture ELISA
Dysentery/enteritis	Stool	Gram stain	Field	Culture
Cholera	Stool	Serum Latex agglutination	Field or reference	Culture
Dengue	Serum	None	Reference	Serology
Diphtheria	Throat swab	Gram stain	Field	Culture
Enteric fevers	Blood, stool, urine	Culture	Reference	Culture
Hepatitis	Urine	Test strip	Field	Serology
Intestinal protozoa	Stool	Microscopy	Field	None
Malaria	Blood	Microscopy	Field	None
Measles	Serum	ELISA	Reference	None
Meningitis	Cerebrospinal fluid	Coagglutination ELISA Latex agglutination Microscopy Gram stain	Reference	Culture
Plague	Aspirate, sputum	Gram stain	Field	Culture
Pneumonia	Sputum	Coagglutination ELISA	Reference	Culture
		Gram stain	Field	
Poliomyelitis	Serum	None	Reference	Culture Serology
Relapsing fever	Blood	Field's stain Giemsa stain Microscopy	Field	None
Tetanus	None	None	NA	NA
Tuberculosis	Sputum	Microscopy Acid fast stain	Field	Culture
Typhus	Serum	Weil Felix Indirect fluorescent antibody	Reference	Serology
Viral illnesses	Serum	Latex agglutination	Reference	Culture Serology
Whooping cough	Nasal aspirate	Fluorescent antibody	Reference	Culture

ELISA, enzyme-linked immunosorbent assay; NA, not applicable.

TABLE 23-2 DIFFERENTIAL DIAGNOSIS TABLES BASED ON SYMPTOM

DIARRHEA (With or without blood)

Bacterial	Parasitic	Viral	Other
Cholera and noncholera *Vibrio*	Malaria	Any viral illness	Lactose intolerance
Typhoid *(Salmonella)*	Schistosomiasis	HIV	Food poisoning
Campylobacter	Giardiasis		Pellagra (niacin deficiency)
Shigellosis	Protozoan (amebiasis— *Entamoeba, Crytosporidium, Balantidium coli*)		
Yersinia	Tapeworm (high concentration of parasites)		
Escherichia coli	Strongyloidiasis		
	Intestinal trematodes (opisthorchiasis, clonorchiasis		

COUGH

Bacterial	Parasitic	Other
Bacterial pneumonia (gram-positive and gram-negative	Flukes *(Paragonimus)*	Fungal *(Aspergillus,* blastomycosis, coccidioidomycosis, histoplasmosis)
Tuberculosis *(Mycobacterium)*	Ascaris	Viral, including HIV with superinfeciton
Chlamydial	Hookworm	
Diphtheria (pharyngitis with membrane)	Hydatid cyst rupture *(Echinococcus)*	
Pertussis *(Bordetella)*		
Inhaled anthrax		

RASH/BUMPS/LUMPS

Bacterial	Parasitic	Viral	Fungal	Other
Leprosy *(Mycobacterium)*	Dracunuliasis	Chicken pox	Ringworm	Arthropod (insect) bites
Meningiococcemia	Swimmer's itch (schistosomiasis)	Measles	Blastomycosis	Scabies
Cutaneous anthrax	Flukes *(Fasciola)*	HIV (Kaposi's sarcoma)	Candidiasis	Pellagra (niacin deficiency)

TABLE 23-2 DIFFERENTIAL DIAGNOSIS TABLES BASED ON SYMPTOM   *(continued)*

RASH/BUMPS/LUMPS *(continued)*

Bacterial	Parasitic	Viral	Fungal	Other
Plague *(Yersinia)*	Enterobiasis (anal pruritis	Rotavirus	Mucormycosis	Zinc deficiency
Yaws *(Treponema)*	Filarial infections *(Onchocerca)*	Dengue	Mycetoma (species varies)	Goiter
Rickettsia/Coxiella	*Trypanosoma* Leishmaniasis			
Chlamydia *Lymphogranuloma Venerum* (LGV)	Hydatid cyst leakage *(Echinococcus)*			

NEUROLOGIC

BACTERIAL	PARASITIC	VIRAL	OTHER
Bacterial meningitis	Cysticercosis (tapeworm)	Encephalitis (various species)	Beriberi (thiamine deficiency)
Tetanus, botulism *(Clostridium)*	Trypanosomiasis (African)	Rabies	Pernicious anemia (Vitamin B_{12} or folate deficiency)
Relapsing fever *(Borrelia,* headache)	Toxoplasmosis	Yellow fever, dengue (headache)	Pellagra (niacin deficiency)
	Acanthamoeba, Naegleria		
	Enterobius (headache)		

JAUNDICE

BACTERIAL	PARASITIC	OTHER
Not too many bacterial infections cause jaundice, unless they cause a fulminant infection/sepsis	Malaria	Viral hepatitis
	Liver flukes	Yellow fever (severe cases)
	Hepatic amebiasis	Liver cancer
	Diphyllobothrium (after long-standing pernicious anemia)	
	Hydatid cyst obstruction of biliary tree *(Echinococcus)*	

TABLE 23-2 DIFFERENTIAL DIAGNOSIS TABLES BASED ON SYMPTOM *(continued)*

SEXUALLY TRANSMITTED DISEASES

BACTERIAL	PARASITIC	VIRAL	OTHER
Gonorrhea (*Neisseria*)	*Trichomonas*	Herpes	Candidiasis
Chlamydia trachomatis	*Entamoeba histolytica*	Hepatitis A and B	Pubic lice
Syphilis (*Treponema pallidum*)	*Giardia*	Cytomegalovirus	Scabies
Chancroid (*Hemophilus ducreyi*)		Human papillomavirus	
Donovanosis (*Calymmatobacterium granulomatis*)			
Neonatal sepsis from group B beta hemolytic streptococcus			
Nongonococcal urethritis (*Ureaplasma urealyticum*)			
Bacterial vaginosis (*Gardnerella vaginalis*, may be associated with multiple organisms)			

BLOOD PARASITES Microscopic examination using Giemsa- or Field-stained specimens can be used to diagnose malaria or relapsing fever.

LEISHMANIASIS Direct serum agglutination is available in some field settings.

SYMPTOM-BASED APPROACH

When practicing in the limited setting, workups may need to be symptom based. Tests are limited, and evaluation for potential illnesses have to be based on these symptoms. For better test selection, patient signs and symptoms may guide your choice of specimens. The above is an abbreviated list of organisms and diseases to consider based on symptom (Table 23-2).

BASIC LABORATORY METHODS IN THE FIELD

The following is a list of the most common and useful diagnostic tests that should be available in a basic field laboratory.

COMPLETE BLOOD COUNT

Complete blood count is a valuable study that evaluates for possible infection, anemia, and other hematologic abnormalities. A CBC includes WBC, RBC, hematocrit, and platelet counts (Table 23-3). A limited CBC may be performed in the field with the following materials (Fig. 23-1):

TABLE 23-3 STEPS IN PERFORMING A COMPLETE BLOOD COUNT

STEP	RED BLOOD CELLS	WHITE BLOOD CELLS	PLATELETS
1	Mix venous blood in EDTA as anticoagulant by inversion	Same	Same
2	Place tip of the Thoma pipette for RBC beneath the surface of the blood, aspirate to the 0.5 mark. Accuracy is important in this step to avoid error.	Same, except use the Thoma WBC pipette and aspirate to the 0.5 mark.	Same, except aspirate to the 1.0 mark.
3	Wipe the tip off, place tip into the diluting fluid (Gower's solution), and draw up to the 101 mark.	Same, except diluting fluid is gentian violet; draw up to the 11 mark.	Same, except diluting fluid is ammonium oxalate, draw up to the 101 mark.
4	Close both ends of the pipette with fingers and shake for 30 s at 90 degree angle (if no special shaking machine is available, shake the pipette for 2–3 m).	Same	Same
5	Discard the first 3–4 drops and gently load the hemocytometer making sure no bubbles are seen and it is not overflowing. Allow the cells to settle for a few minutes in a covered Petri dish on top of a moistened filter paper or equivalent (to prevent drying).	Same	Same
6	Use a microscope, count the five small squares of the center larger square, making sure the cells are not counted twice. Multiply the total by 10,000 to calculate the RBC count (RBCs/μL).	Same, except count the four large squares on the corners. Multiply the average number of cells counted by 200 to calculate the WBC count (WBC/mm^3).	Same as RBC, except count both sides of the hemocytometer. If the total number of platelets counted is less than 100, then more small squares need to be counted. The platelets appear round or oval and frequently contain dendritic processes. The formula is number of cells counted divided by number of squares counted times dilution times 250 (platelets/μL).

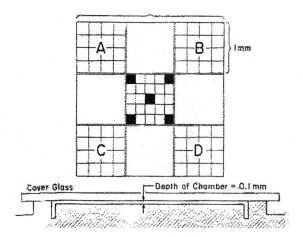

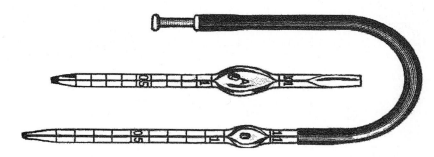

FIGURE 23-1
Picture of
hemocytometer
(with various
counting areas
outlined) and
Thoma RBC and
WBC pipettes.

- Centrifuge
- Capillary tubes
- Hemocytometer
- Thoma RBC pipettes
- WBC pipettes and appropriate diluent

SPUN HEMATOCRIT Fill a capillary tube with blood (approximately three-fourths full) and seal one end with clay. Place the tube in the centrifuge and spin. Measure the hematocrit by placing the tube on a hematocrit capillary tube reader (Fig. 23-2).

RED BLOOD CELL COUNT Reagents used for performing RBC count include the following:

- EDTA (in purple top tube)
- Blood-Gower's solution
- Sodium sulfate
- Glacial acetic acid
- Distilled water

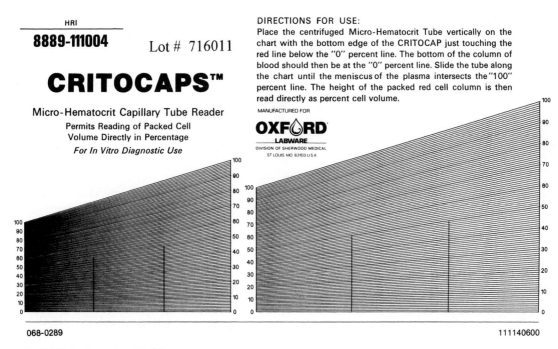

FIGURE 23-2 Hematocrit table.

WHITE BLOOD CELL COUNT Reagents used for performing white blood cell count include the following:

- Diluting fluid (glacial acetic acid and 1% aqueous solution of gentian violet)
- Distilled water
- EDTA (purple top) blood draw tube

PLATELET COUNT Reagents used for performing platelet count include the following:

- EDTA (purple top) blood draw tube
- 1% ammonium oxalate in distilled water

WHITE BLOOD CELL COUNT DIFFERENTIAL To check the differential on the WBC count, take the following steps (Fig. 23-3):

Step 1: Make a smear on a slide and allow to air-dry.
Step 2: Examine the WBCs using Wright's stain (no fixative needed).
Step 3: Cover the slide with plenty of stain and allow to stand for 2 minutes.
Step 4: Add the buffer on top of the stain, and gently blow to mix and make an even distribution. Look for a metallic green scum to appear.

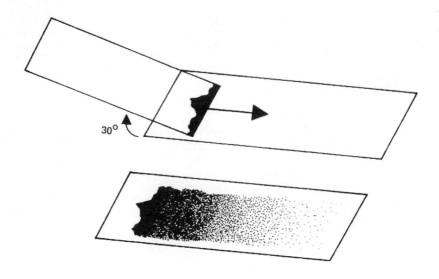

Gently pull the A slide into the blood
allowing it to spread across the edge.
Quickly push it forward.

A smear should form with a thick portion at
the start and a thinner (feather) portion at
the end.

FIGURE 23-3 Method for preparing smear.

Step 5: Rinse gently with distilled water (keeping the slide horizontal) for 15 to
30 seconds. Drain the excess water and allow the slide to air dry. View
under oil immersion.

Step 6: A total of 100 cells are counted; each individual cell type is counted as a
percentage.

The appearance of WBCs for the differential count is described in Table 23-4.

PREGNANCY TESTING

Many urine pregnancy tests are available, including over-the-counter varieties. Each
test requires 2 to 5 minutes for completion. Tests only require the patient to hold the
reaction strip in the urine stream. These strips also can be dipped into a specimen cup
containing the patient's urine. Individually wrapped tests are protected in humid
environments. The test also includes a control test to assure it is being completed
properly. Follow the manufacturer's instructions.

TABLE 23-4 APPEARANCE OF WHITE BLOOD CELLS FOR DIFFERENTIAL

Neutrophil	
Band	
Lymphocyte atypical	
Monocyte	
Eosinopil	
Basophil	
Platelets	

STAINS

GIEMSA STAIN (BLOOD PARASITES) Giemsa is a differential stain for leukocytes, blood parasites, and fecal protozoa. Reagents used for this staining method include the following:

- Giemsa stain
- Methyl alcohol
- Pure glycerol
- Phosphate buffer (pH 6.4)

The procedure is performed as follows:

1. Immerse thick smears in distilled water to hemolyze red blood cells; do not allow to dry. Fix thin smears in absolute methanol for 1 minute and allow thin smears to dry.
2. Flood with Giemsa stain and allow to react for 30 to 60 seconds.
3. Rinse with phosphate buffer (pH 6.4), drain, dry, and examine.

GRAM STAIN Gram stain is used to separate bacteria into two groups and visualize their morphology (Fig. 23-4). Reagents used for this staining procedure include the following:

- Crystal violet
- Ammonium oxalate
- Ethyl alcohol, 95%
- Iodine

GRAM STAIN
↓

Streptococcus	Clostridium	Neisseria	
Enterobacteriacea			
Staphylococcus	Bacillus		Campylobacter
*			
Enterococcus	Nocardia		Pseudomonas
Listeria *	Actinomyces		Vibrio (curved)
Erysipelothrix	Mycobacterium (AFB)		Moraxella
	Lactobacillus		Legionella
			Brucella *
			Haemophilus*
			Bordetella*
			Treponema
			Bacteriodes
			Fusobacterium

* Coccobacillus
AFB   Acid fast bacillus

FIGURE 23-4 Flow chart for gram stain.

- Potassium iodide
- Distilled water
- Acetone (decolorizer, 95% alcohol also may be used but is slower; mixing 1:1 with acetone is more rapid)
- Safranine O

The procedure is performed as follows:

1. Flood smear with crystal violet solution and let stand for 1 minute.
2. Rinse briefly with tap water and drain off excess water.
3. Flood smear with iodine solution and let stand for 1 minute.
4. Rinse briefly with tap water and drain off excess water.
5. Decolorize with solvent until it flows colorlessly from the slide.
6. Counterstain with safranine for 10 seconds.
7. Wash, dry, and examine (gram-positive stain is blue/violet, gram-negative stain is red/pink).

TIPS AND TRICKS:

During gram staining take time to adequately decolorize the specimen; otherwise you will have difficulty identifying gram-negative organisms. To verify that your stain was adequately decolorized, examine the nuclei of PMNs—adequately decolorized nuclei stain pink; inadequately decolorized nuclei stain purple.

ACID-FAST STAIN (AFB, KINYOUN) Acid-fast stain identifies organisms with cell walls resistant to decolorization, particularly mycoplasma. Reagents used for this staining procedure include the following:

- Kinyoun carbolfuchsin
- Basic fuchsin
- Alcohol, 95%
- Phenol crystals
- Distilled water
- Acid-alcohol (hydrochloric acid, concentrated and ethyl alcohol, 95%)
- Methylene blue in distilled water

The procedure is performed as follows:

1. Flood fixed smear with Kinyoun carbolfuchsin; let stand for 2 minutes.
2. Wash with tap water and decolorize by dropping acid-alcohol over the smear until it flows colorlessly.

3. Wash with tap water and counterstain with methylene blue for 20 to 30 seconds.
4. Wash, blot dry, and examine. Acid-fast organisms stain red.

TRICHROME STAIN A procedure using this permanent stain for intestinal parasites can be performed rapidly (within 1 hour). A fresh specimen is best, but specimens preserved in polyvinyl alcohol fixative also may be used (Table 23-5). Reagents used for trichrome staining include the following:

- Schaudinn solution (ethyl alcohol, 95% and mercuric chloride, saturated aqueous)
- Glacial acetic acid and acetic acid
- Iodine
- Trichrome stain
- Carbol-xylene (phenol and xylene)
- Xylene
- Mounting media

TABLE 23-5 TRICHROME STAIN FOR INTESTINAL PARASITES

Fresh Specimen	Preserved Specimen
Flood the fresh specimen with Schaudium fixative for 5 min at 50°C, 1 h at room temperature.	Place two to three drops on slide and allow to dry thoroughly.
Rinse with 70% alcohol with iodine for 1 min.	Rinse in 70% alcohol for 10–20 min.
Repeat 70% alcohol for 1 min.	Repeat alcohol 70% for 3–5 min.
Cover with trichrome stain for 2–8 min (thicker specimens require 8 min).	Trichrome stain for 6–8 min.
Dip in acidified 95% alcohol one drop glacial acetic acid in 10 mL alcohol) for 10–20 s.	Dip in acidified 95% alcohol one drop glacial acetic acid in 10 mL alcohol) for 10–20 s.
Rinse twice with 95% alcohol.	Rinse twice with 95% alcohol and leave the second rinse for 5 min.
Place in 100% alcohol for 3 min.	Carbol-xylene solution for 5–10 min.
Place in xylene for 3 min.	Xylene for 10 min.
Mount with cover slip using mounting media.	Mount with cover slip using mounting media.

BLOOD BANKING

Blood banking capabilities vary in the developing world. Remote hospitals may have blood typing with or without cross-matching capabilities. If you are working in a remote setting, be sure to investigate the options for transfusion.

In some hospital settings the only available blood donors are patient family members who give blood for an acute need. If blood will be used from selected donors in the field, adequate materials must be available for transfusion, and testing capability must be available for determination of type, RH, and HIV and hepatitis B status.

CHEMISTRY

Testing for blood chemistry is usually accomplished using analyzers, with the exception of specific reagent strips, such as those that test for glucose. The function and use of chemistry analyzers is beyond the scope of this chapter.

URINALYSIS

Urinalysis is a basic but extremely important tool used to screen for infection, endocrine or metabolic abnormalities, and renal disease. The ideal container for any specimen is a sterile or chemically clean wide-mouthed bottle. The container must be sterile if a culture is to be performed.

Two types of specimen are used: (a) random mid-stream, which may be used for routine urinalysis and culture, and (b) clean catch mid-stream or catheterized specimen, which is ideal for culture.

The urine should be preserved if analysis is being delayed for 1 or more hours.

- Refrigeration is the most common and acceptable method, but may not be readily available in the field.
- Toluene may be used, but it is flammable and must be pipetted carefully over the urine.
- Thymol is also an alternative, but can interfere with tests for protein using heat and acetic strips.

Table 23-6 summarizes the clinical implications of urine appearance.

Reagent strips are commercially available that test the chemical characteristics of urine without an instrument (Table 23-7). The strips are compared with a color chart located on the reagent bottle (can be read by a non–color-blind person). False-positive and false-negative conditions may occur based on the method used.

Prepare urine for microscopic examination as follows (Table 23-8):

1. Mix the urine specimen; pour 10 mL into a graduated, conical centrifuge tube and centrifuge for 5 minutes at 400× gravity.

TABLE 23-6 CLINICAL IMPLICATIONS OF URINE APPEARANCE

Appearance	Etiology
Colorless	Very dilute urine, diluted urine
Yellow	Normal, B vitamins, nitrofurantoin
Yellow-orange	Concentrated urine, pyridium, bilirubin, urobilinogen
Yellow-green	Biliverdin
Yellow-brown	Biliverdin, bilirubin, senna, rhubarb, cascara
Red	Blood (contamination from menses), hemoglobin, myoglobin, porphyria, beets, amidopyrine, phenindione
Red-pink	(In alkaline urine) rhubarb, senna, cascara, phenophathalein
Red-purple	RBC, hemoglobin, methemoglobin, myoglobin
Brown-black	Methemoglobin, homogentisic acid, melanin, methyldopa, on standing alkaptonuria
Blue-green	*Pseudomonas* infection, indigo
Cloudy	Crystals or amorphous substances, WBCs, RBCs, bacteria, yeast, spermatozoa, prostatic fluid, mucus, feces, x-ray contrast
Milky	Pyuria, fat (lipids, chyle)

2. Decant 9 mL of the supernatant and resuspend the sediment.
3. Place one drop on a glass slide and coverslip, trying not to generate bubbles. Examine the slide under low power (for casts, crystals, other noncellular findings). Report as cells per low-power field (lpf).
4. Switch to high power and examine the slide (for RBCs, WBCs, bacteria, yeast, parasites, sperm, and other cellular findings). Report as cells per high-power field (hpf).

GLUCOSE TESTING

Many types of glucose meters are available. Testing is as easy as placing one drop of blood from a finger stick and waiting 1 to 2 minutes. A full drop of blood should be obtained without excessive trauma or squeezing, which causes cell injury and tissue fluid leakage. Control strips or reagents should be used to ensure that the instrument is functioning properly. Cleaning the instrument following the manufacturer's recommendations reduces the risk of erroneous results. Document the control results for quality improvement.

TABLE 23-7 URINE CHARACTERISTICS AND ASSOCIATED DISEASE STATES

Chemical Characteristics	Associated Disease
pH	Acid: severe diarrhea, dehydration, fever, high-protein diet Alkaline: renal tubular acidosis, severe vomiting, urea-splitting bacteria (*Proteus* species), acute and chronic renal disease, respiratory alkalosis
Specific gravity	Low: diabetes insipidus, use of diuretics, excess water intake High: dehydration, SIADH, x-ray contrast material
Protein	Renal disease, multiple myeloma, macroglobulinemia
Glucose	Diabetes mellitus, rena; glucosuria
Ketone	Fasting or starvation diets, dehydration, carbohydrate metabolism abnormalities
Bilirubin	Jaundice, hepatitis, obstructive biliary tract diseases, liver cell damage, hemolytic anemias tend not to produce bilirubinuria, only when conjugated bilirubin is elevated
Nitrates	Infection
Urobilinogen	Certain liver disease, hemolytic disease
Blood	Gynecologic bleeding or menstruation (poor collection), renal disease, infection, hemoglobinuria (intravascular hemolysis), paroxysmal nocturnal hemoglobinuria lysis of RBCs in urine or from trauma), myoglobinuria (crushing injuries, myocardial infarction)
Leukocyte esterase	Infection (presence of WBCs)

SIADH, (Syndrome of inappropriate secretion of antidiuretic hormone).

MICROBIOLOGY

Samples of blood, urine, cerebrospinal fluid, sputum, stool, and mucous membrane may be examined to diagnose infections from various microorganisms. Choosing the correct samples for each diagnosis is dependent on knowledge of the organisms themselves. In addition to these tissue samples, many serologic tests are being developed for the diagnosis of parasites. Although some serologic tests now available are specific, the use of these tests must be approached with some caution in the developing world because of cost and reliability. Many serologic tests for antibodies do not indicate current activity of infection (they are sensitive but not specific). They cannot specify whether the patient has had a prior infection or has an active infection with the parasite. In this situation, a negative serologic test result is useful to exclude exposure, whereas a positive test result does not establish infection. In those traveling from nonendemic areas to endemic areas with a brief, defined exposure to an organism, positive serology may be helpful.

TABLE 23-8 URINE MICROSCOPIC CHARACTERISTICS OF CLINICAL ENTITIES

Microscopic Characteristics	Diagram	Disease
Mucous strands		Normal
Epithelia cells		Normal
WBC	 granulation Lobulated nucleus	Infection, inflammation
RBC	 crenated	Contamination from gynecologic bleeding, infection, kidney stones, inflammation
Bacteria/yeast/parasites, sperm	Bacteria (rods or cocci) Yeast budding	Infection, sperm may represent recent coitus or retrograde ejaculation
Casts 　Hyaline		Stasis or urine flow, acidic pH, proteinuria
Granular		Inflammatory, renal disease, degradation of cellular cast
WNCs		WBCs into the nephron
RBCs		Always pathologic, renal parenchymal/glomerular basement membrane injury
Crystals	Uric acid Calcium oxalate	Varies

PARASITES

Parasites are organisms that belong to several groups, and include helminths and protozoa. Many parasites can infect humans, but they are difficult to diagnose. Diagnosis is dependent on a number of factors, and patient history is key, including geographic, occupational, immune status, and presenting characteristics. A basic knowledge of the epidemiology and life cycles of parasites assist in making the diagnosis. This knowledge also helps identify what type of tissue sample will yield the diagnosis.

How are parasitic infections diagnosed?

- History: The clinician must rely on a detailed travel, food, transfusion, and socioeconomic history to make the diagnosis of a parasite disease.
- Clinical manifestations: Clinical manifestations of parasitic infections alone are seldom enough to ensure the diagnosis.
- Laboratory: Routine laboratory tests seldom are helpful. Eosinophilia has been recognized as an important clue to some parasitic disease.
- Tissue diagnosis: Once these diseases are considered, the diagnosis is usually straightforward. The diagnosis usually depends on demonstrating and identifying the parasite in stool, urine, sputum, blood, or tissues.

Diagnosis of a parasitic disease depends on demonstrating the parasite in body fluids and tissues. Certain parasites are easily recovered, but others are more difficult to recover. Parasites are commonly recovered in stool, blood, or body tissues. In situations where parasite recovery is uncommon, additional resources may be necessary, including immunodiagnosis, parasite antigens, and DNA probes.

INTESTINAL PARASITES   Many protozoa and helminths are excreted in the feces. When collecting fecal samples, the following precautions should be taken:

- Avoid contamination with water or urine. Collect prior to treatment if possible (antidiarrheal agents change the consistency of the stool).
- Because most parasites shed into the feces in cycles, collect a minimum of three samples on alternate days.
- If specimens are shipped, keep in polyvinyl alcohol to preserve protozoal trophozoites.

When analyzing fecal samples, the following steps should be taken:

- Both macroscopic and microscopic analyses should be performed.
- The microscopic examination focuses on three methods: direct wet mount, concentration techniques, and permanent stains. Ensure that each procedure is performed prior to accepting a negative report for ova and parasite.

Occasionally specimens other than stool must be examined to find intestinal parasites. Duodenal aspirates or small bowel biopsies may be helpful with giardiasis and strongyloidiasis. Proctoscopy or sigmoidoscopy may be needed to find *Entamoeba histolytica* and *Schistosoma mansoni*.

DIRECT WET MOUNT

- Normal saline
- Dilute iodine solution (kills parasites, which eliminates motility)

CONCENTRATION TECHNIQUES Concentration techniques detect a smaller number of protozoan cysts and worm ova. Either formalin-ether sedimentation (all parasites sediment but not all float) or zinc-sulfate flotation may be performed.

PERMANENT STAINS Prepare slides for trophozoites before concentration. Cysts and ova slides can be made from concentrated specimens. Permanently stained smears allow for more definitive identification:

- Iron-hematoxylin stain
- Trichrome stain (can be prepared in approximately 1 hour)

BLOOD AND TISSUE PARASITES Parasites living in the blood and tissues of the host are more difficult to identify.

BLOOD Direct examination of the blood is helpful for diagnosing some parasitic conditions (malaria, leishmania, trypanosomas, micofilaria). Multiple collections of specimens over several days may be required because the organism concentration in the blood may vary.

When analyzing blood samples, the following methods may be used: wet mount, concentrated specimen techniques, and permanent staining. Giemsa or Wright's stain is effective for detecting microfilarial worms and blood protozoa. The most common parasites detected in Giemsa-stained blood smears are plasmodia, microfilariae, and African trypanosomes.

TISSUE PARASITES Choosing a diagnostic technique for tissue parasites can be difficult. Lung flukes and occasionally other helminths may be found in sputum using appropriate concentration techniques. Skin biopsy is an appropriate approach for onchocerciasis, and muscle biopsy can be used for diagnosing trichinosis.

When analyzing tissue samples, the following methods may be used: wet mount, concentrated specimen techniques, and permanent staining. Trichrome/iron hematoxylin is effective for detecting all tissue helminths in body fluids other than blood.

In situations where parasite recovery is uncommon, other techniques are required to make the diagnosis, including immunodiagnostic and nucleic acid hybridization.

Although tests for circulating antibodies for some parasitic diseases have been available for some time, there have been limitations in both sensitivity and specificity. New highly reactive tests along with more purified homologous antigens have significantly increased sensitivity and specificity. Reliable serologic procedures are available for diagnosing the following conditions:

- Amebiasis
- Cysticercosis
- Echinococciasis
- Paragonimiasis
- Schistosomiasis
- Strongyloides
- Toxocariasis
- Toxoplasmosis
- Trichonosis

DNA probes are available for detecting a variety of parasites but have limitations as diagnostic tools relating to the technical aspects of the procedure.

HELMINTHS

NEMATODES (ROUNDWORMS) Humans, the definitive host of medically pertinent species, harbor the adult that produces offspring. The pathogenicity of the intestinal nematodes may be due to migration of larvae through body tissue, piercing of the intestinal wall, blood-sucking activities of the worm, or allergic reaction to substances or the larvae. The pathology of tissue roundworms is primarily due to host responses to parasite secretions and excretions.

UNIQUE CHARACTERISTICS Large numbers of *Ascaris* organisms can form an intestinal obstruction as well as malabsorption. The hookworm has less-severe pulmonary manifestations, and in the intestinal form patients may develop iron-deficiency anemia and hypoalbuminemia due to chronic blood loss (Appendix 23-A).

DIAGNOSIS Direct or concentrated stool specimens can diagnose intestinal nematodes. Fresh stool specimens should be used for *Strongyloides* to avoid confusion with hookworm. (Hookworm eggs may hatch and look like *Strongyloides rhabdiform* larvae.) Do not delay treatment to differentiate between species. Enterobiasis may be found more easily on anal mucosa.

Tissue nematode diagnosis often requires biopsy from a tissue cyst. Presumptive diagnosis may be made by residence in an endemic area, characteristic findings on radiography [calcified cysts in soft tissues on plain radiographs and multiple enhanced/unenhanced lesions on computed tomography (CT) or magnetic resonance imaging (MRI)].

In pulmonary manifestations of ascariasis, larvae and eosinophils may be demonstrated in the sputum. Tissue nematodes are diagnosed with eosinophilia, tissue biopsy, and a number of serologic tests. Positive immunoglobulin G (IgG) antibodies may indicate prior exposure.

FILARIAE Adult filariae live in numerous human tissues requiring an arthropod intermediate host in which the larvae undergo maturation. The microfilariae are more prevalent in peripheral blood at certain times of the day (periodicity) in some species.

UNIQUE CHARACTERISTICS Adult forms reside in human connective tissue or lymphatics (Appendix 23-B).

DIAGNOSIS Diagnosis may be suspected on the basis of travel or exposure history as well as symptoms consistent with filarial infections. The definitive diagnosis depends on recovery of microfilariae or filariae in clinical samples. In lymphatic forms, parasites are recovered from venous blood obtained over a period of several days. Repeated samples are important due to periodicity. Concentrating specimens (by sedimentation or filtration) will increase diagnostic sensitivity. Examine the blood smear for the presence or absence of a sheath and the tail area for presence or absence of cells that exhibit a characteristic pattern of nuclei. In addition, lymphatic parasites can sometimes be found in tissue biopsy samples. If there are no circulating microfilariae, diagnosis depends on clinical symptoms, exposure history, associated laboratory findings, and serology.

CESTODA (TAPEWORMS) Tapeworms are hermaphroditic, long, ribbonlike, and flattened dorsoventrally. Tapeworm parasites divide their life cycle between two or more animal hosts. The adult tapeworm lives in the intestinal tract of the vertebrate host and in the tissue of the intermediate host.

UNIQUE CHARACTERISTICS Humans may serve as either the definitive or intermediate host for different cestode species (Appendix 23-C).

DIAGNOSIS Diagnose intestinal tapeworms by examining the stool for parasite eggs and segments. *T. saginata* eggs may be difficult to differentiate from *T. solium* eggs. Do not delay therapy waiting for speciation. Definitive diagnosis of cystercosis requires examination of biopsy material from a tissue cyst.

Presumptive diagnosis may be made based on a history of residence in an endemic area, characteristic finding on radiographs (calcified cysts in soft tissues), scans (multiple, low-density enhanced/unenhanced lesions on CT or MRI), and suggestive laboratory findings. Suggestive CSF findings in neurocysticercosis include decreased glucose, increased total protein, and lymphocytic and eosinophilic pleocytosis. Serum and CSF enzyme-linked immunosorbent assay and Western blot testing for IgM and IgG anticysticercae antibodies have a sensitivity rate of 75% to 100%. IgG only indicates prior exposure.

TREMATODE Flukes have flattened leaf-shaped bodies with muscular suckers and complex life cycles. Specific freshwater snails are required as an intermediate host for all species. Pathology of schistosomiasis depends on degree of infection, length of infection, reinfection, sensitivity of host, and kinds of tissue infected. A condition known as swimmer's itch occurs with the schistosomes when cercariae of infected animals and birds enter the human skin, causing an allergic dermal response. These do not develop into adults.

UNIQUE CHARACTERISTICS A number of trematodes can cause human disease and infect the human biliary tree, lung, intestinal tract, and blood stream. Each species that infects humans has a specific geographic zone of transmission and is defined by the distribution of the snail vector (Appendix 23-D).

DIAGNOSIS Schistosomiasis requires recovery of characteristic eggs in urine, stool, or a biopsy for definitive diagnosis. Concentration methods may be necessary, and in patients with a low worm load, tissue biopsies may be helpful. Identification of schistosome eggs is based on the characteristic morphology and size. Serologic tests are available but are not very specific.

Liver, lung, and intestinal infections are acquired by eating poorly cooked food containing infectious parasite cysts. Larvae hatch within the intestine and mature there, migrate to the liver, or penetrate the bowel wall and migrate through tissue to the liver or lungs. Liver flukes often present with a triad of fever, hepatomegaly, and eosinophilia. Diagnosis may be made with stool or duodenal aspirate for eggs. In endemic areas, restrict the patient's diet prior to testing to exclude the spurious recovery of eggs in stool.

Because *Paragonimus* eggs are usually absent from sputum during the first 3 months, repeated sputum samples should be obtained. Chest radiography may show patchy infiltrates, ringlike shadows, or pleural thickening. Diagnosis also may be made from pleural fluid and feces. Circulating antibodies may be needed to confirm the diagnosis. Stool specimens or duodenal aspirates may identify clonorchiasis, as well as leukocytosis, eosinophilia, increased alkaline phosphates, and abnormal liver imaging scans (CT and ultrasonography).

PROTOZOA

AMEBAE *Entamoeba histolytica*, the major pathogen in this group, is the causative organism of amebic dysentery. *Dientamoeba fragilis* is also considered mildly pathogenic and does not form cysts. All others are felt to be commensals. Identifying pathogenic versus nonpathogenic forms is key to ensuring proper treatment. Transmission typically occurs via the fecal-oral route.

UNIQUE CHARACTERISTICS It is unknown why this organism is an intestinal commensal in the majority of infected individuals and causes severe disease in others.

DIAGNOSIS Cysts or trophozoites in the stool indicate intestinal manifestations. At least three specimens are necessary to make the diagnosis. Stool specimens may be examined by wet mount, and amebae are identified by the characteristic morphology and linear motion across the microscopic field. Fix the specimens in polyvinyl alcohol for later staining. Permanent staining may be required for identification.

FLAGELLATES The pathogenic protozoa inhabit the gastrointestinal tract, atria, blood stream, or tissue of humans. Many flagellates parasitize humans, although only four (*Giardia lamblia, Trichomonas, Trypanosoma, Leishmania*) commonly induce disease.

DIAGNOSIS In *Trichomonas* infections, motile trophozoites can be seen on a wet mount of vaginal secretions (Appendix 23-F).

Giardia can be diagnosed by the presence of trophozoites or cysts in the stool or duodenal aspirates. Enzyme immunoassay detecting antigens and serologic markers (anti-IgM antibodies) can be helpful. Cultures are available but not widely used. Leishmaniasis can be identified via skin ulceration biopsy and via smear, section, or stain of pathognomonic Leishman-Donovan bodies. Material also should be cultured in a liquid media. In disseminated visceral form, aspirates from bone marrow, liver, spleen, and lymph nodes also may be examined for Leishman-Donovan bodies.

Trypanosoma produces a local chancre at the site of innoculation, which localizes in blood vessels leading to a local vasculitis. Diagnosis can be made by observing lymph node aspirates, blood, and CSF for trypomastigotes with a wet mount or stained smear. If test results are negative, concentrate specimens. IgM antibodies and a sample card agglutination test also can be used.

SPOROZOA This group includes the organisms causing malaria and toxoplasmosis. Most species produce a spore, which after ingestion or injection is infective for the definitive host. Sporozoa are distinguished by alternating cycles of sexual (sporogony) and asexual reproduction, which is completed in different host species.

Of the four species of malaria, *Plasmodium falciparum* is the most deadly. *P. vivax* is the most widely disseminated and prevalent. *Toxoplasma gondii* and *Pneumocystis carinii* are usually held in check by a competent host immune system.

UNIQUE CHARACTERISTICS See Chapter 9

DIAGNOSIS Malarial parasites can be demonstrated in stained smears of peripheral blood in most symptomatic patients. Distinctions between *Plasmodium* species are made by examination of both thick and thin blood smears (Table 23-9).

STAINS

Giemsa and Wright's stains may help to identify erythrocytic parasites. Giemsa is preferred for the following reasons:

TABLE 23-9 DISTINGUISHING SPECIES OF MALARIA

SPECIES	PLASMODIUM FALCIPARUM	PLASMODIUM MALARIAE	PLASMODIUM OVALE	PLASMODIUM VIVAX
Trophozoite				
Schizont		6–12 merozoites		12–24 merozoites
Gametocyte	Crescent shaped	Ovoid	Round	

- High quality
- Suitable for both thick and thin smears
- Stable in tropical climates

The merits of Wright's stain are as follows:

- High quality
- Thin smears
- Deteriorates in the tropics because the methanol base is hygroscopic

BLOOD SMEAR

THIN SMEAR

- Prepare blood exactly like a WBC differential (air dry rapidly, fix with anhydrous methanol, and stain).

■ Examine red cells in the tail of film under oil immersion; report as number of parasitized erythrocytes per 1,000 cells.

THICK SMEAR Erythrocytes are lysed with water before staining, allowing concentration of parasites. This assists in detection of mild parasitemia.

■ Place one drop of blood on the slide and stir in a circular motion to a diameter of 2 cm.
■ Should be an uneven thickness
■ Dry thoroughly and stain without fixing.
■ In a thick-smear layer of erythrocytes, overlap and lyse during staining. This creates a 20- to 40-fold concentration.
■ Both parasites and white cells are counted, and the number of parasites per unit volume is calculated from the leukocyte count.

READING SMEARS

■ Count number of parasitized red cells (per 1,000 RBCs).
■ Note predominant stage of parasite development (prognosis).
■ Count number of neutrophils containing phagocytosed parasite pigment.

Morphologic differences are the primary means of diagnosing *Plasmodium* species infection. The three characteristic features for identification are:

■ Red nuclear chromatin
■ Blue cytoplasm
■ Brownish-black malarial pigment (hemozoin)

Morphology of the parasite and the infected RBC can vary by both stage and species. Morphologic differences between the four *Plasmodium* species allow their speciation on the stained smear. Most importantly, distinguish between *P. falciparum* and the other three *Plasmodium* species. *Plasmodium falciparum* may be identified by the morphology of intraerythrocytic parasites (banana-shaped gametocytes, predominance of small ring forms, and rings with double nuclei) and by erythrocytes (multiply infected erythrocytes, normal-sized erythrocytes, and high parasitemia).

> **DID YOU KNOW?**
>
> The quantity of the parasites in the blood smear can help predict disease severity as well as monitor the treatment response.

Know which of the *Plasmodium* species are endemic in the region in which the exposure took place. Paroxysms vary with species. Parasitemia fluctuates, and the number of organisms increase during paroxysms. Parasites may be difficult to detect during the first few days of an initial attack; therefore, repeat smears must be performed.

DNA probes and antigen detection are available and may play an important role in the future of malaria diagnosis. Available serologic tests are used primarily for epidemiology purposes.

APPENDIX 23-A NEMATODES

SCIENTIFIC (COMMON NAME)	EPIDEMIOLOGY	DISEASE-PRODUCING FORM, AND LOCATION IN HOST	HOW INFECTION OCCURS	MAJOR DISEASE MANIFESTATIONS	DIAGNOSTIC STAGE (SPECIMEN OF CHOICE)
Enterobius vermicularis (pinworm)	Worldwide	Adult worms in colon, eggs on perianal region	Eggs are laid by the female on the perianal skin and transmitted from hand to mouth	Perianal itching	flattened edge↑ **Diagnosis:** eggs found by cellophane test
Trichuris trichiura (whipworm)	Worldwide, especially in warm, moist climate	Adult worms in colon	Ingestion of eggs containing mature larvae from infected soil or food	Light infection may be asymptomatic. Heavy infection causes enteritis, diarrhea, and rectal prolapse.	**(Picture of egg)** hyaline plug at both ↑ **Diagnoses:** eggs in feces
Ascaris lumbricoides (large intestinal roundworm)	Worldwide, especially in warm, moist climate	Larval migration through liver and lungs. Adult worms in small intestine	Ingestion of eggs containing mature larvae from infected soil or food	Light infection may be asymptomatic. Heavy infection causes pneumonia from larval migration. Diarrhea and bowel or appendix obstruction.	Nonfertilized amorphous mass shell albuminous covering **Diagnosis:** eggs (or adults) in feces

SCIENTIFIC (COMMON NAME)	EPIDEMIOLOGY	DISEASE-PRODUCING FORM, AND LOCATION IN HOST	HOW INFECTION OCCURS	MAJOR DISEASE MANIFESTATIONS	DIAGNOSTIC STAGE (SPECIMEN OF CHOICE)
Trichinella spiralis (trichina worm)	Cosmopolitan	Adult worms in small intestine	Ingestion of encysted larvae in undercooked meat (pork or bear)	Gastric distress, fever eye edema, acute muscle pain, eosinophilia	**Diagnosis:** encysted *larvae in muscle* biopsy; serology
Necator americanus (New World hookworm)	United States, West Africa, Asia, South Pacific	Larval migration, ground itch, adult worms in small intestine	Eggs shed in feces, mature in soil, larvae hatch and mature; infective (filariform) larvae penetrate host skin, especially in the feet	Repeated infection results in larval dermatitis with later pulmonary symptoms. Microcytic hypochronic anemia from chronic blood loss if heavy infection and poor diet	2-8 cell stage **Diagnosis:** eggs in feces
Ancylostoma duodenale (Old World hookworm)	Europe, Brazil, Mediterranean area, and Asia	As above	As above	As above	Resembles *Necator americanus*
Strongyloides stercoralis (Threadworm)	Cosmopolitan warm areas	Larval migration, pulmonary signs, adult worms in small intestine	Immature (rhabditiform) larvae shed in feces and mature in soil. Infective (filariform) larvae penetrate host skin, especially feet. Autoinfection by by maturing larvae occurs in intestine.	Repeated infection results in larval dermatitis with later pulmonary symptoms. Heavy infections cause abdominal pain, vomiting, and diarrhea. Moderate eosinophilia; immunosuppressed host may suffer severe symptoms or death from heavy infection as autoinfection can occur.	**Diagnosis:** rhabditiform larvae in feces

787

APPENDIX 23-B FILARIAE

SCIENTIFIC (COMMON NAME)	EPIDEMIOLOGY, PERIODICITY, INTERMEDIATE HOST	DISEASE-PRODUCING FORM, AND LOCATION IN HOST	HOW INFECTION OCCURS	MAJOR DISEASE MANIFESTATIONS	DIAGNOSTIC STAGE (SPECIMEN OF CHOICE)
Wuchereria bancrofti (Bancroft's filaria)	Tropics, nocturnal periodicity, *Culex, Aedes,* and *Anopheles* mosquitoes	Adults live in lymphatics, microfilariae in the blood	Filariform larvae are injected into the blood when the mosquito bites a human	Invades lymphatics and causes granulomatous lesions, chills, fever, eosinophilia and elephantiasis	Sheath present, no nuclei in tail **Diagnosis:** microfilariae in blood, serology
Brugia malay (Malayan filaria)	Far East, nocturnal periodicity, *Anopheles* and *Mansonia* mosquitoes	As above	As above	As above	Sheath present, 2 nuclei in tip of tail

APPENDIX 23-B FILARIAE *(continued)*

SCIENTIFIC (COMMON NAME)	EPIDEMIOLOGY, PERIODICITY, INTERMEDIATE HOST	DISEASE-PRODUCING FORM, AND LOCATION IN HOST	HOW INFECTION OCCURS	MAJOR DISEASE MANIFESTATIONS	DIAGNOSTIC STAGE (SPECIMEN OF CHOICE)
Loa loa (eyeworm)	Africa, diurnal periodicity, *Chrysops* fly	Adults migrate throughout the subcutaneous tissues, microfilariae in the blood	Filariform larvae are injected in the blood when the fly takes a blood meal	Chronic and benign disease; Calabar swelling is a transient subcutaneous swelling	Continuous row of posterior nuclei, sheath present **Diagnosis:** microfilariae in blood serology
Onchocerca volvulus (blinding filaria)	Central America and Africa, no periodicity, *Simuluim* (black fly)	Adult live in fibrotic nodules, microfilariae migrate subcutaneously	As above	Chronic and nonfatal; allergy to microfilariae causes local symptoms—may cause blindness	no sheath, nuclei not terminal **Diagnosis:** adults in excised nodules, microfilariae in tissue scraping of nodule

789

APPENDIX 23-B FILARIAE *(continued)*

SCIENTIFIC (COMMON NAME)	EPIDEMIOLOGY, PERIODICITY, INTERMEDIATE HOST	DISEASE-PRODUCING FORM, AND LOCATION IN HOST	HOW INFECTION OCCURS	MAJOR DISEASE MANIFESTATIONS	DIAGNOSTIC STAGE (SPECIMEN OF CHOICE)
Dracunculus medinensis (Guinea worm)	Africa, Asia, South America, no periodicity, *Cyclops* (crustacean)	Adults live in subcutaneous tissues, females migrate larvae released from skin ulcer	Ingestion of water containing crustaceans infected with larvae	Systemic allergic symptoms and local ulcer formation	**Diagnosis:** adult in skin ulcer larvae released into water

SCIENTIFIC (COMMON NAME)	EPIDEMIOLOGY	DISEASE-PRODUCING FORM, AND LOCATION IN HOST	HOW INFECTION OCCURS	MAJOR DISEASE MANIFESTATIONS	DIAGNOSTIC STAGE (SPECIMEN OF CHOICE)
Hymenolepis nana (dwarf tapeworm)	Worldwide (common in southeastern United States)	Adults live in the small intestine	Egg is ingested by humans via contaminated food or water; autoreinfection is common	Light infection (asymptomatic); heavy infection causes abdominal pain, diarrhea, headaches, and dizziness	Polar thickening / 50μm x 30μm / hooklets **Diagnosis:** eggs in feces
Taenia saginata (beef tapeworm)	Cosmopolitan in beef-eating countries	As above	*Cysticercus bovis* larvae are eaten by humans in undercooked beef	Most people are asymptomatic but can experience abdominal pain, diarrhea, and weight loss	15–30 lateral uterine branches in the gravid proglattid in four suckers in the scolex **Diagnosis:** eggs or proglottid in feces

APPENDIX 23-C CESTODES *(continued)*

SCIENTIFIC (COMMON NAME)	EPIDEMIOLOGY	DISEASE-PRODUCING FORM, AND LOCATION IN HOST	HOW INFECTION OCCURS	MAJOR DISEASE MANIFESTATIONS	DIAGNOSTIC STAGE (SPECIMEN OF CHOICE)
Taenia solium (pork tapeworm, cysticercosis)	Worldwide	As above, *racemose, cysticercus* in brain	*Cysticercus cellulose* larvae are eaten by humans in undercooked pork; accidental ingestion of eggs	As above; if in the brain, may have seizures, or death can occur	Egg is identical to *Taenia saginata* 7–12 lateral uterine branches in the gravid proglattid and four suckers and a crown of hooks in the scolex
Diphyllobothrium latum (broad fish tapeworm	Temperate areas where freshwater fish is eaten	As above	Plerocercoid larvae accidentally ingested by humans in undercooked freshwater fish		 **operculum**
Sparganosis		Pleuroceroid larva in tissues of humans	Human ingests infected copepod crustacean	Inflammatory reaction around pleurocercoid larvae developing in tissues	

APPENDIX 23-D TREMATODES

SCIENTIFIC (COMMON NAME)	EPIDEMIOLOGY	DISEASE-PRODUCING FORM, AND LOCATION IN HOST	HOW INFECTION OCCURS	MAJOR DISEASE MANIFESTATIONS	DIAGNOSTIC STAGE (SPECIMEN OF CHOICE)
Fasciolopsis buski (large intestinal fluke)	Far East	Adults live in the small intestine	Ingestion of encysted metacercariae on raw vegetation	Edema, eosinophilia, diarrhea, malabsorption, and even death in heavy infection	operculum **Diagnosis:** eggs in feces
Fasciola hepatica (sheep liver fluke) Zoonosis	Worldwide; humans are accidental host	Adults live in the bile ducts	As above	Traumatic tissue damage and irritation to the liver and bile ducts jaundice and eosinophilia can occur.	Similar to *F. buski* **Diagnosis:** eggs in feces
Clonorchis sinenesis (Oriental or Chinese liver fluke)	Far East	As above	Ingestion of encysted metacercariae in uncooked fish	Jaundice and eosinophilia in acute phase; long-term heavy infections lead to liver disease	**Diagnosis:** eggs in feces

793

APPENDIX 23-D TREMATODES *(continued)*

SCIENTIFIC (COMMON NAME)	EPIDEMIOLOGY	DISEASE-PRODUCING FORM, AND LOCATION IN HOST	HOW INFECTION OCCURS	MAJOR DISEASE MANIFESTATIONS	DIAGNOSTIC STAGE (SPECIMEN OF CHOICE)
Paragonimus westermani (Oriental lung fluke)	Far East, India, parts of Africa	Adults live encysted in lung	Ingestion of encysted metacercariae in uncooked crab or crayfish	Chronic fibrotic disease resembling tuberculosis cough with blood-tinged sputum	operculum — terminal thickening **Diagnosis:** eggs in *sputum* or feces
Heterophyes heterophyes Metagoniumus yokogawai (the heterophyids)	Far East	Adults live in small intestine	Ingestion of encysted metacercariae in uncooked fish	No intestinal symptoms unless very heavy infection	Less rounded shoulders than *Clonorchis* — knob **Diagnosis:** eggs in feces

APPENDIX 23-D TREMATODES *(continued)*

SCIENTIFIC (COMMON NAME)	EPIDEMIOLOGY	DISEASE-PRODUCING FORM, AND LOCATION IN HOST	HOW INFECTION OCCURS	MAJOR DISEASE MANIFESTATIONS	DIAGNOSTIC STAGE (SPECIMEN OF CHOICE)
Schistosoma mansoni (Manson's blood fluke; Bilharzia; swamp fever)	Africa, Middle East, and South America	Adults in venules of the colon. (Eggs are trapped in liver and other tissues).	Fork-tailed cercarieae burrow into the capillary bed of feet, legs, or arms	Granuloma formation around eggs, toxic, and allergic reactions	large lateral lateral spine **Diagnoses:** eggs in feces
Schistosoma japonicum (Oriental blood fluke)	Far East	As above	As above	As above, except symptoms are more severe due to greater egg production	small lateral spine **Diagnosis:** eggs in feces

APPENDIX 23-D TREMATODES *(continued)*

SCIENTIFIC (COMMON NAME)	EPIDEMIOLOGY	DISEASE-PRODUCING FORM, AND LOCATION IN HOST	HOW INFECTION OCCURS	MAJOR DISEASE MANIFESTATIONS	DIAGNOSTIC STAGE (SPECIMEN OF CHOICE)
Schistosoma haematobium (bladder fluke)	Africa, Middle East, and Portugal	Adults in venules of the bladder and rectum; eggs caught in tissue	As above	Bladder colic with blood and pus, systemic symptoms are mild	 terminal spine **Diagnoses:** eggs live in urine

APPENDIX 23-E PROTOZOA

SCIENTIFIC (COMMON NAME)	EPIDEMIOLOGY	DISEASE-PRODUCING FORM, AND LOCATION IN HOST	HOW INFECTION OCCURS	MAJOR DISEASE MANIFESTATIONS	DIAGNOSTIC STAGE (SPECIMEN OF CHOICE)
Entamoeba histolytica (amebic dysenery)	Worldwide	Trophozoites in large intestinal mucosa, liver, or other tissue	Ingestion of cyst in fecally contaminated food or water	Enteritis with abdominal pain and bloody dysentery	**Diagnosis:** cysts and trophozoites in feces
Dientamoeba fragilis (none)	Worldwide	Trophozoites in large intestine	Ingestion of trophozoite	Diarrhea	**Diagnosis:** trophozoites in feces (no cysts formed)

797

SCIENTIFIC (COMMON NAME)	EPIDEMIOLOGY	DISEASE-PRODUCING FORM, AND LOCATION IN HOST	HOW INFECTION OCCURS	MAJOR DISEASE MANIFESTATIONS	DIAGNOSTIC STAGE (SPECIMEN OF CHOICE)
Balantidium coli (balantidial dysentery)	Worldwide	Trophozoites in large intestinal mucosa	Ingestion of cysts	Moderate or mild dysentery	**Ciliate** Cyst **Diagnosis:** trophozoites or cysts in feces
Acanthamoeba spp, Naeglaria spp, (amebic meningoencephalitis)	Worldwide	Amoebic trophozoites in brain	Accidental entrance through nasopharyngeal mucosa	Rapid death	**Diagnosis:** trophozoites in cerebrospinal fluid (wet mount)
Babesia spp Zoonosis	Worldwide	Trophozoites in red blood cells	Tick bite	Fever; symptoms can resemble malaria	**Diagnosis:** trophozoites in blood smear

APPENDIX 23-F FLAGELLATES

SCIENTIFIC (COMMON NAME)	EPIDEMIOLOGY	DISEASE-PRODUCING FORM, AND LOCATION IN HOST	HOW INFECTION OCCURS	MAJOR DISEASE MANIFESTATIONS	DIAGNOSTIC STAGE (SPECIMEN OF CHOICE)
Giardia lamblia (traveler's diarrhea)	Worldwide	Trophozoites in large intestinal mucosa	Ingestion of cysts in fecally contaminated food or water	Mild to severe dysentery; malabsorption syndrome	"monkey" face **Diagnosis:** cysts and trophozoites in feces

APPENDIX 23-F FLAGELLATES *(continued)*

SCIENTIFIC (COMMON NAME)	EPIDEMIOLOGY	DISEASE-PRODUCING FORM, AND LOCATION IN HOST	HOW INFECTION OCCURS	MAJOR DISEASE MANIFESTATIONS	DIAGNOSTIC STAGE (SPECIMEN OF CHOICE)
Trichomonas vaginalis (trich)	Worldwide	Trophozoites	Sexual contact	Irritating, frothy vaginal discharge, men usually symptomatic	**Undulating membrane** → **Diagnosis:** trophozoites in urine or vaginal smear (no cysts formed)
Leishmania tropica (Oriental sore, Baghdad boil)	Mediterranean area, Asia, Africa, Central America	Leishmania in macrophages in skin lesion	Bite of *Phlebotomus spp* (sand fly)	Self-healing skin lesion	**Diagnosis:** LD bodies in macrophages around lesion

APPENDIX 23-F FLAGELLATES *(continued)*

SCIENTIFIC (COMMON NAME)	EPIDEMIOLOGY	DISEASE-PRODUCING FORM, AND LOCATION IN HOST	HOW INFECTION OCCURS	MAJOR DISEASE MANIFESTATIONS	DIAGNOSTIC STAGE (SPECIMEN OF CHOICE)
Leishmania brazeliensis (New World leishmaniasis, espundia, uta)	Central and South America	Leishmania in macrophages in skin lesion and mucocutaneous tissue	As above	Self-healing skin lesion, later ulceration of cephalic mucocutaneous tissue	**Diagnosis:** recovery of leishmania forms from lesion
Leishmania donovani (kala-azar, dumdum fever),	Mediterranean area, Asia, Africa, South America	Leishmania in macrophages in skin lesion and somatic organs	As above	Initial skin lesion later daily double spiking fever, enlarged liver and spleen, death in late stages.	**Diagnosis:** leishman donovan (LD) bodies in early lesion, organ tissue biopsy later
Trypanosoma gambiense (sleeping sickness)	West Africa	Trypanosomes in blood, lymph nodes, later in central nervous system	Bite of *Glossina spp* (tsetse fly)	Fever, lymphadenopathy (Winterbottom's sign), enlarged spleen and liver, lethargy and death	>30 μm x 1.5 to 3.5 μm **Diagnosis:** trypanosomes in blood, xenodiagnosis

APPENDIX 23-F FLAGELLATES *(continued)*

SCIENTIFIC (COMMON NAME)	EPIDEMIOLOGY	DISEASE-PRODUCING FORM, AND LOCATION IN HOST	HOW INFECTION OCCURS	MAJOR DISEASE MANIFESTATIONS	DIAGNOSTIC STAGE (SPECIMEN OF CHOICE)
Trypanosoma rhodesiense (sleeping sickness)	East Africa	As above	As above	As above, except course more acute and fatal than *T. gambiense*	See above
Trypanosoma cruzi (Chaga's disease)	South America	Early trypanosomal and critidial forms in blood; later LD bodies in heart and other tissue	Infected feces of *Triatoma spp* (kissing bug, reduviid bug) rubbed into bite site	Fever enlarges spleen and liver, Romaña's sign (edema around eyes), chronic damage to heart and digestive tract; acute death especially in children	more "C" shaped **Diagnosis:** trypanosomes in blood, xenodiagnosis

APPENDIX 23-G SPOROZOA

SCIENTIFIC (COMMON NAME)	EPIDEMIOLOGY	DISEASE-PRODUCING FORM, AND LOCATION IN HOST	HOW INFECTION OCCURS	MAJOR DISEASE MANIFESTATIONS	DIAGNOSTIC STAGE (SPECIMEN OF CHOICE)
Toxoplasma gondii (toxoplasmosis)	Worldwide	Trophozoites intracellularly in all organs; pseudocysts in brain and other tissue	Ingestion of oocysts; ingestion of trophozoites or pseudocysts in undercooked meat; congenital passage of trophozoites	Fever, enlarge lymph nodes, in the fetus or neonate can cause damage. Can cause acute infection in the immunosuppressed	**Diagnosis:** serology

CHAPTER 24

Protecting Yourself: Traveling Healthy

Michael J. VanRooyen and C. James Holliman

To be an effective health-care provider in the field, it is essential to pay close attention to your personal health. Keeping healthy while working abroad requires preparing for common health problems and following some simple preventive health guidelines. This chapter provides information about the most common traveler-acquired illnesses and how to prevent them. Also discussed are issues relating to security and injury prevention while working abroad.

EPIDEMIOLOGY OF TRAVEL-RELATED ILLNESSES

The main causes of mortality in travelers are generally the same as those in their countries of origin.

> **KEY POINT:**
>
> Deaths among travelers from exotic infectious illnesses or wildlife are actually very uncommon. The most common causes of death are due to cardiac illness and accidents.

Most foreign travelers die from cardiovascular disease (acute myocardial infarction or sudden cardiac arrest, 42%) or trauma (24%), most commonly as a result of vehicular crashes (6.9%), falls (5.7%), drowning (3.9%), homicide (3.1%), and airplane crashes (2.9%). Nineteen percent of deaths are from medical causes, mostly pneumonia. Higher risk areas for travel-related mortality are Central America and northern South America;

TABLE 24-1 PREVENTION OF TRAVEL-RELATED ILLNESSES

General guidelines for international travel
   Always seek pretravel medical advice.
   Take your malaria prophylaxis as prescribed.
   Take personal precautions against insects.
   Assemble a travel medical kit.
   Be prepared to purify your drinking water.
   Take appropriate dietary precautions.
   Don't walk barefoot out of doors.
   Don't go into potentially schistosomiasis-laden water.
   Avoid exposure to body fluids (take your own syringes for injection
      medications such as insulin).
   Protect yourself from accidental injury.
Constructive behaviors to avoid travel injuries
   Wear bike or motorcycle helmets.
   Use seatbelts.
   Use hired local drivers if possible.
   Know local traffic rules.
   Be aware of hotel fire safety rules and exits.
   Trravel in groups.

the lowest relative risk areas are Canada and Western Europe. Table 24.1 lists some of the simple things you can do to avoid having health problems while working in the field.

PREPARING FOR FOREIGN TRAVEL

Three or four months in advance of your trip you should obtain a passport and check with your travel agent or appropriate embassies regarding the need for a visa. To acquire a visa you may need to visit the embassy or mail your stamped passport to the embassy with the necessary application forms and fees. There also may be a courier service available through your travel agent that will, for a fee, deliver and pick up your passport at the embassy. If you do not already have one, you may want to obtain a credit card for charging your travel expenses, which helps decrease the amount of money you need to carry with you. Credit cards also often offer a better exchange rate. Money access machines are becoming more common (check with your bank regarding fees, services, and liability for lost cards) and offer ready cash in local currency.

United States passport requirements are a birth certificate, current photo ID (driver's license, etc.), two recent color photos (each 4 × 4 cm, which can be obtained at most American Automobile Association offices and many photo supply stores), and completed passport application forms and necessary fees. You can call your local post office for the nearest passport office to obtain the necessary forms and apply for your passport (you must apply for your first passport in person; later renewals can be made by mail).

Travel paperwork to bring along with your passport when traveling includes an International Certificate of Vaccination (filled in with all immunizations recorded by your physician or travel clinic), signed prescriptions or verification letters about prescription medications you are taking, invitation letters from local hosts, and government permits for any special activities you are planning.

If you will be providing health services abroad, be sure to find out if you will need a medical license for the country where you will be working. Be sure to bring copies of medical licenses and diplomas even if there is no formal requirement, in case certification requirements are necessary. It is also helpful to make extra copies of travel documents for yourself and friends or family members before you depart on a trip. Carry a list of emergency contacts and your travel documents with you at all times in the event of an emergency. Copies of your itinerary and local contacts should be left at home. You also may want to update your will and power of attorney prior to departure.

IMMUNIZATIONS

There are several immunizations that should be updated regardless of your travel destination. These include tetanus/diphtheria (safest recommendation is every 5 years), oral polio vaccine, and MMR (measles, mumps, rubella). If you have preexistent cardiopulmonary disease, you should also receive the influenza and pneumococcal vaccines (Table 24.2).

Additional immunizations to consider for rural travel to developing countries or for health-care workers include typhoid vaccine, meningococcal vaccine, hepatitis A and B vaccines (these need to be started at least 3 months in advance of your trip), rabies vaccine, and plague vaccine. Other vaccinations (more related to the countries you will

TABLE 24-2 RECOMMENDED IMMUNIZATION
FOR INTERNATIONAL TRAVEL

VACCINATION	RECOMMENDED, REQUIRED, OR OPTIONAL	SCHEDULE
Yellow Fever	Required	Booster every 10 years
Cholera	Optional	Only for targeted high-risk areas (refugee camps)
Hepatitis A	Recommended	Initial series
Hepatitis B	Recommended	Initial series
Meningococcal meningitis	Recommended	Revaccination 3-4 years after initial dose
Rabies	Recommended	Booster if titer is low after primary course
Polio	Required	Booster for travelers to developing countries
Measles (MMR)	Required	Booster for those born on or after 1957
Japanese encephalitis	Optional	
Tetanus (DPT)	Recommended	dT booster every 10 years
Influenzae		
Haemophiles influenzae	Not recommended	
Influenza vaccine	Optional	High-risk travelers only (>65, chronic illness)
Pneumococcal vaccine	Optional	High-risk travelers only (>65, chronic illness)

be visiting) include yellow fever (equatorial Africa and South America), cholera (India and other countries with current outbreaks), and Japanese encephalitis (rural China and rural Japan). Yellow fever vaccination is required for entry in many countries in East Africa. Some countries also require proof of HIV-negative status for medical workers.

MALARIA PROPHYLAXIS

Malaria prophylaxis is necessary when traveling to endemic regions. There are several options for malaria prophylaxis, depending on the country being visited and the degree of exposure within the country (urban vs. rural). See later section on Malaria.

TABLE 24-3 BASIC TRAVEL MEDICAL KIT

Wound care
  Gauze (4 × 4 and wrap)
  Povodine iodine pads
  Bandages (assorted)
  Sterile strips ("butterflies")
Supplies
  Thermometer
  Elastic wrap
  Plastic bag
  Antibacterial soap
  Insect repellant (with DEET)
  Scissors, tweezers, and tape
Medication
  General
    Acetaminophen tablets
    Acetaminophen with codeine tablets
    Extra personal medication (such as anithypertensives)
    Short-acting benzodiazapine for sleep
    Throat lozenges/cough drops
  Antibiotics
    Malaria prophylaxis/treatment
    Ciprofloxacin 500-mg tablets
    Metronidazole 750-mg tablets
    Triple antibiotic eye ointment
  Gastrointestinal
    Loperamide tablets
    Antacid tablets
    Histamine blocker
  Antiallergy
    Diphenhydramine 25-mg tablets
    EPI-Pen injectable epinephrine
    Prednisone 20-mg tablets
    2% hydrocortisone cream

TABLE 24-4 TRAVEL HEALTH RESOURCES

International Association for Medical Assistance to Travelers: (716) 754-4883 (United States), (519) 836-0102 (Canada). This service can give you the phone number and address of English-speaking physicians in different countries who are available for a fixed fee to see tourists.

CDC Travel Health: Excellent travel health resource www.cdc.gov/travel

Communicable Disease Center: (404) 639-3311, (404) 639-2888 (nights and weekends). Advice on infectious and parasitic diseases.

U.S. Department of State Overseas Citizens' Emergency Center: (202) 647-5226. This number is mainly for notification of legal problems.

Travel Health Online: www.tripprep.com

Travel Medicine Advisor Customer Service: 1 (800) 688-2421.

ADDITIONAL PRETRAVEL PREPARATIONS

Diarrhea prophylaxis should be considered; choose either antibiotics or bismuth subsalicylate (Pepto-Bismol), and take your first dose 1 day before your trip. Obtain supplies of other prescription medications; it is best to leave them in their labeled bottles. Be sure to include sufficient supply to cover a few extra days.

TRAVEL MEDICAL KIT COMPONENTS

Many people consider it helpful to assemble a traveler's medical kit before leaving the country. Most travelers, particularly health workers, tend to pack far too many things in a travel medical kit. Because you will probably want to keep your medical kit with your carry-on luggage, consider limiting its contents to a few essentials (Table 24.3). A more comprehensive kit is described in Appendix 4.

TRAVEL HEALTH CONSULTATION RESOURCES

With the advent of the Internet, there is no shortage of sites available to provide information for the foreign traveler. There are a number of contacts and Web sites available to the international traveler (Table 24.4).

SPECIFIC TRAVEL-RELATED ILLNESSES

TRAVEL-RELATED DIARRHEA

EPIDEMIOLOGY Diarrhea is defined as the passage of at least three unformed stools (stool conforms to container boundaries) in a 24-hour period and the presence of at least one symptom of enteric disease (abdominal pain, nausea, emesis, fever, etc.). A loose stool means one or more unformed evacuations that total less than 100 mL per 24 hours without enteric disease symptoms. Dysentery means frequent small volume stools that are bloody and mucoid.

The incidence of travel-related diarrhea for a person from a developed country traveling in a developing country is 20% to 25% per week (peaking at 60% overall). Intermediate risk areas are the Caribbean, Mediterranean, Japan, Israel, and South Africa. Low-risk areas are the United States, Canada, Northern Europe, and Australia (risk 2% to 5%). The attack rate remains high for a traveler for up to 1 year of residence in a foreign country; it then decreases, but not to the baseline local level. Of all cases of travel-related diarrhea, 10% to 40% are serious enough to interfere with travel plans.

The etiologic pathogens causing travel-related diarrhea include the following:

- Enterotoxigenic *Escherichia coli*: 40%
- *Shigella* species: 15%
- *Salmonella* species: 7% to 10%
- Other *E. coli*: 10% to 15%
- Viruses (Norwalk, etc.): 5% to 10%
- Parasites (*Giardia, Amoeba,* etc.): 5% to 10%
- Uncommon: *Clostridium perfringens, Vibrio cholera, Staphylococcus aureus, Cryptosporidium*

DIAGNOSIS The diagnosis of traveler's diarrhea is made by history alone; that is, diarrhea with enteric symptoms (blood or mucus) and travel exposure. Stool cultures or ova and parasite laboratory examinations are not needed unless the patient is toxic, there is bloody diarrhea (dysentery), or diarrhea has lasted for more than 1 week. Pregnancy, multiple antibiotic allergies, and an immunosuppressed state are also indications for testing. Some physicians use a fecal smear (iodine stain) positive for leukocytes as an indication for workup of a diarrhea patient.

TREATMENT Treatment of traveler's diarrhea first involves assessment for dehydration, and if indicated, treatment with intravenous (IV) fluids or oral rehydration solution. Antimotility agents are safe to use unless abdominal pain, fever, or dysentery is present. The patient should avoid dairy products, caffeine, and alcohol. Nonspecific treatment, such as with Kaopectate or Pepto-Bismol, may be helpful. Antibiotics are clearly effective and are the mainstay of treatment. Table 24.5 outlines suggested treatment regimens for diarrheal illness.

Antibiotics should not be prescribed for all travelers. Problems with extended use of antibiotic prophylaxis include the following:

- Antibiotic-induced diarrhea (possibly 5%–10% with any of the agents)
- Photodermatitis (doxycycline, sulfa)
- Stevens-Johnson syndrome (sulfa)
- Bacterial resistance (doxycycline, amoxicillin)

TABLE 24-5 TREATMENT AND PREVENTION OF DIARRHEAL ILLNESS

Choices for antimotility agents:

1. Loperamide (Imodium): 4 mg orally immediately, then 2 mg per stool, up to 16 mg/day

2. Lomotil (diphenoxalate 2.5 mg and atropine 0.25 mg per tabs or 5 mL): 2 tablets orally immediately then 1 tabs per stool, up to 8 tabs per day

3. Codeine: 15–60 mg orally every 3–4 h as needed

4. Donnatal elixir (phenobarbital 16.2 mg, hyoscyamine sulfate 0.1037 mg, atropine sulfate 0.0194 mg, scopolamine hydrobromide 0.0065 mg per tablet, caplet, or 5 mL): one to two tablespoons or teaspoons orally every 4–6 h as needed

Antimicrobial drug choices for traveler's diarrhea:

1. Trimethoprim-sulfamethoxazole (Bactrim, Septra): 1 DS tablet twice daily for 3 days

2. Ciprofloxacin: 500 mg every 12 h or Noroxacin 400 mg every 12 h for 3 days

3. Doxycycline (Vibramycin): 100 mg twice daily for 3–5 days

4. Metronidazole (Flagyl): 250–500 mg three times daily for 7 days

(Note: Choices 3 and 4 are not as consistently effective as choices 1 and 2.)

Antibiotics that have proven not to be effective:

1. Penicillin V-K and erythromycin, which have limited gram-negative coverage

2. Amoxicillin, which has a high degree of *Escherichia coli* resistance in most areas

3. Amoxicillin-clavulanate (Augmentin), for which the incidence of antibiotic-induced diarrhea is about the same as what you're trying to prevent.

Antibiotics that might be effective (but not reported yet in well-controlled studies) include azithromycin, aztreonam, and cephalosporins.

Antibiotic prophylaxis. The drugs of choice for the prevention of traveler's diarrhea include

Bactrim or Septra: 1 DS tablet per day

Ciprofloxacin: 500 mg/day

Noroxin: 400 mg/day

The effectiveness of these is 50% to 90%.

■ Yeast superinfections (any)
■ Alcohol intolerance (metronidazole)

Prophylaxis with bismuth subsalicylate (Pepto-Bismol) can be used instead of antibiotics. A dose of four tablets twice daily is 41% effective (reduction in incidence). A dose of 2 ounces of the liquid form four times daily is 62% effective. Increasing doses are more effective, but are limited by symptoms of salicylism (tinnitus, gastrointestinal upset, etc.).

Prophylaxis for children is more difficult because some effective medications are contraindicated. These include tetracycline, doxycycline, and quinolones. Trimethoprim/sulfa is safe to use for most children unless they are allergic to sulfa. For children receiving bismuth subsalicylate, reduce the dose to avoid salicylate toxicity; however, it is less effective at lower doses.

Common sense preventive measures to prevent traveler's diarrhea are included in Table 24.6.

MALARIA

BACKGROUND AND EPIDEMIOLOGY There are an estimated 400 million cases of malaria worldwide every year. It causes 2 to 3 million deaths per year. Of the 1,000 U.S. cases reported each year, half occur in foreign civilians.

The relative number of malaria cases caused by the different species distribution are as follows:

- *Plasmodium vivax* (48%)
- *P. falciparum* (39%)
- *P. malariae* (5%)
- *P. ovale* (2%)

Descriptive definitions for malaria are as follows:

- Indigenous: acquired in an area where malaria occurs regularly
- Introduced: acquired from an imported case in an area not harboring malaria
- Imported: acquired outside a specific area or country
- Induced: acquired through artificial means (blood transfusion, contaminated syringes, "malarial therapy" for Lyme disease, etc.)

TABLE 24-6 SIMPLE MEASURES TO PREVENT TRAVELER'S DIARRHEA

Don't drink tap water.
Drink carbonated beverages and/or bottled water.
Don't add ice to drinks.
Wipe bottle or can rim before drinking.
Don't add dairy products to tea or coffee.
Eat only fully cooked food (not handled or left out).
Avoid raw shellfish (and any other raw meat foods).
Don't buy foods from street vendors (especially ice cream).
Don't eat vegetables / fruits that can't be peeled.
Avoid oral contact with shower water.
Use bottled water for tooth brushing.

DIAGNOSIS The incubation of the malaria parasite period after inoculation before symptoms develop is:

- 8 to 30 days for *P. falciparum* and *P. vivax*
- 9 to 20 days for *P. ovale*
- 16 to 28 days for *P. malariae*

Initial symptoms are headache, malaise, anorexia, nausea, and vomiting, which are followed by intermittent chills, fever, and diaphoresis lasting 1 to 8 hours (or up to 36 hours for *P. falciparum*).

Secondary signs and complications include the following:

- Cerebral malaria (*P. falciparum*), with seizures, stupor, psychosis, or coma
- Renal dysfunction (may develop into acute renal failure)
- Pulmonary edema/acute respiratory distress syndrome (uncommon)
- Hypoglycemia (common)
- Hepatosplenomegaly with or without jaundice
- Anemia
- Decreased resistance to other infections
- Occasional splenic rupture

Confirmation of diagnosis involves checking the following:

- Thick blood smear (for low-level parasitemia)
- Thin blood smear (to identify species)
- Serology (not as useful acutely)

It may be important to also check:

- Baseline LFTs and prothrombin time
- Baseline renal function
- Complete blood count, platelets, glucose

TREATMENT The treatment for malaria depends partially on the species. For *P. vivax* or *P. ovale*:

- Chloroquine base (600 mg as soon as possible, then 300 mg in 6 hours, then 300 mg every 24 hours for 2 days)
- Primaquine phosphate (to kill the hypnozoites dormant in the liver), 15 mg every day for 14 days (unless G6PD deficiency)

For emergent treatment of *P. falciparum:*

- Chloroquine base (even if resistant)
- Quinidine gluconate 10 mg/kg IV every hour, followed by continuous infusion of 0.02 mg/kg/min for 3 days

■ Quinine is an alternative but may no longer be available (dose is 650 mg orally of the sulfate form three times daily for 3 days).

Additional agents for chloroquine-resistant *P. falciparum* include the following:

■ Pyrimethamine-sulfadoxine (Fanisidar) 3 tablets orally on day 3 of therapy
■ Tetracycline 250 mg orally four times daily for 7 days
■ Doxycycline 100 mg orally twice daily for 7 days
■ Clindamycin 900 mg orally three times daily for 3 days
■ Mefloquine 1,250 mg once

PREVENTION If you are traveling to a known chloroquine-sensitive area (such as Mexico or the Middle East), use 300 mg of the base form of chloroquine phosphate (500 mg of salt form) orally weekly beginning 1 week before the trip and continuing until 4 weeks after the trip. Be careful that small children do not ingest the adult prophylactic doses (fatalities have been reported).

For chloroquine-resistant areas use mefloquine hydrochloride (Lariam), one 250-mg tablet weekly and doxycycline 200 mg daily. Proguanil (Paludrine) is not available in United States, but is prescribed in Great Britain and other European countries, and is recommended for sub-Saharan Africa (200 mg daily). Malarone (atovaquone and proquanil) is a new agent used for prophylaxis (1 tab daily). It is well tolerated and has reportedly few side effects. The prophylactic doses of the above medications need to be continued for 4 weeks after returning from the malarial area.

DID YOU KNOW?

One of the main reasons for malaria infection in travelers is the failure to complete the course of prophylaxis upon returning home.

Contraindications to mefloquine include the following:

■ History of epilepsy
■ History of psychiatric disorder
■ Need to do fine motor tasks
■ Known hypersensitivity
■ Pregnancy
■ Use of beta blockers, calcium blockers, or quinine or quinidine
■ Weight under 15 kg

Prevention is still the most effective way to avoid getting malaria. Preventive measures to reduce risk of mosquito bites include the following:

■ Remain inside screened areas between dusk and dawn (when mosquitoes are most active).

- Use netting, even around inside sleeping areas.
- Wear clothing that covers as much skin as possible.
- Use insect repellent on exposed skin.
- Use pyrethrum insect spray indoors.
- Spray nearby mosquito breeding areas with insecticide.

AMEBIC DYSENTERY

DID YOU KNOW?

Amebiasis may cause over 50,000 deaths annually worldwide, making it the third leading parasitic cause of death (after malaria and leishmaniasis).

EPIDEMIOLOGY Possibly 10% of the world's population is infected with intestinal amebas. Prevalence in tropical countries is 30%. The prevalence in the U.S. homosexual population is 25%. The fatality rate for amebic dysentery is 2%, and the overall complication rate is 3% to 4%.

Humans are the primary reservoir for the amebic parasite. There are two life cycle forms, as for *Giardia:* the trophozoite, which causes illness, and the cysts, which are passed in stool and are infectious. Transmission is by the fecal-oral route. Most infections are asymptomatic, and attack rates are 5% to 30%. The cysts can remain viable for months in a moist environment, but are sensitive to chlorination, dessication, and boiling.

CLINICAL FEATURES The main pathology is in the colon, with the trophozoites causing initial mucosal inflammation, then mucosal erosions, then ulcers. Extraintestinal spread is blood borne. Large abscesses can develop in the liver, lung, brain, and other tissues. The incubation period is variable, but typically is 5 to 10 days. Symptoms start with crampy abdominal pain, then dysentery with possible weight loss, anorexia, and nausea. The complications are colon perforation, toxic megacolon, formation of an ameboma (an inflammatory mass that may cause bowel obstruction), liver abscess (which may rupture into the pleural or pericardial space), and brain abscess.

DIAGNOSIS Fresh stool or colon mucus shows cysts or trophozoites on saline preparations or with iodine stains. Often three or more stool examinations are required. Serologic tests are important to distinguish amebiasis from ulcerative colitis. Sigmoidoscopy is useful to inspect ulcers and obtain stool or mucus for culture and stain. Abdominal computed tomography if available is useful if liver abscess is suspected.

TREATMENT Two general classes of medications are used:

1. The tissue amebacides combat invasive amebiasis in the bowel and liver. These include metronidazole, emetine, dehydroemetine, and chloroquine.

2. The lumenal drugs kill amebas within the colon. These include iodoquinol, paromomycin, and diloxanide.

Treatment of asymptomatic carriers is recommended for food handlers (always) and for all cases in low-incidence regions (United States, Europe), but is not always recommended for asymptomatic cases in high-incidence tropical countries.

Treatment regimens for asymptomatic carriers include the following:

- Iodoquinol: 650 mg three times daily for 10 days (40 mg/kg/day); side effects mild (nausea, emesis, rash)
- Paromomycin: 500 mg three times daily for 7 to 10 days (30 mg/kg/day); permitted during pregnancy
- Diloxanide furoate (Furamide): 500 mg three times daily for 10 days (20 mg/kg/day); only available in the United States by calling the CDC in Atlanta

Choices for treatment of invasive disease are as follows:

- Metronidazole: 750 mg three times daily for 10 days, followed by iodoquinol 650 mg three times daily for 20 days (or paromomycin 25 to 30 mg/kg/day in three divided doses for 7 days)
- Dehydroemetine: 1 to 1.5 mg/kg/day (maximum 90 mg/day) intramuscularly for up to 5 days following iodoquinol (commonly causes nausea and emesis)
- Tetracycline: 500 mg four times daily for 10 days (indirect amebacidal action)
- Chloroquine phosphate (second-line agent for extraluminal infection): 2 g/day, then 500 mg/day for 2 to 3 weeks

GIARDIASIS

EPIDEMIOLOGY *Giardia* is the most common intestinal protozoan in the United States and the third most common protozoan worldwide. The disease is caused by the protozoan *Giardia lamblia*. It has been reported in 97 countries. Outbreak sites have included Aspen and Vail, Colorado; Rome, New York; Berlin, New Hampshire; St. Petersburg, Russia; and many sites in the Rocky Mountains and Cascade Range.

Risk factors for transmission include poor hygiene, close physical contact, and sexual contact (in male homosexuals). Epidemics and 50% carrier rates occur in day-care centers, institutions for the mentally retarded, and some Native American reservations.

The life cycle of *Giardia* involves trophozoites that inhabit the jejunum and duodenum and cause symptoms. Some trophozoites encyst and then pass in the stool. The cysts are infectious. Ingestion of only a few can cause disease. The cysts are activated (excysted) by passage through the stomach. Some patients may be asymptomatic carriers and cyst passers.

CLINICAL FEATURES The initial infection usually induces acute diarrhea for 2 to 3 days, accompanied by a low-grade fever, anorexia, nausea, and cramping. Later, more chronic symptoms occur, such as diarrhea with foul-smelling stool and flatus, foul-smelling belching, cramping, nausea, anorexia, fatigue, abdominal distention, and sometimes progression to malabsorption, weight loss, and failure to thrive.

DIAGNOSIS A fresh stool examination with iodine or methylene blue stain shows the parasites. Examination yield is better if recent enemas, laxatives, or barium are avoided. The diagnostic yield is 50% to 70% on one stool examination, and 70% to 90% with three stool examinations.

TREATMENT The two most common medications (probably drugs of choice) used are as follows:

- Quinacrine (Atabrine): 100 mg three times daily for 5 to 7 days (7 mg/kg/day). Cure rate is 95%. Side effects are dizziness, toxic psychosis, and metallic taste.
- Metronidazole (Flagyl): 250 mg three times daily for 7 days (21 mg/kg/day). This has a high cure rate, but is still not approved by the U.S. Food and Drug Administration. The side effects are a disulfiram-like reaction if the patient coingests any alcohol.

Other medications include furazolidine and paromomycin. Furazolidine (Furox-one) is given at a dosage of 100 mg four times daily for 7 days (6 mg/kg/day in four divided doses per day for 5–7 days). Its cure rate is 85%. It is usually well tolerated, but may cause nausea or emesis. Paromomycin (Humantin), which is a poorly absorbed aminoglycoside-like antibiotic, also can be used. Its dose is 25 to 30 mg/kg in three divided doses for 5 to 10 days. It is useful for pregnant patients.

SECURITY AND PERSONAL PROTECTION

SECURITY ISSUES AND ESCALATING VIOLENCE AMONG FOREIGN HEALTH WORKERS

Foreign health workers are increasingly serving in politically unstable areas around the world. Assaults and violence against expatriate health workers has increased in the past decade, and foreign volunteers are no longer immune to the dangers of practicing in an unstable setting. It is therefore important to address issues of security and personal safety before going into a potentially dangerous situation. With proper planning, health personnel working abroad can avoid the vast majority of security threats.

BEFORE YOU TRAVEL

Before traveling to any foreign country, become aware of potential dangers and threats. Find out about political instability, threats to certain ethnic groups, urban violence, and military conflicts. If you are in contact with individuals from the country where you plan to travel, discuss security issues with them. Local health-care personnel are some of the best sources of information about the security climate. You can also contact the local embassy or the U.S. Department of State Overseas Security Advisory Council for security concerns in a particular country.

Some of the questions you might ask your local colleagues include the following:

- Are there any obvious security threats?
- Are there any major political changes or elections scheduled?
- Are there certain regions for which travel is not advised?
- Are there any specific threats to foreigners?
- What specific precautions should I take?

If you choose to work in a conflict area or one that has a history of political instability, be sure to obtain as much information about the social and political climate as you can.

SECURITY AWARENESS

Knowledge of potential security threats before traveling is important, but cannot replace common sense and danger avoidance behavior while in the country. Security is an individual responsibility, and you should not blindly depend on the hospital, organization, or institution to provide for your safety. There are several measures that you can take to ensure your own personal security.

GENERAL PERSONAL PRECAUTIONS

General precautions for every travel situation can help you avoid many problems. Your personal safety in any setting can be increased by observing the following simple measures:

- Know where you are going and plan the route. If possible, stay to main roads and avoid side roads or narrow alleys.
- Dress conservatively, giving consideration to local customs. Do not wear expensive jewelry or carry large amounts of cash. Keep cameras and personal electronic equipment discretely out of sight.
- Pick-pockets and thieves work in groups. Be aware of casual contact on the street or jostling crowds. Keep wallets, keys, and money tucked away or in front pockets.
- If you are confronted, always maintain composure. Keep a calm, professional demeanor in potentially hostile situations.
- Travel in groups if possible. This is especially important when traveling at night. Divide your money among friends with whom you are traveling.

■   When walking, travel in groups if possible. Do not walk alone at night. Avoid large shrubs, dense trees, concealed alleys, and building entries.

SAFETY WHILE DRIVING

■   Wear seatbelts at all times while driving. If you are taking a taxi, be sure to use seatbelts.
■   Avoid driving at night when possible.
■   Check for vehicle papers, registration, and documentation before driving.
■   Drive defensively and at a safe speed. Know where you are going and avoid side streets and narrow roads.
■   Keep the doors locked.
■   Be suspicious of people approaching your car or gathered around your vehicle. Most assaults occur when entering or exiting your vehicle.

RECOGNIZING AND MANAGING STRESS

Stress is a common occurrence among health providers in international and remote settings. Working in unfamiliar surroundings and with culturally different groups can lead to a sense of social isolation. It is important to recognize the signs of stress in yourself and in your colleagues. Signs of stress may include the following:

■   Depression
■   Difficulty sleeping
■   Malaise
■   Uncooperative behavior
■   Withdrawal from public activities
■   Decline in work productivity
■   Recurrent illnesses

Stress can be managed and the effects of a stressful environment can be diffused by taking a few precautions:

■   Acknowledge that your work situation is stressful.
■   Make personal time for yourself. This may take the form of meditation, journal writing, or spiritual reflection.
■   Express your fears and stress to others. Take the time to share your common experiences.
■   Maintain physical fitness. Often strenuous physical exercise is the best way to deal with emotional stress.
■   Take breaks. Be sure to allow yourself a day off or an evening out to get away from the workplace.

- Consider counseling if you are having difficulty at work or you are developing symptoms of depression and excess stress.
- Personal health and well-being are paramount to your ability to serve in remote locations. It is important to nurture both your physical and your mental health in the stressful environment of many international settings.

APPENDICES

APPENDIX 1: WHO Common Medications and Doses

1. ANESTHETICS
1.1 General anesthetics and oxygen

ether, anesthetic	Administer until drowsy	inhalation
halothane	Administer until drowsy	inhalation
ketamine	Initial dose 1 mg/kg to 4.5 mg/kg (0.5 to 2 mg/lb). Initial IM dose from 6.5-13 mg/kg (3 to 6 mg/lb).	injection, 50 mg (as hydrochloride)/ml in 10-ml vial
nitrous oxide	Administer until drowsy	inhalation
oxygen	As indicated	inhalation (medicinal gas)
thiopental	1-3 mg/kg IV	powder for injection, 0.5 g, 1.0 g (sodium salt) in ampoule

1.2 Local anesthetics

bupivacaine	Epidural: bupivacaine HCl, 0.5% and 0.75% 3 ml to 5 ml. In obstetrics, use only 0.5% and 0.25%	injection, 0.25%, 0.5% (hydrocholoride) in vial; injection for spinal anesthesia, 0.5% in 4-ml amp to be mixed with 7.5% glucose solution
lidocaine	Retrobulbar Inj: 1.7-3 mg/kg Transtracheal Inj: 2-3 mL injected rapidly	injection, 1%, 2% in vial; injection for spinal anesthesia, 5% in 2-ml ampoule to be mixed with 7.5% glucose solution;
lidocaine + epinephrine (adrenaline)	Max dose of lidocaine HCl with epinephrine should not exceed 7 mg/kg (3.5 mg/lb) or 500 mg.	injection 1%, 2% (hydrochloride)+ epinephrine 1:200 000 in vial
ephedrine	25 to 50 mg (range 10 to 50 mg) SC/IM	injection, 30 mg/ml in 1-ml ampoule (To prevent hypotension in spinal anesthesia during delivery

1.3 Preoperative medication and sedation for short-term procedures

atropine	0.4-0.6 mg IV, IM or SC	injection, 1 mg (sulfate) in 1-ml ampoule
chloral hydrate	Sedative: 250 mg tid po, pc; Hypnotic: 500 mg – 1 g po, 15-30 min before bedtime or 30 min before surgery	syrup, 200 mg/5-ml
diazepam	2-10 min bid to qid po, 2-10 mg IM or IV. Status epilepticus: 5-10 mg IV.	injection, 5 mg/ml in 2-ml ampoule; tablet, 5 mg
promethazine	25 mg po hs, or 12.5 mg po ac & hs	elixir or syrup, 5 mg (hydrochloride)/5-ml

2. ANALGESICS, ANTIPYRETICS, NON-STEROIDAL ANTI-INFLAMMATORY DRUGS (NSAIDs)
2.1 Non-opioids and NSAIDs

acetylsalicylic acid	325-650 mg q 4 h po, prn; max dose is 4000 mg per day po	tablet, 100-500 mg; suppository, 50-150 mg
ibuprofen	200-800 mg q 4-8 h po	tablet, 200 mg, 400 mg
paracetamol	Two 500 mg tablets or capsules every four to six hours.	tablet, 100-500 mg; suppository, 100 mg; syrup, 125 mg/5-ml

APPENDIX 1 *(continued)*

2. ANALGESICS, ANTIPYRETICS, NON-STEROIDAL ANTI-INFLAMMATORY DRUGS (NSAIDs) *(continued)*
2.2 Opioid analgesics

codeine	Analgesia: 15-60 mg q 4-6 h po; Antitussive: 10-20 mg q 4-6 h	tablet, 30 mg (phosphate)
morphine (meperidine)	IV: 2-10 mg/70 kg Oral solution: 10-30 mg q 4 h po prn pain Tablet: 5-30 mg q 4 h po prn pain	injection, 10 mg in 1-ml ampoule (sulfate or hydrochloride); oral solution, 10 mg (sulfate or hydrochloride)/5 ml; tablet, 10 mg (sulfate)
pethidine	50-150 mg IM, SC, or po, every 3 or 4 hours as necessary	injection, 50 mg (hydrochloride) in 1-ml ampoule; tablet, 50 mg, 100 mg

2.3 Drugs used to treat gout

allopurinol	Mild Gout: 200-300 mg daily po Moderately Severe Gout: 400-600 mg daily po	tablet, 100 mg
colchicine	Acute: 1.0-1.2 mg po stat; then 0.5-1.2 mg q 1-2 h po until pain relief or nausea. Prophylaxis: 0.5 or 0.6 mg daily for 3-4 days a wk	tablet, 500 micrograms

2.4 Disease modifying agents used in rheumatoid disorders (DMARDs)

azathioprine	Initially, 1 mg/kg (50 to 100 mg) as a single daily dose or on a bid schedule. Can increase dose after 6-8 weeks.	tablet, 50 mg
methotrexate	Individualize dosage. 10-25 mg once a week po, until response is achieved. May give 2.5 mg q 12 h or 3 doses.	tablet, 2.5 mg (as sodium salt)

3. ANTIALLERGICS AND DRUGS IN ANAPHYLAXIS

chlorphenamine	4 mg q 4-6 h po	tablet, 4 mg (hydrogen maleate); injection, 10 mg (hydrogen maleate) in 1-ml ampoule
dexamethasone	Initial: 0.75-9 mg daily po; Maintenance: Adjust to lowest satisfactory dose	tablet, 500 micrograms, 4 mg; injection, 4 mg dexamethasone phosphate in 1-ml ampoule
epinephrine (adrenaline)	0.2-1.0 mg SC or IM	injection, 1 mg (as hydrochloride or hydrogen tartrate) in 1-ml ampoule
hydrocortisone	For intra-articular injection: Initial dosage: 5-75 mg a day	powder for injection, 100 mg (as sodium succinate) in vial
prednisolone	5-60 mg daily po depending on disease and the patient's response.	tablet, 5 mg

4. ANTIDOTES AND OTHER SUBSTANCES USED IN POISONING
4.1 Non-specific

charcoal, activated	1 gram per kg PO (may use with sorbitol)	powder
ipecac	10-30 cc PO to induce emesis	syrup, containing 0.14% ipecacuanha alkaloids

4.2 Specific

acetylcysteine (N-)	150 mg/kg for acetaminophen/paracetamol overdose	injection, 200 mg/ml in 10-ml ampoule

APPENDIX 1 *(continued)*

4. ANTIDOTES AND OTHER SUBSTANCES USED IN POISONING *(continued)*
4.2 Specific

atropine	0.4-0.6 mg IV, IM or SC	injection, 1 mg (sulfate) in 1-ml ampoule
calcium gluconate	Individualize dose to requirements of patient. Usual IV dose: 500 mg-2 g; must be administered slowly.	injection, 100 mg in 10-ml ampoule
deferoxamine	For patients not in shock (IM): 1.0 g IM. May then take 500 mg q 4 h. Do not exceed 6.0 g in 24 hours.	powder for injection, 500 mg (mesilate) in vial
dimercaprol	Deep IM inj only for arsenic, gold, mercury or lead poisoning 2.5 mg/kg to 5 mg/kg bid to qid.	injection in oil, 50 mg/ml in 2-ml ampoule
methylthioninium chloride (methylene blue)	0.1-0.2 ml/kg. Inject by IV very slowly over several minutes	injection, 10 mg/ml in 10-ml ampoule
naloxone	Opioid overdose: Initially, 0.4-2 mg IV. Dose may be repeated at 2-3 min intervals. Max: 10 mg	injection, 400 micrograms (hydrochloride) in 1-ml ampoule
sodium calcium edetate	Asymptomatic lead poisoning (level <70 mcg/dl but >20 mcg/dl: 1000 mg/m^2/day IV or IM. Lead Nephropathy: 500 mg/m^2 q 24 h for 5 days. Use in conjunction with BAL (dimercaprol).	injection, 200 mg/ml in 5-ml ampoule
sodium thiosulfate	12.5 grams IV given over approx 10 min.	injection, 250 mg/ml in 50-ml ampoule

5. ANTICONVULSANTS/ANTIEPILEPTICS

carbamazepine	Initial: 200 mg bid po; increase weekly by 200 mg/day. Max: 1000 mg/day (age 12-15), 1200 mg/day (age >15).	scored tablet, 100 mg, 200 mg
diazepam	IV: 5-10 mg IV. Rectally: 0.2 mg/kg	injection, 5 mg/ml in 2-ml ampoule (intravenous or rectal)
ethosuximide	Initial: 1 g or less daily po after meals in 4-6 divided doses,	capsule, 250 mg; syrup, 250 mg/5-ml
magnesium sulfate	IM: 4-5 g of a 50% solution q 4 h prn IV: 4 g of a 10-20% IV Infusion: 4-5 g in 250 mL of 5% Dextrose or 0.9 NS	injection, 500 mg/ml in 2-ml ampoule
phenobarbitol	60-200 mg daily po	tablet, 15-100 mg; elixir, 15 mg/5-ml
phenytoin	Tab: Initially 100 mg tid po; adjust dosage prn Inj: Loading dose: of 10-15 mg/kg slow IV (rate not over 50 mg/min). Maintenance dose: 100 mg po or IV q 6-8 h.	capsule or tablet, 25 mg, 50 mg, 100 mg (sodium salt); injection, 50 mg/ml in 5-ml vial
valproic acid	Initially: 15 mg/kg/day po in 2 or 3 divided doses, increasing at 1 week intervals by 5 to 10 mg/kg/day (Max: 60 mg/kg/day)	enteric coated tablet, 200 mg, 500 mg (sodium salt)
clonazepam	Initially: 0.5 mg tid po. May increase dosage in increments of 0.5-1 mg every 3 days. Max: 20 mg per day.	scored tablets 500 micrograms

APPENDIX 1 *(continued)*

6. ANTI-INFECTIVE DRUGS
6.1 Anthelminthics
6.1.1 Intestinal anthelminthics

albendazole	Under 60 kg: 15 mg/kg/day po in bid (Max: 800 mg/day) Over 60 kg: 400 mg bid po with meals. Hydatid Disease: Administer in a 28-day cycle followed by a 14-day albendazole-free interval, for a total of 3 cycles.	chewable tablet, 400 mg
levamisole	Initial Therapy: 50 mg p.o. q8h for 3 days (starting 7-30 days post-surgery) Maintenance: 50 mg p.o. q8h for 3 days every 2 weeks	tablet, 50 mg; 150 mg (as hydrochloride)
mebendazole	Pinworm: 100 mg daily po (1 dose). Common Roundworm, Whipworm, Hookworm: 100 mg bid AM & PM for 3 days po	chewable tablet, 100 mg, 500 mg
niclosamide	As directed	chewable tablet, 500 mg
praziquantel	Three 20 mg/kg doses po for 1 day only	tablet, 150 mg, 600 mg
pyrantel	5 mg/lb (to a maximum of 1 g) as a single dose po	chewable tablet 250 mg (as embonate); oral suspension, 50 mg (as embonate)/ml

6.1.2 Antifilarials

diethylcarbamazine	As directed	tablet, 50 mg, 100 mg (dihydrogen citrate)
ivermectin	Strongyloidiasis: 15-24 kg take 3 mg; 25-35 kg take 6 mg; 36-50 kg take 9 mg; 51-65 kg take 12 mg; 66-79 kg take 15 mg; Onchocerciasis: 15-25 kg take 3 mg; 26-44 kg take 6 mg; 45-64 kg take 9 mg; 65-84 kg take 12 mg; 85 kg take 150 ug/kg	scored tablet, 3 mg, 6 mg

6.1.3 Antischistosomals and anti-trematode drugs

praziquantel	Three 20 mg/kg doses po for 1 day only	tablet, 600 mg
oxamniquine	12-15 mg/kg as a single dose po with food	capsule, 250 mg; syrup, 250 mg/5-ml

6.2 Antibacterials
6.2.1 Beta lactam drugs

amoxicillin	Respiratory Tract: 500 mg q 8 h po or 875 mg q 12 h po. Gonorrheal Infections: 3 g (+ 1 g of probenecid) single dose.	capsule or tablet, 250 mg, 500 mg (anhydrous); powder for oral suspension, 125 mg (anhydrous)/5 ml
ampicillin	Resp. infecitons: Under 40 kg: 25-50 mg/kg/day in equally divided doses at 6-8 h IM or IV; Over 40 kg: 500 mg q 6 h IM or IV. Genitourinary Infections: 50 mg/kg/day divided q 6-8 IM or IV. Bacterial Meningitis: 150-200 mg/kg/day divided q4. Septicemia: 150-200 mg/kg/day divided q4.	powder for injection, 500 mg, 1 g (as sodium salt) in vial

APPENDIX 1 *(continued)*

6.2 Antibacterials *(continued)*
6.2.1 Beta lactam drugs

benzathine benzylpenicillin	Streptococcal URI: single dose 1,200,000 Units IM. Syphilis (Primary, Secondary, and Latent): 2,400,000 Units IM. Syphilis (Late/Tertiary & Neurosyphilis): 2,400,000 Units IM at 7-day intervals for 3 doses.	powder for injection, 1.44 g benzylpenicillin (=2.4 million IU) in 5-ml vial
cloxacillin	Mild to Moderate Infections: 250 mg q 6 h po Severe Infections: 500 mg q 6 h po	capsule, 500 mg, 1 g (as sodium salt); powder for oral solution, 125 mg (as sodium salt)/5 ml; powder for injection, 500 mg (as sodium salt) in vial
Phenoxymethylpenicillin (Penicillin V Potassium)	Streptococcal Infections: 200,000 to 500,000 units every 6 to 8 hours for 10 days.	tablet, 250 mg (as potassium salt); powder for oral suspension, 250 mg (as potassium salt)/5 ml
procaine benzylpenicillin	Streptococcal Group A: Adults and children over 60 lbs. in weight: 2,400,000 units. Pneumococcal: 600,000 units in children and 1,200,000 units in adults, every 2 or 3 days until temp is normal for 48 hours.	powder for injection, 1 g (=1 million IU), 3 g (=3 million IU)
amoxicillin + clavulanic acid	Usual Dosage: 1 tablet q 12 h po Severe Infections & Respiratory Infections: 1 tablet q 8 h po	tablet, 500 mg + 125 mg
ceftazidime	Usual Dosage: 1 g q 8-12 h IV or IM. Urinary Tract Infections: (Uncomplicated) 250 mg q 12 h IV or IM; (Complicated) 500 mg q 8-12 h IV or IM. Bone & Joint Infections: 2 g q 12 h IV\	powder for injection, 250 mg (as pentahydrate) in vial
ceftriaxone	Usual dosage: 1-2 g once daily or in equally divided doses bid IM or IV. Gonococcal Infections, Uncomplicated: 250 mg IM, one dose. Meningitis: 100 mg/kg/day in divided doses q 12 h IM or IV, Surgical Prophylaxis: 1 g IV 30 min-2 h before surgery	powder for injection, 250 mg (as sodium salt) in vial
imipenem + cilastatin	Respiratory, Skin & Gyn (IM): 500 or 750 mg (of impenem) q 12 h IM. Intra-Abdominal Infections (IM): 750 mg q 12 h IM. IV infusion: 250 500 mg dose (of imipenem) over 20-30 min.	powder for injection 250 mg (as monohydrate) + 250 mg (as sodium salt), 500 mg (as monohydrate) + 500 mg (as sodium salt) in vial

6.2.2 Other antibacterial

chloramphenicol	Cpsl: 50 mg/kg/day in divided doses at 6 h intervals po. May increase to 100 mg/kg/day for resistant organisms. Powder for Inj: 50 mg/kg/day in divided doses at 6 h intervals IV	capsule, 250 mg; oral suspension, 150 mg (as palmitate)/5 ml; powder for injection, 1 g (sodium succinate) in vial
ciprofloxacin	UTI: Acute, Uncomplicated: 100 mg q 12 h po for 3 days; Severe/Complicated: 500 mg q 12 h po for 7-14 days; Respiratory: 500 mg q 12 h po for 7-14 days; Bone & Joint: 500-750 mg q 12 h po for 4-6 weeks. Infectious Diarrhea: 500 mg q 12 h po for 5-7 days. Typhoid Fever: 500 mg q 12 h po for 10 days. Gonococcal Infections, Uncomplicated: 250 mg po (single dose)	tablet 250 mg (as hydrochloride)

APPENDIX 1 *(continued)*

6.2.2 Other antibacterial *(continued)*

doxycycline	Usual Dosage: 100 mg q 12 h po for the first day, followed by a maintenance dose of 100 mg/day given as 50 mg q 12 h or 100 mg once daily. Urinary Tract Infections: 100 mg q 12 h po. Malaria Prophylaxis: 100 mg once daily po.	capsule or tablet, 100 mg (hydrochloride)
erythromycin	Usual Dose: 250 mg q 6 h po or 500 mg q 12 h po. Dysenteric Amebiasis: 250 mg qid po for 10 to 14 days. Legionnaires Disease: 1-4 g daily po in divided doses.	capsule or tablet, 250 mg (as stearate or ethyl succinate); powder for oral suspension, 125 mg (as stearate or ethyl succinate); powder for injection, 500 mg (as lactobionate) in vial
gentamicin	Usual Dose: 3 mg/kg/day IM or IV divided in 3 doses at 8-hour intervals. Life-Threatening Infections: Up to 5 mg/kg/day may be administered in 3 or 4 equal doses	injection, 10 mg, 40 mg (as sulfate)/ml in 2-ml vial
metronidazole	Trichomoniasis: 250 mg tid po for 7 days; 375 mg bid po for 7 days; or 2 g as a single dose po. Acute Intestinal Amediasis: 750 mg tid po for 5-10 days. Amebic Liver Abcess: 500-750 mg tid po for 5-10 days. Bacterial Vaginosis: 750 mg q d po for 7 days.	tablet, 200-500 mg; injection, 500 mg in 100-ml vial; suppository, 500 mg, 1 g; oral suspension, 200 mg (as benzoate)/5 ml
nalidixic acid	Initially: 1 g qid po for 1-2 weeks. Prolonged therapy: may reduce dosage to 500 mg qid after initital treatment period.	tablet 250 mg, 500 mg
nitrofurantoin	Usual Dosage: 50-100 mg qid po with food. Urinary Tract Infections (Uncomplicated): 100 mg q 12 h po with food for 7 days.	tablet, 100 mg
spectinomycin	2 g as a single deep IM injection	powder for injection, 2 g (as hydrochloride) in vial
sulfadiazine	Initially: 2 to 4 g. Maintenance: 2 to 4 g, divided into 3 to 6 doses, every 24 hours.	tablet, 500 mg
sulfamethoxazole + trimethoprim	UTI: 800 mg + 160 mg q 12 h po for 10-14 days. Shigellosis and Traveler's Diarrhea: 800 mg + 160 mg q 12 h po for 5 days.	tablet, 100 mg + 20 mg, 400 mg + 80 mg; oral suspension, 200 mg + 40 mg/5 ml; injection, 80 mg + 16 mg/ml in 5-ml and 10-ml ampoules
trimethoprim	100 mg q 12 h po for 10 days, or 200 mg q 24 h po for 10 days	tablet, 100 mg, 200 mg; injection 20 mg/ml in 5-ml ampule
chloramphenicol	50 mg/kg/day in divided doses at 6 h intervals IV	oily suspension for injection 0.5 g (as sodium succinate)/ml in 2-ml ampoule
clindamycin	Serious Infections: 150-450 mg q 6 h po; 600-1200 mg/day IV or IM in 2, 3 or 4 equal doses.	capsule, 150 mg; injection, 150 mg (as phosphate)/ml
vancomycin	2 g daily, divided either as 500 mg q 6 h or 1 g q 12 h, by IV infusion (at a rate no more than 10 mg/min) over at least 60 minutes	powder for injection, 250 mg (as hydrochloride) in vial

6.2.3 Antileprosy drugs

clofazimine	100 mg daily with meals po	capsule, 50 mg, 100 mg
dapsone	100 mg daily po alone or in combination with other leprostatic drugs	tablet, 25 mg, 50 mg, 100 mg

APPENDIX 1 *(continued)*

6.2.3 **Antileprosy drugs** *(continued)*

rifampicin	10 mg/kg daily in a single administration po (1 hour before or 2 hours after a meal), not to exceed 600 mg daily	capsule or tablet, 150 mg, 300 mg

6.2.4 **Antituberculosis drugs**

ethambutol	Initial: 15 mg/kg po as a single dose q 24 h. Retreatment: 25 mg/kg po as a single dose q 24 h. After 60 days, decrease dose to 15 mg/kg po as a single dose q 24 h.	tablet, 100 mg-400 mg (hydrochloride)
isoniazid	300 mg daily po	tablet, 100-300 mg
pyrazinamide	15-30 mg/kg once daily po (Maximum: 2 g/day)	tablet, 400 mg
rifampicin	10 mg/kg daily in a single administration po (1 hour before or 2 hours after a meal), not to exceed 600 mg daily	capsule or tablet, 150 mg, 300 mg
rifampicin + isoniazid	600 mg rifampin, 300 mg isoniazid once daily, administered one hour before or two hours after a meal	tablet, 60 mg + 30 mg; 150 mg + 75 mg; 300 mg + 150 mg; 150 mg + 150 mg *(For intermittent use three times weekly.)*
rifampicin + isoniazid + pyrazinamide	Patients weighing less than 45 kg: 480 mg +240 mg + 1200 mg Patients weighing 45-54 kg: 600 mg + 300 mg +1500 mg Patients weighing over 54 kg: 720 mg + 360 mg + 1800 mg	tablet, 60 mg + 30 mg + 150 mg; 150 mg + 75 mg + 400 mg; 150 mg + 150 mg + 500 mg *(For intermittent use three times weekly.)*
streptomycin	15 mg/kg daily IM up to 1 g or 25-30 mg/kg bid IM (up to 1.5 g) or 25-30 mg/kg two or three times weekly IM (Maximum: 1.5 g)	powder for injection, 1 g (as sulfate) in vial

6.3 **Antifungal drugs**

fluconazole	Vaginal *candidiasis*: 150 mg as a single oral dose. Oropharyngeal *candidiasis*: 200 mg on day 1, then 100 mg q d	capsule 50 mg; injection 2 mg/ml in vial; oral suspension 50 mg/5-ml
griseofulvin	375 mg daily po as a single dose or divided doses	capsule or tablet, 125 mg, 250 mg
nystatin	Tab: 500,000-1,000,000 units tid po. Lozenge: 200,000-400,000 units 4 or 5 times daily po, allow to slowly dissolve in mouth. Pessary: 1 tablet daily intravaginally for 2 weeks.	tablet, 100,000, 500,000 IU; lozenge 100,000 IU; pessary, 100,000 IU

6.4 **Antivirals**
6.4.1 **Antiherpes**

acyclovir	Genital Herpes: 200 mg q 4 h (5 times daily) po for 10 days. Suppressive Therapy: 400 mg bid po for up to 1 year. Herpes zoster: 800 mg q 4 h (5 times daily) po for 7-10 days. Chickenpox: 20 mg/kg (not to exceed 800 mg) qid po for 5 days. Herpes simplex encephalitis: 10 mg/kg IV q 8 h for 10 days.	tablet, 200 mg; powder for injection 250 mg (as sodium salt) in vial

APPENDIX 1 *(continued)*

6.4.2 Antiretrovirals

Adequate resources and specialist oversight are a prerequisite for the introduction of this class of drugs.

nevirapine	tablet 200 mg; oral solution 50 mg/50-mL	
zidovudine	Symptomatic HIV: 100 mg q 4 h po (600 mg total daily dose) Asymptomatic HIV: 100 mg q 4 h po (500 mg/day) Inj: 1-2 mg/kg infused IV over 1 hour q 6 hr	capsules 100 mg, 250 mg; injection, 10 mg/ml in 20-ml vial; oral solution 50 mg/5-ml

6.5 Antiprotozoal drugs
6.5.1 Antiamoebic and antigiardiasis drugs

diloxanide	As directed	tablet, 500 mg (furoate)
metronidazole	As above	tablet, 200-500 mg; injection, 500 mg in 100-ml vial; oral suspension 200 mg (as benzoate)/5 ml

6.5.2 Antileishmaniasis drugs

pentamidine	4 mg/kg once a day for 14 days IV or IM	powder for injection, 200 mg, 300 mg (isethionate) in vial
amphotericin B	3-4 mg/kg/day by slow IV infusion (rate 1 mg/kg/h) in 5% Dextrose (check preparation)	powder for injection, 50 mg in vial

6.5.3 Antimalarial drugs
6.5.3.1 For curative treatment

chloroquine	Inj: 160-200 mg of chloroquine base IM initially, repeat in 6 h if necessary. Tab: Initially, 600 mg of chloroquine base po, followed by 300 mg after 6-8 h and a single dose of 300 mg on each of two consecutive days	tablet 100 mg, 150 mg (as phosphate or sulfate); syrup, 50 mg (as phosphate or sulfate)/5 ml; injection 40 mg (as hydrochloride, phosphate or sulfate)/ml in 5-ml ampoule
primaquine	15 mg (of base) daily po for 14 days	tablet, 7.5 mg, 15 mg (as diphosphate)
quinine	Tab: 260-650 mg tid po for 6-12 days IV unavailable in US, use as directed per local treatment patterns	tablet, 300 mg (as bisulfate or sulfate); injection, 300 mg (as dihydrochloride)/ml in 2-ml ampule
doxycycline	100 mg once daily po	capsule or tablet, 100 mg (hydrochloride) *(For use only in combination with chloroquine).*
mefloquine	1250 mg po as a single dose with food and with at least 8 oz. Water	tablet, 250 mg (hydrochloride)
sulfadoxine + pyrimethamine	Acute malarial attack: 2-3 tab po alone or with quinine. Malarial prophylaxis: 1 tab po once weekly or 2 tab po q 2 weeks 1 to 2 days before departure; continue for 4 to 6 weeks after return	tablet, 500 mg + 25 mg

6.5.3.2 For prophylaxis

chloroquine	300 mg of chloroquine base once weekly po, on the same day each week	tablet, 150 mg (as phosphate or sulfate); syrup 50 mg (as phosphate or sulfate)/5 ml

APPENDIX 1 *(continued)*

6.5.3.2 For prophylaxis *(continued)*

doxycycline	100 mg daily. Prophylaxis should begin 1-2 days before travel to the malarious area and 4 weeks after leaving the malarious area.	capsule or tablet, 100 mg (hydrochloride)
mefloquine	250 mg once weekly po for 4 weeks, then 250 mg every other week. Start 1 week prior to departure to endemic area.	tablet, 250 mg (as hydrochloride)
proguanil		tablet, 100 mg (hydrochloride) *(For use only in combination with chloroquine.)*

6.5.4 Anti-pneumocystosis and anti-toxoplasmosis drugs

pentamidine	4 mg/kg/day	tablet 200 mg, 300 mg
pyrimethamine	25 mg once weekly po	tablet, 25 mg
sulfamethoxazole + trimethoprim	As above	injeciton 80 mg + 16 mg in 5-ml ampoule

6.5.5 Antitrypanosomal drugs
6.5.5 (a) African trypanosomiasis

melarsoprol	As directed	injection, 3.6% solution
pentamidine	4 mg/kg once daily IV (over 60 minutes) or IM for 14 days	powder for injection, 200 mg, 300 mg (isetionate) in vial
suramin sodium	As directed	powder for injection, 1 g in vial
eflornithine	100 mg/kg/dose by IV infusion (over a minimum of 45 minutes) q 6 h for 14 days	injection, 200 mg (hydrochloride)/ml in 100-ml bottles

6.5.5 (b) American trypanosomiasis

benznidazole	As directed	tablet, 100 mg
nifurtimox	As directed	tablet, 30 mg; 120 mg; 250 mg

6.6 Insect repellents

diethyltoluamide	Apply topically	topical solution, 50%, 75%

7. ANTIMIGRAINE DRUGS
7.1 For treatment of acute attack

acetylsalicylic acid	One tablet 3 to 4 times daily. Fatal range overdose: 200-500 mg/kg.	tablet, 300-500 mg
ergotamine	2 mg placed under tongue. Max: 6 mg in any 24-hour period and a max of 10 mg in any one week.	tablet, 1 mg (tartrate)
paracetamol	Two 500 mg tablets or capsules q 4-6 h. Max: 8 tabs in 24 hours.	tablet, 300–500 mg

APPENDIX 1 *(continued)*

7.2 For prophylaxis

propranolol	Initially: 80 mg daily po in divided doses; increase dosage gradually. Maintenance: usually 160-240 mg daily.	tablet, 20 mg, 40 mg (hydrochloride)

8. ANTINEOPLASTIC, IMMUNOSUPPRESSIVES AND DRUGS USED IN PALLIATIVE CARE
8.1 Immunosuppressive drugs

Adequate resources and specialist oversight are a prerequisite for this class of drugs.

8.2 Cytotoxic drugs

Adequate resources and specialist oversight are a prerequisite for this class of drugs.

8.3 Hormones and antihormones

prednisolone	Tab: 5-60 mg/day po depending on illness; IV & IM Inj: Dose varies from 4-6 mg/day q 4-8 h; Intra-articular: usual dose is from 2-10 mg.	tablet, 5 mg; powder for injection, 20 mg in vial, 25 mg (as sodium phosphate or sodium succinate) in vial
tamoxifen	Breast Cancer: 20-40 mg daily bid Prophylaxis in high-risk women: 20 mg daily po for 5 years.	tablet, 10 mg, 20 mg (as citrate)

9. ANTIPARKINSONISM DRUGS

biperiden	Tab: 2 mg tid-qid po Inj: 2 mg q 30 min IM or IV not to exceed 4 doses in 24 hrs	tablet, 2 mg (hydrochloride); injection, 5 mg (lactate) in 1-ml ampoule
levodopa + carbidopa	Usual Initial Dosage: 1 tab of 100 + 10 tid or qid po. Maintenance: (250 + 25)	tablet, 100 mg + 10 mg; 250 mg + 25 mg

10. DRUGS AFFECTING THE BLOOD
10.1 Anti-anemia drugs

ferrous salt	1 tab bid to qid	tablet, 60 mg iron; oral solution, 25 mg iron (as sulfate)/1 ml
ferrous salt + folic acid	1 tab bid to qid (Nutritional supplement for use during pregnancy.)	tablet equivalent to 60 mg iron + 400 micrograms folic acid
folic acid	Usual therapeutic dose: up to 1 mg daily po	injection, 1 mg (as sodium salt) in 1-ml ampoule
hydroxocobalamin	100 mic daily for 6 or 7 days by IM or deep sq injection.	injection, 1 mg in 1-ml ampoule

10.2 Drugs affecting coagulation

desmopressin	Diabetes Insipidus: 10-40 micrograms daily as a single dose or in 2-3 divided doses intranasally	injection, 4 micrograms (acetate)/ml in 1-ml ampoule; nasal spray 10 mic/metered dose
heparin sodium	80 u/kg IV bolus, then IV infusion of 18 u/kg/hr	injection, 1000 IU/ml, 5000 IU/ml, 20,000 IU (acetate)/ml in 1-ml ampoule

APPENDIX 1 *(continued)*

10.2 Drugs affecting coagulation *(continued)*

phytomenadione	As directed	inj. 10 mg/ml in 5-ml ampule; tablet, 10 mg
protamine sulfate	As directed	injection, 10 mg/ml in 5-ml ampoule
warfarin	As directed	tablet, 1 mg, 2 mg and 5 mg (sodium salt)

11. BLOOD PRODUCTS AND PLASMA SUBSTITUTES

12. CARDIOVASCULAR DRUGS
12.1 Antianginal drugs

atenolol	Hypertension/angina: 50 mg once daily po, may increase to 100 mg daily if necessary	tablet, 50 mg, 100 mg
glyceryl trinitrate	Acute: Dissolve 1 tab under tongue at first sign of anginal attack. May repeat approx. every 5 minutes until relief is obtained.	tablet (sublingual), 500 micrograms
isosorbide dinitrate	2.5-10 mg q 2-3 h sublingually	tablet (sublingual), 5 mg
verapamil	Angina: 80-120 mg tid po; Hypertension: 80 mg tid po, adjust dosast up to 360 mg daily	tablet, 40 mg, 80 mg (hydrochloride)

12.2 Antiarrhythmic drugs

atenolol	as indicated above in antianginal drugs	tablet, 50 mg, 100 mg
digoxin	Load with 0.5 mg IV, then bolus .25 mg IV (up to 1 mg total) for rapid atrial fibrillation. Oral dose between .125mg and .5 mg/day.	tablet, 62.5 micrograms, 250 micrograms; oral solution 50 micrograms; injection 250 micrograms/ml in 2-ml ampoule.
lidocaine	IV Inj: 50-100 mg IV bolus at rate of 25-50 mg/min, may repeat in 5 min; IV infusion: following bolus give at a rate of 1-4 mg/min	injection, 20 mg (hydrochloride)/ml in 5-ml ampoule
verapamil	Digitalized Patients with Chronic Atrial Fibrillation: 240-320 mg/day po in 3-4 divided doses; Prophylaxis of PSVT—Non-Digitalized Patients: 240-480 mg/day po in 3-4 divided doses	tablet, 40 mg, 80 mg (hydrochloride); injection, 2.5 mg (hydrochloride)/ml in 2-ml ampoule

Complementary drugs

epinephrine (adrenaline)	0.2-1.0 mg SC or IM	injection 1 mg (as hydrochloride) in 1-ml ampoule
procainamide	Tab: up to 50 mg/kg daily in divided doses q 3 h po; IM: 50 mg/kg daily in divided doses given q 3-6 h. IV: 100 mg q 5 min, rate not to exceed 50 mg/min, until arrhythmia is suppressed or until 500 mg has been given; IV infusion: loading dose of 20 mg/mL (1 g diluted in 50mL of 5% dextrose inj) at rate of 1 mL/min for 25-30 min, then maintenance dose of 2 or 4 mg/mL.	tablet, 250 mg, 500 mg (hydrochloride); injection, 100 mg (hydrochloride)/ml in 10-ml ampoule
quinidine	Atrial Fibrillation/Flutter: 200 mg every 6 hours.	tablet, 200 mg (sulfate)

APPENDIX 1 *(continued)*

12.3 Antihypertensive drugs

atenolol	As indicated above in antianginal drugs	tablet, 50 mg, 100 mg
captopril	Initially, 25 mg bid or tid po, may increase after 1-2 wks to 50 mg bid or tid	scored tablet, 25 mg
hydralazine	Tab: initially 10 mg qid po for 2-4 days, increase to 25 mg qid for rest of week, for subsequent weeks, raise to 50 mg qid; Inj: 20-4-mg IM or IV, repeated as necessary	tablet, 25 mg, 50 mg (hydrochloride); powder for injection, 20 mg (hydrochloride) in ampoule
hydrochlorothiazide	50-100 mg daily po in the AM	scored tablet, 25 mg
methyldopa	Initial: 250 mg bid or tid po for first 48 h, at intervals of 2 or more days; Maintenance: 500 mg-2 g daily po in 2-4 divided doses	tablet, 250 mg
nifedipine	Initially 30-60 mg once daily po, adjust dose over a 7-10 day period	sustained release formulations, tablet 10 mg
reserpine	Initially: 0.5 mg daily po for 1-2 wks; Maintenance: reduce to 0.1-0.25 mg daily	tablet, 100 micrograms, 250 micrograms; injection, 1 mg in 1-ml ampoule
prazosin	1-15 mg/day	tablet, 500 micrograms, 1 mg
sodium nitroprusside	0.5-10.0 mug/kg/min (initial dose 0.25 g/kg/min for eclampsia and renal insufficiency	powder for infusion, 50 mg in ampoule

12.4 Drugs used in heart failure

captopril	6.25 mg twice daily	scored tablet, 25 mg
digoxin	As above	tablet, 62.5 micrograms, 250 micrograms; oral solution, 50 micrograms/ml; injection 250 micrograms/ml in 2-ml ampoule
dopamine	2-10 ug/kg/min by IV infusion	injection, 40 mg (hydrochloride) in 5-ml vial
hydrochlorothiazide	Diuresis: 25-100 mg daily or bid po; Hypertension: 50-100 mg daily po in the AM	tablet, 25 mg, 50 mg

12.5 Antithrombotic drugs

acetylsalicylic acid	Transient Ischemic Attacks: 1300 mg daily po in divided doses; Suspected Acute Myocardial Infarction: 160-162.5 mg po as soon as the infarct is suspected & then daily for at least 30 days	tablet, 100 mg
streptokinase	250,000 IU IV over 30 min. followed by 100,000 IU/h IV. Therapy length determined by condition — Pulmonary Embolism: 24 h (72 h if suspect concurrent deep vein thrombosis); Deep Vein Thrombosis: 72 h; Arterial Thrombosis or Embolism: 24-72 h	powder for injection, 100,000 IU, 750,000 IU in vial

APPENDIX 1 *(continued)*

13. DERMATOLOGICAL DRUGS (topical)
13.1 Antifungal drugs

benzoic acid + salicylic acid	Apply as directed	ointment or cream, 6% + 3%
miconazole	Apply to affected area bid, AM and PM	ointment or cream, 2% (nitrate)
selenium sulfide	Seborrheic Dermatitis and Tinea Versicolor: Apply with water on skin or hair for 10 min., then rinse. Repeat daily for 7 days.	detergent-based suspension, 2%

13.2 Anti-infective drugs

methylrosanilinium chloride (gentian violet)	Apply topically	aqueous solution, 0.5%; tincture, 0.5%
neomycin sulfate + bacitracin	Apply topically	ointment, 5 mg + 500 IU bacitracin zinc/g
potassium permanganate	As directed	aqueous solution 1:10 000
silver sulfadiazine	Apply to a thickness of 1/16 inch once or twice daily	cream, 1%, in 500-g container

13.3 Anti-inflammatory and anitpruritic drugs

betamethasone	Apply topically 1-3 times daily	ointment or cream, 0.1% (as valerate)
calamine lotion	Apply topically	lotion
hydrocortisone	Apply thin film to affected areas bid-qid	ointment or cream, 1% (acetate)

13.4 Astringent drugs

aluminium diacetate	Apply topically as directed	solution, 13% for dilution

13.5 Drugs affecting skin differentiaton and proliferation

benzoyl peroxide	Cleanse affected area, apply topically once or twice daily	lotion or cream, 5%
coal tar	Add 3 to 5 teaspoonfuls of coal tar emulsion to a bath of lukewarm water.	solution, 5%
dithranol	Apply in a thin layer to affected areas once or twice daily, or as directed by a physician	ointment, 0.1%–2%
fluorouracil	Actinic or Solar Keratosis or basal cell carcinoma: Cover lesions bid; continue therapy for at least 2-4 weeks	ointment, 5%
salicylic acid	Apply gel thoroughly to the affected area and occlude tat night.	solution 5%

13.6 Scabicides and pediculicides

benzyl benzoate	Apply as permethrin	lotion, 25%
permethrin	Thoroughly massage into skin from the head to the soles of the feet. Wash off (bath or shower) after 8–14 h.	cream 5%; lotion 1%

APPENDIX 1 *(continued)*

14. DIAGNOSTIC AGENTS
14.1 Ophthalmic drugs

fluorescein	1 to 2 drops (in single instillations) in each eye	eye drops, 1% (sodium salt)
tropicamide	Fundus Examination: Instill 1-2 drops of the 0.5% solution 15-20 minutes prior to the examination	eye drops, 0.5%

14.2 Radiocontrast media

amidotrizoate	For cystography and voiding cystourethrography ranges from 25 to 300 ml depending on the age of the patient	injection, 140-420 mg iodine (as sodium or meglumine salt)/ml in 20-ml ampoule
barium sulfate	As indicated	aqueous suspension
iohexol	As indicated	injection 140-350 mg iodine/ml in 5-ml, 10-ml and 20-ml ampoule

15. DISINFECTANTS AND ANTISEPTICS
15.1 Antiseptics

chlorhexidine	Twice daily oral rinsing for 30 seconds, morning and evening	solution, 5% (digluconate) concentrate for dilution

15.2 Disinfectants

chlorine base compound		powder (0.1% available chlorine) for solution
chloroxylenol		solution, 5%

16. DIURETICS

amiloride	5 mg once daily with food; dosage may be increased to 10 mg daily	tablet, 5 mg (hydrochloride)
furosemide	Diuresis: 20-80 mg daily po (may be repeated q 6-8); 20-40 mg IM or IV (over 1-2 min). Hypertension: 40 mg bid po	tablet, 40 mg; injection, 10 mg/ml in 2-ml ampoule
hydrochlorothiazide	Diuresis: 25-100 mg daily or bid po Hypertension: 50-100 mg daily po in the AM	tablet, 25 mg, 50 mg
spironolactone	Diuresis: Initially, 100 mg po, for at least 5 days; single or divided Hypertension: Initially 50-100 mg po; single or divided doses	tablet, 25 mg
mannitol	50 to 200 g IV in a 24-hour period, adjusted to maintain a urine flow of at least 30 to 50 ml/hr.	injectable solution, 10%, 20%

17. GASTROINTESTINAL DRUGS
17.1 Antacids and other antiulcer drugs

aluminum hydroxide	Tab: 500 mg 5 or 6 times daily, po between meals & hs. Susp: 10 mL (640 mg) 5 or 6 times daily po between meals & hs.	tablet, 500 mg; oral suspension, 320 mg/5 ml
cimetidine	800 mg hs po; or 300 me qid po with meals & hs; or 400 mg bid po 300 mg q 6-8 h IM or IV (infused over 15-20 minutes).	tablet, 200 mg; injection, 200 mg in 2-ml ampoule

APPENDIX 1 *(continued)*

17. GASTROINTESTINAL DRUGS *(continued)*
17.1 Antacids and other antiulcer drugs

magnesium hydroxide	5-15 mL with water up to qid po	oral suspension, 550 mg equivalent to magnesium oxide/10 ml

17.2 Antiemetic drugs

metoclopramide	Gastroesophageal Reflux: 10-15 mg po up to qid 30 minutes	tablet, 10 mg (hydrochloride); injection 5 mg (hydrochloride)/ml in 2-ml ampoule
promethazine	Allergy or nausea and vomiting: 25 mg po hs, or 12.5 mg po ac & hs. By deep IM injection, 25 mg; may repeat once in 2 h,	tablet, 10 mg, 25 (hydrochloride); elixir or syrup, 5 mg (hydrochloride)/5 ml; injection, 25 mg (hydrochloride)/ml in 2-ml ampoule

17.3 Anithaemorrhoidal drugs

local anaesthetic, anti-inflammatory drug	Apply rectally	ointment or suppository

17.4 Anti-inflammatory drugs

hydrocortisone	Insert 1 rectally AM and PM for 2 weeks. In more severe cases, 1 rectally tid or 2 bid	suppository 25 mg; (acetate); retention enema
sulfasalazine	Ulcerative colitis: Initial: 3-4 g daily po in evenly divided doses; Maintenance: 2 g daily po. Rheumatoid arthritis: Initially, 0.5 –1 g daily po; then 2 po in divided doses	tablet, 500 mg; suppository 500 mg; retention enema

17.5 Antispasmodic drugs

atropine	0.4-0.6 mg po, IV, IM or SC	tablet, 0.6 mg (sulfate); injection, 1 mg (sulfate) in 1-ml ampoule

17.6 Laxatives

senna	As directed	tablet, 7.5 mg (sennosides) (or traditional dosage forms)

17.7 Drugs used in diarrhea
17.7.1 Oral rehydration

oral rehydration salts	Mix packet as directed in 1 liter of water	Mix in 1 litre of glucose-electrolyte solution: sodium chloride 3.5 g/1; trisodium citrate dihydrate 2.9 g/1; potassium chloride 1.5 g/1; glucose, anhydrous 20.0 g/1

18 HORMONES, OTHER ENDOCRINE DRUGS AND CONTRACEPTIVES
18.1 Adrenal hormones and synthetic substitutes

dexamethasone	As above	tablet 500 micrograms, 4 mg; injection 4 mg dexamethasone phosphate (as disodium salt) in 1-ml ampoule
hydrocortisone	100-500 mg IM, IV, or by IV infusion. Repeat at 2, 4, or h.	powder for injection, 100 mg (as sodium succinate) in vial

APPENDIX 1 *(continued)*

18 HORMONES, OTHER ENDOCRINE DRUGS AND CONTRACEPTIVES *(continued)*
18.1 Adrenal hormones and synthetic substitutes

prednisolone	Initial dosage varies from 5-60 mg daily po depending on the disease being treated and the patient's response	tablet 1 mg, 5 mg

18.2 Androgens

testosterone	Male hypogonadism: 50-400 mg q 2-4 weeks IM Breast Cancer: 200-400 mg q 2-4 weeks IM	injection, 200 mg (enantate) in 1-ml ampoule

18.3 Contraceptives
18.3.1 Hormonal contraceptives

ethinylestradiol + levonorgestrel	21 day regimen po or 28 day regiment po	tablet, 30 micrograms + 150 micrograms
ethinylestradiol + levonorgestrel	Emergency contraceptive: Two pills taken as soon as possible but within 72 hours of unprotected intercourse, then a second dose of two pills 12 hours later.	tablet, 50 micrograms + 250 micrograms (pack of four)
ethinylestradiol + norethisterone	21 day regimen po or 28 day regimen po	tablet, 35 micrograms + 1.0 mg
levonorgestrel	Emergency contraceptive: 0.75 mg po within 72 h after unprotected intercourse; follow with 0.75 mg 12 h later	tablets, 750 micrograms (pack of two)

18.4 Estrogens

ethinylestradiol	Menopause: 0.2-0.5 mg daily po; Administration should be cyclic (3 weeks on, 1 week off). Prostatic Cancer: 0.15-2.0 mg daily po Breast Cancer: 1.0 mg tid po	tablet, 10 micrograms, 50 micrograms

18.5 Insulins and other antidiabetic agents

glibenclamide	2.5-5 mg/day start dose with breakfast or the first main meal. Daily doses of more than 20 mg are not recommended.	tablets, 2.5 mg, 5 mg.
insulin (soluble)	40 to 60 units, adjust as indicated by response	injection, 40 IU/ml in 10-ml vial, 100 IU/ml in 10 ml vial
intermediate-acting insulin	Start dose of 10 IU once daily, and subsequently adjusted according to the patient's need to a total daily dose ranging from 2-100 IU.	injection, 40 IU/ml in 10 ml vial; 100 IU/ml in 10 ml vial (as compound insulin zinc suspension or isophane insulin)
metformin	Usual starting dose is 500 mg bid po, with am and pm meals Max dose 2500 mg/day.	tablet, 500 mg (hydrochloride)

18.6 Ovulation inducers

clomifene	50 mg daily for 5 days po	tablet, 50 mg (citrate)

APPENDIX 1 *(continued)*

18.7 Progestogens

norethisterone	Amenorrhea: 2.5-10 mg once daily po, for 5-10 days during the second half of the menstrual cycle. Endometriosis: 5 mg once daily po for 2 weeks, with increments of 2.5 ml/day q 2 weeks until 15 mg/day is reached	tablet, 5 mg
medroxyprogesterone acetate	5-10 mg daily po for 5-10 days	tablet, 5 mg

18.8 Thyroid hormones and antithyroid drugs

levothyroxine	Usual Dosage: 50 micrograms daily po with increases 0f 25–50 micrograms at 2-4 week intervals to usual maintenance dosage is 100-200 micrograms daily po.	tablet, 50 micrograms, 100 micrograms (sodium salt)
propylthiouracil	Initial: 300 mg/day po, in 3 equal doses at 8 hour intervals Maintenance: 100-150 mg daily po in 3 doses at 8 hour intervals	tablet, 50 mg

19. IMMUNOLOGICALS
19.1 Diagnostic agents

tuberculin, purified protein derivative (PPD)	The Mantoux test is performed by intracutaneously injecting, with a syringe and needle, 0.1 ml of tuberculin PPD. It is customary to use 5 TU per test dose.	injection

19.2 Sera and immunoglobulins

antitetanus immunoglobulin (human)	As directed	injection, 500 IU in vial
immunoglobulin, human normal	See CDC recommendations	intramuscular injection

19.3 Vaccines (see text for vaccine administering guidelines)
19.3.1 For universal immunization

BCG	Dose of 0.2-0.3 ml is dropped on the cleansed surface of the skin, and the vaccine is administered percutaneously utilizing a sterile multiple-puncture disc.	
hepatitis B	1st Dose: At elected date.; 2nd Dose: 1 month later.; 3rd Dose: 6 months after the first dose.; Recombivax HB is for IM deltoid injection.	
measles	0.5 ml SQ injection	
poliomyelitis	Each sterile immunizing dose (0.5 ml) administer subcutaneously	
tetanus	The immunizing course for all age groups: two (primary) doses of 0.5 ml each, given at an interval of 4 to 8 weeks, followed by a third (reinforcing) dose of 0.5 ml 6 to 12 months later. A booster dose of 0.5 ml should be given at 10-year intervals throughout life	

APPENDIX 1 *(continued)*

19.3.2 For specific groups of individuals

influenza	Dose by age range	
meningitis	Primary Immunization: For both adults and children, vaccine is administered subcutaneously as a single 0.5 ml dose.	
rabies	The potency of one dose (1.0 ml) rabies vaccine is at least 2.5 IU of rabies antigen. The individual dose is 1 ml IM	
rubella	Dose is 0.5 ml, the same for all persons. Inject the total volume of the single dose vial (about 0.5 ml) SQ, the outer upper arm. Do not give immune globulin (IG) concurrently with Meruvax II.	
typhoid	See CDC recommendations	
yellow fever	Primary vaccination. Single SQ injection of 0.5 ml. Booster doses at intervals of 10 years.	

20. MUSCLE RELAXANTS (PERIPHERALLY ACTING) AND CHOLINESTERASE INHIBITORS

neostigmine	15 mg to 375 mg per day. Average dose is 10 tablets (150 mg) over a 24-hour period. Myasthenia Gravis: 0.5 mg SC or IM; Reversal of Neuromuscular Blockade: 0.5-2 mg by slow IV, repeat as required. Also give IV atropine sulfate, 0.6-1.2 mg	tablet, 15 mg (bromide); injection, 500 micrograms in 1-ml ampoule; 2.5 mg (metilsulfate) in 1-ml ampoule
pyridostigmine bromide	Tab: 600 mg (10 tab) daily po in divided doses,	tablet, 60 mg; injection, 1 mg in 1-ml ampoule
suxamethonium bromide	The average dose to produce neuromuscular blockade is 0.6 mg/kg succinylcholine chloride injection IV	injection, 50 mg/ml in 2-ml ampoule; powder for injection
vecuronium bromide	Initially: 0.08-0.1 mg/kg as an IV bolus. Maintenance: doses of 0.010-0.015 mg/kg are usually required within 25-40 min	powder for injection, 10 mg in vial

21. OPHTHALMOLOGICAL PREPARATIONS
21.1 Anti-infective agents

gentamicin	1-2 drops into affected eye(s) q 4 h. Severe infections: May increase to as much as 2 drops once every hour	solution (eye drops), 0.3% (sulfate)
idoxuridine	1 drop in the infected eye(s) every hour during the day. At night the dosage may be reduced to one drop every other hour.	solution (eye drops), 0.1%; eye ointment 0.2%
silver nitrate	2 drops immediately after child is born	solution (eye drops), 1%
tetracycline	Bacterial Infections: 2 drops in the affected eye(s), bid-qid Trachoma: 2 drops in each eye 2-4 times/day for 1-3 months	eye ointment, 1% (hydrochloride)

APPENDIX 1 *(continued)*

21.2 Anti-inflammatory agents

prednisolone	1-2 drops into affected eye(s) up to q h during the day and q 2 h at night. Reduce dosage to 1 drop q 4 when get response.	eye drops, 0.5% (sodium phosphate)

21.3 Local anaesthetics

tetracaine	1-2 drops into eye(s)	solution (eye drops), 0.5% (hydrochloride)

21.4 Miotics and antiglaucoma drugs

acetazolamide	250-1000 mg per day usually in divided doses po	tablet, 250 mg
pilocarpine	1-2 drops in eye(s) up to 6 times daily	solution (eye drops), 2%, 4% (hydrochloride or nitrate)
timolol	1 drop into affected eye(s) bid	solution (eye drops), 0.25%, 0.5% (as maleate)

21.5 Mydriatics

atropine	1-2 drops in eye(s) up to qid	solution (eye drops), 0.1%; solution 0.5%, 1% (sulfate)
epinephrine (adrenaline)	1 drop in eye(s) 1-2 times daily	solution (eye drops), 2% (as hydrochloride)

22. OXYTOCICS AND ANTIOXYTOCICS
22.1 Oxytocics

ergometrine	Usual IM (or emergency IV) dose is 0.2 mg per 1 ml.	tablet, 200 micrograms (hydrogen maleate); injection, 200 micrograms (hydrogen maleate) in 1-ml ampule
oxytocin	Control of Postpartum Uterine Bleeding or incomplete AB: IV (drip method): 10 to 40 u added to IV fluid (maximum 40 units to 1000 ml). IM 10 units after the delivery of the placenta.	injection, 10 IU in 1-ml ampoule

23. PERITONEAL DIALYSIS SOLUTION

intraperitoneal dialysis solution	As directed	parenteral solution

24. PSYCHOTHERAPEUTIC DRUGS
24.1 Drugs used in psychotic disorders

chlorpromazine	Psychoses (inpatient): 25 mg tid po or IM. Increase gradually until the effective dose is reached, usually 400 mg daily. Psychoses (Outpatient): 10 mg tid or qid po; or 25 mg bid to tid po; More Severe Cases: 25 mg tid po. Nausea & Vomiting: Dosage: 10-25 mg q 4-6 h po or 25 mg IM.	tablet, 100 mg (hydrochloride); syrup, 25 mg (hydrochloride)/5 ml; injection, 25 mg (hydrochloride)/ml; in 2-ml ampoule
fluphenazine decanoate	Decanoate: 12.t-25 mg IM or SC Enanthate: 25 mg IM or SC q 2 weeks	injection, 25 mg (decanoate or enanthate) in 1-ml ampoule
haloperidol	Tab: 0.5-5 mg bid to tid po; Inj: 2-5 mg q 4-6 h IM	tablet, 2 mg; injection, 5 mg in 1-ml ampoule

APPENDIX 1 *(continued)*

24.2 Drugs used in mood disorders
24.2.1 Drugs used in depressive disorders

| amitriptyline | Initially: 75 mg daily po in divided doses up to 150 mg daily po in divided doses; Maintenance: dose is 50-100 mg daily po. | tablet, 25 mg (hydrochloride) |

24.2.2 Drugs used in bipolar disorders

carbamazepine	Initial: 200 mg bid po. Maximum: 1000 mg daily (ages 12-15); 1200 mg daily (ages over 15)	scored tablet, 100 mg, 200 mg
lithium carbonate	Usual dosage: 300 mg tid or qid po Acute Mania: 900 mg bid po or 600 mg tid po	capsule or tablet, 300 mg
valproic acid	Initially: 15 mg/kg/day po in 2 or 3 divided doses, increasing at 1 week intervals by 5 to 10 mg/kg/day (Maximum: 60 mg/kg/day)	enteric coated tablet, 200 mg, 500 mg (sodium salt)

24.3 Drugs used in generalized anxiety and sleep disorders

| diazepam | Anxiety and anticonvulsant: 2-10 mg bid to qid po
Muscle Spasms: 2-10 mg tid to qid po | scored tablet, 2 mg, 5 mg |

25. DRUGS ACTING ON THE RESPIRATORY TRACT
25.1 Antiasthmatic drugs

aminophylline	See theophylline	injection, 25 mg/ml in 10 ml ampoule
beclomethasone	As directed	inhalant (aerosol), 50 micrograms per dose (dipropionate); 250 micrograms (dipropionate) per dose
epinephrine (adrenaline)	0.2-1.9 mg SC or IV	injection, 1 mg (as hydrochloride or hydrogen tartrate) in 1-ml ampoule
ipratropium bromide	2 inhalations qid	inhalation, 20 micrograms/metered dose
salbutamol	As directed	tablet, 2 mg, 4 mg; inhalation (aerosol), 100 micrograms per dose; syrup, 2 mg/5ml; solution for use in nebulizers, 5 mg/ml
theophylline	5 mg/kg po (oral loading dose); then, 3 mg/kg q 8 h po	tablet, 100 mg, 200 mg, 300 mg

25.2 Antitussives

| dextromethorphan | 30 mg q 6-8 h po | oral solution, 3.5 mg (bromide)/5 ml |

26. SOLUTIONS CORRECTING WATER, ELECTROLYTE AND ACID-BASE DISTURBANCES (see prior section)

27. VITAMINS AND MINERALS

ascorbic acid	One tab daily as directed	tablet, 50 mg
ergocalciferol	Rickets: 12,000 to 500,000 units daily; Hypoparathyroidism: 50,000 to 200,000 units/d with calcium lactate 4 g, q 6 times/day.	capsule or tablet, 1.25 mg (50,000 IU); oral solution, 250 micrograms/ml (10,000 IU/ml)
iodine	As directed	iodized oil, 0.5 ml (240 mg of iodine/ml), 1 ml (480 mg iodine/1 ml) in ampoule (oral or injectable); solution, 0.57 ml, capsule, 200 mg.

APPENDIX 1 *(continued)*

27. VITAMINS AND MINERALS *(continued)*

pyridoxine	10 to 20 mg daily for 3 weeks.	tablet, 25 mg (hydrochloride)
retinol	100,000 Units IM daily for 3 days, then 50,000 daily for two weeks	10,000 IU (5.5 mg); capsule, 200,000 IU (110 mg); 100,000 IU (55 mg) in 2-ml ampoule
riboflavin	One tab daily as directed	tablet, 5 mg
thiamine	One tab daily as directed	tablet, 50 mg (hydrochloride)

APPENDIX 2: The WHO Emergency Health Kit Basic and Supplemental Units

The World Health Organization (WHO) has compiled an Emergency Health Kit to provide basic medications and supplies for health-care practitioners in large-scale emergencies and humanitarian crisis. The WHO kit provides basic, appropriate generic medications that can be used in most emergency scenarios. For larger-scale emergencies, the Supplemental Units may be obtained as a supplement to the basic unit to provide for 10,000 people for 3 months. The WHO kits may be available from a variety of distributors.

EMERGENCY HEALTH KIT: BASIC UNIT

(EACH UNIT CONTAINS 10 BASIC KITS EACH FOR 1,000 PEOPLE FOR 3 MONTHS)

Drugs
Acetylsalicylic acid, tab 300mg...3000 tab
Aluminum hydroxide, tab 500mg...1000 tab
Benzyl benzoate, lotion 25%..1 liter bottle
Chlorhexidine (5%) ....1 liter bottle
Chloroquine, tab 150mg base ....2000 tab
Ferrous sulfate + Folic acid, tab 200 + 0.25mg ....2000 tab
Gentian violet, powder ....4 units of 25g
Mebendazole, tab 100mg..500 tab
Oral rehydration salts ....200 sachets for 1L
Paracetamol, tab 100mg ....1000 tab
Sulfamethoxazole + Trimethoprim, tab 400 + 80mg (cotrimoxazole)................2000 tab
Tetracycline eye ointment 1% ....50 tubes of 5g each

Renewable supplies
Absorbent cotton wool ....1 kg
Adhesive tape 2.5cm × 5m ....30 rolls
Bar of soap (100-200g)..10 bars
Elastic bandage (crepe) 7.5cm × 10m ....20 units
Gauze bandage 7.5cm × 10m..100 rolls
Gauze compress 10 x 10cm, 12 ply, nonsterile ....500 units
Ballpen, blue or black..10 units
Exercise book A4..4 units
Health card + plastic sachet ....500 units
Small plastic bag for drugs..2000 units
Notepad A6 ....10 units
Thermometer (oral/rectal) Celsius/Fahrenheit ....6 units
Protective glove, nonsterile, disposable...100 units
Treatment guidelines for basic list..2 units

Equipment
Nail brush, autoclavable ....2 units

APPENDIX 2 *(continued)*

Bucket, plastic, approx 20 liters..1 unit
Gallipot, stainless steel, 100ml..1 unit
Kidney dish, stainless steel, approx 26 × 14cm ....1 unit
Dressing set (3 instruments + box) ....2 units
Dressing tray, stainless steel, approx 30 × 15 × 3cm ....1 unit
Drum for compresses, approx 15cm H ....2 units
Foldable jerrycan, 20L...1 unit
Forceps Kocher, no teeth, 12-14cm ....2 units
Plastic bottle, 1L ....3 units
Syringe Luer, disposable, 10ml ....1 unit
Plastic bottle, 125ml..1 unit
Scissors straight/blunt, 12-14cm..2 units

EMERGENCY HEALTH KIT: SUPPLEMENTAL UNIT

(FOR 10,000 PEOPLE FOR 3 MONTHS)

DRUGS

Anesthetics
Ketamine, inj. 50mg/ml ....25 vials of 10 ml each
Lidocaine, inj. 1% ....50 vials of 20 ml each

Analgesics
Pentazocine, inj. 30mg/ml...50 ampules of 1ml each
Probenecid, tab 500mg...500 tab
Recall ASA and paracetamol from basic unit

Anti-allergics
Dexamethasone, inj. 4mg/ml..50 ampules of 1ml each
Prednisolone, tab 5mg...100 tab
Epinephrine (adrenaline), see "respiratory tract"

Anti-epileptics
Diazepam, inj. 5mg/ml..200 ampules of 2ml each
Phenobarbital, tab 50mg...1000 tab

Anti-infective drugs
Ampicillin, tab 250mg (to be used in neonates and pregnant women only) ....2000 tab
Ampicillin, inj. 500mg/vial (to be used in neonates and pregnant women only)...............200 vials
Benzathine benzylpenicillin, inj. 2.4 MIU/vial ....50 vials
Chloramphenicol, caps 250mg ....2000 caps
Chloramphenicol, inj. 1g/vial ....500 vials

APPENDIX 2 *(continued)*

Metronidazole, tab 250mg ....2000 tab
Nystatin, noncoated tablet ....2000 tab of 100,000 IU
Phenoxymethylpenicillin, tab 250mg...4000 tab
Procaine benzylpenicillin, inj. 3-4 MU/vial ....1000 vials
Quinine, inj. 300mg/ml (for cerebral and resistant malaria cases)...........100 ampules of 2ml each
     (Always dilute in 500ml of Glucose 5%)
Quinine sulfate, tab 300mg...3000 tab
Sulfadoxine + pyrimethamine, tab 500mg + 25mg (for resistant malarial strains) ....300 tab
Tetracycline, caps or tab 250mg (for cholera and chlamydial infections) ....2000 units
Recall Mebendazole, Cotrimoxazole, and Chloroquine from basic unit

Blood, drugs affecting the
Folic acid, tab 1mg...5000 tab
Recall iron + folic acid from basic unit

Cardiovascular drugs
Methyldopa, tab 250mg (for hypertension in pregnancy)......................................500 tab
Hydralazine, inj. 20mg/ml ....20 ampules of 1ml each

Dermatological
Polyvidone iodine, 10% sol., 500ml..4 bottles
Zinc oxide, 10% ointment...2 kg
Benzoic acid + salicylic acid, 6% + 3% ointment...1 kg
Recall Tetracycline ointment, Gentian violet, and benzyl benzoate from basic unit

Diuretics
Furosemide, inj. 10mg/ml...20 ampules of 2ml each
Furosemide, tab 40mg...200 tab

Gastrointestinal drugs
Promethazine, tab 25mg...500 tab
Promethazine, inj. 25mg/ml ....50 ampules of 2ml each
Atropine, inj. 1mg/ml.50 ampules of 1ml each
Recall aluminium hydroxide from basic unit

Oxytocics
Ergometrine maleate, inj. 0.2mg/ml...200 ampules of 1ml each

Psychotherapeutic drugs
Chlorpromazine, inj. 25mg/ml..20 ampules of 2ml each

Respiratory tract, drugs acting on
Aminophylline, tab 100mg...1000 tab
Aminophylline, inj. 25mg/ml ....50 ampules of 10ml each
Epinephrine (adrenaline), inj. 1mg/ml.......................................50 ampules of 1ml each

APPENDIX 2 *(continued)*

Solutions correcting water, electrolyte, and acid-base disturbances
Compound solution of sodium lactate (Ringer's lactate),

Inj. sol., with giving set and needle ....200 bags of 500ml each

Glucose, inj. sol. 5%, with giving set and needle ....100 bags of 500ml each

Glucose, inj. sol. 50% ....20 vials of 50ml each

Water for injection ....2000 vials of 10ml each

Recall oral rehydration salts for basic unit

Vitamins
Retinol (Vitamin A), caps 200,000 IU ....4000 caps

Ascorbic acid, tab 250mg ....4000 tab

Renewable supplies
Scalp vein infusion set, disposable, 25G ....300 units

Scalp vein infusion set, disposable, 21G ....100 units

IV placement cannula, disposable, 18G ....15 units

IV placement cannula, disposable, 22G ....15 units

Needle Luer IV, disposable, 19G ....1000 units

Needle Luer IM, disposable, 21G ....2000 units

Needle Luer SC, disposable, 25G ....100 units

Spinal needle, disposable, 20G ....30 units

Spinal needle, disposable, 23G ....30 units

Syringe Luer resterilizable, nylon, 2ml ....20 units

Syringe Luer resterilizable, nylon, 5ml ....100 units

Syringe Luer resterilizable, nylon, 10ml ....40 units

Syringe Luer, disposable, 2ml ....400 units

Syringe Luer, disposable, 5ml ....500 units

Syringe Luer, disposable, 10ml ....200 units

Syringe conic connector (for feeding), 60ml ....20 units

Feeding tube, CH5 (premature baby), disposable ....20 units

Feeding tube, CH8, disposable ....50 units

Feeding tube, CH16, disposable ....10 units

Urinary catheter (Foley), n12,disposable ....10 units

Urinary catheter (Foley), n14,disposable ....5 units

Urinary catheter (Foley), n18,disposable ....5 units

Surgical gloves sterile and resterilizable n6.5 ....50 pair

Surgical gloves sterile and resterilizable n7.5 ....150 pair

Surgical gloves sterile and resterilizable n8.5 ....50 pair

Recall glove, nonsterile, disposable from basic unit

Sterilization test tape (for autoclave) ....2 rolls

Chloramine, tabs or powder ....2.5 kg

Thermometer (oral/rectal) dual Celsius/Fahrenheit ....10 units

Spare bulb for otoscope ....2 units

Batteries R6 alkaline AA size (for otoscope) ....6 units

Urine collecting bag with valve, 2000ml ....10 units

APPENDIX 2 *(continued)*

Finger stall 2 fingers, disposable ....300 units
Suture, synthetic absorbable, braided, size DEC.2(000) with
        Cutting needle curved 3/8, 20mm triangular......................................24 units
Suture, synthetic absorbable, braided, size DEC.3(00) with
        Cutting needle curved 3/8, 30mm triangular......................................36 units
Surgical blade (surgical knives) n22 for handle n4 ....50 units
Razor blade ....100 units
Tongue depressor (wooden), disposable ....100 units
Gauze roll 90m x 0.90m ....3 rolls
Gauze compress 10 x 10cm, 12 ply, sterile ....1000 units

Equipment

Clinical stethoscope, dual cup ....2 units
Obstetrical stethoscope (metal) ....1 unit
Sphygmomanometer (adult) ....1 unit
Razor, nondisposable...2 units
Scale for adult..1 unit
Scale hanging 25kg × 100g (Salter type) + 3 trousers ....3 units
Tape measure ....5 units
Drum for compresses, h:15cm..2 units
Otoscope + disposable set of pediatric speculums ....1 unit
Tourniquet ....2 units
Dressing tray, stainless steel, approx 30 × 15 × 3cm ....1 unit
Kidney dish, stainless steel, approx 26 × 14cm ....1 unit
Scissors straight/blunt, 12-14cm..2 units
Forceps Kocher no teeth, 12-14cm...2 units
Abcess / suture set (7 instruments + box)..2 units
Dressing set (3 instruments + box) ....5 units
Pressure sterilizer, 7.5L (type: Prestige 7506, double rack,
        Ref. UNIPAC 01.571.00) ....1 unit
        Additional rack Public Health Care 2ml/5ml, ref. Prestige 7531 ....2 units
Pressure sterilizer, 20-40L with basket (type UNIPAC 01.560.00)............................1 unit
Kerosene stove, single burner (type UNIPAC 01.700.00) ....2 units
Water filter with candles, 10-20L (type UNIPAC 56.199.02) ....3 units
Nail brush, plastic, autoclavable ....2 units
Portable weight/height chart (UNICEF / SCF)(UNIPAC 01.455.70)......................1 unit

APPENDIX 3: PRESUMPTIVE TREATMENT GUIDELINES FOR COMMON ILLNESSES

Adapted from WHO Treatment Guidelines
and MSF Diagnostic and Treatment Guidelines

SYMPTOM	Wt.	< 4 kg	4–8 kg	8–15 kg	15–35 kg	ADULT
	Age	< 2 months	2 months–1 year	1–5 years	5–15 years	
ANEMIA: **Moderate anemia;** [pallor and weakness]		Refer	ferrous sulphate+ folic acid 1 tab/day for 2 months	ferrous sulphate+ folic acid 2 tab/day for 2 months	ferrous sulphate+ folic acid 3 tab/day for 2 months	ferrous sulphate+ folic acid 3 tab/day for 2 months
Severe anemia; [Edema, dizziness, shortness of breath]		Refer	Refer	Refer	Refer	Refer
PAIN: **Pain;** [Headache, Joint pain, Dental pain]			Paracetamol [100mg] ½ tab × 3	Paracetamol [100mg] 1 tab × 3	Acetylsalicylic* acid (ASA) [300mg] 1 tab × 3	Acetylsalicylic acid (ASA) [300mg] 1 tab × 3
Epigastric (upper) abdominal pain;				Refer	Aluminum Hydroxide ½ tab × 3 for 3 days	Aluminum Hydroxide ½ tab × 3 for 3 days

*For children under 12, paracetamol is to be preferred because of risk of Reye's Syndrome.

APPENDIX 3 *(continued)*

SYMPTOM	Wt.	< 5 kg	5–8 kg	8–11 kg	11–16 kg	16–30 kg	30 kg +
	Age*	< 4 months	4–11 months	12–23 months	2–4 years	5–14 years	15 years or adult
DIARRHEA: *Diarrhea with mild dehydration*	Approximate amount of ORS solution to give in the first 4 hours.						
Quantity Of ORS in mls	200–400	400–600	600–800	800–12,000	1,200–2,200	2,200 4,000	
Diarrhea lasting more than two weeks or in malnourished or poor condition patient.	Give ORS according to dehydration stage and refer.						
*Bloody diarrhea** (dysentery)*	Give ORS according to dehydration stage and refer.						
Diarrhea with severe dehydration	Refer patient for nasogastric tube and / or IV treatment.						
Diarrhea with no dehydration	Continue to feed. Advise the patient to return to the health worker in case of frequent stools, increased thirst, sunken eyes, fever or when patient does not eat or drink normally, or does not get better within three days, or develops blood in stools or repeated vomiting.						

*Age to be used only when weight is not known.
**Protocol to be established according to epidemiological data.

APPENDIX 3 *(continued)*

SYMPTOM	Wt.	> 4 kg	4–8 kg	8–15 kg	15–35 kg	ADULT
	Age	> 2 months	2 months–1 year	1–5 years	5–15 years	
FEVER: *Fever in malnourished or poor condition patient or when in doubt;*		Refer				
Fever with chills; [assuming it's malaria]		Refer	Chloroquine tab 150mg base* ½ tab at once, then ½ tab after 24 hrs, & ½ tab after 48 hours	Chloroquine tab 150mg base 1 tab at once, then 1 tab after 24 hrs, & ½ tab after 48 hours	Chloroquine tab 150mg base 2 tab at once, then 2 tab after 24 hrs, & 1 tab after 48 hours	Chloroquine tab 150mg base 4 tab at once, then 4 tab after 24 hrs, & 2 tab after 48 hours
Fever with cough;		Refer 'see Respiratory tract infections'.				
Fever; [unspecified] *in absence of neck rigidity or confusion*		Refer	paracetamol tab 100mg ½ tab × 3 for 1–3 days	paracetamol tab 100mg 1 tab × 3 for 1–3 days	Acetylsalicylic* acid (ASA) tab 300mg 1 tab × 3 for 1–3 days	ASA tab 300mg 2 tab × 3 for 1–3 days

*Chloroquine 150 base is equivalent to approximately 250 mg chloroquine phosphate or approximately 200mg chloroquine sulfate.

APPENDIX 3 (continued)

DIAGNOSIS	Wt.	> 4 kg	4–8 kg	8–15 kg	15–35 kg	ADULT
	Age	> 2 months	2 months– 1 year	1–5 years	5–15 years	
Respiratory Tract Infections *Severe Pneumonia*		Give first dose of Cotrimoxazole and refer.				
Pneumonia:		Refer	cotrimoxazole tab 400mg SMX +80mg TMP ½ tab × 2 for 5 days	cotrimoxazole tab 400mg SMX +80mg TMP 1 tab × 2 for 5 days	cotrimoxazole tab 400mg SMX +80mg TMP 1 tab × 2 for 5 days	cotrimoxazole tab 400mg SMX +80mg TMP 2 tab × 2 for 5 days
			Reassess after 2 days; continue (breast) feeding, give fluids, clear the nose; return if breathing becomes faster or more difficult, or not able to drink or when condition deteriorates.			
No pneumonia: cough or cold;		Refer	paracetamol tab 100mg ½ tab × 3 for 1–3 days	paracetamol tab 100mg 1 tab × 3 for 1–3 days	Acetylsalicylic* acid (ASA) tab 300mg 1 tab × 3 for 1–3 days	Acetylsalicylic acid (ASA) tab 300mg 2 tab × 3 for 1–3 days
			Supportive therapy; continue (breast) feeding, give fluids, clear the nose; return if breathing becomes faster or more difficult, or not able to drink or when condition deteriorates.			
Prolonged Cough (> 30 days)		Refer				
EAR INFECTIONS: *Acute ear pain and/or ear discharge less than 2 weeks*		Refer	cotrimoxazole tab 400mg SMX +80mg TMP ½ tab × 2 for 5 days	cotrimoxazole tab 400mg SMX +80mg TMP 1 tab × 2 for 5 days	cotrimoxazole tab 400mg SMX +80mg TMP 1 tab × 2 for 5 days	cotrimoxazole tab 400mg SMX +80mg TMP 2 tab × 2 for 5 days
Ear discharge more than 2 weeks, no pain or fever.		Refer				
MEASLES:			Treat respiratory tract disease according to symptoms. Treat conjunctivitis as "Red eyes" Treat diarrhea according to symptoms. Continue breast feeding, give retinol.			

APPENDIX 4: The Mobile Medical Kit

The mobile medical kit is a recommended kit of health providers in the field. This includes personal health items and basic supplies for treating injuries and illnesses in the field. The kit may be used as a template for developing a personalized kit, with medications and supplies specific to the type of travel/work environment.

When designing a mobile medical kit, keep in mind the following:

1. The location and conditions of your destination
2. Endemic diseases specific to the region
3. The number of people you plan to treat or support
4. The duration of travel
5. Preexisting illnesses or specific medical needs of those you will support
6. Weight and space limitations

There are a number of good options for medical kits available. A good resource for personal travel kits is **Adventure Medical Kits, P.O. Box 43309, Oakland, California 94624, (800) 324-3517.**

WOUND CARE ITEMS

20cc syringe for wound irrigation and angiocath
10% Betadine solution
"Butterfly" wound closure strips
Suture kit with hemostats, scissors, and drapes
Sutures for wound closure (nylon)
1% xylocaine for anesthesia
Scalpel
Surgical scrub brush with disinfectant
Calamine lotion
Protective gloves, nonlatex
Foam-padded splints
Cotton-tipped applicators
Cavit temporary filling material
Zinc oxide and eugenol (oil of cloves) mixture for temporary filling
Cotton pledgets
Safety pins
Soap
Duct tape

BANDAGES

Gauze pads (4x4)
Gauze rolls (Kling)
Non-stick dressings (Xeroform, Adaptic)
Bandaids

APPENDIX 4 *(continued)*

Elastic ACE wrap
Moleskin padded adhesive
Tape

OVER-THE-COUNTER MEDICATIONS

ACETAMINOPHEN (TYLENOL)
Indications: For relief of pain and fever. Tylenol has no anti-inflammatory effect.
Dosage: Adults: 1000 mg. Every 4 to 6 hours, children: 15 mg./kg every 4 to 6 hours.

ALUMINUM HYDROXIDE AND SEMETHICONE TABLETS (MYLANTA)
Indications: Each tablet contains both an antacid and an antigas ingredient.
Dosage: Two to four tablets between meals and at bedtime.

DIPHENHYDRAMINE (BENADRYL)
Dosage: Adults: 25 to 50 mg. Every 4 to 6 hours. Children: consult your physician.

HYDROCORTISONE CREAM USP 2%
Indications: For temporary relief of minor skin irritations and allergic reaction.
Dosage: Adults and children 2 years of age and older: apply to affected area three times/day.

IBUPROFEN (MOTRIN)
Dosage: Adults: 400 to 800 mg. Every 8 hours with food
Children: Ibuprofen is available by prescription in a liquid form for children.

ORAL REHYDRATION SALT (ELECTROLYTE SALTS AND GLUCOSE)
Mix with a quart of water for replacing electrolytes and fluids lost during diarrhea illness or
vomiting.

PERMETHRIN 5% CREAM
Indications: Treatment for lice, bedbugs and scabies
Dosage: Apply head to toe, leave on for 12 hours and wash off. Shampoo for head lice.

PRESCRIPTION MEDICATION

Be aware of any contraindications to medication, allergies, or harmful side effects. A physician
should be consulted before any medication is taken by a child, pregnant woman, or nursing
mother.

AMOXICILLIN CLAVULANATE (AUGMENTIN®) 500 MG TABLETS
Indications: Bite wounds, skin infections, pneumonia, urinary tract infections, ear infections,
bronchitis, tonsillitis
Dosage: One tablet every 8 hours, for 7 to 10 days.

APPENDIX 4 *(continued)*

AZITHROMYCIN (ZITHROMAX®) 250 MG CAPSULES
Indications: Tonsillitis, ear infections, bronchitis, pneumonia, sinusitis, traveler's diarrhea, skin infections
Dosage: Take two capsules on the first day, followed by one capsule a day for 4 more days.

CEPHALEXIN (KEFLEX®) 250 TO 500 MG TABLETS
Indications: Skin infections, bronchitis, urinary tract infections, tonsillitis, middle ear infections, some bone infections, bite wounds, tonsillitis, dental infections, sinusitis
Dosage: 250–500 mg. Every six hours.

CIPROFLOXACIN (CIPRO) 500 MG TABLETS
Indications: Diarrhea, pneumonia, urinary tract infections, bone infections.
Dosage: One tablet twice a day, for 3 days. For kidney infections, pneumonia, treat for 7 to 10 days.

COMPAZINE OR PHENERGAN SUPPOSITORIES
Indications: For control of severe nausea and vomiting
Dosage: 25mg. Rectally twice a day.

CORTISPORIN OTIC SUSPENSION
Indications: External ear infections (swimmers ear)
Dosage: Four drops into the affected ear four times a day

EPI E •Z PEN® (EPINEPHRINE AUTO-INJECTOR) & EPI E• Z PEN® JR.
Indications: Emergency treatment of severe allergic reactions (anaphylaxis) to bees, wasps, foods, and other allergens. May also help relieve symptoms of asthma.
Dosage: For adults and children over 66 lbs. Each Epi E•Z Pen® contains 2 ml of epinephrine 1:1000 UPS in a disposable cartridge with a concealed needle to deliver a single dose of 0.3 mg epinephrine IM.

ERYTHROMYCIN 250/500 MG TABLETS
Indications: Bronchitis, tonsillitis, pneumonia, skin infections, sinus infections, ear and eye infections
Dosage: 250–500 mg. Every 6 hours, for 7 to 10 days

IMMODIUM® (DIAMODE) 2 MG CAPSULE (available over-the counter)
Indications: For controlling the abdominal cramping and diarrhea associated with intestinal infections
Dosage: 4 mg initially, followed by one capsule (2mg) after each loose bowel movement; not to exceed 14 mg/day

METRONIDAZOLE (FLAGYL®) 250 MG TABLETS
Indications: Infections with *Giardia* or amoebae; intra-abdominal infections including peritonitis and diverticulitis

APPENDIX 4 (continued)

Dosage: Giardiasis: one tablet three times a day, for 7 days. Amoebiasis: three tablets three times a day, for 5 to 10 days. Other intra-abdominal infections: two tables every 6 hours if the patient is not vomiting.

TRIMETHOPRIM/SULFAMETHOXAZOLE (Bactim, Septra)
Indications: Urinary tract or kidney infections, ear and sinus infections, and bronchitis
Dosage: One tablet twice a day for 5 days for diarrhea and dysentery. Other infections may require 10-day course.

TOBREX® OPHTHALMIC SOLUTION 0.3%
Indications: For external infections of the eye (conjunctivitis or pink eye, or corneal abrasions)
Dosage: One to two drops into the affected eye every 2 hours while awake

VICODIN (hydrocodone 5 mg and acetaminophen 500 mg)
Indications: For relief of pain. Can also be used for relief of diarrhea and suppression of cough.
Dosage: One to two tablets every 4 to 6 hours

APPENDIX 5: Informational Resources

INTERNATIONAL ORGANIZATIONS

International Committee of the Red Cross
17 Avenue de la Paix
CH-1202
Geneva, Switzerland
(telephone) 41.22.7346001
(telex) 22269
(telefax) 41.22.7332057

International Dispensary Association
P.O. Box 3098
1003 AB
Amsterdam, The Netherlands
(telephone) 31.2903.3051
(telex) 13566
(telefax) 31.2903.1854

UNICEF (UNIPAC)
Arhusgade 129
Freeport
DK 2100
Copenhagen, Denmark
(telephone) 45.31.262444
(telex) 19813
(telefax) 45.31.269421

United Nations High Commissioner for Refugees
Palais des Nations
CH-1211
Geneva-10
Switzerland
(telephone) 41.22.7398111
(telex) 27492
(telefax-general) 41.22.7319546
(telefax-supplies) 41.22.7310776

World Health Organization (WHO)
Avenue Appia
CH-1211
Geneva-27
Switzerland
(telephone) 41.22.7912111
(telex) 27821
(telefax) 41.22.7910746

APPENDIX 5 *(continued)*

NONGOVERNMENT ORGANIZATIONS:

Adventure Medicine
Box 1106
Point Reyes Station, CA 94956
FAX: (510) 601-5300
E.Mail: stinsonmd@aol.com

Africare
440 R Street, NW
Washington, DC 20001
Telephone: (202) 462-3614
FAX: (202) 387-1034
Web site: http://www.AFRICARE.org

AID International Inc.
2221 Pea Road
Suite P-30
Atlanta, GA 30309
E.Mail: aidinternational@mindspring.com

American Baptist Churches Board of International Ministries
Box 851
Valley Forge, PA 19482
Telephone: (610) 768-2000
(610) 768-2366
FAX: (610) 768-2088
E.Mail: theresa.randall@abc-usa.org

Americares Foundation
161 Cherry Street
New Canaan, CT 06840
Telephone: (800) 486-4357
Web site: info@americares.org or http://www.americares.org

American Bureau for Medical Advancement in China, Inc.
1216 Fifth Avenue, Room 565
New York, NY 10029
Telephone: (212) 860-1990
FAX: (212) 860-1994
E.Mail: 103644.664@compuserve.com

American Committee for Shaare Zedek Hospital in Jerusalem
49 West 45 Street, Suite 1100
New York, NY 10036
Telephone: (212) 354-8801
FAX: 800-346-1592
Web site: http://www.szmc.org.il

APPENDIX 5 *(continued)*

American College of Emergency Physicians
Section on International Emergency Medicine
American College of Emergency Physicians
PO Box 619911
Dallas, TX 75261-9901
Telephone: 1-800-798-1822, Extension 3250
FAX: (972) 580-2816
E.Mail: twerlinich@acep.org
Web site: www.acep.org

American Medical Student Association
1902 Association Drive
Reston, VA 20191
Telephone: (703) 620-6600, extension 202
E.Mail: amsa@www.amsa.org

American Red Cross
Department of International Services
1601 North Kent Street, 2nd Floor
Arlington, VA 22209
Telephone: (703) 465-4800
Web site: www.redcross.org/intl/index.html

American Refugee Committee
2344 Nicollet Avenue, South
Suite 350
Minneapolis, MN 55404
Telephone: (612) 872-7060
FAX: (612) 607-6499
E.Mail: archq@archq.org
Web site: http://www.archq.org

Amigos de las Americas
5618 Star Lane
Houston, TX 77057
Telephone: (713) 782-5290
E.Mail: info@amigoslink.org
Web site: http://www.amigoslink.org

Archdiocesan HealthCare Network
817 Varnum Street, NE
Washington, DC 20017
Telephone: (202) 636-4306

APPENDIX 5 *(continued)*

Baptist Medical Missions International
Box 193920
Little Rock, AR 72219
Telephone: (501) 455-4977
FAX: (501) 455-2710
E.Mail: bmmi@alpha-net.net

Brethren in Christ World Missions
PO Box 308011
Grantham, PA 17027
Telephone: (717) 697-2634
FAX: (717) 691-6053
E.Mail: bicwm@messiah.edu
Web site: http://www.bic-church.org/wm

Bridges to Community, Inc.
210 Orchard Ridge Road
Chappaqua, NY 10514
Telephone: (914) 238-8354
E.Mail: brdgs2comm@aol.com

Buddhist Tzu Chi Free Clinic
1000 South Garfield Avenue
Alhambra, CA 91801
Telephone: (626) 281-3383

CAM International
8625 La Prada Drive
Dallas, TX 75228
Telephone: (214) 327-8206
Web site: http://www.caminternational.org

Catholic Medical Association
Medical Mission Committee
1 Kingston Manor Drive
St. Louis, MO 63124
Telephone: (314) 997-1025
FAX: (314) 692-7381
E.Mail: dmehan@cathmed.com
Web site: http://www.cathmed.com

APPENDIX 5 *(continued)*

Catholic Medical Mission Board, Inc.
10 West 17 Street
New York, NY 10011
Telephone: (212) 242-7757
(800) 678-5659
FAX: (212) 242-0930
E.Mail: rdecastanzo@cmmb.org
Web site: http://www.cmmb.org

Child Family Health International
2149 Lyon Street, No. 5
San Francisco, CA 94115
Telephone: (415) 206-1905
E.Mail: cfhi@cfhi.orgwww.cfhi.org

Christian Medical & Dental Society/
Global Health Outreach
Box 7500
Bristol, TX 37621
Telephone: (423) 844-1000
E.Mail: gho@christian-doctors.com

Doctors for Global Health (DGH)
Box 1761
Decatur, GA 30031
Telephone and FAX: (404) 377-3566
E.Mail: ccs-dgh@ix.netcom.com
Web site: http://www.dghonline.org

Doctors of the World U.S.A., Inc.
375 West Broadway
Fourth Floor
New York, NY 10012
Telephone: (888) 817-HELP
(212) 226-9890, extension 230
E.Mail: dow@igc.apc.org
Web site: www.doctorsoftheworld.org

Doctors Without Borders USA
11 East 26 Street, Suite 1904
New York, NY 10010
Telephone: (212) 679-6800
Web site: www.dwb.org

APPENDIX 5 *(continued)*

Doctors Without Borders/
Medecins Sans Frontieres (MSF)
6 East 39 Street
Eighth Floor
New York, NY 10016
Telephone: (212) 679-6800
E.Mail: dwb@newyork.msf.org

Emergency International
Suite 105
6600 York Road
Baltimore, MD 21212
Telephone: (410) 377-3828
Web site: www.emgint.org

Fellowship of Associates of Medical Evangelism (FAME)
Box 688
Columbus, IN 47202
Telephone: (812) 379-4351

The Flying Hospital, Inc.
977 Centerville Turnpike
Virginia Beach, VA 23463
Telephone: (757) 226-3902
E.Mail: rosanne.o'connor@flyinghospital.org

Global Response Service Corp.
PO Box 1305
Herndon, VA 22070
Telephone/FAX: (703) 430-4381
Web site: grsc.org

Global Volunteers
375 East Little Canada Road
St. Paul, MN 55117
Telephone: (800) 487-1074
E.Mail: email@globalvolunteers.oeg

Harvard Medical School
Department of Emergency Medicine, PBB-100
Brigham and Women's Hospital
75 Frances Street
Boston, MA 02215
Telephone: (617) 732-8188
E.Mail: mdavis@hms.harvard.edu
Web site: http://smi-nt1:bidmc.harvard.edu/internationalEM

APPENDIX 5 *(continued)*

Health Volunteers Overseas
PO Box 65157
Washington, DC 20035-5157
Telephone: (202) 296-0928
Web site: www.hvousa.org

Helping Hands Health Education
948 Pearl Street
Boulder, CO 80302
Telephone: (303) 449-4279
E.Mail: helpinghands@sannr.com

Helps International
15301 Dallas Parkway, Suite 200
Addison, TX 75001
Telephone: (800) 414-3577
E.Mail: rmartin@helpsintl.org

Himalayan HealthCare, Inc.
565 West End Avenue, Suite 3G
New York, NY 10024
Telephone: (212) 877-6519
E.Mail: lisa.gomer@worldnet.att.net

Hospital Albert Schweitzer-Haiti
150 Kennedy Drive
South Burlington, VT 05403
Telephone: (802) 862-7503
(942) 752-1525
FAX: (802) 658-0725
(941) 752-0755
E.Mail: gfhaiti@bhip.infi.net
Web site: http://www.hashaiti.org

International Hospital Relief Foundation, Inc.
6630 Biscayne Boulevard
Miami, FL 3313
Telephone: (954) 986-7050
E.Mail: intlhospre@aol.com

International Medical Corps
11500 West Olympic Boulevard
Suite 506
Los Angeles, CA 90064
Telephone: (310) 826-7800
FAX: (310) 442-6622
E.Mail: imc@imc-la-org
Web site: http://www.imc-la.org

APPENDIX 5 *(continued)*

International Relief Teams
3547 Camino del Rio South
Suite C
San Diego, CA 92108
Telephone: (619) 284-7979
E.Mail: irteams@aol.com

International Rescue Committee
122 East 42 Street, 12th Floor
New York, NY 10168-3000
Telephone: (212) 551-3082
(212) 551-3000
FAX: (212) 551-3170
Web site: http://www.intrescom.org

Interplast Inc.
300-B Pioneer Way
Mountain View, CA 94041
Telephone: (650) 962-0123
FAX: (650) 692-1619
Web site: http://www.interplast.org

Johns Hopkins University
Center for International Emergency, Disaster, and Refugee Studies
Johns Hopkins Hospital
600 North Wolfe Street
Marburg B186
Baltimore, MD 21287-2080
Telephone: (410) 614-5665
FAX: (410) 955-0141
E.Mail: mvanrooy@jhmi.edu

Loma Linda University International Affairs
11060 Anderson Street
Magan Hall, Suite 105
Loma Linda, CA 92350
Telephone: (909) 558-4420
(909) 824-4420
FAX: (909) 558-0116
E.Mail: jcoggin@univ.ilu.edu

MAP International-Reader's Digest International Fellowship
PO Box 215000
Brunswick, GA 31521-5000
Telephone: (912) 265-6010
FAX: (912) 265-6170
E.Mail: crosser@map.org

APPENDIX 5 *(continued)*

Maryknoll Associate Lay Mission Office
PO Box 307
Maryknoll, NY 10545-0307
Telephone: (888) 828-6623
(800) 818-5276
FAX: (914) 762-7031
E.Mail: bethany@bestweb.net
Web site: http://www.maryknoll.org

Medical Benevolence Foundation
1412 North Sam Houston Parkway, East Suite 120
Houston, TX 77032
Telephone: (281) 590-3591
(800) 547-7627
FAX: (281) 590-3699
E.Mail: lcolman@mbfoundation.org or info@mbfoundation.org
Web site: http://www.mbfoundation.org

Medical International Missionary Aid
Box 7133
Jupiter, FL 33468
Telephone: (561) 747-3334
E.Mail: mariakatalina@msn.com

Medical Ministry International
Box 940207
Plano, TX 75094
Telephone: (972) 437-1995
E.Mail: mmitx@airmail.net

Medical Service Corporation International
1716 Wilson Boulevard
Arlington, VA 22209
Telephone: (703) 276-3000
FAX: (703) 276-3017
E.Mail: msci@iamdigex.net

Medecins Sans Frontieres
8 Rue Saint-Sabin
75011
Paris, France
(telephone) 33.1.40212929
(telex) 214360
(telefax) 33.1.48066868

APPENDIX 5 *(continued)*

Mercy Ships
Box 2020
Lindale, TX 75771
Telephone: (800) 424-7447
FAX: (903) 882-0343
E.Mail: hcsreg@mercyships.org
Web site: http://www.mercyships.org

Mexican Medical Ministries
Box 1847
Spring Valley, CA 91979
Telephone: (619) 660-1106
FAX: (619) 660-1223
E.Mail: mexmedhq@mexicanmedical.com or kristi@mexicanmedical.com

Mission Doctors Association
3424 Wilshire Boulevard
Los Angeles, CA 90010
Telephone: (626) 285-8868
FAX: (626) 309-1716
E.Mail: missiondrs@earthlink.net
Website: http://www.MissionDoctors.org

Missionary Ventures
5528 Commerce Drive
Orlando, FL 32839
Telephone: (407) 859-7322
E.Mail: MVIUSA@aol.com

Moravian Church Board of World Missions
PO Box 1245
Bethlehem, PA 18016
Telephone: (610) 868-1732
FAX: (610) 866-9223

Operation Lifeline International
149 Kearny Avenue
Perth Amboy, NJ 08862
Telephone: (732) 324-2114

Pennsylvania State University
Center for International Emergency Medicine
Emergency Medicine (H043)
Hershey Medical Center
PO Box 850
Hershey, PA 17033-0850
Telephone: (717) 531-8955
FAX: (717) 531-4587
E.Mail: jholliman@psu.edu

APPENDIX 5 *(continued)*

Project HOPE
Carter Hall
Millwood, VA 22646
Telephone: (540) 837-2100

Ronald Reagan Institute of Emergency Medicine
George Washington University
Department of Emergency Medicine
2140 Pennsylvania Avenue, NW
Washington, DC 20037
Telephone: (202) 994-5423
FAX: (202) 994-3924
E.Mail: emdjps@gwumc.edu

Samaritans Purse International Relief
PO Box 3000
Boone, NC 28607
Telephone (828)-262-1980
Email: emergency@samaritan.org

SIM International
Box 7900
Charlotte, NC 28241
Telephone: (704) 587-1479
(704) 588-4300
FAX: (704) 587-1518
E.Mail: info@sim.org
Web site: http://www.sim.org

John Snow, Inc. (JSI)
44 Farnsworth Street
Boston, MA 02210
Telephone: (617) 482-9485
FAX: (617) 482-0617
Web site: http://www.jsi.com
http://www.worlded.com

Southern Baptist Convention International Mission Board
Box 6767
Richmond, VA 23230
Telephone: (804) 353-0151
(800) 888-8657, extension 1575
FAX: (804) 254-8978
E.Mail: van.williams@imb.org

APPENDIX 5 *(continued)*

Surfer's Medical Association
Box 1210
Aptos, CA 95001
Telephone: (831) 684-0916
E.Mail: smacentral@aol.com

Surgical Eye Expeditions International
27 E De la Guerra, Suite C-2
Santa Barbara, CA 93101
Telephone: (805) 963-3303
FAX: (805) 965-3564
Web site: http://www.seeintl.org

TEAM (The Evangelical Alliance Mission)
Box 969
Wheaton, IL 60189
Telephone: (800) 343-3144
E.Mail: rdougherty@TEAMworld.org

United Methodist Church General Board of Global Ministries
475 Riverside Drive
Suite 330
New York, NY 10115
Telephone: (212) 870-3660
(212) 870-3825
FAX: (212) 870-3774
E.Mail: jblanken@gbgm-umc.org
Web site: http://www.gbgm-umc.org

Vellore Christian Medical College Board (USA), Inc.
475 Riverside Drive
Room 243
New York, NY 10115
Telephone: (212) 870-2640
E.Mail: usaboard@vellorecmc.org

VOSH-Volunteer Optometric Service to Humanity
PO Box 310
Rolla, MO 65402
Telephone: (573) 364-1773
FAX: (573) 341-3945

APPENDIX 5 *(continued)*

World Concern
19303 Fremont Avenue North
Seattle, WA 98133
Telephone: (206) 546-7359
FAX: (206) 546-7269
E.Mail: mam@christa.org
Web site: http://www.worldconcern.org

World Gospel Mission
PO Box 948
Marion, IN 46952
Telephone: (765) 664-7331
FAX: (765) 664-7669
E.Mail: wgm@wgm.org
Web site: http://www.wgm.org

World Medical Mission
Box 3000
Boone, NC 28607
Telephone: (828) 262-1980
FAX: (828) 266-1055
Web site: http://www.samaritan.org

World Rehabilitation Fund Inc
386 Park Avenue South, Suite 500
New York, NY 10016
Telephone: (212) 725-7875
FAX: (212) 725-8402
E.Mail: wrfnewyork@msn.com
Web site: http://www.worldrehabfund.org

World Vision International
PO Box 9716
Federal Way, WA 98063
Telephone: (253) 815-2017
FAX: (253) 815-3245
E.Mail: intjobs@worldvision.org
Web site: http://www.worldvision.org

World Witness Associate Reformed Presbyterian Church
1 Cleveland Street
Suite 220
Greenville, SC 29601
Telephone: (864) 233-5226
E.Mail: johnc@worldwitness.org

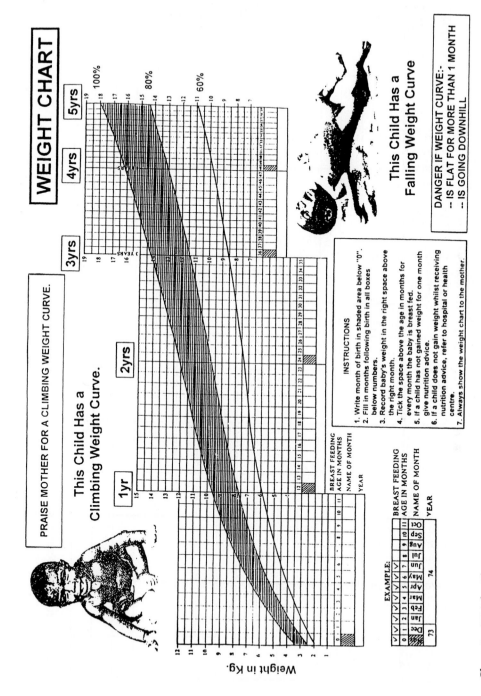

Chart 1: Weight Chart

SOURCE: Standard Treatment for Common Illnesses of Children in Papua, New Guinea. Paediatric Society of Papua, New Guinea, 1986.

Record of prenatal care

Name: _____   Age: _____   Number of children: _____   Ages: _____

Date of last monthly bleeding: _____   Probable due date: _____   Problems with other births: _____

Date of last childbirth: _____

Date of visit	Month of pregnancy	General health and minor problems	Anemia	Risk signs	Swelling Edema (where? how much?)	Pulse	Temp.	Weight (estimate or measure)	Blood Pressure	Protein in urine	Baby's Heart beat	Position of baby in womb	Size of womb (how many fingers above (+) or below (-) the navel?)

Chart 2: Record of Prenatal Care

CHILDHOOD VACCINE ADMINISTRATION RECORD

Name _____   DOB _____   History # _____

1) I have read the information in the Vaccine Information Sheet about the disease(s) and the vaccine(s). I have had the chance to ask questions which were answered to my satisfaction. I believe I understand the benefits and risks of the vaccine(s) and request that the vaccine(s) indicated below be given to the person named above for which I am authorized to make this request.

2) I have asked about immunizations and prior significant reactions. According to the informant, none have occurred.

Immunization		Date	Age	Manufacturer & Lot Number	Route	Site	1) Consent Signature	2) Nurse/MD Signature
Prevnar	1				IM			
Prevnar	2				IM			
Prevnar	3				IM			
Prevnar	4				IM			
DT DTap	1				IM			
DT DTap	2				IM			
DT DTap	3				IM			
DT DTap	4				IM			
*DT DTap	5				IM			
HIB	1				IM			
HIB	2				IM			
HIB	3				IM			
*HIB	4				IM			
OPV IPV	1				PO SQ			
OPV IPV	2				PO SQ			
OPV IPV	3				PO SQ			
*OPV IPV	4				PO SQ			
*MMR	1				SQ			
MMR	2				SQ			
Hep B	1				IM			
Hep B	2				IM			
Hep B	3				IM			
Td	1				IM			
Td	2				IM			
Varicella					SQ			

Circle appropriate response when a choice exists.
*Specific age requirements in effect.   10/00

Chart 3: Childhood Vaccine Administration

Supplemental Vaccine Administration Record

Name_____ DOB_____ History#_____

1) I believe that I understand the benefits and risks of the vaccine (s) and request that the vaccine (s) indicated below be given to the person named above for whom I am authorized to make this request.

2) I have asked about immunizations and prior significant reactions. According to the informant, none have occurred.

Immunization	Date	Manufacturer & Lot Number	Route	Site	1) Consent Signature	2)Nurse/MD Signature
Hep A			IM			
Typhoid			SQ/IM*			
Yellow Fever			SQ			
Cholera			SQ/IM			
Meningococcal			SQ			
Pneumococcal			SQ/IM			
JEV			SQ			
Rabies			IM			
Influenza			IM			

* Route dependent upon type vaccine given.

Sept. 97

Chart 4:   Supplemental Vaccine Administration Record

CHILD HEALTH CHART

CLINIC 1 .... No ....

CLINIC 2 .... No ....

		GIRL
CHILD'S NAME	BIRTH WEIGHT	BOY

DATE OF BIRTH   day   month   year

MOTHER'S NAME

CARETAKER IF NOT THE MOTHER

FATHER'S NAME

WHERE DOES THE CHILD LIVE?

How many children has the mother had? .... Number dead ....

Number alive ....

CARD GIVEN AND MOTHER TAUGHT BY

ASK THE MOTHER ABOUT THESE REASONS FOR GIVING THE CHILD EXTRA CARE *(make a circle round the right answer)*

			TAKE EXTRA CARE
Was the baby less than 2.5 kg at birth.	no	yes	
Is this baby a twin	no	yes	
Is this baby bottle fed	no	yes	
Does the mother need more family support	no	yes	
Are any brothers or sisters underweight	no	yes	
For example – tuberculosis or leprosy or social problems	no	yes	

Remember to discuss child spacing

chart produced by
TALC   TALC P. O. BOX 49, ST. ALBANS, UK.
Training materials are also available

GROWTH CURVE Reference values – WHO recommended 1980
UPPER LINE: 50th CENTILE BOYS LOWER LINE: 3rd CENTILE GIRLS

IMMUNISATIONS   DATE GIVEN

BCG

POLIO
- FIRST DOSE
- SECOND DOSE
- THIRD DOSE
- FOURTH DOSE

DPT
- Diptheria   FIRST DOSE
- Whooping Cough   SECOND DOSE
- Tetanus   THIRD DOSE

MEASLES
- FIRST DOSE

MOTHER'S TETANUS
TOXOID (or one booster)
- SECOND DOSE
- THIRD DOSE

ORAL REHYDRATION
DATES

Taught	
Used	

Date of visit

Kg 17 16 15 14 13 12 11 10 9 8 7 6 5 4 3 2 0

MONTH of birth

3 TO 4 YEARS   4 TO 5 YEARS

YEAR

36 38 40 42 44 46 48 50 52 54 56 58 60

Chart 5:   Childhood Growth Chart

SOURCE: From Werner D et al. Where There Is No Doctor. Rev Ed. Hesperian Foundation, Berkeley, CA, 1992.

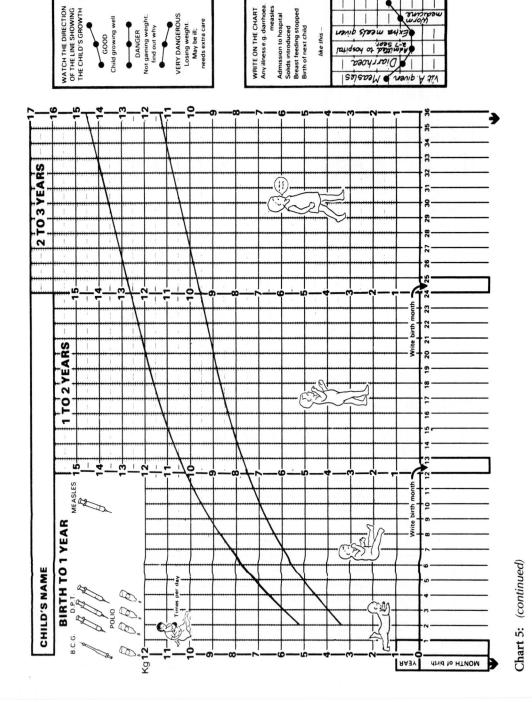

Chart 5: *(continued)*

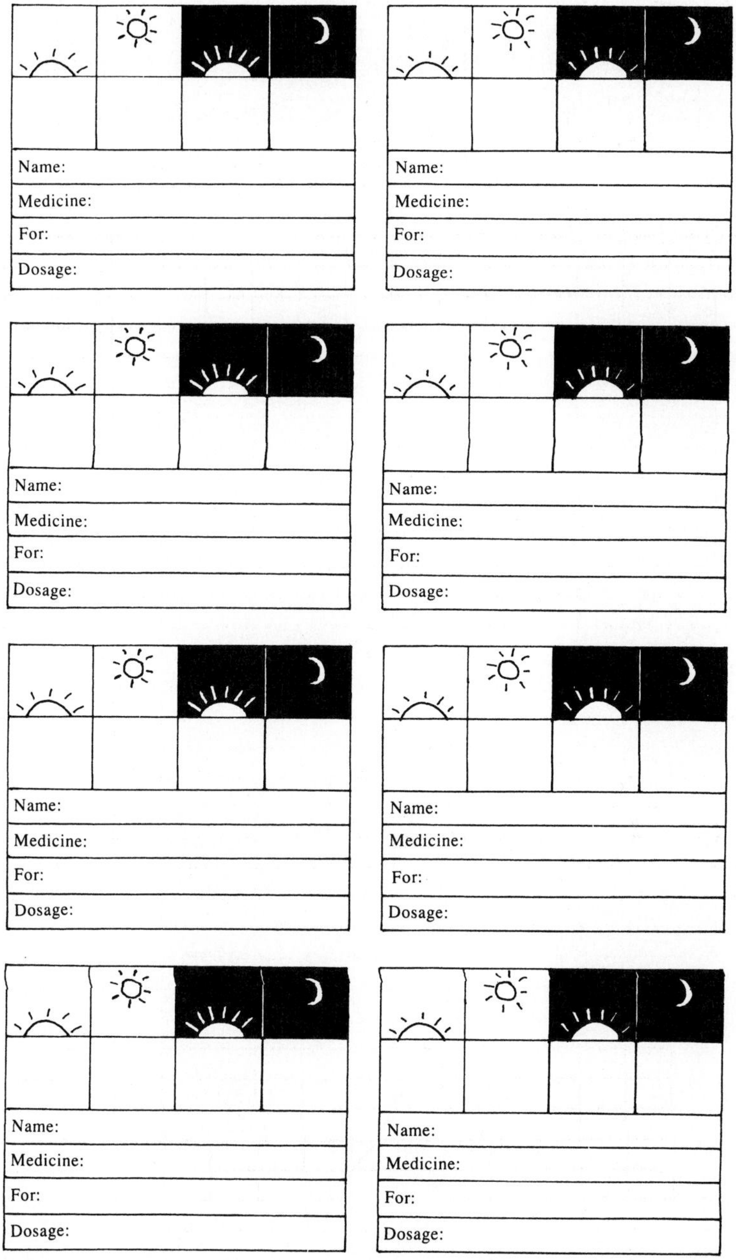

Chart 6: Dosage Blanks for Giving Medications to Those Who Cannot See

Source: From Werner D et al. Where There Is No Doctor. Rev Ed. Hesperian Foundation, Berkeley, CA, 1992.

Index